The Health Professional's Guide to Dietary Supplements

The Health Professional's Guide to Dietary Supplements

Shawn M. Talbott, PhD

Chief Scientific Officer, SupplementWatch, Inc.
Draper, Utah

Kerry Hughes, MSc

President, EthnoPharm
Vallejo, California

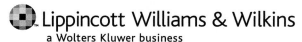
Lippincott Williams & Wilkins
a Wolters Kluwer business
Philadelphia • Baltimore • New York • London
Buenos Aires • Hong Kong • Sydney • Tokyo

Acquisitions Editor: Emily Lupash
Managing Editor: Meredith Brittain
Marketing Manager: Christen Murphy
Production Editor: Eve Malakoff-Klein
Designer: Doug Smock
Compositor: Maryland Composition, Inc.
Printer: R.R. Donnelley & Sons—Crawfordsville

Printed in the United States of America

Library of Congress Cataloging-in-Publication Data

Talbott, Shawn M.
    The health professional's guide to dietary supplements / Shawn M.
    Talbott, Kerry Hughes.
    p. ; cm.
    Includes bibliographical references and index.
    ISBN-13: 978-0-7817-4672-4
    ISBN-10: 0-7817-4672-8
    1. Dietary supplements--Handbooks, manuals, etc. 2. Dietary
supplements--Therapeutic use--Handbooks, manuals, etc. I. Hughes, Kerry.
II. Title.
    [DNLM: 1. Dietary Supplements--Handbooks. QU 39 T142h 2007]
RM258.57.T35 2007
615'.1--dc22

                  2006014283

*The publishers have made every effort to trace the copyright holders for borrowed
material. If they have inadvertently overlooked any, they will be pleased to make
the necessary arrangements at the first opportunity.*

To purchase additional copies of this book, call our customer service
department at **(800) 638-3030** or fax orders to **(301) 223-2320.**
International customers should call **(301) 223-2300.**

Visit Lippincott Williams & Wilkins on the Internet: http://www.LWW.com.
Lippincott Williams & Wilkins customer service representatives are
available from 8:30 am to 6:00 pm, EST.

06 07 08 09 10
1 2 3 4 5 6 7 8 9 10

To Julie Talbott and to my many students over the years who have helped me to take the science behind supplements and answer the question, "So what?" The answer to that question helps to focus us, as educators and health care professionals, on our clients, patients, and students—and most of all, forces us to apply that science in a way that can yield health benefits and promote well-being.
—Shawn Talbott

To my grandmother, Mary Howorth, and her delicious garden of spices and vegetables that was among my first introductions to plants; to my parents, Gary and Ethel Hughes, who are true healers themselves; and to my brother and sister, Owen and Holly, for their many healing laughs through the years. In precious memory of Chief Phil Crazybull, 1949–2006: "Telling people about the healing qualities of plants in any language they can hear."
—Kerry Hughes

Reviewers

Keryn Bickman-Morris, MS, RD, CDE
Clinical Nutritionist
Preferred Nutrition Consultants, LLC
Scottsdale, Arizona

Luke Bucci, PhD, CCN, CNS
Vice President, Research
Schiff Nutrition International
Salt Lake City, Utah

Amy Cifelli, MS, RD, LDN
Manager, Metabolic Diet Study Center
Department of Nutritional Sciences
College of Health and Human Development
Penn State University
University Park, Pennsylvania

Nancy Cotugna, DrPH, RD
Department of Health, Nutrition, and Exercise Sciences
College of Health Sciences
University of Delaware
Newark, Delaware

Ruth DeBusk, PhD, RD
Owner
DeBusk Communications, LLC
Tallahassee, Florida

Constance Grauds, RPh
President
Association of Natural Medicine Pharmacists
San Rafael, California

Mary P. Miles, PhD
Assistant Professor, Movement Science and Nutrition
Department of Health and Human Development
Montana State University
Bozeman, Montana

David Pearson, PhD, CSCS*D
Associate Professor, Physical Education
Director, Strength Research Laboratory
School of Physical Education, Sport, and Exercise Science
Ball State University
Muncie, Indiana

Christopher Rasmussen, MS, CSCS
Research Coordinator, Part-Time Lecturer
Department of Health, Human Performance, and Recreation
Baylor University
Waco, Texas

Jeffrey A. Simancek, BS, CMT, CPT
Chair, Massage Therapy Department
Olympia Career Training Institute
Grand Rapids, Michigan

Lisa Stalans, MPH, ATC, LAT, CSCS
Assistant Athletic Trainer
Women's Soccer, Women's Tennis
University of Texas
Austin, Texas

Kent J. Tagge, BSN, MS
ACSM-, NSCA-, ACE-Certified Personal Trainer
IDEA Elite Personal Fitness Trainer
Owner, KoolerTrek Personal Fitness Studio
Salt Lake City, Utah

Thomas E. Temples, PhD
Coordinator, Physical Education Program
Department of Health and Physical Education
North Georgia College and State University
Dahlonega, Georgia

Annie C. Wetter, PhD, CSCS
Assistant Professor, Nutrition and Dietetics
School of Health Promotion and Human Development
University of Wisconsin
Stevens Point, Wisconsin

Lisa Young, PhD, RD
Adjunct Assistant Professor
Department of Nutrition, Food Studies, and Public Health
Steinhardt School of Education
New York University
New York, New York

Preface

Nearly 2,500 years ago, Hippocrates, the "father of modern medicine," embraced the concept, "Let food be thy medicine and medicine be thy food." Medicinal herbs have been used since time immemorial in all cultures the world over. Even though we know that diet plays a significant role in 5 of the 10 leading causes of death (including coronary heart disease, stroke, certain cancers, type 2 diabetes, and atherosclerosis), the advent of modern pharmaceutical therapy in the nineteenth century caused the unfortunate fall of the "food as medicine" philosophy within the practice of modern medicine.

The passage of the Dietary Supplement Health and Education Act of 1994 (DSHEA) marked a new era for the importance of nutrition in human health. Millions of consumers have embraced the concept of using food, dietary supplements, and herbal extracts to positively affect their health, and the dietary supplement industry has grown from almost zero to more than $20 billion in annual domestic sales, with worldwide sales exceeding $100 million. Although estimates vary, approximately 60% of adults in the United States identify themselves as consumers of dietary supplements; according to the Food and Drug Administration (FDA), close to 200 million Americans consume supplements.

Despite the widespread use of dietary supplements by American consumers, studies show that physicians and other health professionals are both unlikely to ask and unlikely to be told of their patients' use of supplements. This is partly because of the often daunting challenge of determining the proper clinical usage and relevance of dietary supplements.

The broad definition of dietary supplements encompasses a wide variety of plant constituents (roots, leaves, stems, etc.), vitamins, minerals, amino acids, and other ingredients that can have essential or nonessential bioactive constituents with associated health benefits (or risks). Consumers tend to use dietary supplements either as "preventive nutrition" (e.g., a daily vitamin E supplement taken to prevent heart disease) or as "phytomedicine" (e.g., *Ginkgo biloba* used to alleviate mental dysfunction associated with senile dementia). Of course, consumers also use dietary supplements in myriad other ways as promoters of weight loss, to increase energy levels, and to treat specific diseases.

Although the FDA regulates dietary supplements in many of the same ways that it regulates conventional foods, supplement products are required to carry the disclaimer, "This product is not intended to diagnose, treat, cure, or prevent any disease." Like foods, but unlike drugs, most dietary supplements do not require premarketing approval by the FDA, but the FDA has the authority to restrict sales and remove specific supplements from the market if they are shown to pose a public health risk. Because the scientific and medical evidence for the efficacy and safety of dietary supplements is highly variable in terms of both quantity and quality, it is incumbent on health professionals to actively inform patients and clients of the risks and benefits associated with the use of these products. To do that, health professionals need to have a basic understanding of the evidence (for and against) the use of a particular supplement in a given condition or for a given effect.

This book is an effort to do just that: to provide health professionals with the background needed to converse with their patients or clients about the clinical evidence behind a wide variety of dietary supplements. Consumers need to realize that dietary supplements are not panaceas or "magic bullets" that can counteract poor health habits; rather, they are supplements to a comprehensive lifestyle approach to good health that also includes a balanced diet, regular physical activity, stress management, and other positive health practices.

Another purpose of this book is to recognize that the major reason for incorporating herbal medicine in human health is its traditional ethnobotanical use. As consumers in modern societies have become more interested in accessing herbal medicines in trade and through the recommendation of health care professionals, the clinical evidence for herbal medicine has grown significantly. Since the passage of the DSHEA, a tremendous amount of clinical investigation has been conducted into herbal medicine and other dietary supplements. This clinical evidence lessens the validity of doctors and pharmacists not wanting to supervise the use of supplements. It is especially important to recognize the tremendous importance of traditional medicine in developing the safe use of herbs.

The goal of the purely clinical approach taken in evaluating and reviewing dietary supplements in this book is to review dietary supplements only on scientific merit to date. As the scientific community is better able to find appropriate methods of studying the merits of traditional medicine, we expect the use of these substances will become an increasing part of health care maintenance in mainstream medicine, as well as provide further credibility to traditional healing methods.

ORGANIZATIONAL PHILOSOPHY

This volume covers more than 120 supplements in 12 chapters. The chapters group supplements by their major primary effects (e.g., weight loss, heart health, etc.). For many natural products, however, effects may significantly overlap. For example, a supplement that is primarily promoted for and used by consumers for supporting heart health may also have benefits as an antioxidant. We have used our best judgment— based on the clinical evidence, our experience with these ingredients, and traditional use—to place specific supplements within the appropriate chapter. If you do not see a supplement where you expect to find it, please consult the index at the back of the book (which has entries according to supplements' common as well as scientific names) or the List of Supplements at the beginning of the book, which is organized alphabetically by supplement name. A number of other herbal and dietary supplements are on the market today beyond what we have included in this book; we would have liked to include many more into our review but we hope we included those which will be the most helpful to clinicians.

Studies of botanical and herbal supplements are often difficult to evaluate because of inherent variation of natural products from study to study, incomplete description and analysis of the active ingredients, and variations in the dosing, duration, and population being studied. Even considering the large number of supplements covered here (more than 120 entries), readers will notice certain omissions. In determining the supplements to be covered in this book, we focused our efforts on the supplements that we felt would most likely be used by a significant number of consumers, would be encountered in a clinical setting, and would posses a sufficient body of clinical evidence for us to evaluate. We did not attempt to consider in any detail the many laboratory, animal, and epidemiological studies on various supplements; instead, we focused our review and analysis on clinical evidence, with particular focus on prospective feeding studies in clearly defined human populations. We also did not attempt to review the various combinations of supplements that can be encountered in commercial products but instead focused on identifying the specific dosage levels and usage patterns for individual and clearly defined supplements that are associated with efficacy and safety in human populations.

CHAPTER STRUCTURE

This book provides the busy health professional with a quick at-a-glance summary of each supplement, as well as a more comprehensive analysis of the available evidence for those who wish to delve into the details. Features of each chapter include:

- **Alphabetical list of supplements covered.** For handy reference, the first page of each chapter lists alphabetically all the supplements that are discussed in that chapter.
- **Supplement information.** After the alphabetical list of supplements at the beginning of the chapter, each supplement is discussed in turn. The following subsections for each supplement provide easy-to-reference information:
- **Overall Rank.** The supplement in question is given a star ranking— that is, a rating of one to five stars based on the level of scientific substantiation for each of its major effects:

  ★★★★★ = Significant scientific agreement
  ★★★★ = Support, but not conclusive
  ★★★ = Some support, but limited and not conclusive
  ★★ = Very limited preliminary support
  ★ = Theoretical basis, but scientific support nonexistent
  ZERO = No scientific or theoretical support

Although such a ranking is partly a subjective undertaking by the authors, it accurately reflects the quality and quantity of the clinical evidence and traditional usage that exists for the supplement and also weighs both the risk/benefit and impact of conflicting positive and negative data. A given supplement may score three stars for one clinical indication or effect but more or fewer stars for another, depending on the strength of the clinical evidence for each effect. In general, more stars are better in terms of the strength of the clinical evidence for the effect in question, but health professionals will of course need to consider the individual patient or client and his or her specific needs.

When warranted, the "Overall Rank" section also includes any important safety considerations and/or warnings for using the supplement in question (but be sure to also check the "Safety/Dosage" section for each supplement).

- **Overview.** A brief summary of the supplement—its uses and how it works in the body.
- **Comments.** The authors' thoughts on the particular supplement, including the circumstances in which the supplement can be useful.
- **Scientific Support.** A detailed recap and sampling of clinical studies involving the supplement.
- **Safety/Dosage.** Important information about how much of the supplement to take for certain effects. Any crucial safety issues associated with this supplement are noted here.
- **References.** Sources the authors consulted regarding the supplement in this section.
- **Additional Resources.** Other sources of useful information for health professionals wanting to delve deeper into a particular topic.

APPENDIX OF STAR RANKINGS

The appendix to this book presents an alphabetical list of all the supplements in the book accompanied by their star rankings. This quick reference can tell you at a glance the effectiveness of a certain supplement for various effects, but be sure to read the description of that supplement in the text for comprehensive information.

In summary, the *Health Professional's Guide to Dietary Supplements* offers both a quick reference as well as a comprehensive summary of the clinical evidence for a wide range of popular dietary supplements. This book is intended to give health professionals the information they need to actively engage their patients or clients in the important joint decision to incorporate or not to incorporate dietary supplements into a broader lifestyle regimen.

Contents

Contents

List of Supplements

1

Weight Loss Supplements

Bladderwrack (*Fucus vesiculosis*)
Carnitine
Chitosan
Citrus aurantium (Synephrine)
Conjugated Linoleic Acid (CLA)
Guarana (*Paullinia cupana*)

Hydroxycitric Acid (HCA, *Garcinia cambogia*)
Ma Huang (*Ephedra sinensis*, Ephedrine)
Pyruvate
White Willow Bark (*Salix alba*)

BLADDERWRACK (*FUCUS VESICULOSIS*)

Overall Rank

★★★ as a dietary source of iodine
★ for weight loss and "fat burning"
★ for enhancing thyroid function

OVERVIEW

Bladderwrack is rarely used alone as a supplement but is formulated as a support ingredient in various formulations. It is often used in dietary supplement products designed for weight loss, fat burning, enhancing thyroid function, and increasing energy. It is even more common in cosmetic formulations for improving skin tone and health. Like several types of seaweed supplements, bladderwrack is mainly used because of its high iodine content; other reasons include its high trace mineral, fiber, and vitamin B_{12} content. Thus, there are sound theoretical reasons for including such supplements in the diet.

Iodine is necessary in the production of thyroid hormones by the thyroid gland. Low levels of thyroid hormones are associated with reduced energy levels and weight gain. In some cases, people battling for years to control their weight have eventually come to find their thyroid levels are low; with the help of their doctors, they find a solution to maintaining the proper weight by pharmaceutical control of thyroid levels. Although included in weight loss formulations for a similar reason, bladderwrack is only intended as *dietary* support. Additionally, because bladderwrack contains trace minerals, vitamin B_{12}, and fiber, it is often included to support the diet, thereby promoting nutritional balance and benefiting energy levels and overall wellness.

COMMENTS

Although bladderwrack is a confirmed source of iodine, no clinical support yet backs its use as a single "whole herb" ingredient; therefore, its usefulness in providing clinical efficacy in supplement formulations is not known. Because of its lack of clinical support, bladderwrack cannot be recommended as a dietary supplement for its therapeutic indications at this time.

SCIENTIFIC SUPPORT

No clinical studies have been conduced with bladderwrack as a single ingredient. Some preclinical work with bladderwrack has confirmed the following activities: antioxidant, reduction of platelet aggregation, reduction in blood glucose, and inhibition of enzyme activity associated with HIV. One clinical study exists with bladderwrack acting as an antioxidant in a "body-contouring" product and producing favorable results (Reilly and Reeve, 2000).

SAFETY/DOSAGE

Because little work has been done in human clinical studies with bladderwrack, the proper dosage for its indications is still not known. It is commonly suggested to start with a small dosage and increase until the proper dosage is found for the individual. The German Commission E warns that bladderwrack preparations should not provide an excess of 150 µg/day of iodine (Blumenthal et al., 1998). Since bladderwrack has been confirmed as a source of iodine, some concern exists for the possibility of overconsumption, causing thyroid imbalance (Phaneuf et al., 1999).

Depending on the source waters that bladderwrack is harvested from, there is concern for the risk of heavy metal contamination.

REFERENCES

Blumenthal M, Busse WR, Goldberg A, Gruenwald J, Hall T, Riggins CW, Rister RS, eds. The Complete German Commission E Monographs. Austin, TX: American Botanical Council, 1998.

Phaneuf D, Cote I, Dumas P, Ferron LA, LeBlanc A. Evaluation of the contamination of marine algae (seaweed) from the St. Lawrence River and likely to be consumed by humans. Environmental Research 1999;80(2 pt 2):S175–S182.

Reilly W, Reeve V. Body contouring using an oral herbal antioxidant formulation. Centelaplus: a dose controlled observational study. Redox Report 2000;5(2–3):144–145.

ADDITIONAL RESOURCES

Jimenez-Escrig A, Jimenez-Jimenez I, Pulido R, Saura-Calixto F. Antioxidant activity of fresh and processed edible seaweeds. Journal of the Science of Food and Agriculture 2001;81(5):530–534.

CARNITINE

Overall Rank

★★★ for enhancing general heart function (in congestive heart failure and post–myocardial infarction when combined with coenzyme Q_{10})
★★ for weight loss and "fat burning"
★★ for endurance

OVERVIEW

Carnitine is an amino acid found in the diet in meat and dairy products, but it is also synthesized in the liver and kidneys from lysine and methionine. The major function of carnitine is to facilitate the transport and metabolism of long-chain fatty acids into the mitochondria for ß oxidation and energy generation. As a dietary supplement, carnitine is marketed to enhance endurance, increase fat metabolism, lower cholesterol and triglyceride levels, and improve cardiovascular performance (as a general cardioprotective).

Because of the role of carnitine in facilitating fatty acid transport into the mitochondria for ß oxidation, it is possible that elevated carnitine levels would permit a greater or faster transport of fat, leading to increased fat oxidation, which might impact weight loss and/or endurance. A greater reliance on fat for energy might also result in a sparing of muscle glycogen, a reduction of lactic acid production, and a subsequent enhancement of exercise performance. Unfortunately, the existing clinical evidence for a beneficial effect of carnitine supplements in healthy adults is disappointing.

COMMENTS

As a weight loss supplement, carnitine does not appear to be particularly effective for either promoting weight loss or enhancing fat burning. For endurance athletes, carnitine supplements are of little value, except possibly for vegetarians who may not consume adequate levels of carnitine or its precursor amino acids (lysine and methionine) in their diets. For general cardioprotective benefits, carnitine supplementation may be beneficial to help maintain blood lipid profiles and promote fatty acid utilization within heart muscle. The benefits of carnitine supplements on "heart strength" in cases of congestive heart failure and in post–myocardial infarction and postsurgical conditions may be enhanced by combination supplementation with coenzyme Q_{10}.

SCIENTIFIC SUPPORT

Carnitine is thought to be a conditionally essential nutrient for premature infants; evidence points to carnitine supplementation reducing apnea and improving the general metabolic profile of prematurity (O'Donnell et al., 2002). In most cases, however, carnitine is delivered as part of a regimen of total parenteral nutrition to infants housed in neonatal intensive care units, so drawing a direct comparison with daily oral carnitine supplementation for weight loss or fat burning in healthy adults is difficult.

Carnitine supplements (1 g/day for 3–6 months) have been shown to improve muscle strength and subjective measures of vitality, general health, and physical function in patients with end-stage renal failure undergoing hemodialysis (Sloan et al., 1998).

Studies of the role of carnitine as an ergogenic aid have been equivocal, with several trials suggesting a beneficial effect of supplements and others indicating no effect at all. Several early studies suggested an indirect effect of carnitine (2–6 g/day) on endurance performance by showing a reduction in the respiratory exchange ratio, which indicates a greater reliance on fats for energy generation (Huertas et al., 1992). Other studies have failed to indicate any glycogen-sparing effect of carnitine supplements (6 g/day). It has also been shown that with supplements, although blood carnitine levels go up, the acyl-enzyme system for fatty acid transport into the mitochondria is not augmented, suggesting that the body sufficiently "loads" enough carnitine into the mitochondrial membrane without the help of dietary supplements. There is some indication that carnitine supplementation may help to accelerate recovery following exhaustive exercise (Volek et al., 2002)—an effect that could translate into an eventual ergogenic benefit in athletes training or competing over multiday events where postexercise recovery becomes a limiting factor.

In terms of weight loss, the very low calorie diets (less than 800 calories per day) used for intensive obesity treatment have been shown to result in lower levels of carnitine in the blood and tissues, possibly owing to an increase in carnitine excretion (Davis et al., 1990). Because carnitine transports fatty acids into mitochondria for oxidation, any reduction in carnitine status in people trying to lose weight may be viewed as detrimental. A double-blind investigation (Villani et al., 2000) tested the weight loss effects of carnitine in 36 moderately overweight women over 2 months (18 received 4 g/day of carnitine, and 18 received placebo). Subjects also completed 30 minutes of walking exercise (60–70% of maximum heart rate) 4 days/week. Results indicated no significant changes in body weight, fat mass, or the amount of fat oxidation at either rest or during exercise, suggesting that carnitine may not be particularly effective for promoting weight loss.

Supporting the beneficial role of carnitine supplements, however, are studies in kidney dialysis patients showing that low carnitine levels in the dialysate can lead to elevated levels of blood lipids. Likewise, studies of heart disease patients have shown that carnitine supplements (2 g/day over 6 months) can reduce cholesterol and triglyceride levels. Perhaps the most convincing data on the benefits of carnitine as a dietary supplement come from several studies of patients with heart disease. Among persons who had suffered a heart attack, carnitine supplements (2–3 g/day over 4–8 weeks) resulted in a reduction in the amount of damage to the heart muscle and an increase in heart muscle viability (Pichard et al., 1989). Among those suffering from angina (chest pain), carnitine reduces the incidence of angina and cardiac arrhythmias as well as reduces the need for antiangina and antiarrhythmic medications. In addition, carnitine (2 g/day for 6 months) can also increase exercise tolerance in patients with angina, meaning that they can exercise longer and at higher levels before experiencing chest pain.

The available data suggest that although the ergogenic benefits of carnitine supplements for endurance athletes are probably unfounded, or at least hard to measure, the benefits in terms of heart function and blood lipid maintenance are interesting. Under conditions in which the heart muscle is deprived of oxygen (i.e., heart attack and angina), fat breakdown and energy production are reduced. It also appears that carnitine concentrations may be somewhat reduced in cardiac cells undergoing such stress (Pichard et al., 1988). Supplemental levels of carnitine may help replenish the lost carnitine and facilitate a return to adequate levels of fatty acid transport and energy production in the heart muscle.

SAFETY/DOSAGE

Doses of 2–6 g/day over 6 months have been studied with no observed adverse side effects. Doses of 2–6 g/day are typically recommended for cardiovascular, sports performance, and weight loss benefits, although the effectiveness of any dose of carnitine for sports or weight loss effects are not impressive. As a "heart health" nutrient, approximately 2 g/day of carnitine may provide some benefits in terms of promoting general heart function.

It is important to note that some supplemental forms of carnitine actually contain the physiologically inactive form of carnitine (D-carnitine) rather than the form that is active in humans (L-carnitine). Oversaturation of the tissue with D-carnitine could displace the active form of carnitine in tissues and lead to muscle weakness.

REFERENCES

Davis AT, Davis PG, Phinney SD. Plasma and urinary carnitine of obese subjects on very-low-calorie diets. J Am Coll Nutr 1990;9(3):261–264.

Huertas R, Campos Y, Diaz E, Esteban J, Vechietti L, Montanari G, D'Iddio S, Corsi M, Arenas J. Respiratory chain enzymes in muscle of endurance athletes: effect of L-carnitine. Biochem Biophys Res Commun 1992;188(1):102–107.

O'Donnell J, Finer NN, Rich W, Barshop BA, Barrington KJ. Role of L-carnitine in apnea of prematurity: a randomized, controlled trial. Pediatrics 2002;109(4):622–626.

Pichard C, Roulet M, Rossle C, Chiolero R, Schutz Y, Temler E, Boumghar M, Schindler C, Zurlo F, Jequier E, et al. Effects of L-carnitine supplemented total parenteral nutrition on lipid and energy metabolism in postoperative stress. JPEN 1988;12(6):555–562.

Pichard C, Roulet M, Schutz Y, Rossle C, Chiolero R, Temler E, Schindler C, Zurlo F, Furst P, Jequier E. Clinical relevance of L-carnitine-supplemented total parenteral nutrition in postoperative trauma. Metabolic effects of continuous or acute carnitine administration with special reference to fat oxidation and nitrogen utilization. Am J Clin Nutr 1989;49(2):283–289.

Sloan RS, Kastan B, Rice SI, Sallee CW, Yuenger NJ, Smith B, Ward RA, Brier ME, Golper TA. Quality of life during and between hemodialysis treatments: role of L-carnitine supplementation. Am J Kidney Dis 1998;32(2):265–272.

Villani RG, Gannon J, Self M, Rich PA. L-carnitine supplementation combined with aerobic training does not promote weight loss in moderately obese women. Int J Sport Nutr Exerc Metab 2000;10(2):199–207.

Volek JS, Kraemer WJ, Rubin MR, Gomez AL, Ratamess NA, Gaynor P. L-carnitine L-tartrate supplementation favorably affects markers of recovery from exercise stress. Am J Physiol Endocrinol Metab 2002;282(2):E474–E482.

ADDITIONAL RESOURCES

Bonner CM, DeBrie KL, Hug G, Landrigan E, Taylor BJ. Effects of parenteral L-carnitine supplementation on fat metabolism and nutrition in premature neonates. J Pediatr 1995;126(2):287–292.

Davis AT, Albrecht RM, Scholten DJ, Morgan RE. Increased plasma carnitine in trauma patients given lipid-supplemented total parenteral nutrition. Am J Clin Nutr 1988;48(6):1400–1402.

Lolic MM, Fiskum G, Rosenthal RE. Neuroprotective effects of acetyl-L-carnitine after stroke in rats. Ann Emerg Med 1997;29(6):758–765.

Papamandjaris AA, MacDougall DE, Jones PJ. Medium chain fatty acid metabolism and energy expenditure: obesity treatment implications. Life Sci 1998;62(14):1203–1215.

Simoneau JA, Veerkamp JH, Turcotte LP, Kelley DE. Markers of capacity to utilize fatty acids in human skeletal muscle: relation to insulin resistance and obesity and effects of weight loss. FASEB J 1999;13(14):2051–2060.

Stadler DD, Chenard CA, Rebouche CJ. Effect of dietary macronutrient content on carnitine excretion and efficiency of carnitine reabsorption. Am J Clin Nutr 1993;58(6):868–872.

Sulkers EJ, Lafeber HN, Degenhart HJ, Przyrembel H, Schlotzer E, Sauer PJ. Effects of high carnitine supplementation on substrate utilization in low-birth-weight infants receiving total parenteral nutrition. Am J Clin Nutr 1990;52(5):889–894.

Wennberg A, Hyltander A, Sjoberg A, Arfvidsson B, Sandstrom R, Wickstrom I, Lundholm K. Prevalence of carnitine depletion in critically ill patients with undernutrition. Metabolism 1992;41(2):165–171.

CHITOSAN

Overall Rank

★★ for fat absorption
★★ for cholesterol reduction
★ for weight loss

OVERVIEW

Chitosan is made from the shells of shellfish and is a type of dietary fiber called an aminopolysaccharide (a combination of sugar and protein). Because of its positive charge, it has the ability to attract and bind to the negatively charged fatty acids in our diet. When consumed with fatty foods, chitosan has the ability to bind the fats and essentially block their absorption. Chitosan can absorb up to 4–6 times its weight in fat or cholesterol; therefore, for approximately every gram of chitosan consumed, about 4–6 g of fat can be blocked.

COMMENTS

Most of the research on chitosan has been performed on animals and has shown chitosan to effectively block fat from digestion by binding to fats in the digestive system. However, the clinical data have given mixed results. Generally, it is accepted that chitosan works only if it is used in conjunction with a reduced-calorie diet, but clinical data are still needed to prove the best conditions for the use of chitosan and to back up claims of supplements.

SCIENTIFIC SUPPORT

Weight Loss

In a small study conducted by Gades and Stern (2002), seven healthy males were fed a high-fat diet (>120 g/day) for 12 days. Chitosan (5.25 g/day) was administered on days 6–9 before meals and snacks, and charcoal markers were consumed on days 2, 6, and 10 to indicate the baseline and supplement periods. All feces were collected on days 2–12 and analyzed for fecal fat for the 4 baseline and 4 supplement days. Fecal fat content was found unchanged on the days of chitosan administration; therefore, no fat-blocking effect was observed.

Zahorska-Markiewicz et al. (2002) examined the use of chitosan in a complex treatment for obesity involving 6 months in which subjects followed a low-calorie diet (1,000 kcal/day), chitosan or placebo supplementation, and modifications in physical activity and behavior, supported by 2-hour group meetings with a physician, psychologist, and dietician 2 times weekly. The chitosan (750 mg of pure chitosan called Chitinin, 2 tablets 3 times daily before each main meal) was studied using a double-blind, placebo-controlled, randomized design. Significantly greater body weight loss was found in the chitosan group (15.9 kg) versus the placebo group (10.9 kg), and also significantly lower systolic and diastolic blood pressure readings were observed in the chitosan group. No difference in cholesterol (total or low-density lipoprotein [LDL]) levels between groups and no adverse effects were noted.

The fat-blocking effects of prescription orlistat versus chitosan supplementation were compared in a randomized, open-label, two-period, sequential study design. Twelve healthy volunteers followed a standardized diet for the 21-day study and were subjected to a 7-day initial run-in diet. The groups were randomized and given either orlistat (120 mg) or chitosan (890 mg) 3 times daily for 7 days, and then the groups were crossed over for another 7 days of treatment. Fecal fat excretion was measured daily and found to be significantly increased with orlistat and not significantly changed by chitosan (Guerciolini et al., 2001).

In a randomized, double-blind, placebo-controlled study in obese, hypercholesterolemic subjects without dietary restriction, chitosan (as Asorbitol, a commercial chitosan product) or placebo was administered at the dosage of 250 mg 3 times daily. Sixty-eight subjects completed the study, and weight, body mass index, lean body mass, waist, hip, blood pressure, fasting lipids, and insulin levels were taken at the beginning and at weeks 4 and 6 of the study. The only change in the measured parameters was an increase in high-density lipoprotein (HDL) cholesterol in the chitosan group versus a decrease in the placebo group (Ho et al., 2001).

Pittler et al. (1999) examined the use of chitosan for weight loss in a randomized, double-blind, placebo-controlled clinical trial. Thirty-four overweight people were given either a placebo or chitosan (2 g/day) for 28 days. The participants were instructed to maintain their normal diet and to document the types and amounts of foods they consumed. At the end of the study, no significant changes in weight were observed between the treatment and placebo groups, and no changes in the levels of serum cholesterol, body mass index, triglycerides, ß carotene, and vitamins A, D, and E were observed. No serious adverse effects were noted, and the authors concluded that unless accompanied by other dietary alterations, chitosan does not reduce body weight in overweight people.

In a randomized, double-blind, placebo-controlled study of 86 obese people, the effect of a chitosan fiber along with a low-calorie diet was measured on weight loss and lipid-lowering parameters. The chitosan fiber product (Somagril) studied was a mixture of chitosan, guar, ascorbic acid, and other micronutrients, and the treatment group was given 4 tablets/day (unspecified amount of chitosan) for 4 weeks. The results for the chitosan group (C) and the placebo group (P) indicated statistically significant reductions in body weight (9.26% C and 3.60% P), over-weight percentage (11.26% C and 4.14% P), total cholesterol (23.37% C and 10.87% P), LDL cholesterol (27.09% C and 10.94% P), and triglycerides (21.16% C and 11.40% P) in both groups. HDL cholesterol levels increased 13.44% in the C group and 2.27% in the P group. Additionally, to find out whether chitosan was interfering with the absorption of mineral salts or fat-soluble vitamins, blood concentrations of sodium, potassium, calcium, magnesium, zinc, iron, copper, and vitamins A, D, and E were measured and found to have no significant changes between the two groups. Only mild and transient effects were found in both groups, with 5% reporting flatulence in the C group and 18.4% reporting nausea and/or constipation in the P group, with no statistically significant differences between the two groups (Colombo and Sciutto, 1996).

Macchi (1996) studied the effect of a chitosan fiber product (Somagril) plus a low-calorie diet or free diet in 30 obese subjects for the period of 1 month in a randomized, placebo-controlled study. The chitosan group (C) was treated with 4 tablets/day combined with a 1,200-calorie diet, the placebo group (P) was treated with the same low-calorie diet with 4 tablets/day of a placebo, and a third group (F) had no dietary restrictions plus the chitosan treatment. Reductions were found in body weight (4 kg C, 2.6 kg P, and 2.8 kg F); body mass index (1.7 kg/cm^2 C, 0.6 kg/cm^2 P, and 1.1 kg/cm^2 F); body fat (4% C, 1.2% P, and 3.3% F); and skin folds (17 mm C, 5 mm P, and 11 mm F). It is interesting to note the greater reduction in skin folds in both the chitosan groups versus the placebo. The author pointed out that even if the body weight reductions in the placebo and chitosan groups were similar, the groups with the chitosan treatment, with or without the dietary restrictions, produced a greater loss of adipose tissue as reflected by the skin fold data. Diastolic blood pressure was significantly decreased in the C (7 mm Hg) and F (9 mm Hg) groups but not in the P group (1 mm Hg). In all groups, plasma cholesterol and triglyceride levels decreased, but only in the F group was there an increase in HDL. The author noted no significant adverse effects.

In a randomized, double-blind, placebo-controlled study of 90 obese people, the effect of a chitosan fiber along with a low-calorie diet was measured on weight loss and lipid-lowering parameters. The chitosan fiber product (Somagril) studied was given at a dosage of 4 tablets/day (unspecified amount of chitosan). The chitosan group (C) and the placebo group (P) followed a low-calorie diet, and both showed reduction in body weight (7.19 kg C and 3.36 kg P) at the end of the study, with a statistically greater effect found in the chitosan group. Statistically significant reductions in overweight percentage (10.4% C and 3.8% P), arterial systolic (12.1 mm Hg C and 2.8 mm Hg P) and diastolic pressure (12.4 mm Hg C and 3.8 mm Hg P), total cholesterol (25.3% C and 11.1% P), LDL cholesterol (32.1% C and 13.6% P), and triglycerides (22.6% C and 10.1% P) were found. The C group showed a statistically greater effect in the reductions of all parameters. Additionally, HDL increased 11.8% in the C group and 4.6% in the P group. No statistically significant side effects were noted in either group. The authors concluded that the chitosan fiber product plus a low-calorie diet is useful in treating obese patients, with benefits including reduced levels of hypertension and hyperlipoproteinemia (Sciutto and Colombo, 1995).

Giustina and Ventura (1995) studied the combination of a chitosan dietary fiber product (Somagril, 4 tablets/day) and a low-calorie diet for its effects on weight reduction in a randomized, double-blind, placebo-controlled study of 100 obese subjects. Statistically significant reductions in the chitosan group (C) and the placebo group (P) of body weight (83.6 kg C and 76.3 kg P), overweight percentage (from 17.2% to 7.3% C and 16.3% to 12.4% P), arterial systolic pressure (from 145.3 to 135 mm Hg C and 146.0 to 142.9 mm Hg P), arterial diastolic pressure (92.6 mm Hg to 84.2 C and 92.5 to 90.0 P), and respiratory rate (27.6/min to 21.2/min C and 28.1/min to 26.3/min P) were measured. No statistically significant side effects between the two groups were noted, and any adverse effects were mild and transient. The authors concluded that the chitosan fiber product plus a low-calorie diet is useful in the treatment of obesity—better than a low-calorie diet alone and with the side benefits of ameliorating the secondary disorders of hypertension or dyspnea.

Cholesterol Reduction

In a study involving 21 overweight subjects with normal cholesterol levels, 2.4 g of a supplement containing chitosan and glucomannan (1.2 g each) were administered daily for 28 days. Subjects were advised to maintain their normal dietary and activity patterns throughout the study; and it was confirmed in the blood work that caloric intake and intake of fat and dietary fiber (excluding the supplement) did not alter between the beginning and end of the study. At the end of the study, serum total, HDL, and LDL levels were reduced significantly compared with the initial period; however, serum triacylglycerol concentration did not change. Fecal fat excretion did not change between the two periods, but there was a trend toward excretion of neutral sterols and bile acids. Owing to this finding, the authors concluded that the cholesterol lowering properties of chitosan and glucomannan are probably the result of the increase in fecal steroid excretion and not to fat excretion (Gallaher et al., 2002).

Maezaki et al. (1993) found that 3–6 g/day of chitosan reduced total serum cholesterol in eight healthy males and increased HDL levels. The average decrease in LDL was from 189 mg/dL before treatment to 177 mg/dL after 14 days of treatment (three 1-g chitosan biscuits daily for 7 days, and six 1-g biscuits daily for 7 days). Once the supplementation of the biscuits was stopped, the total cholesterol levels increased again to a level not significantly different from the starting value. The serum HDL cholesterol levels increased significantly from 51 mg/dL to 56 mg/dL after treatment with chitosan; likewise, when the treatment was stopped, levels decreased to similar pretreatment levels. Additionally, it was found that the excretion of primary bile acids, cholic acid, and chenodeoxycholic acid were significantly increased by chitosan treatment, whereas the excretion of cholic acid was decreased after treatment stopped. The authors concluded that these findings suggest the mechanism for reducing cholesterol is a reduction of the cholesterol "pool" in the body through the combination and elimination of chitosan with bile acids in the digestive tract.

SAFETY/DOSAGE

The dosage recommendations of chitosan supplements are about 2–6 g/day, in divided 1-g doses with each meal.

Much work has been performed to determine the possible toxicity of chitosan because of its use as a pharmaceutical drug delivery adjunct, and it has been found to be quite safe. However, because it has the ability to absorb fats, it may also absorb fat-soluble vitamins and carotenoids when supplemented at high dosages. Additionally, chitosan may cause gas, bloating, and diarrhea owing to the blockage of fat digestion (Deuchi et al., 1995; Ylitalo et al., 2002).

A warning may be found on many labels of chitosan supplements against use by people with shellfish allergies. However, because chitosan is made from the shells (versus the protein-containing meat) of shellfish, opinion is mixed as to whether someone with a severe allergy could experience problems.

REFERENCES

Colombo P, Sciutto AM. Nutritional aspects of chitosan employment in hypocaloric diet. Acta Toxicol Ther 1996;17(4):287–302.

Deuchi K, Kanauchi O, Shizukuishi M, Kobayashi E. Continuous and massive intake of chitosan affects mineral and fat-soluble vitamin status in rats fed on a high-fat diet. Biosci Biotechnol Biochem 1995;59(7):1211–1216.

Gades MD, Stern JS. Chitosan supplementation does not affect fat absorption in healthy males fed a high-fat diet, a pilot study. Int J Obes Relat Metab Disord 2002;26(1):119–122.

Gallaher DD, Gallaher CM, Mahrt GJ, Carr TP, Hollingshead CH, Hesslink R Jr, Wise J. A glucomannan and chitosan fiber supplement decreases plasma cholesterol and increases cholesterol excretion in overweight normocholesterolemic humans. J Am Coll Nutr 2002;21(5):428–433.

Giustina A, Ventura P. Weight-reducing regimens in obese subjects: effects of a new dietary fiber integrator [in Italian]. Acta Toxicol Ther 1995;SVI:199–214.

Guerciolini R, Radu-Radulescu L, Boldrin M, Dallas J, Moore R. Comparative evaluation of fecal fat excretion induced by orlistat and chitosan. Obes Res 2001;9(6):364–367.

Ho SC, Tai ES, Eng PH, Tan CE, Fok AC. In the absence of dietary surveillance, chitosan does not reduce plasma lipids or obesity in hypercholesterolaemic obese Asian subjects. Singapore Med J 2001;42(1):6–10.

Macchi G. A new approach to the treatment of obesity: chitosan's effects on body weight reduction and plasma cholesterol's levels. Acta Toxicol Ther 1996;17(4):303–320.

Maezaki Y, Tsuji K, Nakagawa Y, Kawai Y, Akimoto M., Tsugita T, Takekawa W, Terada A, Hara H, Mituoka T. Hypocholesterolemic effect of chitosan in adult males. Biosci Biotech Biochem 1993;57(9):1439–1444.

Pittler MH, Abbot NC, Harkness EF, Ernst E. Randomized, double-blind trial of chitosan for body weight reduction. Eur J Clin Nutr 1999;53(5):379–381.

Sciutto AM, Colombo P. Lipid-lowering effect of chitosan dietary integrator and hypocaloric diet in obese subjects [in Italian]. Acta Toxicol Ther 1995;16:215–230.

Ylitalo R, Lehtinen S, Wuolijoki E, Ylitalo P, Lehtimaki T. Cholesterol-lowering properties and safety of chitosan. Arzneimittelforschung 2002;52(1):1–7.

Zahorska-Markiewicz B, Krotkiewski M, Olszanecka-Glinianowicz M, Zurakowski A. Effect of chitosan in complex management of obesity. Pol Merkuriusz Lek 2002;13(74):129–132.

CITRUS AURANTIUM (SYNEPHRINE)

Overall Rank

★★★ for weight loss
★★ for thermogenesis
★ for athletic performance

OVERVIEW

Citrus aurantium (bitter orange extract, or zhi shi) contains an ephedrine alkaloid, synephrine, as its main active ingredient. At the onset of the controversy over ephedra and ephedrine (see the section titled "Ma Huang [*Ephedra sinensis*, Ephedrine]" later in this chapter), companies had already begun searching for alternatives for this potent thermogenic agent. The most obvious and safest alternative seemed to be synephrine, which is a compound in the same group of ephedrine alkaloids as ephedrine. However, although structurally similar, synephrine activity appears to be less potent and somewhat different in its mechanism. *Citrus aurantium* is also beginning to be promoted for athletic perform-ance because of its alleged central nervous system (CNS) stimulant activity.

Because *Citrus aurantium* stimulates the ß-3 adrenergic receptors, but not the ß-1, ß-2, or α-1 adrenergic receptors, it is thought to be free of the negative cardiovascular effects of ephedrine; however, it has still been suggested that it exhibits some negative cardiovascular side effects (Candelore et al., 1999; Chen et al., 1981; Park and Keeley, 1998).

COMMENTS

Synephrine has been found to stimulate the brown adipose tissue of dogs, which indicates it can stimulate thermogenesis, but there is a lack of clinical evidence that it does anything for burning fat in humans. Octopamine, another component of *Citrus aurantium*, may suppress appetite in insects, but does it do anything for humans? More questions than answers surround *Citrus aurantium* at this point.

Another important but not commonly discussed point about this supplement is that the naturally occurring form of synephrine found in *Citrus aurantium* is parasynephrine (p-synephrine). This is often confused with another form, which has different activities and potencies, called phenylephrine (also metasynephrine, or m-synephrine). The p-synephrine in *Citrus aurantium* has a milder potency than phenylephrine and should not be confused.

Overall, synephrine has been promoted widely as an alternative to ephedra, without much clinical science to back that claim. Although clearly safer than ephedra, synephrine is likely not completely without cardiovascular side effects.

SCIENTIFIC SUPPORT

Cardiovascular Effects

Penzak et al. (2001) investigated the concentrations of synephrine and octopamine in Seville orange extract (*Citrus aurantium*) and its effect on causing cardiac disturbances in normotensive humans. In a crossover design, participants consumed 8 oz of *Citrus aurantium* followed by another ingestion 8 hours later. Hemodynamic parameters of heart rate, systolic, diastolic, and mean arterial pressure were measured after ingestion and found not to differ significantly between water and treatment groups. The amount of synephrine in the extract was found to be 56.9 +/- 0.52 µg/mL, and there was no octopamine determined (by high-performance liquid chromatography). The ingestion of *Citrus aurantium* was found to be safe for normotensive people; however, the authors concluded that it is contraindicated for people with cardiac problems, such as severe hypertension and tachyarrhythmias, and narrow-angle glaucoma. Additionally, they added that people on monoamine oxidase inhibitors or taking decongestant-containing cold preparations should also avoid *Citrus aurantium*.

Weight Loss and Thermogenesis

Kalman et al. (2000) studied the effects on body mass, body composition, metabolic variables, and mood states of an ephedrine- and synephrine-based supplement in humans. In a randomized, placebo-controlled design, 30 subjects with body mass indexes over 27 kg/m^2 were given a preparation containing ephedrine alkaloids (20 mg), synephrine (5 mg), caffeine (200 mg), and salicin (15 mg) or a matched placebo 2 times daily for 8 weeks. The diet-and-exercise program prescribed for all participants was a 22-kcal/kg National Cholesterol Education Program Step One diet and a supervised cross-training program 3 days/week. The treatment group experienced a 16% decrease in body fat, whereas the control group had a 1% increase, with a significant difference between the groups. Both groups had a significant decline in fat-free mass, but the reduction was greater in the control than the treatment group, which suggested a muscle-sparing effect in the treatment group. No significant changes in cardiac parameters (blood pressure, serial electrocardiograms, pulse rate), serum chemistry, or caloric intake were found.

SAFETY/DOSAGE

Citrus aurantium standardized to synephrine (3–6%) is recommended owing to its naturally low concentration of this main active ingredient. Approximately 200–600 mg of *Citrus aurantium* extract, providing 4–20 mg synephrine, is the usual suggested dosage.

As noted in the study by Penzak et al. (2001), synephrine products are contraindicated for people with cardiac problems, such as severe hypertension and tachyarrhythmias, and narrow-angle glaucoma. Additionally, anyone using monoamine oxidase inhibitors or decongestant-containing cold preparations should avoid *Citrus aurantium*.

REFERENCES

Candelore MR, Deng L, Tota L, Guan XM, Amend A, Liu Y, Newbold R, Cascieri MA, Weber AE. Potent and selective human beta(3)-adrenergic receptor antagonists. J Pharmacol Exp Ther 1999;290(2):649–655.

Chen X, Liu LY, Deng HW, Fang YX, Ye YW. The effects of Citrus aurantium and its active ingredient N-methyltyramine on the cardiovascular receptors. Yao Hsueh Hsueh Pao 1981;16(4):253–259.

Kalman DS, Colker CM, Shi Q, Swain MA. Effects of a weight-loss aid in healthy overweight adults: double-blind, placebo-controlled clinical trial. Curr Ther Res 2000;61(4):199–205.

Park JH, Keeley LL. The effect of biogenic amines and their analogs on carbohydrate metabolism in the fat body of the cockroach Blaberus discoidalis. Gen Comp Endocrinol 1998;110(1):88–95.

Penzak SR, Jann MW, Cold JA, Hon YY, Desai HD, Gurley BJ. Seville (sour) orange juice: synephrine content and cardiovascular effects in normotensive adults. J Clin Pharmacol 2001;41(10):1059–1063.

CONJUGATED LINOLEIC ACID (CLA)

Overall Rank

★★★★	for fat loss in moderately overweight adults
★	for control of blood lipids
ZERO	for fat loss in trained athletes
ZERO	for anticancer effects in humans

OVERVIEW

Linoleic acid is found in the diet in vegetable oils, whereas the conjugated variety, CLA, is found primarily in meat and dairy products. The form of CLA found most commonly in dietary supplements is manufactured from vegetable oils, such as sunflower oil. It is marketed primarily as a weight loss and muscle-building supplement and also as an "anticancer" agent. Linoleic acid is an ω-6 fatty acid, meaning that it is unsaturated, with a double bond occurring at the sixth carbon atom. CLA is an isomer of linoleic acid, which refers to a slight rearrangement of the molecular structure (conjugation) resulting in a fatty acid with altered chemical functions. The rearrangement in this case is a conjugated double bond occurring at carbons 10 and 12 or at carbons 9 and 11; this may be an important distinction because a number of recent studies have suggested that the two isomers may have different metabolic fates in the body.

COMMENTS

The existing evidence supports a beneficial, but modest, effect of CLA supplements (3–6 g/day for 4–12 weeks) in promoting fat loss in moderately overweight adults. Athletes do not appear to derive the same weight loss or lean-mass-enhancing effects that have been observed in studies of overweight sedentary subjects. Anticancer claims for CLA supplements are based on preliminary laboratory findings and are not supported by convincing clinical evidence.

SCIENTIFIC SUPPORT

Most research on the dietary intake of CLA has been conducted in animals. Weight loss studies in rodents have shown a beneficial effect of CLA feeding, with supplemented rats gaining less body fat but more lean body mass compared with control animals. In livestock studies (cattle, pigs, and chickens), supplemental CLA has been shown to promote growth and prevent muscle wasting, whereas body fat accumulation may be suppressed owing to an increase in energy expenditure. In rabbits with high cholesterol, CLA feeding reduces LDL and triglycerides.

In humans, Noone et al. (2002) showed that blended CLA supplements (3 g of either a 50:50 or 80:20 blend of c9/t11:t10/c12) could reduce fasting plasma triglyceride and cholesterol levels but with no effect on levels of HDL, glucose, or insulin or on body weight in healthy normolipidemic subjects. A similar study by Benito et al. (2001a) found no change in blood levels of cholesterol or triglycerides in normolipidemic subjects consuming 3.9 g/day of CLA for 93 days.

Although little human weight loss data are available, a handful of small studies have shown that sedentary, moderately overweight subjects consuming 3.2–6.8 g/day of CLA for 4–12 weeks show a statistically significant loss of body fat and an increase in lean body mass, whereas body weight may or may not be reduced (Blankson et al., 2000; Riserus et al., 2001; Smedman and Vessby, 2001; Thom et al., 2001). Kreider et al. (2002) have shown that resistance-trained athletes supplemented with 6 g/day of CLA for 28 days derive no significant benefits in terms of body weight, fat mass, or fat-free mass. Likewise, in metabolic ward studies, CLA supplementation has also been shown to have no significant effect on energy expenditure, fat oxidation, or respiratory exchange ratio at rest or during exercise (Zambell et al., 2001).

SAFETY/DOSAGE

Animal data have not suggested any significant side effects associated with CLA supplementation, but recent clinical data may indicate that supplementation with the t10/c12 isomer of CLA (but not a mixture of c9/t11 and t10/c12) can cause insulin resistance and increase both oxidative stress and inflammatory markers in abdominally obese men (Basu et al., 2000a; Riserus et al., 2002). However, no changes in inflammatory or thrombotic markers were noted in subjects taking 3.9 g/day of blended CLA isomers (Tonalin) for 93 days (Benito et al., 2001b; Kelley et al., 2001).

Typical dosage recommendations for CLA supplements used for weight loss are 3–6 g/day. Given the current controversy linking the t10/c12 isomer of CLA with elevated markers of inflammation and oxidative stress, it may be prudent to select supplements containing a blended combination of CLA isomers.

REFERENCES

Basu S, Riserus U, Turpeinen A, Vessby B. Conjugated linoleic acid induces lipid peroxidation in men with abdominal obesity. Clin Sci (Lond) 2000;99(6):511–516.

Benito P, Nelson GJ, Kelley DS, Bartolini G, Schmidt PC, Simon V. The effect of conjugated linoleic acid on plasma lipoproteins and tissue fatty acid composition in humans. Lipids 2001a;36(3):229–236.

Benito P, Nelson GJ, Kelley DS, Bartolini G, Schmidt PC, Simon V. The effect of conjugated linoleic acid on platelet function, platelet fatty acid composition, and blood coagulation in humans. Lipids 2001b;36(3):221–227.

Blankson H, Stakkestad JA, Fagertun H, Thom E, Wadstein J, Gudmundsen O. Conjugated linoleic acid reduces body fat mass in overweight and obese humans. J Nutr 2000;130(12):2943–2948.

Kelley DS, Simon VA, Taylor PC, Rudolph IL, Benito P, Nelson GJ, Mackey BE, Erickson KL. Dietary supplementation with conjugated linoleic acid increased its concentration in human peripheral blood mononuclear cells, but did not alter their function. Lipids 2001;36(7):669–674.

Kreider RB, Ferreira MP, Greenwood M, Wilson M, Almada AL. Effects of conjugated linoleic acid supplementation during resistance training on body composition, bone density, strength, and selected hematological markers. J Strength Cond Res 2002;16(3):325–334.

Noone EJ, Roche HM, Nugent AP, Gibney MJ. The effect of dietary supplementation using isomeric blends of conjugated linoleic acid on lipid metabolism in healthy human subjects. Br J Nutr 2002;88(3):243–251.

Riserus U, Basu S, Jovinge S, Fredrikson GN, Arnlov J, Vessby B. Supplementation with conjugated linoleic acid causes isomer-dependent oxidative stress and elevated C-reactive protein: a potential link to fatty acid-induced insulin resistance. Circulation 2002;106(15):1925–1929.

Riserus U, Berglund L, Vessby B. Conjugated linoleic acid (CLA) reduced abdominal adipose tissue in obese middle-aged men with signs of the metabolic syndrome: a randomised controlled trial. Int J Obes Relat Metab Disord 2001;25(8):1129–1135.

Smedman A, Vessby B. Conjugated linoleic acid supplementation in humans—metabolic effects. Lipids 2001;36(8):773–781.

Thom E, Wadstein J, Gudmundsen O. Conjugated linoleic acid reduces body fat in healthy exercising humans. J Int Med Res 2001;29(5):392–396.

Zambell KL, Horn WF, Keim NL. Conjugated linoleic acid supplementation in humans: effects on fatty acid and glycerol kinetics. Lipids 2001;36(8):767–772.

ADDITIONAL RESOURCES

Basu S, Smedman A, Vessby B. Conjugated linoleic acid induces lipid peroxidation in humans. FEBS Lett 2000;468(1):33–36.

Herbel BK, McGuire MK, McGuire MA, Shultz TD. Safflower oil consumption does not increase plasma conjugated linoleic acid concentrations in humans. Am J Clin Nutr 1998;67(2):332–337.

Zambell KL, Keim NL, Van Loan MD, Gale B, Benito P, Kelley DS, Nelson GJ. Conjugated linoleic acid supplementation in humans: effects on body composition and energy expenditure. Lipids 2000;35(7):777–782.

GUARANA (*PAULLINIA CUPANA*)

Overall Rank
(as an herbal source of caffeine)

★★★ for energy
★★ for athletic and mental performance
★★ for weight loss
★ for aphrodisiac properties

OVERVIEW

Guarana is a Brazilian herb that may be found in supplements and foods (because it is generally recognized as safe). It has become a popular addition to energy drinks owing to its high caffeine content. Traditionally, guarana has been used as a mental, physical, and sexual stimulant. Today, guarana is mostly used for energy, for athletic performance, and in weight loss formulations, but preclinical studies are exploring its effects on increasing sexual function. No clinical work has been performed on guarana as a single ingredient, so its use as a supplement relies on its traditional medicinal use and the strength of the research behind caffeine for inducing alertness, suppressing the appetite, and promoting thermogenesis. Although caffeine is accepted as the major active ingredient, other important compounds in guarana are under ongoing investigation, including polyphenols and saponins (Henman, 1982).

COMMENTS

No clinical studies have been performed with guarana as a single supplement in humans; therefore, even though there is much clinical support for the use of caffeine on the claims of mental and physical performance, claims for the use of guarana as a whole herb remain largely unfounded.

SCIENTIFIC SUPPORT

Weight Loss
Although guarana has been tested in studies of weight loss, it is formulated with other herbs, so these studies were not included in this review (Andersen and Fogh, 2001; Bouthegourd et al., 2002). Guarana is sometimes formulated with ephedra or supplements containing ephedrine alkaloids to trigger the well-known and studied synergistic effect between caffeine and ephedrine alkaloids (Nasser et al., 1999). Boozer et al. (2001) found that ephedra (ma huang) and guarana produced fat and weight loss. Another study of the impact on obesity of a formulation containing several herbs, including guarana, found favorable results on weight loss. The formulation contained the standardized ingredients of ephedra, caffeine, and chromium picolinate from the herbal mixture (Woodgate and Conquer, 2001).

Athletic Performance
The use of guarana for athletic performance has been tested in mice on measures of exercise-induced hypoglycemia and in physical and cognitive tests with favorable results. Additionally, a mixture of herbs including guarana was found to relax rabbit corpus cavernosum (Antunes et al., 2001; Espinola et al., 1997).

SAFETY/DOSAGE

The dosage of guarana is from 200–2,000 mg/day, in divided doses, of an extract standardized to 5.5–10% of caffeine (providing 11–200 mg of caffeine per serving). A dosage of more than 200 mg of caffeine per serving (in supplement, food, or beverage) is not recommended.

The safety concerns of guarana are mainly owing to the caffeine content. Persons who are caffeine sensitive may be overstimulated at higher doses, with possible symptoms of related insomnia, restlessness, anxiety, high blood pressure, irritability, headaches, and heart palpitations. Guarana is not recommended for pregnant women or children. The American Herbal Products Association (AHPA) has given guarana a Class 2 rating: "not recommended for excessive or long term use" (McGuffin et al., 1997).

Another concern for guarana toxicity is for formulations containing ephedra (ephedrine alkaloids). Consumption of ephedrine alkaloids and caffeine have well-known and serious cardiovascular risks (Haller et al., 2002).

REFERENCES

Andersen T, Fogh J. Weight loss and delayed gastric emptying following a South American herbal preparation in overweight patients. J Hum Nutr Diet 2001;14(3):243–250.

Antunes E, Gordo WM, de Oliveira JF, Teixeira CE, Hyslop S, De Nucci G. The relaxation of isolated rabbit corpus cavernosum by the herbal medicine Catuama and its constituents. Phytother Res 2001;15(5):416–421.

Boozer CN, Nasser JA, Heymsfield SB, Wang V, Chen G, Solomon JL. An herbal supplement containing ma huang-guarana for weight loss: a randomized, double-blind trial. Int J Obes Relat Metab Disord 2001;25(3):316–324.

Bouthegourd JC, Martin JC, Gripois D, Roseau S, Blouquit MF, Even PC, Tome D, Quignard-Boulange A. Efficacy of dietary CLA and CLA+guarana (ADI pill) on body adiposity, and adipocytes cell number and size. FASEB J 2002;16(4).

Espinola EB, Dias RF, Mattei R, Carlini EA. Pharmacological activity of guarana (Paullinia cupana Mart.) in laboratory animals. J Ethnopharmacol 1997;55(3):223–229.

Haller CA, Peyton J III, Benowitz NL. Pharmacology of ephedra alkaloids and caffeine after single-dose dietary supplement use. Clin Pharmacol Ther 2002;71(6):421–432.

Henman AR. Guarana (Paullinia cupana var. sorbilis): ecological and social perspectives on an economic plant of the central Amazon basin. J Ethnopharmacol 1982;6(3):311–338.

McGuffin M, Hobbs C, Upton R, Goldberg A. American Herbal Products Association's Botanical Safety Handbook. Boca Raton, FL: CRC Press, 1997.

Nasser JA, Wang V, Chen GC, Solomon JL, Heymsfield SB, Boozer CN. Efficacy trial for weight loss of an herbal supplement of ma huang and guarana. FASEB J 1999;13(5 pt 2).

Woodgate DE, Conquer JA. Double-blind study evaluating the effects of a novel herbal supplement on weight loss in overweight adults. FASEB J 2001;15(4).

Hydroxycitric Acid (HCA, GARCINIA CAMBOGIA)

Overall Rank

★★★ for appetite suppression
★★   for weight loss and "fat burning"

OVERVIEW

Garcinia cambogia is a small fruit that contains the active ingredient hydroxycitric acid (HCA); the abbreviation (-)HCA is also used. One of the main theories of how garcinia and HCA work is through the inhibition in cells of citrate lyase, which is needed for the conversion of carbohydrates to fat. Prevention of carbohydrate conversion to fat is thought to induce the body to oxidize the excess carbohydrates, leading to fully loaded glycogen stores, which in turn may play a part in suppressing the appetite. Preclinical studies have confirmed body weight loss in rats fed HCA, and HCA's activity of suppressing the appetite and reducing food intake was confirmed. Clinically, however, HCA has failed to perform well. This may be the result of citrate lyase being important only in very high carbohydrate diets, a type of diet that most studies do not prescribe, along with other variables (a high-fiber diet can bind to HCA and block it).

COMMENTS

The theory behind the use of HCA and *Garcinia cambogia* seems to be sound, but clinical studies have still to prove under which conditions HCA is best used. To date, many of the herbal supplements containing HCA are probably not effective because they lack the correct conditions of use.

SCIENTIFIC SUPPORT

Appetite Suppression

In a randomized, placebo-controlled, single-blind, crossover study, 24 overweight men and women were administered HCA for 2 weeks. After 2 weeks of treatment, the study subjects' 24-hour energy intakes (EIs), appetite profiles, hedonics, moods, and possible changes in dietary restraint were assessed in a laboratory restaurant. EIs were decreased by 15–30%, and body weight tended to decrease during the HCA treatment period without changes in other factors. It was concluded that EI was reduced with HCA treatment, while satiety remained the same (Westerterp-Plantenga and Kovacs, 2002).

In a double-blind, placebo-controlled, randomized, crossover study, the effects of the ingestion of HCA alone and combined with medium-chain triglycerides on satiety and food intake was investigated. Twenty-one normal to moderately obese subjects participated in the study, which consisted of three 2-week intervention periods separated by washouts of 2 or 6 weeks. A significant loss in body weight was found in all groups, but no differences were found among the groups. The 24-hour EI and appetite-related parameters were similar for all treatments. Neither HCA alone nor HCA combined with medium-chain triglycerides produced changes in food intake or satiety (Kovacs et al., 2001a).

In a double-blind, placebo-controlled, randomized, crossover study, the effects of the ingestion of HCA alone and combined with medium-chain triglycerides on satiety, fat oxidation, energy expenditure, and body weight was investigated. Eleven males participated in the study, which consisted of three intervention periods separated by washout periods of 4 weeks. Body weight was significantly reduced in all three groups but was not found to be different among the groups. Likewise, the appetite parameters and energy expenditures were not different among treatments. Neither HCA alone nor HCA combined with medium-chain triglycerides resulted in increased satiety, fat oxidation, 24-hour EI, or body weight loss compared with placebo (Kovacs et al., 2001b).

Mattes and Bormann (2000) studied the effect of HCA in promoting weight loss through appetite suppression. In a double-blind, placebo-controlled study, 89 mildly overweight women were prescribed 5,020-kJ diets for 12 weeks, and either 400 mg of *Garcinia cambogia* (2.4 g/day of garcinia and 1.2 g/day of HCA) or a placebo 30–60 minutes before meals. Weight and body composition was measured every other week for 12 weeks. Both groups showed a loss in body weight, with the treatment group showing significantly greater reduction. The HCA, however, had no effect on appetite-related variables.

Weight Loss

Preuss et al. (2002) studied the efficacy of *Garcinia cambogia*-derived HCA (HCA-SX from Super CitriMax) in suppressing appetite and inhibiting fat synthesis in a study involving 48 moderately obese adults. Both the HCA group (2,800 mg/day) and the placebo group were treated 30 minutes before meals for 8 weeks. A diet of approximately 2,000 kcal and a walking program supervised by a trainer were prescribed to both groups. Losses of body weight of 3.3% (after 4 weeks) and 4.8% (after 8 weeks) were observed in the treatment group. Triglyceride, LDL, and total cholesterol levels were all reduced in the treatment groups as well. The authors concluded that HCA-SX could be useful in weight management.

To test the theory that HCA increases fatty acid oxidation by reducing the malonyl–coenzyme A concentrations, 10 cyclists were studied after ingestion of an HCA supplement or placebo. The cyclists ingested either 3.1 mL/kg body weight of an HCA solution or a placebo 45 and 15 minutes before exercise and 30 and 60 minutes after the start of exercise. During rest and after 2 hours of exercise at 50% of their maximal work output, the cyclists were measured for their total fat and carbohydrate oxidation rates. Blood samples were collected at rest and during 15-minute intervals of exercise. No significant changes were found in total fat and carbohydrate oxidation rates between the groups. Even when ingested in large quantities, HCA did not increase total fat oxidation in vivo in endurance-trained athletes (van Loon et al., 2000).

In a double-blind, placebo-controlled, randomized, crossover study, HCA was tested for effects on metabolic parameters in humans. With or without moderately intense exercise over four laboratory visits, energy expenditure, respiratory quotient (following an overnight fast), and blood samples (for glucose, insulin, flucagon, lactate, and ß hydroxybu-yrate) were measured. Treatment with HCA did not affect energy expend-iture either with the exercise or at rest. Blood parameters did not differ significantly between treatments through the course of the study, and respiratory quotient was not significantly lowered at rest or during exer-cise compared with a placebo. The authors concluded that the hypothesis that HCA could affect the fat oxidation in fasting or moderately exercising humans with a typical Western diet was not supported (Kriketos et al., 1999).

In a randomized, double-blind, placebo-controlled clinical study, HCA was tested for its efficacy in lowering body weight and fat mass loss in overweight humans. Over the course of 12 weeks, participants were given either 1,500 mg/day of HCA or placebo and prescribed a high-fiber, low-energy diet. Every other week, body weight was measured, and fat mass measurements were taken at 0 and 12 weeks. No significant weight loss or fat mass loss was observed in this study by treatment of HCA compared with placebo (Heymsfield et al., 1998).

Roman et al. (1996) investigated the efficacy of *Garcinia cambogia* in promoting weight loss, and reducing cholesterolemia and triglyceridemia in overweight subjects. In a randomized, placebo-controlled design, 40 participants were given either an extract of *Garcinia cambogia* (500 mg) or placebo before each meal for 8 weeks. The treatment group showed a significant reduction in the amount of overweight and in cholesterol and triglycerides compared with the placebo group.

SAFETY/DOSAGE

Garcinia cambogia products vary in their amounts of standardized HCA, but it is rare to find any product claiming less than 50% HCA. Two to three divided doses of *Garcinia cambogia*, 750–1,500 mg each, may be taken before mealtime (30–60 minutes).

No serious side effects have been noted. The acute LD50 of HCA-SX is more than 5,000 mg/kg (orally in rats), and no gross toxicological pathology was found on autopsy, indicating the safety of this product (Ohia et al., 2002).

There have been safety concerns with ephedra-containing supplements, and HCA is a common component combined with ephedra formulations designed for bodybuilding and weight loss.

REFERENCES

Heymsfield SB, Allison DB, Vasselli JR, Pietrobelli A, Greenfield D, Nunez C. Garcinia cambogia (hydroxycitric acid) as a potential antiobesity agent: a randomized controlled trial. JAMA 1998;280(18):1596–1600.

Kovacs EM, Westerterp-Plantenga MS, de Vries M, Brouns F, Saris WH. Effects of 2-week ingestion of (-)-hydroxycitrate and (-)-hydroxycitrate combined with medium-chain triglycerides on satiety and food intake. Physiol Behav 2001a;74(4–5):543–549.

Kovacs EM, Westerterp-Plantenga MS, Saris WH. The effects of 2-week ingestion of (--)-hydroxycitrate and (--)-hydroxycitrate combined with medium-chain triglycerides on satiety, fat oxidation, energy expenditure and body weight. Int J Obes Relat Metab Disord 2001b;25(7):1087–1094.

Kriketos AD, Thompson HR, Greene H, Hill JO. (-)-Hydroxycitric acid does not affect energy expenditure and substrate oxidation in adult males in a post-absorptive state. Int J Obes Relat Metab Disord 1999;23(8):867–873.

Mattes RD, Bormann L. Effects of (-)-hydroxycitric acid on appetitive variables. Physiol Behav 2000;71(1–2):87–94.

Ohia SE, Opere CA, LeDay AM, Bagchi M, Bagchi D, Stohs SJ. Safety and mechanism of appetite suppression by a novel hydroxycitric acid extract (HCA-SX). Mol Cell Biochem 2002;238(1–2):89–103.

Preuss HG, Bagchi D, Rao CVS, Echard BW, Satyanarayana S, Bagchi M. Effect of hydroxycitric acid on weight loss, body mass index and plasma leptin levels in human subjects. FASEB J 2002;16(5):A1020.

Roman RR, Flores SJ, Alarcon A. Control of obesity with Garcinia cambogia extract <original> extracto de Garcinia cambogia en el control de la. Investigacion Medica Internacional 1996;22:97–100.

van Loon LJ, van Rooijen JJ, Niesen B, Verhagen H, Saris WH, Wagenmakers AJ. Effects of acute (-)-hydroxycitrate supplementation on substrate metabolism at rest and during exercise in humans. Am J Clin Nutr 2000;72(6):1445–1450.

Westerterp-Plantenga MS, Kovacs EM. The effect of (-)-hydroxycitrate on energy intake and satiety in overweight humans. Int J Obes Relat Metab Disord 2002;26(6):870–872.

MA HUANG (*EPHEDRA SINENSIS*, EPHEDRINE)

Overall Rank

 WARNING: Banned for sale as a dietary supplement in the United States.

★★★★ for weight loss
★★★ for thermogenesis
★★ for athletic performance

OVERVIEW

The ephedrine alkaloids are by far the most popular supplements on the market for weight loss (at least until their ban from the U.S. market), with the top being ephedrine. Ephedrine is available in a purified form (as pseudoephedrine) in some over-the-counter medicines or as a more crude herbal medicine in the form of an extract, tea, or dried plant material of ma huang (*Ephedra sinensis*) or one of about 40 other plant species that contain ephedrine, such as *Sida cordifolia*. Ephedrine is a general sympathomimetic agent, which means that it stimulates the central nervous system by mimicking the effects of many of the body's own sympathetic hormones (e.g., adrenaline and norepinephrine). Ephedrine is used mostly for its stimulating (alertness and energy) effects, as an appetite suppressant in weight loss, and as a decongestant. Its role in weight loss is primarily as a thermogenic agent (Bukowiecki et al., 1982).

Although ephedrine is known to be an effective bronchodilator and an increasing amount of clinical evidence shows that it is beneficial in the treatment of obesity, ephedrine's track record for safety has caused much controversy (Tinkelman and Avner, 1977). The controversy concerns the question of whether ephedra should be allowed as a dietary supplement, which claims are allowed for its use, what warnings should products carry, and how responsible manufacturers should be in the adverse effects of ephedra use. Because of the legal risk surrounding ephedra, many companies are now looking to replace or deemphasize ephedrine in their weight loss supplement formulations.

COMMENTS

This supplement has been the most controversial of all the herbs and supplements on the market and has caused much concern over the regulation of all supplements. However, as with most diet drugs, ephedra seems to be dangerous mainly when it is combined with other drugs (adrenergic), when it is taken at higher-than-recommended dosages, and when people who take it have certain cardiovascular risks. Reviews are ongoing about who is most susceptible to ephedra-related risks, and current thought is that personal aberrations in adrenoceptors are key factors. What is certain is that ephedra and ephedrine are powerful enough to produce an immediate effect, and with any drug capable of such an effect, adverse effects may accompany it.

Many of the studies quoted here focus on a combination of ephedra and caffeine, which is representative of how ephedra is typically used. Aspirin is also commonly combined with ephedra, and although aspirin alone is not used as a weight loss aid, its combination with ephedrine and caffeine is a powerful thermogenic stimulant. Salicylic acid and the salicylates are natural forms of aspirin that can also be found in the traditional herbal supplement called white willow bark, or *Salix alba* (discussed later in this chapter). The combination of ephedrine, caffeine, and aspirin—known as ECA stack—has become one of the most popular weight loss supplements on the market. In dietary supplement formulations, caffeine source plants, white willow bark, or other plants with salicylates may be used as combination products to stimulate thermogenesis with ephedra.

SCIENTIFIC SUPPORT

Athletic Performance

Bell et al. (2001) noted that both caffeine and ephedrine singularly and in combination are known to improve athletic performance in high-intensity aerobic activity that lasts 10–20 min. In this first study, exercise performance was improved by both caffeine and ephedrine, with ephedrine stimulating the CNS and caffeine stimulating the skeletal muscle. In an effort to investigate whether this effect was sustained after 20 min, 12 subjects who were running a 10-km run were given (90 minutes before the run began) either a placebo (P), caffeine (C, 4 mg/kg), ephedrine (E, 0.8 mg/kg) or ephedrine plus caffeine (E+C). The run times for the ephedrine-containing trials (E and E+C) were significantly reduced compared with the C and P trials. Heart rate and pace (in the last 5 km) for the ephedrine-containing trials (E and E+C) were significantly reduced compared with the C and P trials. The ratings of perceived exertion were similar for all trials. Caffeine was found to increase epinephrine and norepinephrine response and blood lactate, glucose, and glycerol levels, whereas ephedrine reduced the epinephrine response and increased dopamine levels (Bell et al., 2002).

Bell et al. (2000) examined the effect of reducing the dosage of combined ephedrine and caffeine administration in athletes on limiting the negative side effects of vomiting and nausea (experienced by 25% of subjects) reported in earlier studies. They found that 4–5 mg of caffeine per kilogram combined with 0.8–1 mg of ephedrine per kilogram resulted in the maintenance of ergogenic effect while reducing the negative side effects. The lowest-dose combination caused no incidence of vomiting or nausea.

Thermogenesis

In a randomized, double-blind, crossover study, 10 volunteers were given ephedra (50 mg 3 times daily) or a placebo to determine 24-hour energy expenditure, mechanical work, and urinary catecholamines (Shannon et al., 1999). The treatment with ephedra resulted in a 3.6% increase in energy expenditure. The authors noted that from the data on urinary excretion, ephedra probably induces its thermogenic effect from direct ß-1 and ß-2 adrenoceptor agonism.

Liu et al. (1995) studied which ß adrenoceptors were involved in sympathetic stimulation of thermogenesis by ephedrine in combination with a nonselective ß-adrenoceptor agonist, nadolol. Nine healthy subjects were given a placebo, ephedra or ephedrine, and three doses (2.5, 5, and 10 mg) of nadolol. Energy expenditure, respiratory quotient, heart rate, blood pressure, and plasma variables (potassium, glucose, lactate, glycerol, nonesterified fatty acids, and triglycerides) were measured. The doses of nadolol were given to determine what fraction of the thermogenic response to ephedrine (30 mg) remained after inhibition of ß-1 and ß-2 adrenoceptor–mediated responses. All three ß-adrenoceptor subtypes (1, 2, and 3) were presumed to be involved, and it was estimated that at least 40% of the thermogenic response by ephedrine was mediated by the ß-3 adrenoceptor.

In a randomized, double-blind, crossover design, the effect of ephedrine (50 mg orally 3 times daily) and a very low calorie diet (1965 kJ) on energy expenditure, protein metabolism, and hormone levels was studied in 10 obese people. The study lasted for 6 weeks with a treatment period during weeks 2–5. Both groups followed the prescribed very low calorie diet. No differences were found between the ephedrine and placebo groups for weight loss. Ephedrine treatment partially prevented the fall in resting metabolic rate and improved nitrogen balance during the diet. The authors concluded that ephedrine treatment (chronic administration of adrenoceptor agonists) could be used to help obese patients in weight loss programs who have decreased capacity for energy expenditure (Pasquali et al., 1992).

Astrup (1986) investigated the possible role of brown adipose tissue (BAT) in humans in the process of thermogenesis. It had been known that BAT in rodents is the main site of nonshivering thermogenesis and facultative thermogenesis, and that BAT is mediated by the sympathetic nervous system. However, the role of BAT in stimulation of thermogenesis in humans was unknown. Humans are known to have BAT in the interscapular subcutaneous tissue, and an ephedrine-induced thermogenesis response in humans had been observed. Therefore, BAT was theorized to play a significant role in temperature regulation, and it was thought that BAT in obese adults might have a diminished thermogenic ability. In a first study, the interscapular tissue was examined for thermogenic response after ephedrine stimulation, and it was found to be no different in heat production to white adipose tissue in the lumbar area. In a second study, perirenal BAT was examined for thermogenic response and found to be active only in one subject of five. In the single subject, it was estimated that BAT thermogenesis could account for 15% of the ephedrine-induced increase in the body's oxygen consumption.

As a follow-up to the 1985 study, Astrup et al. (1986) investigated the effect of ß-adrenergic stimulation to glucose (or diet)-induced thermogenesis. The oxygen consumption reflected by 3 months of ephedrine treatment by five female subjects was sustained at a 10% elevated level. Additionally, the thermogenesis induced by glucose was increased during treatment compared with control (the group that was studied after termination of 3 months treatment). The respiratory quotient also indicated that more lipid was oxidized in the treatment group.

The thermogenic effect of ephedrine was studied in five overweight women. A single oral dose of 1 mg/kg body weight was given to the five women and studied by indirect calorimetry before, during, and 2 months after chronic treatment of ephedrine (20 mg perorally 3 times daily). The extra consumption of oxygen caused by the single dose of ephedrine was 1.31 before treatment, 7.0 after 4 weeks of treatment, 6.91 after 12 weeks of treatment, and 1.21 after treatment stopped. The serum T3:T4 ratio increased significantly after 4 weeks of treatment but decreased below the starting value after 12 weeks of treatment. The body weight of the five women participating in the study declined significantly after treatment (2.5 kg at 4 weeks and 5.5 kg at 12 weeks). The sustained increases in oxygen consumption after a single dose of ephedrine at 4 and 12 weeks of treatment shows an increased thermogenic response from an acute dose during chronic administration of ephedra (Astrup et al., 1985).

Weight Loss

Boozer et al. (2002) studied the long-term safety of a supplement containing ephedra (80 mg/day ephedrine alkaloids) and kola nut (192 mg/day caffeine) in a 6-month, randomized, double-blind, placebo-controlled study. In the treatment group, small changes in blood pressure and increased heart rate were noted, without increased cardiac arrhythmias. Dry mouth, heartburn, and insomnia were reported more often in the treatment group. The authors concluded that the supplement containing ephedra and caffeine was able to promote weight loss without significant adverse effects.

Boozer et al. (2001) performed an 8-week, randomized, double-blind, placebo-controlled clinical study on the short-term safety and efficacy for weight loss of a supplement containing ephedra (ma huang) and guarana (containing caffeine). Sixty-seven overweight participants were given either a placebo or the supplement and monitored at the end of the study. Weight and fat loss, hip circumference, and serum triglycerides were all reduced in the treatment group. The common reported side effects were dry mouth, insomnia, and headache. The authors mentioned that the long-term safety of this supplement needed further investigation.

Zahorska-Markiewicz et al. (2001) performed a study on adrenergic drugs to find out if they were able to change the concentrations of serum neuropeptide Y in obese women. The concentrations of neuropeptide Y is postulated to be a counter-regulatory factor that can prevent weight increase. The adrenergic drugs selected for the study were ephedrine and caffeine or combinations of ephedrine, caffeine, and yohimbine. The 13 obese participants were instructed to follow a very low calorie diet along with either a placebo or one of the treatments. Physical examination, heart rate, blood pressure, heart rate variability, and neuropeptide Y serum tests were measured for all the participants. No serious side effects were observed from treatment, and the authors concluded that this was because they used such low concentrations of the adrenergic drugs. Further, the low concentrations of treatment drugs resulted in no change of plasma neuropeptide Y or cardiovascular changes being observed.

Molnar et al. (2000) performed the first clinical study of a caffeine–ephedrine combination in adolescents. Either a placebo or a caffeine–ephedrine mixture (300 mg of caffeine and 30 mg of ephedrine daily for those under 80 kg; and a 600 mg–60 mg combination daily for those over 80 kg) was given to the adolescents for 20 weeks. Body weight decreased by more than 5% in 81% of the treatment group and in 31% of the control group. Adverse events did not differ between groups.

Pasquali and Casimirri (1993) reviewed the results of ephedrine treatment in different groups: in unselected obese subjects, low-energy adapted obese women, ephedrine combined with caffeine, and ephedrine with underfeeding. In their studies they did not find a synergistic advantage in using ephedra with caffeine as other studies have noted. However, they did conclude that ephedrine either alone or with caffeine could promote fat loss while preserving free fatty mass and therefore is useful to a large population of obese subjects in weight loss treatment. The purpose of this study was to examine the cases of ephedrine use to elucidate the population that benefits most from ephedrine treatment and which other treatment regimens (e.g., caffeine, low-calorie diets) should be combined.

SAFETY/DOSAGE

The AHPA recommends that the daily dosage should be no more than 100 mg in four divided doses of not more than 25 mg ephedrine alkaloids. The German Commission E recommends a single dosage of 15–

30 mg. For children over the age of 6, the recommended dosage is 0.5 mg total ephedrine alkaloids per kilogram of body weight (maximum daily dosage of 2 mg/kg).

Warnings have been issued by both the U.S. Food and Drug Administration (FDA) and Health Canada on the use of ephedra-containing supplements, and ephedra supplements are largely banned for sale in the United States (certain low-dose "raw" ephedra supplements were not part of the ban and can be found in some health food stores). Possible side effects listed by the German Commission E are tachycardia, restlessness, irritability, insomnia, urinary disturbances, nausea, and vomiting. Higher dosages or overdose may cause dependency, significant increase in blood pressure, and cardiac arrhythmia (Blumenthal et al., 1998).

Clinical studies have been performed to determine the cardiovascular effects of ephedra. Kalman et al. (2002) found that a 14-day period of ingestion of a supplement containing ephedra and caffeine (under the recommended dosage) produced no noticeable cardiovascular effects. However, Haller and Benowitz (2000) were requested by the FDA to review 140 adverse events involving ephedra reported between June 1, 1997, and March 31, 1999. Of the reviewed reports, 31% were found to be "definitely" or "probably" related to ephedra use, and another 31% were found to be "possibly" related. Cardiovascular effects were thought to be the primary cause of the adverse reactions in those cases found to be "definitely," "probably," or "possibly" related. The authors concluded that ephedra may cause a health risk to some people and indicated a need for better understanding of individual risk.

In a study of nasal and oral doses of ephedrine and ephedrine-like compounds, low doses were found to decrease tiredness, and the authors pointed to significant and substantial increases in blood pressure and orthostatic hypotension as the causes of increasing the cardiovascular risk during physical exercise. No dependency was found in this study (Berlin et al., 2001). Toubro et al. (1993) also performed a clinical study on the safety and efficacy of long-term treatment with ephedrine and found ephedrine and caffeine to be effective, with mild and transient side effects and no withdrawal symptoms.

Numerous case histories have been published of adverse events involving ephedra alkaloids. Of the cases published, the outcomes have varied from mild side effects, cardiovascular effects, death, disability, and even acute psychosis (McKenna et al., 2002; Tormey and Bruzzi, 2001).

REFERENCES

Astrup A. Thermogenesis in human brown adipose tissue and skeletal muscle induced by sympathomimetic stimulation. Acta Endocrinol Suppl (Copenh) 1986;278:1–32.

Astrup A, Lundsgaard C, Madsen J, Christensen NJ. Enhanced thermogenic responsiveness during chronic ephedrine treatment in man. Am J Clin Nutr 1985;42(1):83–94.

Astrup A, Madsen J, Holst JJ, Christensen NJ. The effect of chronic ephedrine treatment on substrate utilization, the sympathoadrenal activity, and energy expenditure during glucose-induced thermogenesis in man. Metabolism 1986;35(3):260–265.

Bell DG, Jacobs I, Ellerington K. Effect of caffeine and ephedrine ingestion on anaerobic exercise performance. Med Sci Sports Exerc 2001;33:1399–1403.

Bell DG, Jacobs I, McLellan TM, Zamecnik J. Reducing the dose of combined caffeine and ephedrine preserves the ergogenic effect. Aviat Space Environ Med 2000;71:415–419.

Bell DG, McLellan TM, Sabiston CM. Effect of ingesting caffeine and ephedrine on 10-km run performance. Med Sci Sports Exerc 2002;34:344–349.

Berlin I, Warot D, Aymard G, Acquaviva E, Legrand M, Labarthe B, Peyron I, Diquet B, Lechat P. Pharmacodynamics and pharmacokinetics of single nasal (5 mg and 10 mg) and oral (50 mg) doses of ephedrine in healthy subjects. Eur J Clin Pharmacol 2001;57:447–455.

Blumenthal M, Busse WR, Goldberg A, Gruenwald J, Hall T, Riggins CW, Rister RS, eds. The Complete German Commission E Monographs. Austin, TX: American Botanical Council, 1998.

Boozer CN, Daly PA, Homel P, Solomon JL, Blanchard D, Nasser JA, Strauss R, Meredith T. Herbal ephedra/caffeine for weight loss: a 6-month randomized safety and efficacy trial. Int J Obes Relat Metab Disord 2002;26:593–604.

Boozer CN, Nasser JA, Heymsfield SB, Wang V, Chen G, Solomon JL. An herbal supplement containing ma huang-guarana for weight loss: a randomized, double-blind trial. Int J Obes.Relat Metab Disord 2001;25:316–324.

Bukowiecki L, Jahjah L, Follea N. Ephedrine, a potential slimming drug, directly stimulates thermogenesis in brown adipocytes via beta-adrenoreceptors. Int J Obes Relat Metab Disord 1982;6(4):343–350.

Haller CA, Benowitz NL. Adverse cardiovascular and central nervous system events associated with dietary supplements containing ephedra alkaloids. N Engl J Med 2000;343:1833–1838.

Kalman D, Incledon T, Gaunaurd I, Schwartz H, Krieger D. An acute clinical trial evaluating the cardiovascular effects of an herbal ephedra-caffeine weight loss product in healthy overweight adults. Int J Obes Relat Metab Disord 2002;26:1363–1366.

Liu YL, Toubro S, Astrup A, Stock MJ. Contribution of beta 3-adrenoceptor activation to ephedrine-induced thermogenesis in humans. Int J Obes Relat Metab Disord 1995;19:678–685.

McKenna D, Jones K, Hughes K, Humphrey S. Botanical Medicines: The Desk Reference for Major Herbal Supplements. New York: Haworth Press, 2002.

Molnar D, Torok K, Erhardt E, Jeges S. Safety and efficacy of treatment with an ephedrine/caffeine mixture. The first double-blind placebo-controlled pilot study in adolescents. Int J Obes Relat Metab Disord 2000;24:1573–1578.

Pasquali R, Casimirri F. Clinical aspects of ephedrine in the treatment of obesity. Int J Obes Relat Metab Disord 1993;17(suppl 1):S65–S68.

Pasquali R, Casimirri F, Melchionda N, Grossi G, Bortoluzzi L, Morselli Labate AM, Stefanini C, Raitano A. Effects of chronic administration of ephedrine during very-low-calorie diets on energy expenditure, protein metabolism and hormone levels in obese subjects. Clin Sci (Lond) 1992;82(1):85–92.

Shannon JR, Gottesdiener K, Jordan J, Chen K, Flattery S, Larson PJ, Candelore MR, Gertz B, Robertson D, Sun M. Acute effect of ephedrine on 24-h energy balance. Clin Sci (Lond) 1999;96(5):483–491.

Tinkelman DG, Avner SE. Ephedrine therapy in asthmatic children. Clinical tolerance and absence of side effects. JAMA 1977;237(6):553–557.

Tormey WP, Bruzzi A. Acute psychosis due to the interaction of legal compounds—ephedra alkaloids in "Vigueur Fit" tablets, caffeine in "Red Bull" and alcohol. Med Sci Law 2001;41:331–336.

Toubro S, Astrup A, Breum L, Quaade F. The acute and chronic effects of ephedrine/caffeine mixtures on energy expenditure and glucose metabolism in humans [discussion S82]. Int J Obes Relat Metab Disord 1993;17 (suppl 3):S73–S77.

Zahorska-Markiewicz B, Obuchowicz E, Waluga M, Tkacz E, Herman ZS. Neuropeptide Y in obese women during treatment with adrenergic modulation drugs. Med Sci Monit 2001;7:403–408.

ADDITIONAL RESOURCES

Meston CM, Heiman JR. Ephedrine-activated physiological sexual arousal in women. Arch Gen Psychiatry 1998;55(7):652–656.

PYRUVATE

Overall Rank

★★★   for weight loss
  ★★   for athletic performance

OVERVIEW

Pyruvate supplements are typically marketed to enhance weight loss and increase energy levels. Pyruvate is a salt form of pyruvic acid—a three-carbon molecule derived from the breakdown of glucose. The form of pyruvic acid found in dietary supplements is combined with various minerals such as sodium, calcium, magnesium, and potassium to improve stability. In the body, glucose (six carbons) is split into two pyruvic acid molecules (three carbons each) in the end stages of cellular glycolysis. When enough oxygen is present, pyruvic acid can be converted into acetyl coenzyme A in the mitochondrion of the cell to produce energy. Because glucose (the chief sugar used by cells for energy) is broken down in the body into pyruvic acid, an increased level of pyruvic acid in the body is theorized to enhance a cell's ability to generate energy.

COMMENTS

Clinical data, though limited, supports the effect of pyruvate as an effective supplement for weight loss. The problem, however, is that most commercial products contain less than 1 g of pyruvate per serving—or about 20–50 times less than the levels shown to be effective in the available clinical studies. Even in the studies of multigram feeding that show a benefit in pyruvate supplements, the more than 20 g of pyruvate used was only marginally effective in inducing weight loss.

SCIENTIFIC SUPPORT

In general, the clinical support for pyruvate as either a weight loss aid or a way to boost energy levels is weak. A handful of human studies from the same laboratory (Stanko et al., 1992a, 1992b, 1994, 1996) have shown that daily consumption of 22–44 g of pyruvate over 3–4 weeks can help improve loss of body fat and body weight and may help to slow weight regain and reaccumulation of body fat following a weight loss diet. Overall, the difference in weight loss between the pyruvate supplement and placebo groups was not large, amounting to approximately 1.1–1.6 kg (about 2–3 lb) additional weight loss in the pyruvate groups.

SAFETY/DOSAGE

No significant side effects are expected with the levels of pyruvate found in most commercially available dietary supplements (which is typically quite low). In some studies, subjects consuming relatively large doses of pyruvate have reported minor gastrointestinal disturbances such as diarrhea and flatulence.

Although 1–5 g/day of pyruvate are typically recommended, that dosage is primarily a marketing consideration (people will actually pay for products with that much pyruvate). Most commercial preparations contain 500 mg to 1 g of pyruvate, with 2–3 servings/day recommended. Existing clinical studies have used daily doses of more than 20 g of pyruvate (which would be far too expensive to sell as a dietary supplement).

REFERENCES

Stanko RT, Arch JE. Inhibition of regain in body weight and fat with addition of 3-carbon compounds to the diet with hyperenergetic refeeding after weight reduction. Int J Obes Relat Metab Disord 1996;20(10):925–930.

Stanko RT, Reynolds HR, Hoyson R, Janosky JE, Wolf R. Pyruvate supplementation of a low-cholesterol, low-fat diet: effects on plasma lipid concentrations and body composition in hyperlipidemic patients. Am J Clin Nutr 1994;59(2):423–427.

Stanko RT, Tietze DL, Arch JE. Body composition, energy utilization, and nitrogen metabolism with a 4.25-MJ/d low-energy diet supplemented with pyruvate. Am J Clin Nutr 1992a;56(4):630–635.

Stanko RT, Tietze DL, Arch JE. Body composition, energy utilization, and nitrogen metabolism with a severely restricted diet supplemented with dihydroxyacetone and pyruvate. Am J Clin Nutr 1992b;55(4):771–776.

ADDITIONAL RESOURCES

Bryson JM, King SE, Burns CM, Baur LA, Swaraj S, Caterson ID. Changes in glucose and lipid metabolism following weight loss produced by a very low-calorie diet in obese subjects. Int J Obes Relat Metab Disord 1996;20(4):338–345.

Sukala WR. Pyruvate: beyond the marketing hype. Int J Sport Nutr 1998;8(3):241–249.

WHITE WILLOW BARK (SALIX ALBA)

Overall Rank

★ for weight loss (when combined with ephedrine and caffeine as the A in ECA stacks)
★ for pain control
ZERO for weight loss (as a stand-alone supplement)

OVERVIEW

The bark of the white willow tree (*Salix alba*) is a source of salicin and other salicylates—compounds similar in structure to aspirin (acetylsalicylic acid). Native Americans are thought to have used ground willow bark and bark steeped for tea as medicinal remedies for everything from pain to fevers. Today, white willow bark is often used as a natural alternative to aspirin, but perhaps the most common use in dietary supplements is as an adjunct for weight loss (as the A in ECA stacks containing ephedra or synephrine and caffeine in the form of pure caffeine from herbal sources such as guarana or kola nut).

Because of the chemical similarities with aspirin, white willow bark extract is often promoted as an "all natural" alternative—but rarely with adequate levels of salicin to impact headaches, inflammation, or fevers.

As a weight loss aid, white willow bark extract offers little to no benefits by itself. In combination with other dietary supplements, however, white willow bark is thought to extend or increase the activity of several therm-ogenic ingredients (e.g., *Citrus aurantium*, green tea, guarana, and others) in elevating energy expenditure and promoting fat metabolism.

COMMENTS

White willow bark is a common minor ingredient in several weight loss formulations because of the anti-inflammatory properties it derives from inhibiting prostaglandins. A side effect of blocking prostaglandin activity is an inhibition of norepinephrine breakdown; thus, the ultimate effect of white willow bark supplements (when used for weight loss) is to have more norepinephrine around. Norepinephrine is known to interact with a special kind of receptor found on fat cells (ß-3 receptor) to stimulate the breakdown of fat. Because white willow bark appears to increase norepinephrine levels, it might also stimulate fat metabolism, which might lead to enhanced weight loss (Daly et al., 1993; Dulloo and Miller, 1987, 1989; Geissler, 1993; Krieger et al., 1990). Without more definitive findings, however, white willow bark cannot be consid-ered effective on its own as a weight loss agent.

If you have a pounding headache that you want to go away quickly, chances are you will experience better results with regular aspirin from your local pharmacy or grocery store (at a better price than white willow bark). For those looking for a "gentler" approach to either temporary inflammation or weight management (thermogenesis), lower-dose white willow bark might be an effective alternative to aspirin.

SCIENTIFIC SUPPORT

The primary active compound in white willow bark is salicin (which can also be found in other plants and herbs such as meadow sweet). In the body, salicin can be converted into salicylic acid, which has powerful effects as an anti-inflammatory and pain reliever. Until synthetic aspirin (acetylsalicylic acid) could be produced in large quantities, white willow bark was the treatment of choice for reducing fever, relieving headache and arthritis pain, and controlling swelling, and it remains a popular and approved option in Germany and other European countries (Levesque and Lafont, 2000). Although synthetic aspirin is clearly a more effective pain reliever and anti-inflammatory agent compared with the weaker natural bark extract, white willow bark can also serve as a source of tannins, a combination that might provide a synergistic action in elevating energy expenditure by interfering with the prostaglandin production and inhibiting norepinephrine breakdown (Norton and Meisinger, 1977). This mild effect on keeping norepinephrine concentrations elevated would not be expected to significantly elevate resting energy expenditure on its own, but its effect appears to be enough, when used in combination with other thermogenic supplements, to help promote increased fat oxidation (examples include ma huang (now banned in the United States), synephrine, green tea, guarana, and others).

SAFETY/DOSAGE

Stomach ulcers and other gastrointestinal complaints (nausea and diarrhea) are common side effects of prolonged high-dose consumption of either synthetic aspirin or white willow bark extracts. Long-term use of high doses of either salicin source is not recommended, although the natural bark extract is often tolerated much better than the more powerful synthetic aspirin (Toubro et al., 1993). People concerned about blood clotting and bleeding time should use aspirin and white willow bark with caution, because both have the potential to interfere with platelet aggregation and prolong bleeding time (i.e., a blood-thinning effect).

Standardized extracts of white willow bark are available, with total salicin intake typically 60–120 mg per day for relief of acute pain, fever, or inflammation. For longer-term consumption as an adjunct to weight management and thermogenesis, smaller doses are generally tolerated much better (Toubro et al., 1993)

REFERENCES

Daly PA, Krieger DR, Dulloo AG, Young JB, Landsberg L. Ephedrine, caffeine and aspirin: safety and efficacy for treatment of human obesity. Int J Obes Relat Metab Disord 1993;17(suppl 1):S73–S78.

Dulloo AG, Miller DS. Aspirin as a promoter of ephedrine-induced thermogenesis: potential use in the treatment of obesity. Am J Clin Nutr 1987;45(3):564–569.

Dulloo AG, Miller DS. Ephedrine, caffeine and aspirin: "over-the-counter" drugs that interact to stimulate thermogenesis in the obese. Nutrition 1989;5(1):7–9.

Geissler CA. Effects of weight loss, ephedrine and aspirin on energy expenditure in obese women. Int J Obes Relat Metab Disord 1993;17(suppl 1):S45–S48.

Krieger DR, Daly PA, Dulloo AG, Ransil BJ, Young JB, Landsberg L. Ephedrine, caffeine and aspirin promote weight loss in obese subjects. Trans Assoc Am Physicians 1990;103:307–312.

Levesque H, Lafont O. Aspirin throughout the ages: a historical review. Rev Med Interne 2000;21(suppl 1):8s–17s.

Norton WL, Meisinger MA. An overview of nonsteroidal anti-inflammatory agents. Inflammation 1977;2(1):37–46.

Toubro S, Astrup AV, Breum L, Quaade F. Safety and efficacy of long-term treatment with ephedrine, caffeine and an ephedrine/caffeine mixture. Int J Obes Relat Metab Disord 1993;17(suppl 1):S69–S72.

ADDITIONAL RESOURCES

Chrubasik S, Eisenberg E, Balan E, Weinberger T, Luzzati R, Conradt C. Treatment of low back pain exacerbations with willow bark extract: a randomized double-blind study. Am J Med 2000;109(1):9–14.

2

Sports Supplements (Ergogenic Aids)

Amino Acids and Protein
  Supplements
Androstenedione
Branched-Chain Amino Acids (BCAAs)
Carnosine
Cordyceps Mushroom (*Cordyceps
  sinensis*)
Creatine
DHEA (Dehydroepiandrosterone)

Glycerol
HMB (ß-Hydroxy-ß-Methylbutyrate)
Medium-Chain Triglycerides (MCTs)
Protein (Casein, Whey, Soy, Collagen,
  Colostrum)
Proteolytic Enzymes
Ribose
Tribulus (*Tribulus terrestris*)

AMINO ACIDS AND PROTEIN SUPPLEMENTS

Overall Rank

★★★★★ for soy protein and heart health
 ★★★★ for whey protein, muscle synthesis, and exercise recovery
 ★★★★ for soy protein and menopausal benefits
 ★★★★ for branched-chain amino acids (BCAAs) and endurance
  ★★★ for colostrum and exercise recovery
  ★★★ for hydrolyzed collagen protein (HCP) and joint health
  ★★★ for glutamine and immune support
  ★★★ for arginine and blood flow

OVERVIEW

Amino Acids

Amino acids are the basic building blocks of protein and can be obtained in an almost endless variety of supplemental forms, including capsules, tablets, bars, and powders. Some available products provide a foodlike mixture of all 20 nutritionally important amino acids, while other products focus on the specific characteristics of isolated amino acids. The evidence for the health and performance benefits of isolated amino acids is mixed at best. Only in limited circumstances do these supplements represent a valuable approach for athletes. The reader is referred to separate entries in this chapter providing scientific evidence suggesting that an isolated amino acid supplement may be useful for promoting health or performance (i.e., BCAAs, carnitine, glutamine, ß-hydroxy-ß-methylbutyrate [HMB], etc.).

Protein (Casein, Whey, Soy, Collagen, Colostrum)

Discussions of the value of protein supplements have become increasingly complicated in the last several years. The primary cause of debate is not the question of whether athletes require greater dietary protein intakes compared with their sedentary counterparts (the consensus suggests that they do) but rather the explosion in marketing of various forms of protein fractions like casein, whey, soy, colostrum, collagen, and others. The protein debate has slowly changed from "How much?" to "Which is best?" with no shortage of opinions and isolated studies but no clear consensus to guide decision making.

The evidence is strong that protein needs are elevated by exercise training, infection, and other periods of acute and chronic stress. Some of the best evidence comes from studies of competitive athletes, in whom protein needs are nearly doubled during periods of intense training and competition. Athletes competing in power or strength sports probably require about 1.6 g of protein per kilogram of body weight, and endurance athletes may need about 1.3 g/kg.

COMMENTS

Undeniably, protein is a vitally important nutrient for general health and hundreds of specific functions in the body. The recommended dietary allowance (RDA) for protein is 0.8 g/kg of body weight for adults (0.36 g/lb), with growing children, adolescents, and both power and endurance athletes needing slightly more. By RDA standards, an adult weighing 70 kg (154 lb) needs 56 g/day (about the amount provided in 8 oz of lean meat).

In most cases, the scientific evidence for a performance-enhancing effect of amino acids and/or protein comes from studies of using protein supplements to ensure adequate dietary protein intake. In a limited number of examples, isolated amino acid supplements provide additional performance and/or health effects, such as those noted for branched-chain amino acids for delaying fatigue, HMB and glutamine for inhibiting muscle loss, arginine for promoting blood flow, and cysteine for increasing cellular glutathione levels. In most other cases in which isolated amino acids have been used as dietary supplements, however, benefits in health and performance have been disappointing.

Protein is one of the primary nutrients involved in the growth, development, and repair of virtually all tissues in the body. Aside from simply ensuring adequate dietary protein requirements, supplemental protein can also be beneficial following strenuous exercise (by enhancing repair and regeneration of damaged tissues) and as a weight loss aid (because of the low glycemic index and heightened sense of satiety provided by a protein meal compared with meals higher in carbohydrates).

SCIENTIFIC SUPPORT

Isolated Amino Acids

Amino acids are typically categorized by their nutritional role as essential or nonessential. Essential amino acids are not produced in the body and therefore must be obtained from dietary sources. Nonessential amino acids can be either manufactured directly by the body or obtained by conversion from another amino acid. It is important to keep in mind that *nonessential* does not mean that these amino acids are not important. Rather, it simply means that under ideal circumstances, there are routes other than the diet through which these amino acids can be obtained. Several of the nonessential amino acids are considered "conditionally essential," meaning that under certain conditions, such as injury, disease, increased stress, or intense physical activity, the body's metabolic machinery is unable to generate adequate levels, and supplemental dietary sources are required.

A growing body of evidence suggests that specialized amino acid mixtures based on essential or semiessential amino acids can be especially beneficial for promoting postexercise recovery (Volek et al., 2002—2 g of carnitine for 3 weeks); increasing collagen deposition and wound healing (Williams et al., 2002—14 g of arginine, 3 g of HMB, and 14 g of glutamine for 7–14 days); and stimulating muscle growth (Rasmussen et al., 2000; Tipton et al., 2001—6 g of essential amino acids plus 35 g of sucrose). Considerable debate on this issue continues, however, because not all studies support a benefit of amino acid supplementation for enhancing muscle metabolism or exercise performance (Lambert et al., 1993—single 4.2-g dose of arginine, lysine, ornithine, and tyrosine; Vukovich et al., 1997—2.9 g of leucine, isoleucine, valine, glutamine, and carnitine for 7 days).

Whey Protein

Whey is one of two proteins found in milk (the other is casein). Whey protein accounts for only about 20% of the total protein found in milk, while casein makes up about 80% of milk protein. Long considered a useless byproduct of dairy (cheese) manufacturing, whey protein is enjoying an increased interest as a protein supplement. Because whey protein includes a variety of immunoglobulin compounds (α lactalbumin; ß lactoglobulin; lactoferrin; albumin; and immunoglobulins A, G, and M), whey supplements are often touted as effective in boosting immune protection and enhancing postexercise recovery. It is important to note that commercial products vary widely in their content of immunoglobulins and other immune-active protein fractions, and much of the difference among products is related to different manufacturing processes.

Whey protein also contains approximate 20–30% of its amino acid content as BCAAs (leucine, isoleucine, and valine), which can be readily oxidized by the muscle as energy and may be associated with a delay in fatigue during long-duration exercise, especially in the heat.

In addition to its high content of immunoglobulins and BCAAs, whey protein is a rich source of cysteine, an important amino acid constituent of the cellular antioxidant glutathione. Intense exercise is known to reduce cellular glutathione levels; thus, high-cysteine whey protein supplementation may be an effective approach to restoring glutathione levels in the body.

It is important to note that commercial whey proteins can differ dramatically depending on the processing method and the total protein content. For example, whey protein can exist as simple whey powder (30% or less total protein content), whey protein concentrate (30–85% protein content) or whey protein isolate (90% or higher protein content). In the case of whey protein isolates (the most expensive type), two key processing methods—ion exchange filtration and cross-flow microfiltration—can remove different components of the total whey protein, resulting in end products with different tastes, textures, and functional properties. Whey proteins processed using the ion exchange methodology appear to retain most of the functional benefits associated with immune system maintenance. Enhanced resistance to infection and a 25–44% increase in glutathione levels (an antioxidant enzyme containing cysteine) have been noted in HIV-positive subjects consuming concentrated whey protein (Micke et al., 2001). Whey protein also contains lactoferrin, a protein that has been shown to possess bacteriostatic and bactericidal activity against microorganisms that can cause gastroenteric infections and food poisoning.

Whey protein has been used in a number of animal and human feeding studies that have shown its benefits in promoting weight gain, elevating glutathione levels, and preventing metabolic acidosis (although this effect can be claimed for virtually any high-quality protein source). Whether or not the minor content differences between various whey proteins actually result in any appreciable differences in muscle gain or exercise performance in humans has never been convincingly demonstrated.

Soy Protein

Soy protein has been criticized by some nutritionists as being an "inferior" dietary source of protein, but such criticisms are unfounded for the more modern purified soy protein isolates (90–97% protein) that are currently marketed as dietary supplements. Soy protein has primarily been studied for its benefits in reducing hyperlipidemia, slowing bone loss, alleviating menopausal symptoms (hot flashes), and preventing cancers of the breast and prostate. Some, but not all, of the beneficial effects of soy protein appear to be caused by the presence of estrogen-like phytonutrients called isoflavones (primarily daidzein and genistein).

Soy protein is considered to be quite safe, with as much as 60 g of protein containing 90 mg of isoflavones used with no adverse effects in studies of up to one year. Soy protein and soy foods (such as roasted soybeans) consumed during lactation can contain up to 40 mg of isoflavones and still result in 4–6 times lower isoflavone concentration in breast milk compared with amounts provided by soy-based infant formula.

Because most studies have investigated the effects of soy protein on indices of heart disease and osteoporosis, see "Soy" in Chapter 7.

Colostrum
Bovine colostrum, another form of dairy protein, has recently become a popular dietary supplement among both strength and endurance athletes. A handful of studies have shown a performance benefit (e.g., improved power output during cycling, enhanced vertical jump capacity) following supplementation with 20–60 g/day of colostrum protein for 8 weeks (Coombes et al., 2002). Other studies of colostrum supplementation have investigated benefits on immune system activity and gastrointestinal function and permeability (Playford et al., 2001); see "Colostrum" in Chapter 8.

Gelatin and Hydrolyzed Collagen Protein (HCP)
Gelatin is a form of protein extracted from the bones/hides of cows and pigs. Long used in the pharmaceutical industry to produce gelatin capsules, gelatin is used in some dietary supplements as an inexpensive protein source. From a muscle-building perspective, gelatin does not appear to be an especially good choice because it lacks several essential amino acids required for maintenance of muscle tissue. On the other hand, as a dietary supplement for enhancing connective tissue health, a handful of studies suggest that 7–10 g/day of gelatin, as hydrolyzed collagen protein, can have a positive benefit on osteoarthritis and osteoporosis. For additional information on gelatin and HCP for joint support, see "Hydrolyzed Collagen Protein (HCP, Gelatin)" in Chapter 5.

SAFETY/DOSAGE

There are no adverse side effects associated with protein supplements (Poortmans and Dellalieux, 2000), aside from the obvious potential for allergic and digestive reactions to supplements containing whey, colostrum, or casein in persons sensitive to dairy products.

Excess protein intake could lead to imbalances in other macronutrients (carbohydrate and fat) and associated micronutrients. Protein intake should probably be kept below 2.0 g/kg of body weight because no scientific evidence supports beneficial effects above that level.

Concerns have been raised for several years regarding the possible "strain" put on the liver and kidneys by excessive protein intake. Although this may be a very real concern for people at risk for liver or kidney disease (for whom high-protein diets may accelerate tissue damage), there is no convincing evidence indicating a safety concern for healthy persons.

Dosage recommendations for dietary protein (Lemon, 1991) in sedentary persons are RDA levels of 0.8 g/kg of body weight, while endurance athletes need somewhat more (1.3 g/kg) and strength athletes still more (1.6 g/kg).

REFERENCES

Coombes JS, Conacher M, Austen SK, Marshall PA. Dose effects of oral bovine colostrum on physical work capacity in cyclists. Med Sci Sports Exerc 2002;34(7):1184–1188.

Lambert MI, Hefer JA, Millar RP, Macfarlane PW. Failure of commercial oral amino acid supplements to increase serum growth hormone concentrations in male body-builders. Int J Sport Nutr 1993;3(3):298–305.

Lemon PW. Effect of exercise on protein requirements. J Sports Sci 1991;9(spec no):53–70.

Micke P, Beeh KM, Schlaak JF, Buhl R. Oral supplementation with whey proteins increases plasma glutathione levels of HIV-infected patients. Eur J Clin Invest 2001;31(2):171–178.

Playford RJ, MacDonald CE, Calnan DP, Floyd DN, Podas T, Johnson W, Wicks AC, Bashir O, Marchbank T. Co-administration of the health food supplement, bovine colostrum, reduces the acute non-steroidal anti-inflammatory drug-induced increase in intestinal permeability. Clin Sci (Lond) 2001;100(6):627–633.

Poortmans JR, Dellalieux O. Do regular high protein diets have potential health risks on kidney function in athletes? Int J Sport Nutr Exerc Metab 2000;10(1):28–38.

Rasmussen BB, Tipton KD, Miller SL, Wolf SE, Wolfe RR. An oral essential amino acid-carbohydrate supplement enhances muscle protein anabolism after resistance exercise. J Appl Physiol 2000;88(2):386–392.

Tipton KD, Rasmussen BB, Miller SL, Wolf SE, Owens-Stovall SK, Petrini BE, Wolfe RR. Timing of amino acid-carbohydrate ingestion alters anabolic response of muscle to resistance exercise. Am J Physiol Endocrinol Metab 2001;281(2):E197–E206.

Volek JS, Kraemer WJ, Rubin MR, Gomez AL, Ratamess NA, Gaynor P. L-carnitine L-tartrate supplementation favorably affects markers of recovery from exercise stress. Am J Physiol Endocrinol Metab 2002;282(2):E474–E482.

Vukovich MD, Sharp RL, Kesl LD, Schaulis DL, King DS. Effects of a low-dose amino acid supplement on adaptations to cycling training in untrained individuals. Int J Sport Nutr 1997;7(4):298–309.

Williams JZ, Abumrad N, Barbul A. Effect of a specialized amino acid mixture on human collagen deposition. Ann Surg 2002;236(3):369–374; discussion 374–375.

ADDITIONAL RESOURCES

Antonio J, Street C. Glutamine: a potentially useful supplement for athletes. Can J Appl Physiol 1999;24(1):1–14.

Barth CA, Behnke U. Nutritional physiology of whey and whey components. Nahrung 1997;41(1):2–12.

Blomstrand E, Hassmen P, Ekblom B, Newsholme EA. Administration of branched-chain amino acids during sustained exercise—effects on performance and on plasma concentration of some amino acids. Eur J Appl Physiol Occup Physiol 1991;63(2):83–88.

Buchman AL, O'Brien W, Ou CN, Rognerud C, Alvarez M, Dennis K, Ahn C. The effect of arginine or glycine supplementation on gastrointestinal function, muscle injury, serum amino acid concentrations and performance during a marathon run. Int J Sports Med 1999;20(5):315–321.

Davis JM, Welsh RS, De Volve KL, Alderson NA. Effects of branched-chain amino acids and carbohydrate on fatigue during intermittent, high-intensity running. Int J Sports Med 1999;20(5):309–314.

di Luigi L, Guidetti L, Pigozzi F, Baldari C, Casini A, Nordio M, Romanelli F. Acute amino acids supplementation enhances pituitary responsiveness in athletes. Med Sci Sports Exerc 1999;31(12):1748–1754.

Doi T, Matsuo T, Sugawara M, Matsumoto K, Minehira K, Hamada K, Okamura K, Suzuki M. New approach for weight reduction by a combination of diet, light resistance exercise and the timing of ingesting a protein supplement. Asia Pac J Clin Nutr 2001;10(3):226–232.

Elam RP, Hardin DH, Sutton RA, Hagen L. Effects of arginine and ornithine on strength, lean body mass and urinary hydroxyproline in adult males. J Sports Med Phys Fitness 1989;29(1):52–56.

Gardner CD, Newell KA, Cherin R, Haskell WL. The effect of soy protein with or without isoflavones relative to milk protein on plasma lipids in hypercholesterolemic postmenopausal women. Am J Clin Nutr 2001;73(4):728–735.

Lemon PW. Is increased dietary protein necessary or beneficial for individuals with a physically active lifestyle? Nutr Rev 1996;54(4 pt 2):S169–S175.

Lemon PW. Protein and amino acid needs of the strength athlete. Int J Sport Nutr 1991;1(2):127–145.

Lemon PW, Proctor DN. Protein intake and athletic performance. Sports Med 1991;12(5):313–325.

Markus CR, Olivier B, Panhuysen GE, Van Der Gugten J, Alles MS, Tuiten A, Westenberg HG, Fekkes D, Koppeschaar HF, de Haan EE. The bovine protein alpha-lactalbumin increases the plasma ratio of tryptophan to the other large neutral amino acids, and in vulnerable subjects raises brain serotonin activity, reduces cortisol concentration, and improves mood under stress. Am J Clin Nutr 2000;71(6):1536–1544.

Mero A. Leucine supplementation and intensive training. Sports Med 1999;27(6):347–358.

Millward DJ. Optimal intakes of protein in the human diet. Proc Nutr Soc 1999;58(2):403–413.

Olson GB, Savage S, Olson J. The effects of collagen hydrolysate on symptoms of chronic fibromyalgia and temporomandibular joint pain. Cranio 2000;18(2):135–141.

Tarnopolsky MA, Atkinson SA, MacDougall JD, Chesley A, Phillips S, Schwarcz HP. Evaluation of protein requirements for trained strength athletes. J Appl Physiol 1992;73(5):1986–1995.

Tarnopolsky MA, Bosman M, Macdonald JR, Vandeputte D, Martin J, Roy BD. Postexercise protein-carbohydrate and carbohydrate supplements increase muscle glycogen in men and women. J Appl Physiol 1997;83(6):1877–1883.

Wagenmakers AJ. Amino acid supplements to improve athletic performance. Curr Opin Clin Nutr Metab Care 1999;2(6):539–544.

ANDROSTENEDIONE

Overall Rank

 WARNING: Banned for sale as a dietary supplement in the United States.

★ for promoting muscle growth and accelerating fat loss

OVERVIEW

Androstenedione is the steroid hormone that is a direct precursor to both estrone and testosterone. Androstenedione levels peak in a person's mid-20s and decline steadily after age 30. Androstenedione supplements are marketed as alternatives to anabolic steroids with common claims for boosting testosterone levels, increasing libido, and accelerating gains in muscle mass and strength.

In the body, androstenedione becomes active on conversion to testosterone—the major "male" hormone responsible for muscle growth and other male characteristics such as growth of facial hair and development of a deep voice. Higher levels of testosterone are thought to help athletes exercise more intensely and recover faster, but supplementation with androstenedione results in only a transient rise in serum testosterone levels (and estrogen levels) that has not been shown to provide any measurable gains in muscle mass, strength, or postexercise recovery. Two areas of concern are that androstenedione supplements appear to downregulate endogenous synthesis of testosterone and reduce high-density lipoprotein (HDL) levels. Many commercial products combine androstenedione with alleged herbal inhibitors of aromatase and 5-α-reductase (e.g., tribulus, saw palmetto, chrysin, indoles) as a way to prevent conversion of androstenedione to estrogen and to inactive metabolites of testosterone. Studies of these combination products, however, have not shown them to be effective in this regard.

COMMENTS

Because of the lack of positive research findings in the area of muscle building and the potential for serious health risks associated with anabolic steroids, androstenedione supplements are not considered safe or effective, and they should be avoided.

SCIENTIFIC SUPPORT

Supplement makers claim that a 300-mg dose of androstenedione increases testosterone levels by 300% over 2–4 hours. The most recent studies suggest that although androstenedione supplementation (200–300 mg/day for 4–12 weeks) is able to transiently increase testosterone levels in healthy young men (Brown et al., 2001a; Brown et al., 2001b), it also leads to an increase in estrogen levels that is not inhibited by herbal inhibitors of aromatase and 5-α-reductase. In studies that include resistance training (8–12 weeks), androstenedione supplements (100–300 mg/day) resulted in no differences in terms of muscle strength, lean body mass, or fat mass (Ballantyne et al., 2000; Broeder et al., 2000). In the androstenedione groups, however, the blood level of estradiol was elevated by 83%, HDL was reduced by 5%, and luteinizing hormone was reduced 18–70% (suggesting a downregulation of endogenous testosterone production).

Overall, well-designed clinical studies clearly show that androstenedione supplementation only transiently elevates serum testosterone levels (16–38%), does not enhance muscle strength in healthy men aged 30–65 years of age, and may result in adverse health consequences (increased estrogen levels and reduced HDL).

SAFETY/DOSAGE

Although no long-term studies have been conducted on the safety of androstenedione as a dietary supplement, a fairly substantial body of literature confirms the adverse effects associated with other anabolic steroids. In particular, prolonged use of steroids can result in dangerous side effects that include blood lipid abnormalities (elevated low-density lipoprotein [LDL] and reduced HDL cholesterol) and may increase the risk of heart disease, hormone-sensitive cancers such as breast and prostate cancer, and various liver abnormalities.

Typical dosage recommendations for androstenedione are in the range of 50–300 mg/day, but those levels have not been associated with benefits in terms of muscle gain, fat loss, or physical performance. Competitive athletes should be aware of the potential for androstenedione supplementation to alter the testosterone-epitestosterone ratio so it exceeds the 6:1 limit set by both the International Olympic Committee (IOC) and the National Collegiate Athletic Association (NCAA) in their screening for testosterone doping.

REFERENCES

Ballantyne CS, Phillips SM, MacDonald JR, Tarnopolsky MA, MacDougall JD. The acute effects of androstenedione supplementation in healthy young males. Can J Appl Physiol 2000;25(1):68–78.

Broeder CE, Quindry J, Brittingham K, Panton L, Thomson J, Appakondu S, Breuel K, Byrd R, Douglas J, Earnest C, Mitchell C, Olson M, Roy T, Yarlagadda C. The Andro Project: physiological and hormonal influences of androstenedione supplementation in men 35 to 65 years old participating in a high-intensity resistance training program. Arch Intern Med 2000;160(20):3093–3104.

Brown GA, Vukovich MD, Martini ER, Kohut ML, Franke WD, Jackson DA, King DS. Effects of androstenedione-herbal supplementation on serum sex hormone concentrations in 30- to 59-year-old men. Int J Vitam Nutr Res 2001a;71(5):293–301.

Brown GA, Vukovich MD, Martini ER, Kohut ML, Franke WD, Jackson DA, King DS. Endocrine and lipid responses to chronic androstenediol-herbal supplementation in 30- to 58-year-old men. J Am Coll Nutr 2001b;20(5):520–528.

ADDITIONAL RESOURCES

Brown GA, Martini ER, Roberts BS, Vukovich MD, King DS. Acute hormonal response to sublingual androstenediol intake in young men. J Appl Physiol 2002;92(1):142–146.

Brown GA, Vukovich MD, Reifenrath TA, Uhl NL, Parsons KA, Sharp RL, King DS. Effects of anabolic precursors on serum testosterone concentrations and adaptations to resistance training in young men. Int J Sport Nutr Exerc Metab 2000;10(3):340–359.

King DS, Sharp RL, Vukovich MD, Brown GA, Reifenrath TA, Uhl NL, Parsons KA. Effect of oral androstenedione on serum testosterone and adaptations to resistance training in young men: a randomized controlled trial. JAMA 1999;281(21):2020–2028.

Leder BZ, Longcope C, Catlin DH, Ahrens B, Schoenfeld DA, Finkelstein JS. Oral androstenedione administration and serum testosterone concentrations in young men. JAMA 2000;283(6):779–782.

BRANCHED-CHAIN AMINO ACIDS (BCAAs)

Overall Rank

★★★★ for enhancing endurance exercise performance
★★★★ for enhancing postexercise recovery

OVERVIEW

The branched-chain amino acids are a group of three essential amino acids: leucine, valine, and isoleucine. The recommended dietary intake for BCAAs is about 3 g/day, an amount that should be easily obtained from protein foods. Supplemental levels of around 5–20 g/day have been used to increase endurance, delay fatigue, and improve mental performance during prolonged exercise.

COMMENTS

For endurance athletes, particularly those competing in longer races (more than 2 hours) such as marathons, triathlons, road cycling, back-packing, and orienteering, BCAA supplements can help delay central fatigue and maintain mental performance. Participation in shorter-duration events is unlikely to result in substantial changes in blood levels of BCAAs, tryptophan, or fatty acids, so BCAA supplementation is not needed.

SCIENTIFIC SUPPORT

The idea behind BCAA supplements relates to a phenomenon known as central fatigue, which holds that mental fatigue in the brain can adversely affect physical performance in endurance events. The central fatigue hypothesis suggests that low blood levels of BCAAs may accelerate the production of serotonin, a key neurotransmitter in the brain, and prematurely lead to fatigue (Blomstrand et al., 1988). Tryptophan, an amino acid that circulates in the blood, is a precursor of serotonin and can be more easily transported into the brain to increase serotonin levels when BCAA levels in the blood are low, because high blood levels of BCAAs can block tryptophan transport into the brain (Castell et al., 1999). During exercise, as muscle and liver glycogen are depleted for energy, blood levels of BCAAs also decrease while fatty acid levels increase to serve as an additional energy source (Davis, 1995). The problem with extra fatty acids in the blood is that they need to attach to albumin as a carrier protein for proper transport. In doing so, the fatty acids displace tryptophan from its place on albumin and facilitate the transport of tryptophan into the brain for conversion into serotonin (Hassmen et al., 1994). Therefore, the combination of reduced BCAAs and elevated fatty acids in the blood causes more tryptophan to enter the brain and more serotonin to be produced, leading to central fatigue (Tanaka et al., 1997). Supplementing the diet with additional levels of BCAA is thought to block the tryptophan transport and therefore delay fatigue (Blomstrand et al., 1997).

In addition to their effects on prolonging endurance and delaying central fatigue, BCAA supplements have been associated with a reduced rate of protein and glycogen breakdown during exercise and an inhibition of muscle breakdown following exhaustive exercise (Blomstrand et al., 1991; Gastmann et al., 1998).

Although the general theory of central fatigue and BCAA supplementation is sound, not all research findings have been positive. In general, acute BCAA supplementation (immediately before or during exercise) has been shown to increase mental performance, improve cycling endurance, and reduce the time to complete a marathon (Davis et al., 1999; Hassmen et al., 1994). Chronic BCAA supplementation (2 weeks) has also been shown to be effective in improving time-trial performance in trained cyclists (Mittleman et al., 1998). A number of studies in trained and untrained subjects, however, have shown no effect of BCAA supplements on exercise performance or mental performance (van Hall et al., 1995). In some cases, BCAAs have been compared with carbohydrate supplementation during exercise, with results showing that both delay fatigue to similar degrees (Davis et al., 1992).

SAFETY/DOSAGE

Supplemental intakes of BCAAs have been studied in the range of 3–25 g/day in tablet and liquid form with no adverse side effects. Higher intakes should be avoided because of the possibility of competitive inhibition of the absorption of other amino acids from the diet and the risk of gastrointestinal distress. Effective doses are in the range of 3–20 g/day taken before or during exercise for delaying fatigue or immediately following exercise as an aid to recovery.

REFERENCES

Blomstrand E, Celsing F, Newsholme EA. Changes in plasma concentrations of aromatic and branched-chain amino acids during sustained exercise in man and their possible role in fatigue. Acta Physiol Scand 1988;133(1):115–121.

Blomstrand E, Hassmen P, Ek S, Ekblom B, Newsholme EA. Influence of ingesting a solution of branched-chain amino acids on perceived exertion during exercise. Acta Physiol Scand 1997;159(1):41–49.

Blomstrand E, Hassmen P, Ekblom B, Newsholme EA. Administration of branched-chain amino acids during sustained exercise—effects on performance and on plasma concentration of some amino acids. Eur J Appl Physiol Occup Physiol 1991;63(2):83–88.

Castell LM, Yamamoto T, Phoenix J, Newsholme EA. The role of tryptophan in fatigue in different conditions of stress. Adv Exp Med Biol 1999;467:697–704.

Davis JM. Carbohydrates, branched-chain amino acids, and endurance: the central fatigue hypothesis. Int J Sport Nutr 1995;5(suppl):S29–S38.

Davis JM, Bailey SP, Woods JA, Galiano FJ, Hamilton MT, Bartoli WP. Effects of carbohydrate feedings on plasma free tryptophan and branched-chain amino acids during prolonged cycling. Eur J Appl Physiol Occup Physiol 1992;65(6):513–519.

Davis JM, Welsh RS, De Volve KL, Alderson NA. Effects of branched-chain amino acids and carbohydrate on fatigue during intermittent, high-intensity running. Int J Sports Med 1999;20(5):309–314.

Gastmann UA, Lehmann MJ. Overtraining and the BCAA hypothesis. Med Sci Sports Exerc 1998;30(7):1173–1178.

Hassmen P, Blomstrand E, Ekblom B, Newsholme EA. Branched-chain amino acid supplementation during 30-km competitive run: mood and cognitive performance. Nutrition 1994;10(5):405–410.

Mittleman KD, Ricci MR, Bailey SP. Branched-chain amino acids prolong exercise during heat stress in men and women. Med Sci Sports Exerc 1998;30(1):83–91.

Tanaka H, West KA, Duncan GE, Bassett DR Jr. Changes in plasma tryptophan/branched chain amino acid ratio in responses to training volume variation. Int J Sports Med 1997;18(4):270–275.

van Hall G, Raaymakers JS, Saris WH, Wagenmakers AJ. Ingestion of branched-chain amino acids and tryptophan during sustained exercise in man: failure to affect performance. J Physiol 1995;486(pt 3):789–794.

ADDITIONAL RESOURCES

Davis JM, Alderson NL, Welsh RS. Serotonin and central nervous system fatigue: nutritional considerations. Am J Clin Nutr 2000;72(2 suppl):573S–578S.

Yamamoto T, Castell LM, Botella J, Powell H, Hall GM, Young A, Newsholme EA. Changes in the albumin binding of tryptophan during postoperative recovery: a possible link with central fatigue? Brain Res Bull 1997;43(1):43–46.

Yamamoto T, Newsholme EA. Diminished central fatigue by inhibition of the L-system transporter for the uptake of tryptophan. Brain Res Bull 2000;52(1):35–38.

CARNOSINE

Overall Rank

★★   as a broad-spectrum antioxidant
 ★   for enhancing exercise performance

OVERVIEW

Carnosine is a dipeptide compound composed of alanine and histidine. Carnosine is found in high concentrations in skeletal and heart muscles, and although no definite metabolic role has been ascribed to carnosine, it has been implicated in a variety of physiological processes. Perhaps the best-described function of carnosine is as a "broad-spectrum" antioxidant, where it has been shown to interact with several free-radical species, including singlet oxygen, hydrogen peroxide, and both peroxyl and hydroxyl radicals. In addition, carnosine is able to inhibit cellular damage induced by iron, copper, and zinc. Carnosine also appears to play a role in activating the enzymes responsible for generating muscle contractions (myofibrillar adenosine triphosphatase) as well as serving as an intramuscular buffering agent to retard accumulation of lactic acid.

Of the potential therapeutic actions of carnosine, including antihypertensive effects, immunomodulation, wound healing, and antitumor/chemopreventive effects, there is some laboratory and preclinical evidence to suggest benefits, but most of these claims have not been convincingly documented nor subjected to rigorous clinical evaluation. Another possible benefit of carnosine is in the general area of "antiaging" because of the findings that carnosine levels may be reduced in concert with elevations in advanced glycosylation end products. If supplemental carnosine can reduce protein glycosylation, it may have therapeutic benefit in diabetes and other conditions in which glycosylated proteins lead to neuropathy and tissue dysfunction.

COMMENTS

Given the potential physiological benefits of carnosine just outlined, its use as a dietary supplement is generally slanted toward sports nutrition, heart health, and antiaging. Its possible roles in delaying fatigue, reducing stress, buffering acid buildup, healing wounds, improving muscle contraction, and protecting cells from oxidative damage tend to position carnosine as both an ergogenic aid and a general tonic. Unfortunately, much of what is know about carnosine is limited to laboratory and animal studies, and there is simply no convincing clinical evidence that dietary supplements containing carnosine can deliver anything beyond a modest antioxidant effect.

SCIENTIFIC SUPPORT

Carnosine is absorbed intact in the small intestine (jejunum) by a specific active transport mechanism. It circulates in the blood for transport to the kidney, liver, and muscle (where the highest concentrations are found). Carnosine is either used by these tissues or hydrolyzed (broken down) into alanine and histidine by the enzyme carnosinase found in the blood, liver, and kidney (Quinn et al., 1992).

As a water-soluble antioxidant, carnosine is capable of decreasing cell membrane oxidation caused by iron, zinc, copper, hydrogen peroxide, singlet oxygen, and both peroxyl and hydroxyl free radicals (Decker et al., 2000). The antioxidant effect of carnosine appears to be far greater than the individual or combined activity of its constituent amino acids, indicating that the peptide linkage between alanine and histidine is involved in some unique way in the overall antioxidant activity of carnosine (Quinn et al., 1992). In animal and test-tube experiments, carnosine has been shown to inhibit oxidation of LDL cholesterol and reduce development of breast cancer in rodents. High doses of carnosine may also possess some immune-stimulating activity, as shown by animal experiments in which very large doses of 50–200 mg/kg per day improved survival time by 50% in x-ray irradiated mice (Quinn et al., 1992). Carnosine appears to promote wound healing, as shown by animal experiments in which 6–20 mg/kg per day for 2 weeks reduced the size and depth of gastric ulcers and accelerated regeneration of the damaged tissue (Alabovskii et al., 1999).

In humans, we know that topical administration of carnosine (in the form of 1% N-acetylcarnosine in eye drops) is effective in treating cataracts (Babizhayev et al., 2002). Although much has been made in marketing material for carnosine-containing supplements (lactate-buffering capacity, carnosine capacity of muscle biopsies, etc.), there is a distinct lack of clinical data to support any of the many alleged benefits of oral carnosine consumption. One of the only published studies in humans shows that high-intensity exercise (strength or endurance training) has no appreciable effect on muscle carnosine concentration (Mannion et al., 1994).

SAFETY/DOSAGE

Although no long-term safety studies have been conducted in humans, carnosine is not expected to result in any significant side effects when consumed at levels found in most commercial dietary supplements. Rodent experiments have noted no adverse toxic effects even at doses up to 500 mg/kg of body weight (about 35 g for an average-sized man). The average daily intake of carnosine from foods is probably in the range of 50–250 mg (based on a diet containing at least one serving, or 3–4 oz, of beef, pork, or chicken).

Carnosine is fairly well absorbed (up to 15% of ingested dose); circulates in the blood; and is quickly used by peripheral tissues, metabolized to its constituent amino acids (alanine and histidine), or filtered to the urine by the kidneys. Therefore, supplements should be consumed in several divided doses throughout the day to maximize absorption. Oral doses of 1–3 g/day are typically recommended, but convincing clinical benefits are lacking.

REFERENCES

Alabovskii VV, Boldyrev AA, Vinokurov AA, Gallant S, Chesnokov DN. Comparison of protective effects of carnosine and acetylcarnosine during cardioplegia. Biull Eksp Biol Med 1999;127(3):290–294.

Babizhayev MA, Deyev AI, Yermakova VN, Semiletov YA, Davydova NG, Doroshenko VS, Zhukotskii AV, Goldman IM. Efficacy of N-acetylcarnosine in the treatment of cataracts. Drugs R D 2002;3(2):87–103.

Decker EA, Livisay SA, Zhou S. A Re-evaluation of the antioxidant activity of purified carnosine. Biochemistry (Mosc) 2000;65(7):766–770.

Mannion AF, Jakeman PM, William PL. Effects of isokinetic training of the knee extensors on high-intensity exercise performance and skeletal muscle buffering. Eur J Appl Physiol Occup Physiol 1994;68(4):356–361.

Quinn PJ, Boldyrev AA, Formazuyk VE. Carnosine: its properties, functions and potential therapeutic applications. Mol Aspects Med 1992;13(5):379–444.

ADDITIONAL RESOURCES

Gutierrez A, Anderstam B, Alvestrand A. Amino acid concentration in the interstitium of human skeletal muscle: a microdialysis study. Eur J Clin Invest 1999;29(11):947–952.

Roberts PR, Zaloga GP. Cardiovascular effects of carnosine. Biochemistry (Mosc) 2000;65(7):856–861.

Stuerenburg HJ. The roles of carnosine in aging of skeletal muscle and in neuromuscular diseases. Biochemistry (Mosc) 2000;65(7):862–865.

CORDYCEPS MUSHROOM (*CORDYCEPS SINENSIS*)

Overall Rank

★★★★ for enhancing endurance and exercise performance
★★★★ for enhancing overall lung function (measured by maximal oxygen consumption)
★★★ for direct energy-promoting and antifatigue benefits

OVERVIEW

Cordyceps is a Tibetan mushroom used in Traditional Chinese Medicine for lung protection and reproductive invigoration as well as to balance chi—the fundamental "energy of life." In Western terminology, cordyceps is also used as a traditional remedy for ailments of the immune, endocrine, cardiovascular, respiratory, renal, and hepatic systems. The available clinical data published in English provide evidence for a beneficial effect of cordyceps in relieving asthma, increasing lung function (in frail older people or sedentary adults and in endurance athletes), and boosting libido (in frail older persons).

COMMENTS

Many of the claims for cordyceps parallel those of ginseng due to its reported effects on increasing energy levels, sex drive, and endurance. Although the pharmacologically active components of cordyceps remain unknown, at least two chemical constituents—cordycepin (deoxyadenosine) and cordycepic acid (mannitol)—have been identified and suggested as being the active compounds in improving lung function and increasing energy levels and sex drive. Cordyceps is available as a standardized supplement (usually 1–4% mannitol as a marker), with doses of 2–4 g/day providing clinically meaningful benefits in most studies.

SCIENTIFIC SUPPORT

Much of the scientific evidence for the physiological effects of the cordyceps mushroom comes from the wide variety of animal studies available in translations from the Chinese journals in which they are published. Those studies show that cordyceps is effective for controlling blood levels of insulin, glucose, and corticosterone, as well as increasing numbers and activity of many immune cell fractions, including T-helper cells and natural killer cells (Bao et al., 1988; Kuo et al., 1996; Dai et al., 2001). In animal studies, cordyceps feeding increased the ratio of adenosine triphosphate (ATP) to inorganic phosphate in the liver by about 50%, resulting in an ability to use oxygen more efficiently (30–50% increase), better tolerate acidosis and hypoxia (lack of oxygen) and live 2–3 times longer than a control group exposed to a low-oxygen environment (Dai et al., 2001).

In the few clinical studies available, cordyceps-treated subjects showed significant improvements in their level of fatigue (Cooper et al., 1999), memory and cognitive capacity (Zhu et al., 1998a), sex drive (Zhu et al., 1998b), oxygen uptake (Cooper et al., 1999; Talbott et al., 2002), and endurance exercise performance (Nicodemus et al., 2001). One human study (Zhu et al., 1998b) suggests that the increased libido reported in elderly subjects may result from DHEA (dehydroepiandrosterone) levels increasing from low to normal.

SAFETY/DOSAGE

Dietary supplementation with cordyceps is not associated with any significant side effects, but a theoretical possibility exists for adenosine-containing supplements to induce a slight "blood-thinning" effect. Typical doses used in clinical studies have ranged from 2–6 g/day for benefits associated with increased energy levels, reduced fatigue, and an enhanced ability to use oxygen.

REFERENCES

Bao TT, Wang GF, Yang JL. Pharmacological actions of Cordyceps sinensis. Chung Hsi I Chieh Ho Tsa Chih 1988;8(6):352–354, 325–326.

Cooper C, Zhu J, et al. Elevated VO2max in frail elderly subjects. Med Sci Sports Exerc 1999;31:S174.

Dai G, Bao T, Xu C, Cooper R, Zhu JS. CordyMax Cs-4 improves steady-state bioenergy status in mouse liver. J Altern Complement Med 2001;7(3):231–240.

Kuo YC, Tsai WJ, Shiao MS, Chen CF, Lin CY. Cordyceps sinensis as an immunomodulatory agent. Am J Chin Med 1996;24(2):111–125.

Nicodemus K, Hagan D, Zhu J. Supplementation with cordyceps Cs-4 fermentation product enhanced exercise performance and fat oxidation in athletes. Med Sci Sports Exerc 2001;33:S164.

Talbott SM, Zhu JS, Rippe JM. CordyMax enhances endurance in sedentary individuals. Med Sci Sports Exerc 2001;33.

Zhu JS, Halpern GM, Jones K. The scientific rediscovery of an ancient Chinese herbal medicine: Cordyceps sinensis, part I. J Altern Complement Med 1998a;4(3):289–303.

Zhu JS, Halpern GM, Jones K. The scientific rediscovery of a precious ancient Chinese herbal regimen: Cordyceps sinensis, part II. J Altern Complement Med 1998b;4(4):429–457.

ADDITIONAL RESOURCES

Bucci LR. Selected herbals and human exercise performance. Am J Clin Nutr 2000;72(2 suppl):624S–636S.

CREATINE

Overall Rank

★★★★★ for enhancing muscle building and improving muscular power
★★ for enhancing endurance exercise performance (by enhancing glycogen storage)

OVERVIEW

Normally, about 1–2 g/day of creatine are produced in the body from arginine, glycine, and methionine. Dietary sources, including meat and fish, add another 1–2 g/day of creatine, although overcooking destroys most of the creatine (the 1 g of creatine in an 8-oz steak may fall to zero if that steak is well done). In the body, creatine plays a vital role in cellular energy production as creatine phosphate (phosphocreatine) in regenerating ATP in skeletal muscle. Oral administration of creatine in supplement form elevates muscle creatine stores, increases muscular strength, and improves exercise performance in short-duration, sprint-type sports. Thus, creatine supplements are typically marketed as body-building and "strength-boosting" supplements to enhance muscle growth and power output.

COMMENTS

Creatine has become one of the hottest sports supplements for one major reason—it works. Creatine is effective in specific situations: high-intensity activities that require short bouts of repeated explosive activity (e.g., weight lifting, football, sprinting). Athletes in other sports might achieve an indirect benefit because creatine supplements possibly allow more intense levels of weight training, with the strength and power benefits of higher-intensity training transferring to their sports.

SCIENTIFIC SUPPORT

Creatine is stored in muscle cells as phosphocreatine and is used to help generate cellular energy for muscle contractions. It also may increase the amount of water that each muscle cell holds, thus increasing the size of the muscle (and possibly its function). Although it has not been studied extensively, there may also be a role for creatine in maintaining muscle mass and preventing the muscle wasting that occurs as a result of aging and in chronic conditions such as AIDS and heart failure (Terjung et al., 2000).

At this writing, more than 2-dozen well-controlled clinical studies exist to support the efficacy of creatine supplements in improving performance in high-intensity, repeated-bout activities (e.g., weight lifting, sprinting, jumping). Creatine supplements do not appear to enhance physical performance among subjects performing lower-intensity endurance activities like cycling and running (Vandebuerie et al., 1998), although there is limited evidence that creatine supplements enhance the ability of skeletal muscles to store glycogen (a potential endurance benefit). Increased muscle mass might enhance endurance performance, but the weight gain from water and muscle could actually result in a decline in performance.

The benefits of creatine are likely to be at least partly the result of the person's ability to train harder and thus increase strength. This might be good news to athletes who are training intensely, but it means that creatine alone (without exercise) probably has little effect on the muscle mass of sedentary persons (Bermon et al., 1998). A significant gain in physical performance in high-intensity exercise has been shown with creatine doses of 20–30 g/day, but more recent research indicates that similar performance benefits are possible with much lower doses in the range of 2–5 g/day taken over a longer period (Terjung et al., 2000).

Daily creatine supplements (5–10 g/day for 5–12 days) also seem to increase balance and muscle strength in the legs, hands, and feet of patients with muscular dystrophy (Terjung et al., 2000). Such patients usually have lower creatine levels than do healthy people, so boosting muscle stores might help augment cellular energy production and support muscular contraction. Although this may be considered a relatively small gain, it could be very important to the person who can now pick up a glass of water, button a shirt, or walk unaided across a room.

SAFETY/DOSAGE

Although the long-term effects of prolonged creatine use have not been examined, no obvious adverse effects have been linked to use of creatine as a dietary supplement for periods exceeding 5 years (Graham et al., 1999; Poortmans et al., 1999; Volek et al., 2000). Side effects reported anecdotally include gastrointestinal distress, nausea, dehydration, and muscle cramping, but none of these effects has been documented in scientific studies. A cautionary note is in order for people with kidney disorders and for those at risk for dehydration (e.g., athletes exercising in extreme heat or reducing weight for wrestling or lightweight crew).

The most common regimen for creatine supplementation follows a 2-phase cycle: a loading phase of 5–10 days (20–25 g/day) followed by a variable-length maintenance phase (2–5 g/day) to maintain muscle saturation. Creatine absorption appears to be enhanced when the supplement is taken with a high-carbohydrate drink such as fruit juice (Tarnopolsky et al., 2001). It is unclear, however, whether the loading phase is actually needed to achieve the observed benefits on muscle size and power, and lower-dose regimens using the maintenance phase only (2–5 g/day) appear to deliver the same benefits in a slightly longer period.

REFERENCES

Bermon S, Venembre P, Sachet C, Valour S, Dolisi C. Effects of creatine monohydrate ingestion in sedentary and weight-trained older adults. Acta Physiol Scand 1998;164(2):147–155.

Graham AS, Hatton RC. Creatine: a review of efficacy and safety. J Am Pharm Assoc (Wash) 1999;39(6):803–810.

Poortmans JR, Francaux M. Long-term oral creatine supplementation does not impair renal function in healthy athletes. Med Sci Sports Exerc 1999;31(8):1108–1110.

Tarnopolsky MA, Parise G, Yardley NJ, Ballantyne CS, Olatinji S, Phillips SM. Creatine-dextrose and protein-dextrose induce similar strength gains during training. Med Sci Sports Exerc 2001;33(12):2044–2052.

Terjung RL, Clarkson P, Eichner ER, Greenhaff PL, Hespel PJ, Israel RG, Kraemer WJ, Meyer RA, Spriet LL, Tarnopolsky MA, Wagenmakers AJ, Williams MH. American College of Sports Medicine roundtable. The physiological and health effects of oral creatine supplementation. Med Sci Sports Exerc 2000;32(3):706–717.

Vandebuerie F, Vanden Eynde B, Vandenberghe K, Hespel P. Effect of creatine loading on endurance capacity and sprint power in cyclists. Int J Sports Med 1998;19(7):490–495.

Volek JS, Duncan ND, Mazzetti SA, Putukian M, Gomez AL, Kraemer WJ. No effect of heavy resistance training and creatine supplementation on blood lipids. Int J Sport Nutr Exerc Metab 2000;10(2):144–156.

ADDITIONAL RESOURCES

Aaserud R, Gramvik P, Olsen SR, Jensen J. Creatine supplementation delays onset of fatigue during repeated bouts of sprint running. Scand J Med Sci Sports 1998;8(5 pt 1):247–251.

Archer MC. Use of oral creatine to enhance athletic performance and its potential side effects. Clin J Sport Med 1999;9(2):119.

Becque MD, Lochmann JD, Melrose DR. Effects of oral creatine supplementation on muscular strength and body composition. Med Sci Sports Exerc 2000;32(3):654–658.

Casey A, Greenhaff PL. Does dietary creatine supplementation play a role in skeletal muscle metabolism and performance? Am J Clin Nutr 2000;72(2 suppl):607S–617S.

Feldman EB. Creatine: a dietary supplement and ergogenic aid. Nutr Rev 1999;57(2):45–50.

Jones AM, Atter T, Georg KP. Oral creatine supplementation improves multiple sprint performance in elite ice-hockey players. J Sports Med Phys Fitness 1999;39(3):189–196.

Juhn MS, Tarnopolsky M. Oral creatine supplementation and athletic performance: a critical review. Clin J Sport Med 1998;8(4):286–297.

Leenders NM, Lamb DR, Nelson TE. Creatine supplementation and swimming performance. Int J Sport Nutr 1999;9(3):251–262.

Mujika I, Padilla S, Ibanez J, Izquierdo M, Gorostiaga E. Creatine supplementation and sprint performance in soccer players. Med Sci Sports Exerc 2000;32(2):518–525.

Rawson ES, Clarkson PM. Acute creatine supplementation in older men. Int J Sports Med 2000;21(1):71–75.

Robinson TM, Sewell DA, Casey A, Steenge G, Greenhaff PL. Dietary creatine supplementation does not affect some haematological indices, or indices of muscle damage and hepatic and renal function. Br J Sports Med 2000;34(4):284–288.

DHEA (DEHYDROEPIANDROSTERONE)

Overall Rank

★★★★ for restoring DHEA and DHEA-S levels in elderly men and women and in overtrained athletes

★★ for building muscle and reducing fat in healthy young athletes

★★ for boosting testosterone levels and enhancing sexual function

OVERVIEW

DHEA is an androgenic hormone produced in the adrenal glands. In the body, DHEA is converted into other hormones such as testosterone, estrogen, progesterone, or cortisol. DHEA levels are known to decrease with age, particularly after the age of 40 years but perhaps as early as 20–30 years. Because DHEA levels decline with age (reducing up to 90%) and DHEA functions as a direct precursor to testosterone and estrogen, it is often promoted as a "fountain of youth" or "antiaging" supplement. The theory is that by boosting blood DHEA levels, sex hormone levels can be elevated and alleviate some of the conditions associated with aging. Muscle wasting, bone loss, and reduced sex drive are among the potential targets for DHEA supplementation.

COMMENTS

DHEA supplements tend to be relatively inexpensive and widely available from a number of manufacturers. Low-dose DHEA (20–50 mg/day for 12 months) in elderly men and women has been shown to improve bone density, skin thickness, and general feelings of well-being (Labrie et al., 1997) by restoring DHEA-S (the storage form of DHEA) to levels comparable in young adults. Athletes with normal testosterone and DHEA-S levels are unlikely to benefit from DHEA supplementation, but athletes undergoing intense training or at risk for overtraining might benefit from 25–100 mg/day of DHEA to restore DHEA-S levels (Wallace et al., 1999).

SCIENTIFIC SUPPORT

DHEA supplements, at 50–100 mg/day, have been shown to increase muscle mass and improve overall feelings of well-being among a group of 40- to 70-year-old subjects who took the supplements for 6 months. Another small study (nine elderly men) showed a link between 5 months of DHEA supplementation (50 mg/day) and improvements in markers of immune system function (lymphocytes, natural killer cells, and immunoglobulins). Several studies have shown increased serum testosterone levels following regular DHEA supplementation (50–100 mg/day), and anorexic young women may be able to slow bone loss with DHEA supplements (Brown et al., 1999; Wallace et al., 1999).

Supplementation with DHEA (100 mg/day for 12 weeks) in a group of healthy men (average age of 48 years) with normal testosterone levels resulted in only a modest increase in lean body mass and muscle strength (Wallace et al., 1999) and no significant elevation in serum testosterone levels.

SAFETY/DOSAGE

DHEA has the potential to interfere with drugs metabolized by cytochrome P450 3A—a long list that includes Xanax, BuSpar, Celexa, Zoloft, Allegra, Mevacor, Zocor, Meridia, and Viagra, among many others. Although it is difficult to show clear side effects from DHEA supplements, several publications have raised concerns regarding altered hormone profiles, liver abnormalities, increased cancer risk (prostate in men and breast in women), and other steroidlike effects (e.g., increased facial hair, acne, mood swings). Because DHEA is converted into testosterone, theoretical concerns have been suggested (but not documented) that chronic use in men might worsen prostate hyperplasia or even promote prostate cancer. Of the potential adverse effects associated with high-dose DHEA supplements, virilization in women may result from increased testosterone levels, while gynecomastia may result in men from an elevation in estrogen levels. Because of these potential adverse effects, DHEA dosages should be limited to between 25 and 100 mg/day, and then only used by people with a known or elevated risk for suppressed DHEA and DHEA-S levels. It is important to emphasize that although these safety concerns are certainly possible and logical, they are only suspected risks that may not apply to all persons who may derive benefits from DHEA supplements. Competitive athletes should be aware of the potential for DHEA supplementation to alter the testosterone-epitestosterone ratio, causing it to exceed the 6:1 limit set by both the IOC and the NCAA in their screening for testosterone doping (Dehennin et al., 1998).

REFERENCES

Brown GA, Vukovich MD, Sharp RL, Reifenrath TA, Parsons KA, King DS. Effect of oral DHEA on serum testosterone and adaptations to resistance training in young men. J Appl Physiol 1999;87(6):2274–2283.

Dehennin L, Ferry M, Lafarge P, Peres G, Lafarge JP. Oral administration of dehydroepiandrosterone to healthy men: alteration of the urinary androgen profile and consequences for the detection of abuse in sport by gas chromatography-mass spectrometry. Steroids 1998;63(2):80–87.

Labrie F, Belanger A, Cusan L, Candas B. Physiological changes in dehydroepiandrosterone are not reflected by serum levels of active androgens and estrogens but of their metabolites: intracrinology. J Clin Endocrinol Metab 1997;82(8):2403–2409.

Wallace MB, Lim J, Cutler A, Bucci L. Effects of dehydroepiandrosterone vs androstenedione supplementation in men. Med Sci Sports Exerc 1999;31(12):1788–1792.

ADDITIONAL RESOURCES

Alen M, Pakarinen A, Hakkinen K, Komi PV. Responses of serum androgenic-anabolic and catabolic hormones to prolonged strength training. Int J Sports Med 1988;9(3):229–233.

Brown GA, Vukovich MD, Reifenrath TA, Uhl NL, Parsons KA, Sharp RL, King DS. Effects of anabolic precursors on serum testosterone concentrations and adaptations to resistance training in young men. Int J Sport Nutr Exerc Metab 2000;10(3):340–359.

Filaire E, Duche P, Lac G. Effects of amount of training on the saliva concentrations of cortisol, dehydroepiandrosterone and on the dehydroepiandrosterone:cortisol concentration ratio in women over 16 weeks of training. Eur J Appl Physiol Occup Physiol 1998;78(5):466–471.

Filaire E, Le Scanff C, Duche P, Lac G. The relationship between salivary adrenocortical hormones changes and personality in elite female athletes during handball and volleyball competition. Res Q Exerc Sport 1999;70(3):297–302.

GLYCEROL

Overall Rank

★★★ for enhancing hydration status
★★★ for improving endurance performance in hot environments

OVERVIEW

Glycerol, also known as glycerin, is an alcohol compound that is most commonly found in the diet as a component of fat or triglycerides and serves as the backbone onto which fatty acid molecules are attached. Glycerol is marketed as a dietary aid for "hyperhydrating" the body by increasing blood volume and helping to delay dehydration. Therefore, endurance athletes training and competing in hot, humid environments might be interested in the common claims for glycerol that it can increase blood volume, enhance temperature regulation, reduce dehydration, and improve exercise performance in the heat.

COMMENTS

For endurance athletes engaged in strenuous training or competition in hot environments, consumption of glycerol-containing beverages may help hydrate tissues, increase blood volume, and delay the fatigue and exhaustion associated with dehydration.

SCIENTIFIC SUPPORT

Several studies support the theory that glycerol added to fluids will increase tissue hydration compared with drinking fluid without glycerol added. Following glycerol consumption, heart rate and body core temperature are lower during exercise in the heat (Jimenez et al., 1999), suggesting an ergogenic (performance-enhancing) effect. In long-duration activities, such as running and cycling in the heat, a larger supply of stored water may lead to a delay in dehydration and exhaustion (Wagner, 1999). Both laboratory and field studies confirm the modestly ergogenic effects of glycerol on endurance performance (Inder et al., 1998; Meyer et al., 1995; Montner et al., 1996). It is important to note that these benefits, although noted for trained endurance athletes exercising in hot, humid environments, are not necessarily observed in athletes who are less well trained or are exercising in more temperate climates (Arnall and Goforth, 1993; Wagner, 1999).

SAFETY/DOSAGE

No significant adverse side effects are associated with glycerin diluted with fluids, but some subjects may experience headaches, nausea, and diarrhea following glycerol consumption (Wagner, 1999). In patients for whom increased blood volume may be undesirable, including those with conditions such as pregnancy, high blood pressure, diabetes, or kidney disease, glycerol supplementation should be avoided. Because the recommended dose of glycerol relates to the amount of total body water, larger people typically require more glycerol to obtain the desired hydration effects. Approximately 1 g of glycerin per kilogram (2.2 lb) of body weight is diluted in 20–25 mL of liquid. A 70-kg man (154 lb) therefore would need 70 g of glycerin diluted in 1,400–1,750 mL of fluid (about 1–2 L). The mixture should be consumed slowly over the course of 1–2 hours before exercising in the heat.

REFERENCES

Arnall DA, Goforth HW Jr. Failure to reduce body water loss in cold-water immersion by glycerol ingestion. Undersea Hyperb Med 1993;20(4):309–320.

Inder WJ, Swanney MP, Donald RA, Prickett TC, Hellemans J. The effect of glycerol and desmopressin on exercise performance and hydration in triathletes. Med Sci Sports Exerc 1998;30(8):1263–1269.

Jimenez C, Melin B, Koulmann N, Allevard AM, Launay JC, Savourey G. Plasma volume changes during and after acute variations of body hydration level in humans. Eur J Appl Physiol Occup Physiol 1999;80(1):1–8.

Meyer LG, Horrigan DJ Jr, Lotz WG. Effects of three hydration beverages on exercise performance during 60 hours of heat exposure. Aviat Space Environ Med 1995;66(11):1052–1057.

Montner P, Stark DM, Riedesel ML, Murata G, Robergs R, Timms M, Chick TW. Pre-exercise glycerol hydration improves cycling endurance time. Int J Sports Med 1996;17(1):27–33.

Wagner DR. Hyperhydrating with glycerol: implications for athletic performance. J Am Diet Assoc 1999;99(2):207–212.

HMB (ß-HYDROXY-ß-METHYLBUTYRATE)

Overall Rank

★★★★ for reducing muscle catabolism during intense exercise training
★★★★ for slowing muscle loss from wasting associated with cancer or AIDS

OVERVIEW

ß-Hydroxy-ß-methylbutyrate is a metabolite of the amino acid leucine and is found in the diet in small amounts in protein-rich foods like fish and milk. Depending on total protein and leucine intake, HMB production in the body may average about 0.25 to 1 g/day. Because HMB is thought to be the active form of leucine, it is promoted as a supplement to help regulate protein metabolism and reduce muscle breakdown during intense exercise.

COMMENTS

Athletes trying to minimize protein losses and muscle breakdown may want to consider HMB, particularly during high-intensity periods of resistance and endurance training and following long-duration competitions such as marathon running. The primary drawback of HMB is the large amount needed (3–6 g/day) to slow muscle loss and its high cost at those doses.

SCIENTIFIC SUPPORT

There is some evidence that HMB reduces muscle catabolism and may protect against muscle damage in various situations, including cancer-related wasting (May et al., 2002), AIDS-related wasting (Clark et al., 2000), resistance and weight training (Jowko et al., 2001; Panton et al., 2000), and prolonged running (Knitter et al., 2000). Studies suggest no benefit of HMB supplements in reducing muscle damage and loss (Paddon-Jones et al., 2001). In most studies, indicators of postexercise muscle damage, such as blood creatine kinase levels, are typically reduced in subjects consuming HMB. This may indicate a reduced level of muscle damage and could lead to improved muscle function. Research in animals (cattle, pigs, and poultry) and humans suggest that inhibition of muscle damage by HMB increases muscle mass and strength.

One study (Panton et al., 2000) looked at HMB supplements (versus placebo) in 39 men and 36 women (aged 20–40 years). Subjects received 3 g/day of HMB while training 3 times per week for 4 weeks. In the HMB group, blood levels of creatine phosphokinase (an indicator of muscle damage) were reduced compared with the placebo group, and both upper-body strength and fat-free mass were increased. Overall, the study shows that a short-term period of HMB supplementation can increase upper-body strength and minimize muscle damage when combined with an exercise program in both men and women. Other studies have replicated these findings in subjects ranging from 18 to 70 years of age who undergo muscle-damaging exercise for periods of 3–8 weeks (Vukovich at el., 2001).

SAFETY/DOSAGE

No side effects have been reported in animal studies (which have used large doses of HMB for several weeks) or in human studies using as much as 6 g/day (Gallagher et al., 2000a, 2000b). The recommended dose is based on the effective levels noted in clinical studies and ranges from 3–6 g/day taken in two or three divided doses.

REFERENCES

Clark RH, Feleke G, Din M, Yasmin T, Singh G, Khan FA, Rathmacher JA. Nutritional treatment for acquired immunodeficiency virus-associated wasting using beta-hydroxy beta-methylbutyrate, glutamine, and arginine: a randomized, double-blind, placebo-controlled study. JPEN 2000;24(3):133–139.

Gallagher PM, Carrithers JA, Godard MP, Schulze KE, Trappe SW. Beta-hydroxy-beta-methylbutyrate ingestion, part I: effects on strength and fat free mass. Med Sci Sports Exerc 2000a;32(12):2109–2115.

Gallagher PM, Carrithers JA, Godard MP, Schulze KE, Trappe SW. Beta-hydroxy-beta-methylbutyrate ingestion, part II: effects on hematology, hepatic and renal function. Med Sci Sports Exerc 2000b;32(12):2116–2119.

Jowko E, Ostaszewski P, Jank M, Sacharuk J, Zieniewicz A, Wilczak J, Nissen S. Creatine and beta-hydroxy-beta-methylbutyrate (HMB) additively increase lean body mass and muscle strength during a weight-training program. Nutrition 2001;17(7–8):558–566.

Knitter AE, Panton L, Rathmacher JA, Petersen A, Sharp R. Effects of beta-hydroxy-beta-methylbutyrate on muscle damage after a prolonged run. J Appl Physiol 2000;89(4):1340–1344.

May PE, Barber A, D'Olimpio JT, Hourihane A, Abumrad NN. Reversal of cancer-related wasting using oral supplementation with a combination of beta-hydroxy-beta-methylbutyrate, arginine, and glutamine. Am J Surg 2002;183(4):471–479.

Paddon-Jones D, Keech A, Jenkins D. Short-term beta-hydroxy-beta-methylbutyrate supplementation does not reduce symptoms of eccentric muscle damage. Int J Sport Nutr Exerc Metab 2001;11(4):442–450.

Panton LB, Rathmacher JA, Baier S, Nissen S. Nutritional supplementation of the leucine metabolite beta-hydroxy-beta-methylbutyrate (hmb) during resistance training. Nutrition 2000;16(9):734–739.

Vukovich MD, Stubbs NB, Bohlken RM. Body composition in 70-year-old adults responds to dietary beta-hydroxy-beta-methylbutyrate similarly to that of young adults. J Nutr 2001;131(7):2049–2052.

ADDITIONAL RESOURCES

Kreider RB, Ferreira M, Wilson M, Almada AL. Effects of calcium beta-hydroxy-beta-methylbutyrate (HMB) supplementation during resistance-training on markers of catabolism, body composition and strength. Int J Sports Med 1999;20(8):503–509.

Nissen S, Sharp RL, Panton L, Vukovich M, Trappe S, Fuller JC Jr. beta-hydroxy-beta-methylbutyrate (HMB) supplementation in humans is safe and may decrease cardiovascular risk factors. J Nutr 2000;130(8):1937–1945.

Nissen S, Sharp R, Ray M, Rathmacher JA, Rice D, Fuller JC Jr, Connelly AS, Abumrad N. Effect of leucine metabolite beta-hydroxy-beta-methylbutyrate on muscle metabolism during resistance-exercise training. J Appl Physiol 1996;81(5):2095–2104.

Papet I, Ostaszewski P, Glomot F, Obled C, Faure M, Bayle G, Nissen S, Arnal M, Grizard J. The effect of a high dose of 3-hydroxy-3-methylbutyrate on protein metabolism in growing lambs. Br J Nutr 1997;77(6):885–896.

Slater GJ, Jenkins D. Beta-hydroxy-beta-methylbutyrate (HMB) supplementation and the promotion of muscle growth and strength. Sports Med 2000;30(2):105–116.

Slater G, Jenkins D, Logan P, Lee H, Vukovich M, Rathmacher JA, Hahn AG. Beta-hydroxy-beta-methylbutyrate (HMB) supplementation does not affect changes in strength or body composition during resistance training in trained men. Int J Sport Nutr Exerc Metab 2001;11(3):384–396.

Vukovich MD, Dreifort GD. Effect of beta-hydroxy beta-methylbutyrate on the onset of blood lactate accumulation and VO(2) peak in endurance-trained cyclists. J Strength Cond Res 2001;15(4):491–497.

MEDIUM-CHAIN TRIGLYCERIDES (MCTs)

Overall Rank

★★★ for modestly increasing metabolic rate compared with long-chain triglycerides

★★ for promoting weight loss

★ for enhancing endurance exercise performance

OVERVIEW

Medium-chain triglycerides (MCTs) are fats that contain 6, 8, 10, or 12 carbons. The number of carbons distinguishes them from long-chain (14 or more carbons) or short-chain (two or four carbons) fats. The length of the carbon chain affects the overall function in the body. MCTs are absorbed rapidly and burned for immediate energy, whereas other fats are absorbed and metabolized more slowly. Thus, most of the clinical evidence for MCTs added to the diet exists for the treatment of various fat malabsorption syndromes, but MCT supplements are typically sold to athletes as flavored or unflavored MCT oil with claims of improving endurance performance, promoting fat burning, sparing muscle glycogen, and maintaining or enhancing muscle mass.

It is theorized that because MCTs are rapidly absorbed and metabolized, the athlete who ingests them acquires a fuel source that helps to spare the use of muscle glycogen (stored carbohydrate). Because depletion of muscle glycogen is a factor in fatigue, ingestion of MCT oil could provide the body with an immediate source of fat that is rapidly broken down for energy; thus, muscle glycogen stores are not used up as quickly and the onset of fatigue is delayed.

MCTs are also thought to increase metabolic rate. Assuming that diet (calorie intake) and exercise (calorie output) remain the same, any increase in metabolic rate could result in a small, slow reduction in body fat. MCTs are thought to be burned immediately for energy rather than being stored as body fat and used for energy at a later time. In theory, MCTs could help to maintain muscle mass because they produce ketone bodies that are used for energy before amino acids drawn from muscle tissue are used for energy.

COMMENTS

Although a handful of early studies seemed promising, the results of recent well-controlled studies on MCT supplements suggest that they are not effective in increasing endurance performance. In the absence of convincing scientific studies of bodybuilders or weight lifters, MCT supplements cannot be recommended as an effective supplement for reducing body fat or maintaining muscle mass. Likewise, the results of recent well-controlled studies in endurance athletes do not support the use of MCT oil to spare muscle glycogen or enhance performance. A notable exception are extreme endurance athletes, such as cyclists in multistage races (e.g., Tour de France) and participants in multiday "adventure race" events (e.g., the 7-day Eco-Challenge), who may have difficulty consuming enough calories and may find that 1 tablespoon of MCT oil provides approximately 110 easily absorbed calories to augment energy needs.

SCIENTIFIC SUPPORT

Because the length of the carbon chain affects absorption and MCTs are rapidly absorbed, they are transported directly to the liver and are quickly oxidized. Their rapid transport and oxidation is more similar to carbo-hydrate than to other fats, and MCTs have a somewhat reduced tendency to be stored as body fat (thus their questionable marketing as weight loss aids). In contrast, the long-chain fats, the most prevalent type of fat in the diet, are slowly absorbed and oxidized and often stored as body fat. Most MCTs are metabolized by the liver and provide energy, although some ketone bodies will also be produced from MCT metabol-ism. Ketone bodies may be eliminated in the urine or used as an alternat-ive fuel source by the muscles and the brain during starvation and extremes of endurance exercise.

Other than studies of various fat malabsorption syndromes, most studies of MCTs as dietary supplements have looked at endurance run-ners and cyclists to determine effectiveness in increasing endurance per-formance. Researchers have studied both the use of muscle glycogen when MCTs are consumed and the effect that MCTs have on running or cycling times. In these studies, the endurance cyclists engage in moder-ate to intense exercise while ingesting an MCT supplement, an MCT supplement plus a carbohydrate supplement, or a placebo. The results of these studies suggest that MCT oil does not reduce the use of muscle glycogen or improve endurance performance (Angus et al., 2000; Horow-itz et al., 2000; Misell et al., 2001).

Despite the frequent claims for the benefits of MCTs in bodybuilding (increased metabolic rate, reduced body fat, and preserved muscle mass), no published scientific studies have examined MCT use by bodybuilders. One study, however, showed that MCT supplements (2 mg/kg of body weight) reduced whole-body leucine flux (a marker of protein break-down) by 20% in healthy sedentary men (Keller et al., 2002), and another study showed that septic and hypercatabolic patients receiving an MCT emulsion recovered faster than those receiving long-chain fatty acids (Garnacho-Montero et al., 2002). Most product claims for commer-cial MCT supplements are based on studies showing that overall meta-bolic rate is moderately increased 20–30% with MCT ingestion (30–40% energy as fat with 50–80% of fat as MCT or LCT) compared with long-chain triglycerides (Jiang et al., 2001; Matsuo et al., 2001a, 2001b; Papamandjaris et al., 2000; Tsuji et al., 2001). Not all studies, however, have shown an effect on metabolic rate or rate of weight gain or loss (Kovacs et al., 2001).

SAFETY/DOSAGE

Consumption of MCT oil by humans is safe up to levels of 1 g/kg of body weight. A byproduct of MCT metabolism is ketone bodies, and the use of MCT oil by diabetics is not recommended unless it is part of a medically supervised treatment. People with liver disease should not use MCT oil because MCTs are delivered rapidly to the liver and their presence could put additional stress on that organ. MCT supplements do not contain any essential fatty acids, but this would not present a problem unless MCTs were the only source of fat in the diet. In some studies, large doses of MCT oil (70–90 g) are associated with intestinal cramping, whereas smaller quantities of MCT oil tend not to influence gastrointestinal function. Typical doses are 1–2 tablespoons per day (14–28 g of total fat) consumed "straight" or added to food or beverages. Initial doses should be small (i.e., ½ tablespoon per day) to make sure there are no gastrointestinal side effects.

REFERENCES

Angus DJ, Hargreaves M, Dancey J, Febbraio MA. Effect of carbohydrate or carbohydrate plus medium-chain triglyceride ingestion on cycling time trial performance. J Appl Physiol 2000;88(1):113–119.

Horowitz JF, Mora-Rodriguez R, Byerley LO, Coyle EF. Preexercise medium-chain triglyceride ingestion does not alter muscle glycogen use during exercise. J Appl Physiol 2000;88(1):219–225.

Keller U, Turkalj I, Laager R, Bloesch D, Bilz S. Effects of medium- and long-chain fatty acids on whole body leucine and glucose kinetics in man. Metabolism 2002;51(6):754–760.

Garnacho-Montero J, Ortiz-Leyba C, Jimenez-Jimenez FJ, Garcia-Garmendia JL, Jimenez-Jimenez LM, Garnacho-Montero MC, Barrero-Almodovar A. Clinical and metabolic effects of two lipid emulsions on the parenteral nutrition of septic patients. Nutrition 2002;18(2):134–138.

Jiang ZM, Zhang SY, Wang XR, Yang NF, Zhu Y, Wilmore D. A comparison of medium-chain and long-chain triglycerides in surgical patients. Ann Surg 1993;217(2):175–184.

Kovacs EM, Westerterp-Plantenga MS, Saris WH. The effects of 2-week ingestion of (--)-hydroxycitrate and (--)-hydroxycitrate combined with medium-chain triglycerides on satiety, fat oxidation, energy expenditure and body weight. Int J Obes Relat Metab Disord 2001;25(7):1087–1094.

Matsuo T, Matsuo M, Kasai M, Takeuchi H. Effects of a liquid diet supplement containing structured medium- and long-chain triacylglycerols on body fat accumulation in healthy young subjects. Asia Pac J Clin Nutr 2001a;10(1):46–50.

Matsuo T, Matsuo M, Taguchi N, Takeuchi H. The thermic effect is greater for structured medium- and long-chain triacylglycerols versus long-chain triacylglycerols in healthy young women. Metabolism 2001b;50(1):125–130.

Misell LM, Lagomarcino ND, Schuster V, Kern M. Chronic medium-chain triacylglycerol consumption and endurance performance in trained runners. J Sports Med Phys Fitness 2001;41(2):210–215.

Papamandjaris AA, White MD, Raeini-Sarjaz M, Jones PJ. Endogenous fat oxidation during medium chain versus long chain triglyceride feeding in healthy women. Int J Obes Relat Metab Disord 2000;24(9):1158–1166.

Tsuji H, Kasai M, Takeuchi H, Nakamura M, Okazaki M, Kondo K. Dietary medium-chain triacylglycerols suppress accumulation of body fat in a double-blind, controlled trial in healthy men and women. J Nutr 2001;131(11):2853–2859.

ADDITIONAL RESOURCES

Bach AC, Ingenbleek Y, Frey A. The usefulness of dietary medium-chain triglycerides in body weight control: fact or fancy? J Lipid Res 1996;37:708–726.

Goedecke JH, Elmer-English R, Dennis SC, Schloss I, Noakes TD, Lambert EV. Effects of medium-chain triacylglycerol ingested with carbohydrate on metabolism and exercise performance. Int J Sport Nutr 1999;9:35–47.

Jeukendrup, AE, Saris WH, Schrauwen P, Brouns F, Wagenmakers AJ. Metabolic availability of medium-chain triglycerides coingested with carbohydrates during prolonged exercise. J Appl Physiol 1995;79:756–762.

Jeukendrup AE, Thielen JJ, Wagenmakers AJ, Brouns F, Saris WH. Effect of medium-chain triacylglycerol and carbohydrate ingestion during exercise on substrate utilization and subsequent cycling performance. Am J Clin Nutr 1998;67:397–404.

Seaton TB, Welle SL, Warenko MK, Campbell RG. 1986. Thermic effect of medium-chain and long-chain triglycerides in man. Am J Clin Nutr 1986;44:630–634.

Traul KA, Driedger A, Ingle DL, Nakhasi D. 2000. Review of the toxicologic properties of medium-chain triglycerides. Food Chem Toxicol 2000;38:79–98.

Van Zyl CG, Lambert EV, Hawley JA, Noakes TD, Dennis SC. 1996. Effects of medium-chain triglyceride ingestion on fuel metabolism and cycling performance. J Appl Physiol 1996;80:2217–2225.

PROTEIN (CASEIN, WHEY, SOY, COLLAGEN, COLOSTRUM)

See "Amino Acids and Protein Supplements."

PROTEOLYTIC ENZYMES

Overall Rank

★★★★ for reducing inflammation and pain associated with tissue trauma and injury
★★★★ for enhancing postexercise recovery

OVERVIEW

The term *proteolytic* is a catch-all term referring to enzymes that digest protein. Supplemental forms can incorporate any of a wide variety of enzymes, including trypsin, chymotrypsin, pancreatin, bromelain, papain, and a range of fungal proteases. In the body, proteolytic digestive enzymes are produced in the pancreas, but supplemental forms of enzymes may come from fungal or bacterial sources, extraction from the pancreas of livestock animals (trypsin and chymotrypsin) or extraction from plants (e.g., papain from papayas and bromelain from pineapples). The primary uses of proteolytic enzymes in dietary supplements are as digestive enzymes, anti-inflammatory agents, and pain relievers, and to accelerate recovery or wound healing after exercise.

COMMENTS

A compelling body of scientific evidence supports the use of proteolytic enzyme supplements for enhancing digestive function, speeding recovery from injury or surgery, and reducing swelling or bruising. Much of this research, however, is quite dated (1970s) clinical evidence from German and Czechoslovakian researchers (for anti-inflammatory and analgesic effects), whereas more recent data primarily concern the use of orally delivered enzymes for digestive benefits. Benefits claimed for enzymes used in treating autoimmune diseases and food allergies are not convincing and await further study. Thus, proteolytic enzymes used as dietary supplements by athletes wishing to enhance recovery from exercise or injury and for patients recovering from surgery appears to be warranted.

SCIENTIFIC SUPPORT

It is quite logical that proteolytic enzymes would help alleviate a suboptimal production of the body's own digestive enzymes (which can occur in various pancreatic conditions). Supplemental enzymes can help alleviate gastrointestinal complaints such as gas and bloating, diarrhea, and cramps associated with inefficient or incomplete digestion. Additionally, some evidence indicates that a small percentage of supplemental enzymes may be absorbed intact (and active) into the systemic circulation, where they appear to have anti-inflammatory and pain-relieving actions that can be of benefit to athletes recovering from exercise or injury and to patients recovering from surgery.

Several clinical trials show the benefit of using oral proteolytic enzymes as a digestive aid. Proteolytic enzymes are also theorized to help reduce symptoms of food allergies and as a treatment for rheumatoid arthritis and other autoimmune diseases (which are thought by some alternative medicine practitioners to be caused by whole proteins from foods leaking into the blood and causing an immune reaction—sometimes called leaky gut). Unfortunately, there is not a great deal of scientific evidence, either from laboratory or clinical studies, to support the use of enzymes for treating allergies or autoimmune conditions.

Perhaps the strongest evidence for benefits of proteolytic enzyme supplements comes from the numerous European studies showing various enzyme blends to be effective in accelerating recovery from exercise and injury in sports participants as well as promoting tissue repair in patients following surgery. In one study of football players suffering from ankle injuries, those receiving proteolytic enzyme supplements experienced accelerated healing and returned to the field about 50% faster than did athletes assigned to receive a placebo tablet (Buck and Phillips, 1970; Craig, 1975). A handful of other small trials have shown that athletes taking proteolytic enzymes benefited from reduced inflammation, faster healing of bruises and other tissue injuries (including fractures), and reduced overall recovery time compared with athletes taking a placebo. In patients recovering from facial and various reconstructive surgeries, treatment with proteolytic enzymes significantly reduced swelling, bruising, and stiffness compared with placebo (Adamek et al., 1997).

In several double-blind studies, the pain-relieving and anti-inflammatory effects of an enzyme blend (Wobenzym) was compared with a common analgesic drug (Diclofenac) in patients suffering from osteoarthritis of the knee, tendon injuries, or neck pain (Strafun and Tovmasian, 2000; Tilscher et al., 1996). Following 4–8 weeks of supplementation, pain measurements (at rest, on motion, on walking, and at night) showed a similar significant improvement after treatment in both groups. Similar findings have been reported for other painful or inflammatory conditions, including numerous studies of postsurgical recovery (Duskova and Wald, 1999; Gal et al., 1998; McCue et al., 1972; Neverov and Klimov, 1999).

SAFETY/DOSAGE

Proteolytic enzymes are generally considered to be quite safe, although some people may experience mild gastrointestinal side effects (heartburn). Persons at risk for gastric or duodenal ulcers might want to avoid enzyme supplements, which have the potential for aggravating ulcerated tissues. In addition, because proteolytic enzyme supplements tend to produce a modest anticoagulant (blood-thinning) effect, they should be used with caution when combined with other blood-thinning agents, including nonsteroidal anti-inflammatory drugs.

The dosage or "strength" of an enzyme supplement is typically expressed in "activity units" that refer to the enzyme's ability to digest a certain amount of protein. Because the same milligram amount of a particular enzyme may have different activity units based on its processing and blending, it is advisable to select a clinically validated enzyme supplement (such as Wobenzym or Phlogenzym) or at least one that contains a combination of enzymes with activity at different pH levels. Preferred brands are enteric coated, meaning that the formulations are protected from digestion in the stomach for optimal delivery of the enzymes to the intestines where they can perform their actions.

REFERENCES

Adamek J, Prausova J, Wald M. Enzyme therapy in the treatment of lymphedema in the arm after breast carcinoma surgery. Rozhl Chir 1997;76(4):203–204.

Buck JE, Phillips N. Trial of Chymoral in professional footballers. Br J Clin Pract 1970;24(9):375–377.

Craig RP. The quantitative evaluation of the use of oral proteolytic enzymes in the treatment of sprained ankles. Injury 1975;6(4):313–316.

Duskova M, Wald M. Orally administered proteases in aesthetic surgery. Aesthetic Plast Surg 1999;23(1):41–44.

Gal P, Tecl F, Skotakova J, Mach V. Systemic enzyme therapy in the treatment of supracondylar fractures of the humerus in children. Rozhl Chir 1998;77(12):574–576.

McCue FC III, Webster TM, Gieck J. Clinical effects of proteolytic enzymes after reconstructive hand surgery. A double-blind evaluation of oral trypsin-chymotrypsin. Int Surg 1972;57(6):479–482.

Neverov VA, Klimov AV. The pathogenetic basis for and clinical use of systemic enzyme therapy in traumatology and orthopedics. Vestn Khir Im I I Grek 1999;158(1):41–44.

Strafun SS, Tovmasian VV. The use of Wobenzym in the comprehensive treatment of patients with digital flexor tendon injury. Klin Khir 2000;(4):39–40.

Tilscher H, Keusch R, Neumann K. Results of a double-blind, randomized comparative study of Wobenzym-placebo in patients with cervical syndrome. Wien Med Wochenschr 1996;146(5):91–95.

ADDITIONAL RESOURCES

Desser L, Rehberger A, Kokron E, Paukovits W. Cytokine synthesis in human peripheral blood mononuclear cells after oral administration of polyenzyme preparations. Oncology 1993;50(6):403–407.

RIBOSE

Overall Rank

★★★★ for prevention of exercise-induced ischemia in cardiac disease
★★★ for enhancement of endurance exercise performance
★★ for improvement of muscle strength and power

OVERVIEW

Ribose is a five-carbon simple sugar (a pentose) that forms the carbohydrate portion, or backbone, of RNA and DNA molecules. When combined with adenine, ribose produces adenosine, one of the components of the energy currency of the cell, ATP. Ribose is used in the body in several specific ways. It can be converted into pyruvate and enter into the pathways of energy metabolism, or it can be used to manufacture nucleotides, the primary building blocks for important structures in the body such as RNA, DNA, and ATP. As a result, ribose supplements are typically marketed for increasing energy levels, exercise endurance, and muscular power output.

COMMENTS

Clearly, anybody concerned with managing diminished blood flow to the heart or muscle tissues would be interested in ribose supplementation. In particular, people who experience chest pain, shortness of breath, or leg pain during exercise may want to consider ribose as a daily dietary supplement. The casual or occasional exerciser is unlikely to benefit from ribose supplements except in the case of several back-to-back days of intense exercise. For the "weekend warrior," who probably has enough time between exercise sessions to fully recover ATP levels, supplemental ribose is not recommended. Competitive athletes, who may be training once or more per day, could notice very modest benefits such as increased power output and increased time to exhaustion with regular ribose supplementation (because of enhanced ATP resynthesis following exercise-induced depletion); required doses, however, are large (more than 10 g/day) and expensive.

SCIENTIFIC SUPPORT

Because ribose can serve as a precursor to adenosine (the A in ATP) and seems to stimulate the production of ATP (in laboratory studies), the theory behind ribose supplementation is that it maximizes ATP stores and therefore increases cellular energy stores for improved exercise performance and fatigue prevention.

In the cell, ATP loses its phosphate groups to generate energy. Losing one phosphate turns ATP (triphosphate) into ADP (diphosphate) and finally into AMP (monophosphate). Adenine or adenosine (no phosphates) can either be converted back to AMP or lost from the cell. The conversion back to AMP/ADP/ATP or the "salvage" of adenosine requires a ribose-containing molecule known as 5-phosphororibosyl-1-pyrophosphate (PRPP). If this salvage does not take place, the adenosine is lost and must be converted "from scratch"—a process known as de novo synthesis, which again requires the ribose-containing PRPP.

Ribose has been under study as a therapy for cardiac ischemia (reduced blood flow to the heart) for a number of years (Pasque and Wechsler, 1984). The data from those studies clearly indicate that ribose can help improve heart function during and following periods of reduced blood flow and oxygen delivery (Erickson, 1990). Under conditions of constricted blood and oxygen flow to heart and muscle tissue, ATP levels have been shown to decrease by as much as 50%. This finding is not unexpected, but the fact that creatine phosphate levels recover relatively quickly while ATP levels may remain depressed for several days suggests that adenosine levels may not be adequately maintained. In animal studies, supplemental ribose permits recovery of approximately 85% of normal ATP levels within 24 hours following restricted circulation.

In patients with coronary artery disease, supplemental ribose allows subjects to exercise for significantly longer periods than they could before they consumed ribose and longer than subjects who consumed a placebo supplement (Pliml et al., 1992). During intense exercise, ATP levels are reduced 10–20%, which may be attributed to the loss of adenosine and inadequate resynthesis of ATP (Wagner et al., 1991). In some muscle fibers, complete resynthesis of ATP may require 24–96 hours (1–4 days) to fully recover from exhaustive exercise. Supplemental ribose has the potential to increase the rate of adenosine production and ATP synthesis following exhaustive exercise by approximately 3–4 times, meaning that recovery of ATP stores can be reduced from 1–4 days to 6–24 hours (Wagner et al., 1991).

SAFETY/DOSAGE

Because ribose is found in all cells of the body, it is generally recognized as a nontoxic substance. Supplemental doses of as much as 60 g/day have been given with no significant side effects (Erickson, 1990). At such high levels, the possible occurrence of gastrointestinal distress, diarrhea, and hypoglycemia are more likely. For purposes of maintaining elevated levels of ribose in the blood, smaller doses of 3–10 g/day of ribose are common in commercial dietary supplements, but as noted earlier, the clinical evidence for energy or endurance benefits of such doses in healthy subjects has been disappointing.

REFERENCES

Erickson D. Sugar fix? A simple sugar may help hearts heal. Sci Am 1990;263(6):119, 122.

Pasque MK, Wechsler AS. Metabolic intervention to affect myocardial recovery following ischemia. Ann Surg 1984;200(1):1–12.

Pliml W, von Arnim T, Stablein A, Hofmann H, Zimmer HG, Erdmann E. Effects of ribose on exercise-induced ischemia in stable coronary artery disease. Lancet 1992;340(8818):507–510.

Wagner DR, Gresser U, Zollner N. Effects of oral ribose on muscle metabolism during bicycle ergometer in AMPD-deficient patients. Ann Nutr Metab 1991;35(5):297–302.

ADDITIONAL RESOURCES

De Jong JW, Van der Meer P, Owen P, Opie LH. Prevention and treatment of ischemic injury with nucleosides. Bratisl Lek Listy 1991;92(3–4):165–173.

TRIBULUS (*TRIBULUS TERRESTRIS*)

Overall Rank

★★★ for sexual performance
★★ for athletic performance

OVERVIEW

Tribulus is a traditional Chinese medicinal herb that has gained attention lately for its uses in enhancing sexual and athletic performance and treating painful urination and as a general tonic (Anand et al., 1994). The main active components in tribulus appear to be steroidal saponins and protodioscin. Tribulus has been proven to improve sexual desire and erectile function by converting protodioscin to DHEA. Both phytochemicals have been shown in preclinical tests to stimulate sexual desire and function (Adaikan et al., 2000; Gauthaman et al., 2002; Zarkova, 1992).

COMMENTS

Few well-designed studies have been conducted on *Tribulus terrestris* for its primary indications of sexual performance and athletic performance. Of the few human clinical studies involving treatment with only tribulus, the results were favorable. A few other studies exist in the areas of sexual performance and athletic performance, but they used tribulus in a mixture with other supplements, and it is not known how much the tribulus contributed to the clinical results (Antonio et al., 2000; Brown et al., 2000, 2001a, 2001b, 2001c; Street et al., 2000). Of note, a heart drug made from *Tribulus terrestris saponins* is being recommended for clinical therapy and prevention of atherosclerosis in Russia (Kemertelidze et al., 1982). Overall, even though tribulus is one of the most popular ingredients in supplements for bodybuilding, clinical support to back up its claims is still lacking.

SCIENTIFIC SUPPORT

Sexual Performance

Nikolova and Stanislavov (2000) performed a clinical study involving 51 patients using an extract of *Tribulus terrestris* (Tribestan) and found statistically significant improvement in parameters to measure infertility. The use of tribulus treatment over 3 months produced reductions in the leukocyte count and the locally secreted immunoglobulins, elevation of α-amylase levels, and normalization of seminal parameters. The authors noted that the treatment with *Tribulus terrestris* extract had a side benefit of improving overall male health, indicated by decreased cholesterol and triglyceride levels and elevated levels of lipoproteins by the end of the study.

Stanislavov and Nikolova (2000) reported that in 15% of the infertile couples in Russia, 9% of males and 15% of women showed signs of infertility that might have been the result of immunological health. In a study of a cohort of this group, *Tribulus terrestris* extract (Tribestan) was chosen because of the presence of furostanol compounds in the plant and the absence of reported toxicity in humans. As a result of treatment, conception was reportedly good in these couples, especially when the males had high titers of sperm antibodies. The authors noted that due to the good results, they recommended treatment in similar cases in practice.

In a double-blind study with *Tribulus terrestris*, 45 men with fertility problems (moderate idiopathic oligozoosperms) were given a dry-powder extract or a placebo. After 3 months of treatment, 7 of the 36 men treated successfully conceived with their wives. In the treatment groups, significant increases in normal acrosome morphology and acrosome reaction test were found (Adimoelja et al., 1978).

Athletic Performance

Ten highly trained cyclists were given a supplement of *Tribulus terrestris* and ipriflavone or a placebo for 38 days. Cyclists in the active group improved hormonal markers of overtraining and performance during the period of intense training and competition (McGregor et al., 2000).

Street et al. (2000) gave capsules containing 250 mg of *Tribulus terrestris*, 100 mg of 7-ispropoxyisofavone, 100 mg of *Avena sativa*, and 50 mg of saw palmetto to two bodybuilders to determine the effect of the supplement on plasma testosterone and luteinizing hormone. As part of the normal weight-lifting regime, the supplements were administered for 2 weeks, 8 capsules 2 times daily. The luteinizing hormone and plasma testosterone levels were found not to change within the period of supplementation, nor were biochemical measures of liver function changed.

SAFETY/DOSAGE

For a standardized extract (60% saponins), the dosage is 100–500 mg 3 times daily; an unspecified preparation of tribulus was used in a couple of clinical studies at the dosage of 750–1,350 mg/day along with other supplements (Brown et al., 2000, 2001a, 2001b, 2001c).

The only reported side effect of tribulus is frequent urination, and because of its diuretic properties, tribulus is not recommended in cases of dehydration (Singh and Sisodia, 1971). There are no known drug interactions with tribulus.

Possible association with hepatotoxicity, photosensitization, and a disease called geeldikkop have been made with the ingestion of large amounts of tribulus by sheep but have never been confirmed (Bourke, 1984; Glastonbury, 1984).

REFERENCES
Adaikan PG, Gauthaman K, Prasad RNV, Ng SC. Proerectile pharmacological effects of Tribulus terrestris extract on the rabbit corpus cavernosum. Annals Academy of Medicine Singapore 2000;29(1): 22–26.

Adimoelja FXA, Tanojo TD, Surjaatmaja S. Phytopharmaca, an alternative treatment for male subfertility. Int J Androl 1997;20(suppl 1):39.

Anand R, Patnaik GK, Srivastava S, Kulshreshtha DK, Dhawan BN. Evaluation of antiurolithiatic activity of Tribulus terrestris. International Journal of Pharmacognosy 1994;32(3):217–224.

Antonio J, Uelmen J, Ehler L, Raether J, Sanders M. Influence of a Tribulus-containing supplement on body composition and strength in football players and bodybuilders. Med Sci Sports Exerc 2000;32(5 suppl):S61.

Bourke CA. Staggers in sheep associated with the ingestion of Tribulus terrestris. Aust Vet J 1984;61(11):360–363.

Brown GA, Kohut ML, Franke WD, Jackson D, Vukovich MD, King DS. Serum hormonal and lipid responses to androgenic supplementation in 30- to 59-year-old men. Med Sci Sports Exerc 2000;32(5 suppl):S122.

Brown GA, Vukovich MD, Martini ER, Kohut ML, Franke WD, Jackson DA, King DS. Effects of androstenedione-herbal supplementation on serum sex hormone concentrations in 30- to 59-year-old men. Int J Vitam Nutr Res 2001a;71(5):293–301

Brown GA, Vukovich MD, Martini ER, Kohut ML, Franke WD, Jackson DA, King DS. Endocrine and lipid responses to chronic androstenediol-herbal supplementation in 30- to 58-year-old men. J Am Coll Nutr 2001b;20(5):520–528.

Gauthaman K, Adaikan PG, Prasad RN. Aphrodisiac properties of Tribulus Terrestris extract (Protodioscin) in normal and castrated rats. Life Sci 2002;71(12):1385–1396.

Glastonbury JR, Doughty FR, Whitaker SJ, Sergeant E. A syndrome of hepatogenous photosensitisation, resembling geeldikkop, in sheep grazing Tribulus terrestris. Aust Vet J 1984;t;61(10):314–316.

Kemertelidze EP, Pkhidze TA, Kachukahashvili TN, Umikashvili RS, Turova AD, Sokolova LN. The new anti sclerotic drug Tribusponin. Khimiko-Farmatsevticheskii Zhurnal 1982;16(1):119–122.

McGregor SJ, Sayder AR, Pizza FX. Herbal supplementation in highly trained cyclists during a period of intensified competition. Med Sci Sports Exerc 2000;32(5 suppl):S117.

Nikolova V, Stanislavov R. Tribulus terrestris and human reproduction clinical laboratory data. Dokladi na B"lgarskata Akademiya na Naukite 2000;53(12):113–116.

Singh RCP, Sisodia CS. Effect of Tribulus terrestris fruit extracts on chloride and creatinine renal clearances in dogs. Indian J Physiol Pharmacol 1971;15(3):93–96.

Stanislavov R, Nikolova V. Tribulus terrestris and human male fertility: I. Immunological aspects. Dokladi na B"lgarskata Akademiya na Naukite 2000;53(10):107–110.

Street C, Antonio J, Scally MC. The effects of Tribulus terrestris on endocrine status in recreational bodybuilders: A preliminary report. Med Sci Sports Exerc 2000;32(5 suppl):S61.

Zarkova, S. Steroid saponins of Tribulus terrestris having a stimulant effect on the sexual functions. Revista Portuguesa de Ciencias Veterinarias 1992;79(470):117–126.

3

Energy
Supplements

Bee Products (Bee Pollen, Propolis,
Royal Jelly)
Brewer's Yeast *(Saccharomyces
cerevisiae)*
Ginseng
Inosine

NADH (Nicotinamide Adenine
Dinucleotide)
Rhodiola
Sea Buckthorn *(Hippophae
rhamnoides)*
Vitamin B$_1$ (Thiamin)
Vitamin B$_2$ (Riboflavin)

BEE PRODUCTS (BEE POLLEN, PROPOLIS, ROYAL JELLY)

Overall Rank

★★★ for stimulating the immune system
★★★ for reducing cholesterol
★★★ as an overall tonic
★★ as an antibiotic
★★ for treating and preventing herpes
★★ for treating and preventing premenstrual syndrome (PMS)
★ for boosting energy levels

OVERVIEW

Bee products commonly used as dietary supplements are bee pollen, propolis, and royal jelly. They are all included in one review because they contain many overlapping constituents and claims and are often used in formulations together, making them difficult to narrowly define in terms of content.

Bee pollen is difficult to characterize specifically because products sold as "bee pollen" are made up of a variable content of vitamins, minerals, amino acids, carbohydrates, and trace minerals. The plants the pollen was harvested from and under what conditions also vary. Typical claims

73

for bee pollen include use as an energizer and for athletic endurance, although clinical studies are lacking to confirm these claims.

Royal jelly is the food the worker bees bring to fortify the queen bee, and it is fed to bee larvae in their first few days of life. It is a secretion that comes from the head of the worker bee and contains flower nectar, sugars, and proteins. As an overall tonic and energizer, royal jelly is generally used for people who need something to make them thrive and feel younger.

Propolis, sometimes called "nature's penicillin," is a complex mixture of mostly pollen and waxes that bees collect from plants and then use to sterilize, cement, and varnish the hives. It is rich in amino acids, trace minerals, flavonoids, and vitamin K. Although in preclinical studies propolis has been confirmed to be effective as an antibacterial, antifungal, and anti-inflammatory, clinical studies are needed to confirm these roles and determine the therapeutic dosages and conditions for which it is best suited (Dobrowolski et al., 1991).

COMMENTS

Overall, some evidence exists to support the claims of these bee products, but much more clinical work is needed, and certainly an effort to define and characterize products would help our understanding. Considering the other natural alternatives with more clinical substantiation that exist for many of the claims of propolis, it may be best to limit the use of propolis until further clinical work is performed. The most exciting and promising uses seem to be as an alternative antibiotic and to treat inflammation, especially considering the negative issues that exist for drugs on the market in those categories and the apparent lack of serious negative side effects with bee products (in nonallergic persons).

SCIENTIFIC SUPPORT

Bee Pollen and Royal Jelly

PREMENSTRUAL SYNDROME. In a randomized, double-blind, placebo-controlled, crossover trial, a preparation (Femal) composed of bee pollen extract, pollen and pistil extract, and royal jelly was tested in women with PMS. During 2 months of treatment, the efficacy of the Femal preparation was tested with well-established questionnaires and daily measurements of body weight. Overall symptom scores were reduced significantly in the treatment group, and the authors noted evidence of a slow onset of benefits to treatment. PMS-related weight gain was reduced by 50% by treatment compared with placebo. No adverse effects were reported in the study (Winther and Christer, 2002).

ATHEROSCLEROSIS. A statistical review on the published human and clinical studies involving royal jelly estimated that the use of 50–100 mg royal jelly daily could reduce total serum cholesterol levels by 14% and total serum lipids by about 10% (Vittek, 1995).

MALNUTRITION. In an uncontrolled clinical trial, royal jelly (Royal Peking Jelly, 800 mg daily) was given to patients with malnutrition secondary to various diseases. Through clinical and biochemical evaluation, promising results were found with respect to body weight, gut proteins, plasma aldosterone concentration, and nitrogen balance (Foppiani, 1984).

Propolis

HERPES. Three groups of 30 people with herpes simplex virus (HSV) type 2 participated in a study comparing propolis to acyclovir and placebo in a randomized, masked-investigator, controlled, multicenter clinical study. Treatment began in the blister phase (ointment was applied 4 times daily topically to blisters, or inserted on tampons if the blisters were vaginal or on the cervix), and the participants were examined at days 3, 7, and 10 of treatment. The clinical symptoms and the number and size of blisters were recorded. The healing process was found to be faster in the propolis group, with the number of patients healed on day 10 being 24, 14, and 12, and the number of patients healed on day 7 being 10, 4, and 3 out of 30 in the propolis, acyclovir, and placebo groups, respectively. In addition, among the women with vaginal infections of microbial pathogens, propolis was found to normalize vaginal flora in 55% of the women, while the acyclovir and placebo groups had no effect. Propolis was also found to be more effective at reducing local symptoms (Vynograd et al., 2000).

IMMUNE STIMULATION. The immune-stimulating effect of a prophylactic propolis treatment was studied in an open prospective clinical study. Propolis XNP was given (500 mg in the morning for 13 days), and cytokine secretion capacity was studied during and after treatment. The cytokine secretion capacity (but not the cytokine plasma levels) increased significantly during the treatment period in a time-dependent manner. The authors concluded that propolis was able to elicit an enhanced immune reactivity without side effects (Bratter et al., 1999).

INFLAMMATORY RESPIRATORY DISEASE. An aqueous propolis extract (Nivcrisol) was studied for the treatment of chronic inflammatory diseases of the upper airways in preschool and school children during the cold season of 1994–1995. Beneficial results found for the propolis extract include decreased numbers of acute and chronic symptoms and a decrease or suppression of the viral-microbial flora in the upper airways. The authors concluded that the propolis extract preparation was a good adjuvant medication for the treatment of some forms of acute or chronic rhinopharyngeal diseases, because they found good clinical results and the preparation was well tolerated and economical (Crisan et al., 1995).

PERIODONTOPATHIES. Propolis has been found beneficial in the treatment of gingivitis and oral ulcers in several small case studies and pilot clinical studies (Goranov et al., 1979; Magro-Filho and de Carvalho, 1994; Martinez Silveira et al., 1988; Mitroi et al., 1987; Neumann et al., 1986; Schmidt et al., 1980). In addition to their use in treating periodontopathies, preparations with propolis have been found to be antimicrobial, anti-inflammatory, and highly antimycotic (against *Candida albicans*) and to have antiscar effects (Gafar et al., 1989; Kosenko and Kosovich, 1990; Vitoria et al., 1999).

GIARDIASIS. In a study of propolis extract ("bee glue" or Propolisina) for the treatment of giardiasis, 138 people were divided into two groups and given either propolis or an imidazole derivative (tinidazole). The propolis extract treatment resulted in a 52% cure in children using a 10% concentrated extract and a comparable efficacy in adults with a 20% concentrated extract. In adults who undertook treatment with a 30% concentrated extract, there was higher efficacy than tinidazole (60% versus 40%, respectively). The authors concluded it to be a good treatment that is economical, which is important for people in developing countries (Miyares et al., 1988).

ANTIBIOTIC. Beyond the clinical antibiotic effects previously discussed, propolis has been confirmed to exhibit antimicrobial activity in various clinical settings (Bekemeier et al., 1973; Chlorazak et al., 1971; Porkhun and Borovaia, 1970).

SAFETY/DOSAGE

Dosage for the various bee products seem to be dependent on the preparation, use, and manufacturer. Allergic reactions to bee products have been reported, as have allergic reactions to royal jelly in persons also allergic to the composite plant family (Lombardi et al., 1998; Shaw et al., 1997). Reports of bronchospasm, asthma, and anaphylaxis have been linked to ingestion of royal jelly (Leung et al., 1995; Thien et al., 1996). A case of hemorrhagic colitis has been reported to be associated with royal jelly intake (Yonei et al., 1997).

REFERENCES

Bekemeier H, Braun W, Friedrich E, Kala H, Metzner J, Schneidewind E, Schwaiberger R, Wozniak KD. Microbiological, pharmacological and clinical studies on the efficiency of propolis. Dermatol Monatsschr 1973;159(4):443–449.

Bratter C, Tregel M, Liebenthal C, Volk HD. Prophylactic effectiveness of propolis for immunostimulation: a clinical pilot study. Forsch Komplementarmed 1999;6(5):256–260.

Chlorazak T, Szaflarski J, Seferowicz E, Scheller S. Preliminary evaluation of clinical usefulness of propolis (beeswax) preparations. Przegl Lek 1971;28(12):828–831.

Crisan I, Zaharia CN, Popovici F, Jucu V, Belu O, Dascalu C, Mutiu A, Petrescu A. Natural propolis extract Nivcrisol in the treatment of acute and chronic rhinopharyngitis in children. Rom J Virol 1995;46(3–4):115–133.

Dobrowolski JW, Vohora SB, Sharma K, Shah SA, Naqvi SAH, and Dandiva PC. Antibacterial, antifungal, antiamebic, antiinflammatory and antipyretic studies on propolis bee products. J Ethnopharmacol 1991;35(1):77–82.

Foppiani E. Preliminary studies on Peking Queen Bee PAP as a food for subjects with calorie-protein malnutrition. Clinica Dietologica 1984;11(3):375–384.

Gafar M, Dumitriu H, Dumitriu S, Guti L. Apiphytotherapeutic original preparations in the treatment of chronic marginal parodontopathies. A clinical and microbiological study. Rev Chir Oncol Radiol O R L Oftalmol Stomatol Ser Stomatol 1989;36(2):91–98.

Goranov K, Zarankova V, Velcheva M. Clinical results of the treatment of parodontosis with propolis and lincomycin. Stomatologiia (Sofiia) 1979;61(1):18–22.

Kosenko SV, Kosovich TI. The treatment of periodontitis with prolonged-action propolis preparations (clinical x-ray research). Stomatologiia (Mosk) 1990;69(2):27–29.

Leung R, Thien FC, Baldo B, Czarny D. Royal jelly-induced asthma and anaphylaxis: clinical characteristics and immunologic correlations. J Allergy Clin Immunol 1995;96(6 pt 1):1004–1007.

Lombardi C, Senna GE, Gatti B, Feligioni M, Riva G, Bonadonna P, Dama AR, Canonica GW, Passalacqua G. Allergic reactions to honey and royal jelly and their relationship with sensitization to compositae. Allergol Immunopathol (Madr) 1998;26(6):288–290.

Magro-Filho O, de Carvalho AC. Topical effect of propolis in the repair of sulcoplasties by the modified Kazanjian technique. Cytological and clinical evaluation. J Nihon Univ Sch Dent 1994;36(2):102–111.

Martinez Silveira G, Gou Godoy A, Ona Torriente R, Palmer Ortiz MC, Falcon Cuellar MA. Preliminary study of the effects of propolis in the treatment of chronic gingivitis and oral ulceration. Rev Cubana Estomatol 1988;25(3):36–44.

Mitroi NM, Luchian S, Kozma A, Marin L. Clinical and therapeutic results obtained in the treatment of affections of the buccal mucosa with an adhesive apiphytotherapeutic preparation, "Propovit MSK". Rev Chir Oncol Radiol O R L Oftalmol Stomatol Ser Stomatol 1987;34(4):261–264.

Miyares C, Hollands I, Castaneda C, Gonzalez T, Fragoso T, Curras R, Soria C. Clinical trial with a preparation based on propolis "propolisina" in human giardiasis [in Spanish]. Acta Gastroenterol Latinoam 1988;18(3):195–201.

Neumann D, Gotze G, Binus W.Clinical study of a test of the plaque- and gingivitis-inhibiting effects of propolis. Stomatol DDR 1986;36(12):677–681.

Porkhun FT, Borovaia AI. Bactericidal effect of propolis and its use in clinical practice. Voen Med Zh 1970;9:65–66.

Schmidt H, Hampel CM, Schmidt G, Riess E, Rodel C. Double-blind trial of the effect of a propolis-containing mouthwash on inflamed and healthy gingival. Stomatol DDR 1980;30(7):491–497.

Shaw D, Leon C, Kolev S, Murray V. Traditional remedies and food supplements. A 5-year toxicological study (1991–1995). Drug Saf 1997;17(5):342–356.

Thien FC, Leung R, Baldo BA, Weiner JA, Plomley R, Czarny D. Asthma and anaphylaxis induced by royal jelly. Clin Exp Allergy 1996;26(2):216–222.

Vitoria PAR, Chinalli KM, Celia CR, Cristiane S, Hanaoka CRF. Candida sp in the oral cavity with and without lesions: Maximal inhibitory dilution of propolis and periogard. Revista de Microbiologia 1999;30(4):335–341.

Vittek J. Effect of royal jelly on serum lipids in experimental animals and humans with atherosclerosis. Experientia 1995;51(9–10):927–935.

Vynograd N, Vynograd I, Sosnowski Z. A comparative multi-centre study of the efficacy of propolis, acyclovir and placebo in the treatment of genital herpes (HSV). Phytomedicine 2000;7(1):1–6.

Winther K, Christer H. Assessment of the effects of the herbal remedy Femal on the symptoms of premenstrual syndrome: A randomized, double-blind, placebo-controlled study. Current Therapeutic Research, Clinical & Experimental 2002;63(5):344–353.

Yonei Y, Shibagaki K, Tsukada N, Nagasu N, Inagaki Y, Miyamoto K, Suzuki O, Kiryu Y. Case report: haemorrhagic colitis associated with royal jelly intake. J Gastroenterol Hepatol 1997;12(7):495–499.

ADDITIONAL RESOURCES

Giurcaneanu F, Crisan I, Esanu V, Cioca V, Cajal N. Treatment of herpes infection of the skin and zona zoster with Nivcrisol-D. Revue Roumaine de Medecine Virologie 1988;39(1):21–24.

BREWER'S YEAST (*SACCHAROMYCES CEREVISIAE*)

Overall Rank

★★★★ as a source of B vitamins
★★★★ as a source of "biologically active" chromium
★★★★ for reducing blood sugar
★★ for reducing cholesterol
★★ for preventing acne
★ for increasing energy
★ for enhancing exercise performance
★ for cardiovascular health

OVERVIEW

Brewer's yeast is not the same as the baker's yeast that makes bread rise or the yeast that causes yeast infections. It is just what it sounds like it should be—the yeast used in making beer. Because of the different methods used in its culture, it can vary in its nutritional profile; however, it tends to be a good source of several B vitamins and a few minerals: thiamin (B_1), riboflavin (B_2), niacin (B_3), folic acid, pyridoxine (B_6), B_{12}, chromium (known as glucose tolerance factor [GTF]), copper, iron, and zinc.

COMMENTS

Most of the clinical work that has been performed on brewer's yeast has been for its potential use as a source of organic chromium, which has been theorized and confirmed in several studies to improve glucose control and lipid values. It is this application that has led to claims about brewer's yeast being good for reducing blood sugar and cholesterol. One study suggests its beneficial role in athletic recovery. The energy claims made on brewer's yeast are yet unfounded by clinical research.

One product made from brewer's yeast that is not included in this review is called brewer's yeast cell wall. It is a byproduct of producing brewer's yeast extracts and is being promoted as a functional food for modulating the immune system, controlling cholesterol, and promoting healthy intestinal flora (Tomohiko et al., 2000, 2001).

SCIENTIFIC SUPPORT

Acne

Weber et al. (1989) studied the effects of a maximum of 5 months of brewer's yeast supplementation (*Saccharomyces cerevisiae* Hansen CBS 5926 [Perenterol]) in 139 patients with acne. Physicians' rating of the results on the treatment group was very good or good in 74% of the patients versus 21.7% in the placebo group. In the treatment group that was rated very good or good, 80% of the patients were considered healed or very much better compared with only 26% of the placebo group that was rated very good or good.

Athletic Recovery and Antioxidant

In a nonblinded, controlled study, the effect of an undefined yeast cell preparation (high in antioxidant vitamins, antioxidant enzymes, trace elements, and minerals) on the stress reaction and antioxidant status of nine highly trained athletes was studied. Venous blood samples were drawn and tested in the resting state after an overnight fast followed by a 15-km cross-country race. The treatment with the yeast cell preparation gave an improvement in the systemic and muscular stress reaction, reflected by a lower soluble interleukin-2 receptor and plasma fibrinogen and higher plasma fibronectin in the resting state, and a significant difference in fibrogen and fibronectin 1 hour after the race. Myoglobin, CKMM3, and mangan superoxide dismutase were reduced, reflecting a decrease in free-radical stress (Konig et al., 1999).

Blood Sugar and Diabetes

The effect of daily chromium supplementation (either brewer's yeast containing 23.3 µg of chromium, or carbon tetrachloride providing 200 µg of chromium) was tested on glucose tolerance, serum lipids, and drug dosage in 78 type 2 diabetes patients. The study was a double-blind, placebo-controlled, crossover design that lasted 32 weeks. The authors concluded that the supplementation with chromium resulted in better control of glucose and lipid variables, with decreases of drug dosages (to the point that some subjects no longer needed insulin). The brewer's yeast supplementation of chromium increased the time chromium was retained in the body and extended the beneficial effects as a result (Bahijiri et al., 2000).

The effect on serum glucose and lipids of brewer's yeast supplementation (10 g/day for 12 weeks) was studied in a controlled (torula yeast) study of 22 Chinese adults. Blood was drawn before the glucose load and at 30-, 60-, 90-, and 120-minute intervals after. The treatment group resulted in decreases in serum triacylglycerol values and in 60- and 90-minute values of oral glucose tolerance testing (Li, 1994).

Rabinowitz et al. (1983) studied the effect of chromium supplementation on carbohydrate utilization in a double-blind, random, crossover trial involving 43 men. This study was conducted because of the observation of diabetes resulting from chromium deficiency in experimental animals and humans during long-term parenteral nutrition. The groups were given either inorganic chromium (chromium trichloride), a brewer's yeast containing GTF (an organic form of chromium), a brewer's yeast not containing GTF, or a placebo. The patients were further split into subgroups of 21 ketosis-prone men, 7 ketosis-resistant nonobese men, and 15 ketosis-resistant obese men. Chromium levels were found to increase in the body pools of the men from treatment with either organic or inorganic forms of chromium by about 25%. Additionally, in the ketosis-resistant subgroups, there was a significant increase in postprandial insulin from treatment with brewer's yeast that contained GTF. No effects were found, however, on carbohydrate metabolism in any of the groups.

In one study of 23 elderly people, the effect on glucose tolerance, insulin, cholesterol, and triglycerides of 200 μg of chromium (from chromic chloride), 5 g of brewer's yeast, or placebo supplementation was studied. After 10 weeks, no differences were found among the groups on the measured parameters. Plasma chromium content, however, rose after the supplementation with chromic chloride, but not with brewer's yeast. The authors concluded that age was not a factor leading to chromium deficiency (Offenbacher et al., 1985).

Saner et al. (1983) conduced a study of the effect of chromium supplementation (with 30 g/day of brewer's yeast containing 50 μg of chromium) for 8 weeks on patients with Turner syndrome, which is characterized by a high incidence of diabetes. Chromium- and lipid-value testing suggested that the study patients had chromium deficiencies and that these deficiencies could have a role in the abnormal glucose tolerance tests found in many Turner syndrome patients.

In a small pilot study involving 10 patients with type 2 diabetes, the effect of brewer's yeast supplementation was studied. Eight of the 10 patients showed improvement in glucose tolerance. No significant changes in serum insulin, total cholesterol, or triglycerides were found (Bialkowska et al., 1981).

Glucose control and lipid values were compared after the daily ingestion of either 9 g of chromium-rich brewer's yeast or chromium-poor torula yeast for 8 weeks. The 24 participants in the study were older (mean age of 78 years) and were divided into normal and diabetic subgroups. In the brewer's yeast group, glucose tolerance improved significantly and insulin output was reduced after supplementation. Additionally, cholesterol and total lipids fell after supplementation in this group, with higher decreases in the hypercholesterolemic people. The torula yeast group showed no significant changes in glucose control, insulin, or lipids. Cholesterol was found to have significantly decreased in the subgroup of nondiabetics but not in the diabetic group. The authors concluded that this study supported the theory that elderly people have low levels of chromium that could be increased by supplementation (Offenbacher and Pi-Sunyer, 1980).

Cardiovascular Health

A review of yeast-derived fiber products has suggested that they are a better source of ß-glucan (a dietary fiber) than are oat products because they are more concentrated; therefore, yeast products may be better dietary additions to lower serum cholesterol levels (Bell et al., 1999). Apart from being a ß-glucan source, brewer's yeast and chromium is known to improve blood lipid values, cholesterol, and triglycerides. Several of these studies have been cited here.

SAFETY/DOSAGE

It is important to look at the nutritional content of the brewer's yeast product to verify that it contains GTF (or chromium) if its intended use is for chromium supplementation. Some people report mild gastrointestinal (GI) upsets when first taking brewer's yeast. Starting with small amounts (1/4 teaspoon daily) and increasing as desired (to 1-3 tablespoons daily) can help patients avoid GI upsets. In clinical studies for blood sugar control, from 5-30 g of GTF-containing brewer's yeast was taken daily with beneficial results. No other serious side effects have been noted.

REFERENCES

Bahijiri SM, Mira SA, Mufti AM, Ajabnoor MA. The effects of inorganic chromium and brewer's yeast supplementation on glucose tolerance, serum lipids and drug dosage in individuals with type 2 diabetes. Saudi Med J 2000;21(9):831–837.

Bell S, Goldman VM, Bistrian BR, Arnold AH, Ostroff G, Forse RA. Effect of beta-glucan from oats and yeast on serum lipids. Crit Rev Food Sci Nutr 1999;39(2):189–202.

Bialkowska M, Bruce A, Magnusson K, Lithell H. The effect of brewer's yeast on glucose tolerance and serum insulin, triglyceride and cholesterol levels in patients with adult onset diabetes. Zywienie Czlowieka 1981;8(2):129–138.

Konig D, Keul J, Northoff H, Halle M, Berg A. Effect of 6-week nutritional intervention with enzymatic yeast cells and antioxidants on exercise stress and antioxidant status. Wien Med Wochenschr 1999;149(1):13–18.

Li YC. Effects of brewer's yeast on glucose tolerance and serum lipids in Chinese adults. Biol Trace Elem Res 1994;41(3):341–347.

Offenbacher EG, Pi-Sunyer FX. Beneficial effect of chromium-rich yeast on glucose tolerance and blood lipids in elderly subjects. Diabetes 1980;29(11):919–925.

Offenbacher EG, Rinko CJ, Pi-Sunyer FX. The effects of inorganic chromium and brewer's yeast on glucose tolerance, plasma lipids, and plasma chromium in elderly subjects. Am J Clin Nutr 1985;42(3):454–461.

Rabinowitz MB, Gonick HC, Levin SR, Davidson MB. Effects of chromium and yeast supplements on carbohydrate and lipid metabolism in diabetic men. Diabetes Care 1983;6(4):319–327.

Saner G, Yuzbasiyan V, Neyzi O, Gunoz H, Saka N, Cigdem S. Alterations of chromium metabolism and effect of chromium supplementation in Turner's syndrome patients. Am J Clin Nutr 1983;38(4):574–578.

Tomohiko N, Kazue A, Satoshi N, Yoshiharu S, Hisakazu L, Takanori T, Toshiaki A. Effects of fermented milk supplemented with brewer's yeast cell wall on constipation and fecal microflora in healthy adults. Oyo Yakuri 2000;59(3–4):47–55.

Tomohiko N, Yoshiharu S, Takashi T, Hiroyuki S. Effect of brewer's yeast cell wall administration on levels of blood lipids in hypercholesterolemic male adults. Oyo Yakuri 2001;61(4–5):237–243.

Weber G, Adamczyk A, Freytag S. Treatment of acne with a yeast preparation. Fortschr Med 1989;107(26):563–566.

GINSENG

Overall Rank

★★★★ for increasing energy levels
★★★★ for relieving stress (adaptogenic effect)
★★★★ for enhancing athletic performance
★★★ for controlling blood sugar
★★★ for improving mental function
★★★ for promoting general well-being (tonic effect)
★★ for enhancing sexual performance
★★ for enhancing immune system function

OVERVIEW

Ginseng refers to a group of adaptogenic herbs from the plant family *Araliacae*. Commonly, the term *ginseng* refers to "true" ginseng (*Panax ginseng* C.A. Meyer), as well as to a related plant called Siberian ginseng (*Eleutherococcus senticosus*, or eleuthero for short). Medicinal preparations are made from the roots of the plants. *Panax ginseng* has been used in Traditional Chinese Medicine (TCM) for thousands of years as a tonic indicated for its beneficial effects on the central nervous system, protection from stress, antifatigue action, enhancement of sexual function, and acceleration of metabolism.

Siberian ginseng did not come into the picture as a botanical remedy until the twentieth century. Found in the northern regions of the former Soviet Union, the roots of *Eleutherococcus senticosus* were sought out as a cheaper substitute for the expensive Oriental ginsengs. Soviet researchers found Siberian ginseng to be an excellent tonic to enhance athletic performance as well as to strengthen the body during times of stress.

Several other "ginsengs" are used as adaptogenic tonics throughout the world; among them are *Panax quinquefolium* (or *Panax quinquefolius*, also known as American ginseng, with a rich history of use by Native Americans) and ashwagandha, sometimes called Indian ginseng (not a true ginseng but with a long history of medicinal use by ayurvedic healers in India). American ginseng is the most similar to the true *Panax ginseng* and is highly prized in the Orient, where it is thought to provide a "cooler" invigoration than the native *Panax ginseng* (considered "warming" by traditional Chinese healers).

In general, the various ginseng supplements available in the U.S. market are claimed to increase energy levels, relieve stress, enhance athletic performance, enhance immune system function, control blood sugar, improve mental function, and promote general well-being. In most of these functions, ginseng, whether Siberian, *Panax ginseng*, or one of the other varieties, is often termed an adaptogen—a therapeutic and restorative tonic generally thought to produce a "balancing" effect on the body. The properties typically attributed to adaptogens are a nonspecific increase in resistance to a wide range of stressors (including physical, chemical, and biological factors) as well as a "normalizing" action irrespective of the direction of the pathological changes. In general, an adaptogen can be thought of as a substance that helps the body adapt to stress.

COMMENTS

Among the many herbs promoted as energy boosters, Asian ginseng is by far the most popular. Although the term *ginseng* actually encompasses a family of roots, *Panax ginseng*, the type grown in China, Korea, and Japan, is the type generally known for its energetic and antistress properties. In TCM, *Panax ginseng* is used as a tonic herb with adaptogenic properties. In general terms, an adaptogen is a substance that boosts energy and aids in combatting stress and remaining calm. The research on ginseng's benefits as a tonic and energy booster is equivocal. Some studies have shown benefits in increasing energy levels in fatigued subjects (Vogler et al., 1999; Wang et al., 1983), but most studies on ginseng as an aid to athletic performance have shown no effect (Bahrke and Morgan, 2000). The differences among study findings may have been the result of many commercially available ginseng supplements actually containing little or no ginseng at all; many researchers often take it for granted that a given product selected off the shelf for study will actually contain what it claims (not always a good assumption). The clearest indication that a supplement contains something other than real ginseng is the price; ginseng root is a very expensive ingredient, and "bargain" ginseng products may not contain real ginseng, enough ginseng, or the active saponin compounds that are thought to deliver ginseng's antifatigue and adaptogenic effects.

Siberian ginseng (eleuthero), is not truly ginseng (it is a shrub rather than a root) but it is a close enough cousin (same botanical family but different genus) to deliver some of the same energetic benefits. Eleuthero is also known as ciwujia in popular sports products. The Siberian form of ginseng is generally a less expensive alternative to true Asian or *Panax ginseng*, though it may have more of a stimulatory effect rather than an adaptogenic effect (not necessarily a bad thing if you just need a boost). Often promoted as an athletic performance enhancer, eleuthero may also possess mild-to-moderate benefits in promoting recovery following intense exercise, perhaps the result of an enhanced delivery of oxygen to recovering muscles.

Ashwagandha is an herb from India that is sometimes called Indian ginseng, not because it is part of the ginseng family but to suggest energy-promoting and stress-reducing benefits similar to those attributed to the more well-known Asian and Siberian ginsengs. Although there has been very little human research done on ashwagandha, herbalists and natural medicine practitioners often recommend the herb to combat stress and fatigue, and it does appear to be particularly suited as a relaxant following stressful events.

Although the scientific evidence for the benefits of ginseng and its mechanisms of action can be considered inconclusive, the adaptogenic role of the various ginseng strains have proven beneficial for many thousands of years and may therefore prove valuable as normalizing substances during stressful conditions.

SCIENTIFIC SUPPORT

The active components in *Panax ginseng* and American ginseng are thought to be a family of triterpenoid saponins that are collectively referred to as ginsenosides. In general, most of the top-quality ginseng products, whether whole root or extract, are standardized for ginsenoside content. The active components in Siberian ginseng are considered to be a group of related compounds called eleutherosides. It has been theorized that ginseng's action in the body is the result of its interaction within the hypothalamic-pituitary axis to balance secretion of adrenal corticotropic hormone (ACTH). ACTH has the ability to bind directly to brain cells and can affect a variety of stress-related processes in the body. These behaviors might include motivation, vitality, performance, and arousal.

In a widely cited, though poorly conducted, study of student nurses on night duty, 1,200 mg/day of *Panax ginseng* appeared to improve general indices of stress and mood disturbances (Coleman et al., 2003). Levels of free fatty acids, testosterone, and blood sugar, which were all elevated by night work, were significantly reduced to the levels observed under day work. In another study, 2,700 mg/day of *Panax quinquefolius* was able to reduce blood sugar levels and insulin requirements in a group of diabetic subjects following 3 months of supplementation (Vuksan et al., 2000). One study of the effects of 200 mg/day of *Panax ginseng* extract for 12 weeks showed improvements over baseline values of mental performance: attention, mental processing, logical deduction, and both motor function and reaction time (Kennedy and Scholey, 2003).

Over a period of several decades, German and Soviet researchers have studied the effects of ginseng extract, typically standardized to 4% ginsenosides, on the performance of athletes. One study compared 200 mg/day of eleuthero versus a placebo in 14 highly trained male athletes (Dowling et al., 1996). The ginseng group showed an increase in maximum oxygen uptake compared with the placebo group as well as a statistically significant improvement in recovery time and lower serum lactate values. Other studies in various groups of young athletes have shown ginseng extract to provide statistically significant improvements in performance measures, such as forced vital capacity and maximum breathing capacity, compared with the placebo groups (Pieralisi et al., 1991; Ziemba et al., 1999).

In a double-blind, placebo-controlled, crossover study (8 weeks on treatment, 2 weeks of washout, and 8 weeks on treatment), 45 patients were given 900 mg of ginseng 3 times a day. Mean International Index of Erectile Function scores were significantly higher in patients treated with the ginseng than those who received a placebo. The authors concluded that ginseng may be an effective alternative for treating male erectile dysfunction (Hong et al., 2002).

An open study consisting of 36 children ranging from 3 to 17 years old were given a combination product containing *Panax quinquefolium* (200 mg) and *Ginkgo biloba* extract (50 mg) to be taken twice daily for 4 weeks. At the beginning of the study, after 2 weeks, and then at week 4, parents completed the Conners' Parent Rating Scale. After 4 weeks of treatment, the proportion of subjects exhibiting improvements ranged from 44% for the social problems attribute to 74% for the Conners' attention-deficit/hyperactivity disorder (ADHD) index and the *Diagnostic and Statistical Manual of Mental Disorders, Fourth Edition* (*DSM-IV*) hyperactive-impulsive attribute. The authors concluded that the combination treatment may improve symptoms of ADHD and that further research on the combination should be done (Lyon et al., 2001).

Unfortunately, the scientific evidence for ginseng is far from definitive. For every study showing a positive benefit in terms of energy levels and/ or physical or mental performance, there is at least one other study showing no benefits (Bahrke and Morgan, 2000). Part of the discrepancy in results from well-controlled studies may have to do with differences among the ginseng extracts used in various studies (nonstandardized extracts with unknown quantities of active components).

SAFETY/DOSAGE

For the most part, plants in the ginseng family are generally considered to be quite safe. There are no known drug interactions, contraindications, common allergic reactions, or toxicity to Siberian ginseng, *Panax ginseng*, or American ginseng, although it is recommended that a course of treatment with ginseng not exceed 3 months—or at least that prolonged use of ginseng be accompanied by a schedule of on/off cycles (2 months on the supplement followed by 1 month off). A word of caution is given to persons with hypertension, because the stimulatory nature of some ginseng preparations have been reported to increase blood pressure (Coon and Ernst, 2002). Additionally, people prone to hypoglycemia (low blood sugar) should use ginseng with caution because of the reported ability of ginseng to reduce blood sugar levels (Vuksan et al., 2000).

Ginseng is one of the many herbal supplements that can be purchased readily as a whole root, a dried powder, or a standardized extract. The most precise approach is to use a standardized extract to ensure that you are getting an effective product. Products should be standardized to contain 4–5% ginsenosides (for *Panax ginseng* and American ginseng) and 0.5–1.0% eleutherosides (for Siberian ginseng). Daily intake of 100–300 mg for 3–6 weeks is recommended to produce adaptogenic and energetic benefits. As a dried root, 1–2 g/day should be used in the case of American ginseng or *Panax ginseng*, or 2–3 g/day of Siberian ginseng.

REFERENCES

Bahrke MS, Morgan WP. Evaluation of the ergogenic properties of ginseng. Sports Med 2000;29(2):113–133.

Coleman CI, Hebert JH, Reddy P. The effects of Panax ginseng on quality of life. J Clin Pharm Ther 2003;28:5–15.

Coon JT, Ernst E. Panax ginseng: a systematic review of adverse effects and drug interactions. Drug Saf 2002;25(5):323–344.

Dowling EA, Redondo DR, Branch JD, Jones S, McNabb G, Williams MH. Effect of Eleutherococcus senticosus on submaximal and maximal exercise performance. Med Sci Sports Exerc 1996;28(4):482–489.

Hong B, Ji YH, Hong JH, Nam KY, Ahn TY. A double-blind crossover study evaluating the efficacy of Korean red ginseng in patients with erectile dysfunction: a preliminary report. J Urol 2002;168:2070–2073.

Kennedy DO, Scholey AB. Ginseng: potential for the enhancement of cognitive performance and mood. Pharmacol Biochem Behav 2003;75:687–700.

Lyon MR, Cline JC, Totosy de Zepetnek J, Shan JJ, Pang P, Benishin C. Effect of the herbal extract combination Panax quinquefolium and Ginkgo biloba on attention-deficit hyperactivity disorder: a pilot study. J Psychiatry Neurosci 2001;26(3):221–228.

Pieralisi G, Ripari P, Vecchiet L. Effects of a standardized ginseng extract combined with dimethylaminoethanol bitartrate, vitamins, minerals, and trace elements on physical performance during exercise. Clin Ther 1991;13(3):373–382.

Vogler BK, Pittler MH, Ernst E. The efficacy of ginseng: a systematic review of randomized clinical trials. Eur J Clin Pharmacol 1999;55:567–575.

Vuksan V, Sievenpiper JL, Koo VY, Francis T, Zdravkovic UB, Xu Z et al. American ginseng (Panax quinquefolius) reduces postprandial glycemia in nondiabetic subjects and subjects with type 2 diabetes mellitus. Arch Internal Med 2000;160:1009–1013.

Wang BX, Cui JC, Liu AJ, Wu SK. Studies on the anti-fatigue effect of the saponins of stems and leaves of Panax ginseng (SSLG). J Tradit Chin Med 1983;3(2):89–94.

Ziemba AW, Chmura J, Kaciuba-Uscilko H, Nazar K, Wisnik P, Gawronski W. Ginseng treatment improves psychomotor performance at rest and during graded exercise in young athletes. Int J Sport Nutr 1999;9(4):371–377.

ADDITIONAL RESOURCES

Attele AS, Wu JA, Yuan CS. Ginseng pharmacology: multiple constituents and multiple actions. Biochem Pharmacol 1999;58(11):1685–1693.

Grandhi A, Mujumdar AM, Patwardhan B. A comparative pharmacological investigation of ashwagandha and ginseng. J Ethnopharmacol 1994;44(3):131–135.

INOSINE

Overall Rank

★★ for improving energy metabolism and endurance performance

OVERVIEW

Inosine is part of a chemical family called purine nucleotides and acts as a precursor to adenosine, an important molecule for cellular energy. Inosine can be found in brewer's yeast and organ meats, such as liver and kidney, and is available as a supplement in its purified form.

Dietary supplements containing inosine are often marketed with claims for increased energy levels and endurance performance, enhanced adenosine triphosphate (ATP) production, improved heart function, and reduced lactic acid accumulation during intense exercise.

Many of the effects attributed to inosine stem from its potential role in increasing levels of a compound known as 2,3 diphosphoglycerate (DPG) in red blood cells. An enhanced 2,3 DPG level would ease the release of oxygen from the blood cells to the tissues and, in theory, enhance energy generation, promote lactic acid removal, and improve exercise performance overall.

COMMENTS

Because there are no convincing studies demonstrating the beneficial effects of inosine as a dietary supplement, it is not recommended as a stand-alone dietary aid. Inosine is commonly contained as part of an overall mixture of ingredients in dietary supplements that may contribute to energy metabolism.

SCIENTIFIC SUPPORT

Several studies have investigated the effects of inosine supplementation on aerobic performance in athletes, yet none have shown convincing benefits associated with the supplement. In at least two studies, a potential for inosine to *interfere* with energy metabolism was suggested, particularly in high-intensity sprint-type events.

Inosine has many possible metabolic roles in the body. Preliminary information suggests that inosine might stimulate axon growth from healthy nerve cells to injured nerve cells in the brain and spinal cord of the central nervous system (Bianchi et al., 1999). It penetrates the cell walls of both cardiac and skeletal muscles, where it promotes the generation of ATP, the energy substance that allows muscles to contract (Febbraio and Dancey, 1999; Norman, 1995). It also serves as a precursor for the formation of hypoxanthine, which may be phosphorylated into the nucleotide inosine monophosphate (IMP). IMP is claimed to be an important regulator between adenine and guanine nucleotide synthesis and may lead to the formation of ATP. Increased production of ATP leads to improved respiration and oxygen transport and serves to enhance all athletic performance, whether aerobic or anaerobic in nature. IMP also helps to maintain glycogen breakdown by activating phosphorylase b and increasing the formation of uric acid. Inosine also contributes to erythrocyte metabolism by promoting the production of 2,3 DPG, which is necessary for the transport of oxygen molecules from the red blood cells to the cell for energy. Both inosine and hypoxanthine are believed to be vasodilating agents, which may enhance blood flow to the heart and skeletal muscles and lead to improvement of various heart conditions (Iwasa et al., 1997; Kipshidze et al., 1978).

A double-blind, placebo-controlled, crossover trial was conducted on 9 highly trained endurance runners to investigate the ergogenic effect of oral inosine supplementation on a 3-mile run time and oxygen uptake (VO_2) peak. Each patient underwent four trials, which followed the same protocol and measured three separate tests within each trial: a 13-minute submaximal treadmill warm-up, a 3-mile treadmill run test, and a maximal treadmill run to test VO_2 peak. Patients were instructed to prepare for each trial as if preparing for a race. The patients were given 6,000 mg (3 doses of 2,000 mg) of inosine per day for 2 days or matching placebo prior to testing. The last dose was taken within 2 hours of testing. The results showed no significant effect of inosine in the 3-mile treadmill run test or in the maximal VO_2 peak test (Williams et al., 1989).

Another randomized, double-blind, placebo-controlled, crossover trial was conducted in 7 healthy male volunteers to evaluate the use of inosine over a period of 5–10 days at a dosage of 10,000 mg/day on measures associated with aerobic and anaerobic performance. All patients completed three trial sessions, which included a series of three stationary cycling performance tests; a 5–6-second sprint, a 30-second sprint, and a 20-minute time trial. These trial sessions were completed prior to the study (at baseline), on days 6 and 11. Patients completed the performance tests after supplementation with inosine (two equal doses taken early morning and late afternoon, dissolved in orange juice) or a placebo. Each trial was separated by a 6-week washout period. The results showed no significant differences for any of the variables measured. It was concluded that inosine has no ergogenic effects, does not improve performance, and may cause possible health problems if taken over long periods (McNaughton et al., 1999).

A similar double-blind, placebo-controlled, crossover trial was performed on 10 competitive male cyclists. These patients completed a bike test, a 30-minute self-paced cycling performance, and a supramaximal cycling sprint following 5 days of oral supplementation with 5,000 mg/day of inosine and a matching placebo. The results showed no differences between the inosine and placebo groups within each test performed

(Starling et al., 1996). These findings demonstrate that prolonged inosine supplementation does not appear to improve aerobic performance and short-term power production during cycling.

Another 8-week, double-blind, placebo-controlled, crossover trial was conducted to examine the effects of the Coenzyme Athletic Performance System (CAPS) on endurance performance to exhaustion. Eleven highly trained male triathletes were given 3 daily doses of CAPS or a matching placebo for two 4-week periods. CAPS consisted of 100 mg of coenzyme Q10, 500 mg of cytochrome C, 100 mg of inosine, and 200 IU of vitamin E. A 4-week washout period separated the two treatment groups. After each treatment period, an exhaustive performance test consisting of a 90-minute treadmill run followed by cycling until exhaustion was performed. The results showed that the mean time to exhaustion and blood parameters for the patients using CAPS were not significantly different from the placebo group. In conclusion, CAPS had no apparent benefit on exercise to exhaustion (Snider et al., 1992).

The overall results obtained from these trials suggest that the anecdotal effects of inosine as stated by athletes and manufacturers hold little weight when tested in the laboratory. Therefore, inosine supplementation has no athletic performance benefit and may be detrimental to general health.

According to Japanese researchers, inosine may be used as a treatment for various heart conditions. A study was performed to evaluate the effect of the nucleoside inosine on the intracardiac hemodynamics and the contraction and relaxation of a diseased myocardium. The study included 102 patients with a macrofocal myocardial infarction. Twenty-two patients received inosine by intravenous drip in a single dose of 200 mg in the acute stage of infarction, 60 patients were given inosine pills in a daily dose of 800 mg in the restoration period for 1 month, and 20 patients were given a placebo. Comparative appraisal of treatments showed prevailing improvement in the condition of patients treated with inosine. These patients had positive ECG dynamics, increased cardiac output, and decreased peripheral resistance. Inosine achieved maximum effect by 60–90 minutes after the beginning of the infusion (Yabe and Yoshimura, 1981).

Another study administered 200 mg of inosine through a central vein to 16 patients with various cardiac diseases, including effort angina pectoris, myocardial infarction, valvular disease, idiopathic cardiomyopathy, and congenital heart disease. Left ventricular performance was assessed by the time course of various hemodynamic parameters, including ejection fraction. The results demonstrated that inosine caused a significant decrease in pulmonary wedge pressure, left ventricular end-diastolic pressure, and systolic left ventricular pressure. Inosine caused increases in all of the other hemodynamic parameters, such as cardiac output and ejection fraction. Quantitative evaluation disclosed the beneficial effects of inosine on the left ventricular function through the remarkable load-reducing effect and the unequivocal positive inotropic effects (Iwasa et al., 1997).

SAFETY/DOSAGE

In general, supplemental inosine appears to be safe at doses of as much as 5–6 g for several weeks. In susceptible people, however, inosine supplementation may lead to buildup of uric acid levels. Uric acid is a byproduct of inosine metabolism and may lead to painful symptoms of gout, such as arthritic joints and toes caused by deposits of uric acid crystals.

REFERENCES

Bianchi GP, Grossi G, Bargossi AM, Fiorella PL, Marchesini G. Can oxypurines plasma levels classify the type of physical exercise? J Sports Med Phys Fitness 1999;39(2):123–127.

Febbraio MA, Dancey J. Skeletal muscle energy metabolism during prolonged, fatiguing exercise. J Appl Physiol 1999;87(6):2341–2347.

Iwasa Y, Iwasa M, Omori Y, Toki T, Yamamoto A, Maeda H, Kume M, Ogoshi S. The well-balanced nucleoside-nucleotide mixture "OG-VI" for special medical purposes. Nutrition 1997;13(4):361–364.

Kipshidze NN, Korotkov AA, Chapidze GE, Marsagishvili LA, Todua EI. Indications for the use of inosine in myocardial infarct. Kardiologiia 1978;18(3):18–28.

McNaughton L, Dalton B, Tarr J. Inosine supplementation has no effect on aerobic or anaerobic cycling performance. Int J of Sports Nutr 1999;9:333–344.

Norman B. Inosine monophosphate accumulation in energy-deficient human skeletal muscle with reference to substrate availability, fibre types and AMP deaminase activity. Scand J Clin Lab Invest 1995;55(8):733–741.

Snider IP, Bazzarre TL, Murdoch SD, Goldfarb A. Effects of coenzyme athletic performance system as an ergogenic aid on endurance to exhaustion. Int J Sport Nutr 1992;2:272–286.

Starling RD, Trappe TA, Short KR, Sheffield-Moore M, Jozsi AC, Fink WJ, Costill DL. Effect of inosine supplementation on aerobic and anaerobic cycling performance. Med Sci Sports Exerc 1996;28(9):1193–1198.

Williams MH, Kreider RE, Hunter DW, Somma CT, Shall LM, Woodhouse ML et al. Effect of inosine supplementation on 3-mile treadmill run performance and VO peak. Med Sci Sports Exerc 1989;22(4):517–522.

Yabe Y, Yoshimura S. Effect of inosine on left ventricular performance and its clinical significance. Japanese Heart Journal 1981;22(6):915–928.

ADDITIONAL RESOURCES

Norman B, Sollevi A, Kaijser L, Jansson E. ATP breakdown products in human skeletal muscle during prolonged exercise to exhaustion. Clin Physiol 1987;7(6):503–510.

Pouw EM, Schols AM, van der Vusse GJ, Wouters EF. Elevated inosine monophosphate levels in resting muscle of patients with stable chronic obstructive pulmonary disease. Am J Respir Crit Care Med 1998;157(2):453–457.

Sahlin K, Broberg S. Adenine nucleotide depletion in human muscle during exercise: causality and significance of AMP deamination. Int J Sports Med 1990;11(suppl 2):S62–S67.

NADH (NICOTINAMIDE ADENINE DINUCLEOTIDE)

Overall Rank

★★★ for jet lag
  ★★ for chronic fatigue syndrome (CFS)
    ★ for increased energy levels

OVERVIEW

NADH is the abbreviation for nicotinamide adenine dinucleotide, with the *H* indicating the reduced form that has an extra hydrogen atom. NADH functions as a coenzyme, meaning that it is a required cofactor for a metabolic process. In the case of NADH, coenzyme functions include roles in energy generation and the production of neurotransmitters such as dopamine and norepinephrine. Thus, NADH supplements are generally promoted for increasing energy levels, reducing CFS, treating jet lag, and enhancing memory and cognitive function.

COMMENTS

NADH supplements typically cost about $1 per 5-mg dose; therefore, an effective dose of the supplement may cost between $2 and $4 per day. Because of the nonexistence of any reliable treatment for chronic fatigue syndrome, the preliminary antifatigue benefits of NADH are promising. Nevertheless, the preliminary nature of these results also means that NADH may be most useful as an adjunct to more established antifatigue supplements such as cordyceps, rhodiola, and ginseng.

SCIENTIFIC SUPPORT

The precise cause of CFS is unknown (Calabrese et al., 1992). Symptoms include prolonged and debilitating fatigue, inability to concentrate, flu-like symptoms, muscle weakness, joint pain, headaches, and sleep disturbances (Chester, 1997; Komaroff and Buchwald, 1991). CFS affects about 500,000 Americans, but no effective treatment is known (Gantz and Holmes, 1989; Houde and Kampfe-Leacher, 1997). Researchers theorize that CFS stems from a lack of the chemical responsible for cellular energy, ATP (Klonoff, 1992). One theory is that both infections and stress deplete cellular ATP levels and lead to chronic fatigue, and that supplemental levels of NADH can stimulate ATP production and provide benefits to people suffering from fatigue and cognitive dysfunction (Colquhoun and Senn, 2000). Further benefits from NADH may stem from its role in stimulating the production of the neurotransmitters dopamine and norepinephrine (involved in brain function and memory) as well as from the stimulation of tyrosine hydroxylase, an enzyme involved in synthesizing neurotransmitters (Birkmayer et al., 2002).

Among the dozen or so clinical reports of NADH supplementation, however, only two are randomized, double-blind, placebo-controlled trials (Birkmayer et al., 2002; Forsyth et al., 1999). Of the many open-label studies of NADH administration to patients with Alzheimer disease, dementia, or Parkinson disease, most of the studies showing a positive effect come from the same clinic in Austria (Birkmayer et al., 2002), and the dosing regimens include oral as well as intravenous, parenteral, and intramuscular routes of administration. The positive benefits of NADH supplementation in these open-label studies have not been duplicated by other clinics or laboratories, and some open-label studies have shown no benefit of NADH supplements (10 mg/day for 3 months) in cases of mild-to-moderate Alzheimer disease (Rainer et al., 2000).

In the two existing well-controlled studies of NADH supplementation, 10–20 mg of NADH showed some promising antifatigue effects. In one study (Forsyth et al., 1999), 10 mg/day of NADH for 4 weeks was effective in alleviating generalized symptoms of CFS in about one third of patients. In another study (Birkmayer et al., 2002), a 20-mg acute dose of a sublingual form of NADH improved cognitive function, mood, and sleepiness in subjects suffering from jet lag.

SAFETY/DOSAGE

Some people report mild side effects such as nervousness and loss of appetite in the first few days of taking NADH. No serious side effects are documented, and animal studies have shown no problems associated with NADH supplementation (Birkmayer and Nadlinger, 2002). Commercial NADH supplements are generally available in 2.5-mg and 5-mg tablets, with suggested dosages ranging from 2.5–15 mg/day, depending on individual requirements (e.g., therapy or maintenance).

REFERENCES

Birkmayer GD, Kay GG, Vurre E. Stabilized NADH (ENADA) improves jet lag-induced cognitive performance deficit. Wien Med Wochenschr 2002;152(17–18):450–454.

Birkmayer JG, Nadlinger K. Safety of stabilized, orally absorbable, reduced nicotinamide adenine dinucleotide (NADH): a 26-week oral tablet administration of ENADA/NADH for chronic toxicity study in rats. Drugs Exp Clin Res 2002;28(5):185–192.

Calabrese L, Danao T, Camara E, Wilke W. Chronic fatigue syndrome. Am Fam Physician 1992;45(3):1205–1213.

Chester AC. Chronic fatigue syndrome criteria in patients with other forms of unexplained chronic fatigue. J Psychiatr Res 1997;31(1):45–50.

Colquhoun D, Senn S. Is NADH effective in the treatment of chronic fatigue syndrome? Ann Allergy Asthma Immunol 2000;84(6):639–640.

Forsyth LM, Preuss HG, MacDowell AL, Chiazze L Jr, Birkmayer GD, Bellanti JA. Therapeutic effects of oral NADH on the symptoms of patients with chronic fatigue syndrome. Ann Allergy Asthma Immunol 1999;82(2):185–191.

Gantz NM, Holmes GP. Treatment of patients with chronic fatigue syndrome. Drugs 1989;38(6):855–862.

Houde SC, Kampfe-Leacher R. Chronic fatigue syndrome: an update for clinicians in primary care. Nurse Pract 1997;22(7):30, 35–36, 39–40 passim.

Klonoff DC. Chronic fatigue syndrome. Clin Infect Dis 1992;15(5):812–823.

Komaroff AL, Buchwald D. Symptoms and signs of chronic fatigue syndrome. Rev Infect Dis 1991;13(suppl 1):S8–S11.

Rainer M, Kraxberger E, Haushofer M, Mucke HA, Jellinger KA. No evidence for cognitive improvement from oral nicotinamide adenine dinucleotide (NADH) in dementia. J Neural Transm 2000;107(12):1475–1481.

ADDITIONAL RESOURCES

Kuhn W, Muller T, Winkel R, Danielczik S, Gerstner A, Hacker R, Mattern C, Przuntek H. Parenteral application of NADH in Parkinson's disease: clinical improvement partially due to stimulation of endogenous levodopa biosynthesis. J Neural Transm 1996;103(10):1187–1193.

RHODIOLA

Overall Rank

★★★ for stress control (adaptogenic effects)
★★★ for endurance performance
★★★ as a physical and mental tonic (adaptogenic effects)

OVERVIEW

Rhodiola comprises more than 200 related species of plants in the Crassulacea family and is generally found in the arctic mountain regions of Siberia (Kelly, 2001). Of the many species of rhodiola, only two have been studied at any appreciable level in humans: *Rhodiola rosea* and *Rhodiola crenulata* ("Rhodiola rosea," 2002) The root of the plant is used medicinally and is also known as arctic root, golden root (for rosea), and more recently, crenulin (for *crenulata*). Rhodiola has been used for centuries to increase the body's resistance to physical and mental stresses (Zhang et al., 1989). As a modern-day dietary supplement, rhodiola is typically promoted for boosting energy levels, relieving stress and anxiety, and enhancing athletic performance.

COMMENTS

Rhodiola rosea extract appears to be valuable as an adaptogen, increasing the body's ability to deal with a number of psychological and physiological stresses. Of particular value is the theoretical role of rhodiola in increasing the body's ability to take up and use oxygen, an effect similar to that of cordyceps, which may explain some of the nonstimulant "energizing" effects attributed to the plant. Rhodiola is often called the "poor man's" cordyceps based on ancient stories in which "commoners" used rhodiola for energy because the plants grew wild throughout the countryside, while only the emperor and his immediate family (and concubines) were allowed access to the rare cordyceps mushroom (from the high-elevation Tibetan plateau).

SCIENTIFIC SUPPORT

Rhodiola is typically considered an adaptogen (like ginseng) and is believed to invigorate the body and mind to increase resistance to a multitude of stresses. The key active constituents in rhodiola are believed to be rosavin, rosarin, rosin, and salidroside (Kelly, 2001), which are reported in animal studies to influence levels of neurotransmitters (serotonin, dopamine, and norepinephrine), catecholamines, and free radicals (Maslova et al., 1994; Ohsugi et al., 1999; Rege et al., 1999)

Unfortunately, most of what we know about the clinical effects of rhodiola supplementation comes from a handful of small studies in which standardized extracts of both *Rhodiola rosea* and *Rhodiola crenulata* have been shown to increase cognitive function and mental concentration while reducing feelings of general fatigue (Darbinyan et al., 2000, Spasov et al., 2000a, 2000b). One of the theoretical mechanisms of action for rhodiola's antifatigue effects is an enhancement of oxygen efficiency; although some studies have observed this effect (Ha et al., 2002), other studies have not (Wing et al., 2003). A possible reason for the discrepancy in these results is study design, with positive-effect studies tending to have larger numbers of subjects, longer durations of supplementation, and more complete characterizations of study materials (standardized *Rhodiola* extracts).

For example, one study of rhodiola followed 15 subjects supplemented with rhodiola for 7 days under simulated high-altitude conditions (4,600 meters) and found a reduction in hypoxia-induced oxidative stress but no change in hemoglobin saturation or blood oxygen levels (Wing et al., 2003). In contrast, a similar study (Ha et al., 2002) of 24 subjects living at a higher altitude (5,380 meters) for a longer duration (1 year) showed a beneficial effect of rhodiola supplementation on blood oxygen levels when rhodiola was given over a longer period (24 days).

Another significant factor among the handful of clinical studies on rhodiola is the material being studied, with well-characterized extracts (standardized to salidroside, rosavin, and other active/marker compounds) showing significant beneficial effects, while less well-characterized material (nonstandardized extracts and raw rhodiola root) tending to show modest or no beneficial effects. For example, three well-controlled studies of a standardized extract of *Rhodiola rosea* have shown benefits in reducing mental and physical fatigue in physicians working night duty (Darbinyan et al., 2000) and students under stress (Spasov et al., 2000a, 2000b).

SAFETY/DOSAGE

Rhodiola rosea extract is thought to be quite safe. There are no known contraindications or interactions with other drugs or herbs, but there are anecdotal reports of mild allergic reactions (rashes) in some persons. General dosage recommendations for extracts of both *Rhodiola rosea* and *Rhodiola crenulata* are typically in the range of 100–600 mg/day. Ideally, a standardized *Rhodiola* extract is preferred, with the best efficacy demonstrated for extracts with active/marker compounds in the ranges of 3–6% rosavin and 1–2% salidroside (Kelly, 2001).

REFERENCES

Darbinyan V, Kteyan A, Panossian A, Gabrielian E, Wikman G, Wagner H. Rhodiola rosea in stress induced fatigue—a double blind cross-over study of a standardized extract SHR-5 with a repeated low-dose regimen on the mental performance of healthy physicians during night duty. Phytomedicine 2000;7(5):365–371.

Ha Z, Zhu Y, Zhang X, Cui J, Zhang S, Ma Y, Wang W, Jian X. The effect of rhodiola and acetazolamide on the sleep architecture and blood oxygen saturation in men living at high altitude. Zhonghua Jie He He Hu Xi Za Zhi 2002;25(9):527–530.

Kelly GS. Rhodiola rosea: a possible plant adaptogen. Altern Med Rev 2001 Jun;6(3):293–302.

Maslova LV, Kondrat'ev BIu, Maslov LN, Lishmanov IuB. The cardioprotective and antiadrenergic activity of an extract of Rhodiola rosea in stress. Eksp Klin Farmakol 1994;57(6):61–63.

Ohsugi M, Fan W, Hase K, Xiong Q, Tezuka Y, Komatsu K, Namba T, Saitoh T, Tazawa K, Kadota S. Active-oxygen scavenging activity of traditional nourishing-tonic herbal medicines and active constituents of Rhodiola sacra. J Ethnopharmacol 1999;67(1):111–119.

Rege NN, Thatte UM, Dahanukar SA. Adaptogenic properties of six rasayana herbs used in Ayurvedic medicine. Phytother Res 1999;13(4):275–291.

Rhodiola rosea [monograph, no authors listed]. Altern Med Rev 2002 Oct;7(5):421–3.

Spasov AA, Mandrikov VB, Mironova IA. The effect of the preparation rodakson on the psychophysiological and physical adaptation of students to an academic load. Eksp Klin Farmakol 2000a;63(1):76–78.

Spasov AA, Wikman GK, Mandrikov VB, Mironova IA, Neumoin VV. A double-blind, placebo-controlled pilot study of the stimulating and adaptogenic effect of Rhodiola rosea SHR-5 extract on the fatigue of students caused by stress during an examination period with a repeated low-dose regimen. Phytomedicine 2000b;7(2):85–89.

Wing SL, Askew EW, Luetkemeier MJ, Ryujin DT, Kamimori GH, Grissom CK. Lack of effect of Rhodiola or oxygenated water supplementation on hypoxemia and oxidative stress. Wilderness Environ Med 2003;14(1):9–16.

Zhang ZH, Feng SH, Hu GD, Cao ZK, Wang LY. Effect of Rhodiola kirilowii on preventing high altitude reactions. A comparison of cardiopulmonary function in villagers at various altitudes. Zhongguo Zhong Yao Za Zhi 1989;14(11):687–690, 704.

ADDITIONAL RESOURCES

Bucci LR. Selected herbals and human exercise performance. Am J Clin Nutr 2000;72(2 suppl):624S-636S.

Linh PT, Kim YH, Hong SP, Jian JJ, Kang JS. Quantitative determination of salidroside and tyrosol from the underground part of Rhodiola rosea by high performance liquid chromatography. Arch Pharm Res 2000;23(4):349–352.

Zhang S, Wang J, Zhang H. Chemical constituents of Tibetan medicinal herb Rhodiola kirilowii. Chung Kuo Chung Yao Tsa Chih 1991;16(8):483, 512.

SEA BUCKTHORN (*HIPPOPHAE RHAMNOIDES*)

Overall Rank

★★★ as an antioxidant
★★★ for cardiovascular health
★★★ for wound healing and dermatitis
★ as an energizer

OVERVIEW

Sea buckthorn is a small shrub that produces berries used in Traditional Chinese Medicine and known since ancient Greek times for its ability to enhance energy, promote weight gain, and heal the skin and make it look younger. In more modern times, studies have found that it may be a good antioxidant and that it contains palmitoleic acid, a rare fatty acid that is a component of our skin and promotes skin health. Other uses for sea buckthorn include promoting cardiovascular health, healing ulcers, and protecting the skin against damage from the sun's ultraviolet rays. Sea buckthorn oil is high in vitamin E, carotenoids, sterols, and the fatty acids: palmitic (16:0), oleic (18:1n-9), palmitoleic (16:1n-7), linoleic (18:2n-6), and α-linolenic (18:3n-3; Johansson et al., 2000).

COMMENTS

Clinical research has not substantiated the claims for sea buckthorn as an energizer; however, experimental and clinical studies have found that it shows promise for promoting cardiovascular health, antioxidant functions (antiaging, cardiovascular), and as a wound and tissue healer.

SCIENTIFIC SUPPORT

Wound Healing and Dermatitis Treatment

A synthetic preparation of sea buckthorn oil (Aekol) was compared in a clinical setting on the treatment of 41 patients with natural sea buckthorn and standard wound-healing remedies. The patients studied exhibited various wound-healing complications, including open injuries on their limbs, pyoderma or necrosis from skeletal trauma, and tissue necrosis after operations. From the study of various clinical and biochemical parameters for wound healing, it was concluded that Aekol exhibited a similar efficacy as natural sea buckthorn extract and far exceeded the traditional remedies (Kostrikova et al., 1990).

Yang et al. (2000) conducted a placebo-controlled parallel study to examine the effect of the daily ingestion of 5 g of sea buckthorn seed oil compared with pulp oil or paraffin oil for 4 months. The outcome measure was the fatty acid composition of skin glycerophospholipids in patients with atopic dermatitis before and after treatment. The seed oil ingestion caused only a slight increase in docosapentaenoic acid (22:5n-3) and a decrease in palmitic acid (16:0). The authors concluded that the composition of glycerophospholipids in the skin is well buffered and not significantly affected by short-term dietary changes.

Yang et al. (1999) studied the effect of daily supplementation for 4 months of 5 g of either sea buckthorn seed oil, pulp oil, or paraffin oil on atopic dermatitis. In a placebo-controlled, double-blind study, the clinical evaluation of each treatment on atopic dermatitis was evaluated, as well as changes in plasma and skin lipid content. The sea buckthorn seed oil was characterized as high in linoleic (34%), α-linolenic (25%), and oleic (19%) fatty acids, whereas the pulp oil was high in palmitic (33%), oleic (26%), and palmitoleic (25%) fatty acids. Significant improvements were observed for dermatitis symptoms in the groups treated with pulp oil and paraffin oil, but no changes in the seed oil group were noted. No changes were detected in levels of triacylglycerols, serum total, or specific immunoglobulin E in either of the groups.

Cardiovascular Health

Johansson et al. (2000) studied the effect of sea buckthorn berry oil (supercritical carbon dioxide extracted) on risk factors of cardiovascular disease in a pilot clinical study. After a treatment period of 4 weeks, the ingestion of 5 g of sea buckthorn oil was found to have no effect on phospholipid fatty acids, plasma lipids, or glucose. The treatment group, however, did show a marked decrease in the rate of adenosine-5'-diphosphate-induced platelet aggregation and maximum aggregation.

The effect of supplementation of the total flavone fraction of sea buckthorn was studied on the sympathetic nerve activity in hypertensive patients. Specifically, the authors were investigating whether this fraction was able to exert an inhibitory effect on sympathetic activity after supine isometric exercise. The 88 participants were given the sea buckthorn flavone extract, nifedipine, or verapamil. After 8 weeks of treatment, the sea buckthorn flavone extract was found not to alter the sympathetic activity in the treatment of hypertension, but it did exhibit an inhibitory effect on the sympathetic activity after supine isometric exercise. The authors noted that for this reason, sea buckthorn flavones might provide a clinical benefit (Zhang et al., 2001).

Eccleston et al. (2002) studied the antioxidant profile of sea buckthorn juice and its effect on various biochemical markers in cardiovascular health: plasma lipids, low-density lipoprotein (LDL) oxidation, platelet aggregation, and plasma soluble cell adhesion protein concentration. This study was in response to the growing evidence that antioxidant nutrients were able to affect cell response and gene expression relating to the oxidative processes that contribute to atherogenesis. After 8 weeks of treatment with sea buckthorn juice, there were no significant changes in plasma total cholesterol, LDL-C, platelet aggregation, or plasma intracellular adhesion molecule 1 levels from placebo. There was a trend (not significant) in a decreased susceptibility of LDL to oxidation, a 20% increase in plasma HDL-C, and a 17% increase in triacylglycerol concentrations.

A flavone fraction from sea buckthorn was studied for its effect on cardiac performance and hemodynamics in a double-blind, placebo-controlled study. The groups consisted of 44 participants who were administered either a placebo or flavone extract (10 mg). The authors found that the flavone extract could strengthen the myocardial contractility and pump functions of the heart and reduce the peripheral vascular resistance while increasing vascular elasticity (Wang et al., 1993).

SAFETY/DOSAGE

Because few clinical studies have been performed on sea buckthorn, and because it has a diversity of potential uses, the optimal dosage recommendations are difficult to ascertain. Generally, it is taken orally, about 250–500 mg/day as an energy promoter, and up to 1 g or more as a topical skin protector or wound healer.

REFERENCES

Eccleston C, Baoru Y, Tahvonen R, Kallio H, Rimbach GH, Minihane AM. Effects of an antioxidant-rich juice (sea buckthorn) on risk factors for coronary heart disease in humans. J Nutr Biochem 2002;13(6):346–354.

Johansson AK, Korte H, Yang B, Stanley JC, Kallio HP. Sea buckthorn berry oil inhibits platelet aggregation. J Nutr Biochem 2000;11(10):491–495.

Kostrikova EV, Goridova LD, Gusak IV. Application of "Aekol" preparation for combined treatment of open injuries. Ortop Travmatol Protez 1990;(12):42–47.

Wang B, Feng Y, Yu Y, et al. The effects of total flavones of Hippophae rhamnoides L. (TFH) on cardiac performance and hemodynamics of normal subjects. Journal of Xi'An Medical University 1993;14(2):138–140.

Yang B, Kalimo KO, Mattila LM, Kallio SE, Katajisto JK, Peltola OJ, Kallio Heikki P. Effects of dietary supplementation with sea buckthorn (Hippophae rhamnoides) seed and pulp oils on atopic dermatitis. Journal of Nutritional Biochemistry 1999;10(11):622–630.

Yang B, Kalimo KO, Tahvonen RL, Mattila LM, Katajisto JK, Kallio HP. Effect of dietary supplementation with sea buckthorn (Hippophae rhamnoides) seed and pulp oils on the fatty acid composition of skin glycerophospholipids of patients with atopic dermatitis. J Nutr Biochem 2000;11(6):338–340.

Zhang X, Zhang M, Gao Z, Wang J, Wang Z. Effect of total flavones of Hippophae rhamnoides L. on sympathetic activity in hypertension. Journal of West China University of Medical Sciences 2001;32(4):547–550.

VITAMIN B$_1$ (THIAMIN)

Overall Rank

★★★★★ for correcting nutrient deficiency
★★★ during stress
★★ for an energy boost

OVERVIEW

Thiamin is a water-soluble vitamin. The active variety is a phosphorylated form called thiamin pyrophosphate, which functions in carbohydrate metabolism to help convert pyruvate to acetyl coenzyme A for entry to the Krebs cycle and subsequent steps to generate ATP. Thiamin also functions in maintaining the health of the nervous system and the heart muscle. Food sources include nuts, liver, brewer's yeast, and pork. Dietary supplements containing thiamin are frequently marketed with claims of increased energy production, maintenance of memory, and improved carbohydrate tolerance.

COMMENTS

This chapter on energy supplements contains information on vitamins B$_1$ and B$_2$. Other B vitamins, such as niacin, folic acid, B$_6$, and B$_{12}$, are covered in the "B-Complex Vitamins (B$_6$, B$_{12}$, Folic Acid, Niacin)" section of Chapter 7.

Because exercise and stress can tax the metabolic pathways that depend on thiamin and riboflavin, it is logical that the requirements for these vitamins may be increased in athletes, active people, and persons exposed to acute or chronic stressors. In these groups, marginally low intakes of thiamin and riboflavin can be corrected easily and safely by supplements containing the recommended dietary allowance (RDA) of these nutrients; for such purposes, a balanced multivitamin is the best approach.

SCIENTIFIC SUPPORT

The term *B complex* simply refers to a mixture or combination of the eight essential B vitamins: thiamin (B$_1$), riboflavin (B$_2$), niacin (B$_3$), pyridoxine (B$_6$), pantothenic acid, folic acid, cyanocobalamin (B$_{12}$), and biotin. Most of the B vitamins play a critical role as cofactors in cellular energy metabolism. Cofactors can be thought of as "helper nutrients" that assist chemical reactions. For example, the process of glycolysis, which converts energy stored as glycogen into glucose molecules, requires vitamin B$_6$ and biotin. The conversion of pyruvate (a metabolite of glucose) to acetyl coenzyme A (the first step in the Krebs cycle in energy metabolism) requires pantothenic acid, and further metabolism requires biotin, riboflavin, and niacin. Lack of any of the B vitamins can cause fatigue and lethargy, which is why B-complex supplements are often promoted as "energy boosters" and "stress formulas."

Because of thiamin's role in carbohydrate metabolism and nerve function, supplements have been promoted for increasing energy and maintaining memory. It is well known that thiamin deficiency (beriberi) is associated with generalized muscle weakness and mental confusion. Although beriberi is rare in industrialized countries, there continue to be reports of the condition in the medical literature. For example, thiamin insufficiency has been reported in Chinese prisoners (Chen et al., 2003), surgical patients (Nakasaki et al., 1997), rural Cubans (Marcais-Matos et al., 1996), Gambian children (Bates et al., 1987), alcoholics (Waldenlind et al., 1981), and older women (Wouters-Wesseling et al., 2002). In addition to these populations, which may be "expected" to have deficient thiamin intakes, other populations that have been shown to have marginal or suboptimal thiamin intake include female collegiate volleyball players (Papadopoulou et al., 2002), collegiate wrestlers (Williams, 1989), and other athletes who may be restricting energy and/or food intake (Manore, 2000; van der Beek et al., 1994). Luckily, inadequate thiamin status is easily and rapidly corrected by thiamin supplements in the range of 50–100 mg/day (Descombes et al., 2000; Nakasaki et al., 1997; Powers et al., 1985; Waldenlind et al., 1981).

Thiamin appears to be involved in the release of acetylcholine, a neurotransmitter, from nerve cells—a fact that may account for isolated studies showing thiamin supplementation to benefit cognitive functioning (Benton et al., 1995). As a coenzyme for carbohydrate and branched-chain amino acid metabolism, thiamin has been touted as both a performance and an energy supplement, but supplementation studies of subjects already at normal thiamin status have not shown a beneficial effect. Because dietary thiamin requirements are based on caloric intake, people who consume more calories, such as athletes, are likely to require higher-than-average intakes of thiamin to help process the extra carbohydrates into energy. In persons who consume "whole" forms of carbohydrates, intakes of thiamin and other B vitamins will increase along with carbohydrate intake.

During acute periods of stress, including exercise, thiamin needs may be temporarily elevated, but outright thiamin deficiencies are rare except in persons consuming a severely restricted diet. On the basis of metabolic studies (Manore, 2000), there is biochemical evidence that riboflavin and/or thiamin status is poorer in persons who exercise moderately (2–5 hours/week) and who diet (restrict their food intake for weight loss). Suboptimal dietary intakes of thiamin, riboflavin, vitamin B_6, and vitamin C are known to compromise physical performance with reductions in mitochondrial metabolism and aerobic power (van der Beek et al., 1994). In one study, subjects consuming a diet low in thiamin and riboflavin (55% of RDA for 11 weeks) showed 7–11% reductions in oxygen uptake and power output (van der Beek et al., 1994). Exercise has also been shown to compromise riboflavin status—an effect that may be compounded and more severely affect performance when dietary intake is marginal (Soares et al., 1993; Winters et al., 1992).

SAFETY/DOSAGE

No adverse side effects are known with thiamin intakes at RDA levels or even at levels several times the RDA. The daily value (DV) for thiamin is 1.5 mg (RDA is 1.2 mg/day for men, 1.1 mg/day for women). The Food and Nutrition Board (FNB) has not established an upper-limit intake level for thiamin, but a level of 50 mg has been established by the Council for Responsible Nutrition as the NOAEL (no observed adverse effect level). Virtually every multivitamin contains thiamin at 100% DV levels (1.5 mg) or higher. Isolated supplements of thiamin are not necessary.

When it comes to defining optimal amounts of vitamins and minerals, confusion is more the rule than the exception. Before 1997, the benchmark of nutritional adequacy was the RDA, established by the FNB, which is part of the National Academy of Sciences. In general, the RDAs have always been viewed (as judged by the FNB) "to be adequate to meet the known nutrient needs of practically all healthy persons." Because scientific knowledge regarding the roles of nutrients, and their role in health and disease, has expanded dramatically since the inception of the RDAs, a new set of terminology—dietary reference intakes (DRIs)—has been established. The DRIs are based on contemporary scientific studies related to the role of nutrients in reducing the risk of osteoporosis, cancer, cardiovascular disease, and other chronic conditions. *DRI* is a generic term used to refer to the following reference values:

- **Estimated average requirement (EAR):** the intake value that meets the nutrient requirements of 50% of an age- and gender-specific population.
- **Recommended dietary allowance (RDA):** the intake value that meets the nutrient requirements of nearly all people in an age- and gender-specific group.
- **Upper intake (UL):** maximum intake of a specific nutrient that is unlikely to pose health risks.
- **Adequate intake (AI):** suggested levels of nutrient intake that are established when insufficient data exist to establish a true RDA.

REFERENCES

Benton D, Haller J, Fordy J. Vitamin supplementation for 1 year improves mood. Neuropsychobiology 1995;32(2):98–105.

Bates CJ, Powers HJ, Lamb WH, Gelman W, Webb E. Effect of supplementary vitamins and iron on malaria indices in rural Gambian children. Trans R Soc Trop Med Hyg 1987;81(2):286–291.

Chen KT, Twu SJ, Chiou ST, Pan WH, Chang HJ, Serdula MK. Outbreak of beriberi among illegal mainland Chinese immigrants at a detention center in Taiwan. Public Health Rep 2003 Jan-Feb;118(1):59–64.

Descombes E, Boulat O, Perriard F, Fellay G. Water-soluble vitamin levels in patients undergoing high-flux hemodialysis and receiving long-term oral postdialysis vitamin supplementation. Artif Organs 2000;24(10):773–778.

Manore MM. Effect of physical activity on thiamine, riboflavin, and vitamin B-6 requirements. Am J Clin Nutr 2000;72(2 suppl):598S–606S.

Macias-Matos C, Rodriguez-Ojea A, Chi N, Jimenez S, Zulueta D, Bates CJ. Biochemical evidence of thiamine depletion during the Cuban neuropathy epidemic, 1992-1993. Am J Clin Nutr 1996;64(3):347–353.

Nakasaki H, Ohta M, Soeda J, Makuuchi H, Tsuda M, Tajima T, Mitomi T, Fujii K. Clinical and biochemical aspects of thiamine treatment for metabolic acidosis during total parenteral nutrition. Nutrition 1997;13(2):110–117.

Papadopoulou SK, Papadopoulou SD, Gallos GK. Macro- and micro-nutrient intake of adolescent Greek female volleyball players. Int J Sport Nutr Exerc Metab 2002;12(1):73–80.

Powers HJ, Bates CJ, Lamb WH, Singh J, Gelman W, Webb E. Effects of a multivitamin and iron supplement on running performance in Gambian children. Hum Nutr Clin Nutr 1985;39(6):427–437.

Soares MJ, Satyanarayana K, Bamji MS, Jacob CM, Ramana YV, Rao SS. The effect of exercise on the riboflavin status of adult men. Br J Nutr 1993;69(2):541–551.

van der Beek EJ, van Dokkum W, Wedel M, Schrijver J, van den Berg H. Thiamin, riboflavin and vitamin B6: impact of restricted intake on physical performance in man. J Am Coll Nutr 1994;13(6):629–640.

Waldenlind L, Borg S, Vikander B. Effect of peroral thiamine treatment on thiamine contents and transketolase activity of red blood cells in alcoholic patients. Acta Med Scand 1981;209(3):209–212.

Williams MH. Vitamin supplementation and athletic performance. Int J Vitam Nutr Res Suppl 1989;30:163–191.

Winters LR, Yoon JS, Kalkwarf HJ, Davies JC, Berkowitz MG, Haas J, Roe DA. Riboflavin requirements and exercise adaptation in older women. Am J Clin Nutr 1992;56(3):526–532.

Wouters-Wesseling W, Wouters AE, Kleijer CN, Bindels JG, de Groot CP, van Staveren WA. Study of the effect of a liquid nutrition supplement on the nutritional status of psycho-geriatric nursing home patients. Eur J Clin Nutr 2002;56(3):245–51.

ADDITIONAL RESOURCES

Fogelholm M. Micronutrient status in females during a 24-week fitness-type exercise program. Ann Nutr Metab 1992;36(4):209–218.

Fogelholm M, Rehunen S, Gref CG, Laakso JT, Lehto J, Ruokonen I, Himberg JJ. Dietary intake and thiamin, iron, and zinc status in elite Nordic skiers during different training periods. Int J Sport Nutr 1992;2(4):351–365.

Fogelholm M, Ruokonen I, Laakso JT, Vuorimaa T, Himberg JJ. Lack of association between indices of vitamin B1, B2, and B6 status and exercise-induced blood lactate in young adults. Int J Sport Nutr 1993;3(2):165–176.

Gleeson M, Bishop NC. Elite athlete immunology: importance of nutrition. Int J Sports Med 2000;21(suppl 1):S44–S50.

Kopp-Woodroffe SA, Manore MM, Dueck CA, Skinner JS, Matt KS. Energy and nutrient status of amenorrheic athletes participating in a diet and exercise training intervention program. Int J Sport Nutr 1999;9(1):70–88.

Manore MM. Vitamin B6 and exercise. Int J Sport Nutr 1994;4(2):89–103.

Suzuki M, Itokawa Y. Effects of thiamine supplementation on exercise-induced fatigue. Metab Brain Dis 1996;11(1):95–106.

VITAMIN B_2 (RIBOFLAVIN)

Overall Rank

★★★★★ for correcting nutrient deficiency
★★★   during stress
★★   for an energy boost

OVERVIEW

Vitamin B_2, or riboflavin, is a water-soluble vitamin. It functions primarily as a coenzyme for many metabolic processes in the body, such as red blood cell formation and nervous system function. Riboflavin is involved in energy production as part of the electron transport chain that produces cellular energy. As a building block for flavin adenine dinucleotide (FAD), riboflavin is a crucial component in converting food into energy. FAD is required for electron transport and ATP production in the Krebs cycle. FAD is also the cofactor for methylenetetrahydrofolate reductase, the enzyme that catalyzes the formation of 5-methyltetrahydrofolate and acts as a methyl donor for homocysteine remethylation. Through this methylation pathway, riboflavin supplementation, together with folate, may act to reduce plasma levels of homocysteine.

Liver, dairy products, dark green vegetables, and many seafoods are good sources of riboflavin. Dietary supplements containing riboflavin, in addition to being marketed as general nutrients, will frequently contain claims for increased energy levels, treatment of chronic fatigue, improved concentration and mood, reduced plasma homocysteine, and promotion of heart health.

COMMENTS

The term *B complex* simply refers to a mixture or combination of the eight essential B vitamins: thiamin (B_1), riboflavin (B_2), niacin (B_3), pyridoxine (B_6), pantothenic acid, folic acid, cyanocobalamin (B_{12}), and biotin. Most of the B vitamins play a critical role as cofactors in cellular energy metabolism. Cofactors can be thought of as "helper nutrients" that assist chemical reactions. For example, the process of glycolysis, which converts energy stored as glycogen into glucose molecules, requires vitamin B_6 and biotin. The conversion of pyruvate (a metabolite of glucose) to acetyl coenzyme A (the first step in the Krebs cycle in energy metabolism) requires pantothenic acid, and further metabolism requires biotin, riboflavin, and niacin. Lack of any of the B vitamins can cause fatigue and lethargy, which is why B-complex supplements are often promoted as "energy boosters" and "stress formulas."

Virtually every multivitamin/mineral supplement available contains the full complement of B-complex vitamins at RDA or higher levels. It is often a better value to get B vitamins through a multivitamin supplement than as a separate B-complex supplement. This chapter on energy supplements contains information on vitamins B_1 and B_2, while other B vitamins, such as niacin, folic acid, B_6, and B_{12}, are covered in the "B-Complex Vitamins (B_6, B_{12}, Folic Acid, Niacin)" section of Chapter 7.

SCIENTIFIC SUPPORT

Requirements for riboflavin, like most B vitamins, are related to calorie intake; therefore, the more food consumed, the more riboflavin needed to support the metabolic processes that convert food into usable energy. Women should be aware that riboflavin needs are elevated during pregnancy and lactation as well as by the use of oral contraceptives (birth control pills). Athletes may require more riboflavin because of both increased caloric intake and increased needs of exercise.

In cases of subclinical (biochemically defined) riboflavin deficiency, daily supplementation of diets with riboflavin (with or without other B vitamins) resulted in an increase in physical work capacity (Suboticanec et al., 1990). In other studies, adding riboflavin to an antianemia regimen (dietary changes plus ferrous sulphate) resulted in a significant increase in circulating plasma iron and in iron stores (hemoglobin) compared with iron supplements alone (Powers et al., 1987). As expected, riboflavin supplements have no effect on physical performance when added to a riboflavin-adequate diet (Manore, 2000).

There is no strong support for the efficacy of isolated riboflavin supplements in promoting health besides correcting a nutrient deficiency. Despite the role of riboflavin in a variety of energy-generating processes, the role for a supplement in directly improving energy levels in a well-nourished person is unlikely.

SAFETY/DOSAGE

Isolated riboflavin supplements are not necessary. Virtually all multivitamins and B-complex formulas contain riboflavin at RDA or higher levels. When it comes to supplementing with B-complex vitamins, isolated single-vitamin supplements are not recommended. A more balanced approach is to supplement with the entire B-complex spectrum simultaneously, or at least with several of the B vitamins in the same supplement. High-dose supplementation with any single B-complex vitamin can interfere with the absorption of another. For example, a folic acid supplement of 400 µg/day (a common level) has been shown to exacerbate a riboflavin deficiency and elevate plasma homocysteine levels (Moat et al., 2003). Likewise, studies of combined B-vitamin supplementation (folate plus B_6 plus riboflavin) generally show that this approach has a more pronounced effect on metabolic parameters, such as plasma homocysteine levels, than supplementing with any single B vitamin (Jacques et al., 2001).

No serious side effects have been reported for supplementation with riboflavin at levels several times above the DV of 1.7 mg. Because the body excretes excess riboflavin in the urine, high supplemental levels are likely to result in brightly colored urine (fluorescent yellow).

The DV for riboflavin is 1.7 mg (RDA is 1.3 mg/day for men, 1.1 mg/day for women). The Food and Nutrition Board sets no UL intake of riboflavin, but as much as 200 mg/day of riboflavin is considered safe (the NOAEL set by the Council for Responsible Nutrition).

When it comes to defining optimal amounts of vitamins and minerals, confusion is more the rule than the exception. Before 1997, the benchmark of nutritional adequacy was the RDA established by the FNB. In general, the RDAs have always been viewed (as judged by the FNB) "to be adequate to meet the known nutrient needs of practically all healthy persons." Because scientific knowledge regarding the roles of nutrients, and their role in health and disease, has expanded dramatically since the inception of the RDAs, a new set of terminology (the DRIs) has been established. The DRIs are based on contemporary scientific studies related to the role of nutrients in reducing the risk of osteoporosis, cancer, cardiovascular disease and other chronic conditions. *DRI* is a generic term used to refer to the following reference values:

- **Estimated average requirement (EAR):** the intake value that meets the nutrient requirements of 50% of an age- and gender-specific population.
- **Recommended dietary allowance (RDA):** the intake value that meets the nutrient requirements of nearly all people in an age- and gender-specific group.
- **Upper intake (UL):** maximum intake of a specific nutrient that is unlikely to pose health risks.
- **Adequate intake (AI):** suggested levels of nutrient intake that are established when insufficient data exist to establish a true RDA.

REFERENCES

Jacques PF, Bostom AG, Wilson PW, Rich S, Rosenberg IH, Selhub J. Determinants of plasma total homocysteine concentration in the Framingham Offspring cohort. Am J Clin Nutr 2001;73(3):613–621.

Manore MM. Effect of physical activity on thiamine, riboflavin, and vitamin B-6 requirements. Am J Clin Nutr 2000;72(2 suppl):598S-606S.

Moat SJ, Ashfield-Watt PA, Powers HJ, Newcombe RG, McDowell IF. Effect of riboflavin status on the homocysteine-lowering effect of folate in relation to the MTHFR (C677T) genotype. Clin Chem 2003;49(2):295–302.

Powers HJ, Bates CJ, Eccles M, Brown H, George E. Bicycling performance in Gambian children: effects of supplements of riboflavin or ascorbic acid. Hum Nutr Clin Nutr 1987;41(1):59–69.

Suboticanec K, Stavljenic A, Schalch W, Buzina R. Effects of pyridoxine and riboflavin supplementation on physical fitness in young adolescents. Int J Vitam Nutr Res 1990;60(1):81–88.

ADDITIONAL RESOURCES

Belko AZ, Meredith MP, Kalkwarf HJ, Obarzanek E, Weinberg S, Roach R, McKeon G, Roe DA. Effects of exercise on riboflavin requirements: biological validation in weight reducing women. Am J Clin Nutr 1985;41(2):270–277.

Belko AZ, Obarzanek E, Kalkwarf HJ, Rotter MA, Bogusz S, Miller D, Haas JD, Roe DA. Effects of exercise on riboflavin requirements of young women. Am J Clin Nutr 1983;37(4):509–517.

Belko AZ, Obarzanek E, Roach R, Rotter M, Urban G, Weinberg S, Roe DA. Effects of aerobic exercise and weight loss on riboflavin requirements of moderately obese, marginally deficient young women. Am J Clin Nutr 1984;40(3):553–561.

Fogelholm M. Micronutrient status in females during a 24-week fitness-type exercise program. Ann Nutr Metab 1992;36(4):209–218.

Fogelholm M, Ruokonen I, Laakso JT, Vuorimaa T, Himberg JJ. Lack of association between indices of vitamin B_1, B_2, and B_6 status and exercise-induced blood lactate in young adults. Int J Sport Nutr 1993;3(2):165–176.

Garry PJ, Goodwin JS, Hunt WC. Nutritional status in a healthy elderly population: riboflavin. Am J Clin Nutr 1982;36(5):902–909.

Kopp-Woodroffe SA, Manore MM, Dueck CA, Skinner JS, Matt KS. Energy and nutrient status of amenorrheic athletes participating in a diet and exercise training intervention program. Int J Sport Nutr 1999;9(1):70–88.

Powers HJ, Bates CJ, Prentice AM, Lamb WH, Jepson M, Bowman H. The relative effectiveness of iron and iron with riboflavin in correcting a microcytic anaemia in men and children in rural Gambia. Hum Nutr Clin Nutr 1983;37(6):413–425.

Rokitzki L, Sagredos A, Keck E, Sauer B, Keul J. Assessment of vitamin B_2 status in performance athletes of various types of sports. J Nutr Sci Vitaminol (Tokyo) 1994;40(1):11–22.

Roughead ZK, McCormick DB. Urinary riboflavin and its metabolites: effects of riboflavin supplementation in healthy residents of rural Georgia (USA). Eur J Clin Nutr 1991;45(6):299–307.

van der Beek EJ, van Dokkum W, Wedel M, Schrijver J, van den Berg H. Thiamin, riboflavin and vitamin B_6: impact of restricted intake on physical performance in man. J Am Coll Nutr 1994;13(6):629–640.

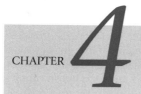

Bone Support Supplements

Boron
Calcium
Magnesium

Vitamin D (Calciferol, Cholecalciferol)
Vitamin K (Phylloquinone,
Menaquinone)

BORON

Overall Rank

★★★★★ for correcting nutrient deficiency
★★★ for promoting bone and joint health
★★ for maintaining testosterone levels (in postmenopausal women)

OVERVIEW

Boron is a trace element that influences calcium and magnesium metabolism. Although it is found in most tissues, boron is concentrated in the bone, spleen, and thyroid, indicating boron's functions in bone metabolism and suggesting a potential role for boron in reproductive and metabolic hormone regulation. Because of the supposed role of boron in hormone metabolism, dietary supplements containing boron are frequently promoted to boost testosterone production, increase muscle mass and strength, improve calcium absorption, and maintain bone density.

COMMENTS

Low-boron diets have been associated with reduced testosterone levels, and boron supplements have been shown to increase serum levels of testosterone (and estradiol) in postmenopausal women. A number of boron supplements target athletes and bodybuilders and tout the benefits of boron for boosting testosterone levels, strength, and muscle mass. As part of a balanced multivitamin/mineral supplement, boron may have beneficial effects on maintaining adequate calcium and magnesium metabolism for optimal bone health. Athletes looking to boron supplements to increase serum testosterone levels and improve muscle mass and strength should look elsewhere.

SCIENTIFIC SUPPORT

The most dramatic effects of boron supplementation on bone metabolism appear in cases of deficient intake of other bone-active nutrients, such as vitamin D, calcium, and magnesium (Meacham et al., 1994; Schaafsma et al., 2001). Perhaps the best-documented beneficial effect of boron is on calcium metabolism or utilization, which in turn benefits bone calcification and maintenance (Nielsen, 1998), although not all studies have demonstrated a beneficial effect of boron supplementation on bone metabolism. One study looked at the benefits of boron supplements (3 mg/day for 3 weeks) on bone health and found no effect on urinary markers of bone breakdown (pyridinium crosslinks) but an increase in calcium absorption (Beattie and Peace, 1993).

Other effects of boron are related to lipid metabolism, energy utilization, immune function, and brain and psychological function (Penland, 1998). It is known from animal studies that boron is essential (Sutherland et al., 1998) and that boron deprivation results in decreased brain electrical activity (Penland, 1998). In humans, assessment of cognitive and psychomotor function has shown that boron deprivation results in poorer performance on tasks related to motor speed and dexterity, attention, and short-term memory, suggesting that adequate boron nutriture is important for brain and psychological function (Benderdour et al., 1998; Penland, 1998).

Claims that boron supplements can boost testosterone were based on a study by the U.S. Department of Agriculture (USDA) of boron-deprived postmenopausal women, in whom boron supplements (3 mg/day) reduced calcium and magnesium excretion while elevating serum levels of testosterone and estradiol (Nielsen et al., 1987). Serum testosterone levels in postmenopausal women, however, are more than 10 times lower than those found in normal men and in strength athletes.

No studies suggest that boron supplementation alone will augment testosterone production or promote muscle growth in healthy athletic men. In one study of healthy sedentary male subjects (Naghii and Samman, 1993), boron supplementation at 10 mg/day for 4 weeks increased testosterone and estradiol and suggested a potential role for the supplement in preventing atherosclerosis. A related study of boron supplementation (3 mg/day for 49 days) in middle-aged men and postmenopausal women showed a higher level of erythrocyte superoxide dismutase, suggesting an increase in cellular antioxidant potential subsequent to boron supplementation (Nielsen, 1994).

A number of studies have shown that boron supplementation reduces urinary losses of calcium, zinc, and magnesium (Benderdour et al., 1998; Meacham et al., 1995; Sutherland et al., 1998), leading to suggestions that boron supplementation may play a role in modulating the demineralization of bone seen in osteoporosis and certain cases of osteoarthritis (Helliwell et al., 1996; Naghii and Samman, 1993), as well as strengthening the mechanical properties of existing bone (McCoy et al., 1994). Epidemiologic evidence suggests that chronically low intakes of boron (1 mg/day or less) may contribute to higher rates of arthritis (20–70% incidence) compared with populations with higher boron intakes (3–10 mg/day intake with 0–10% arthritis incidence; Newnham, 1994).

SAFETY/DOSAGE

Although no recommended dietary allowance (RDA) or adequate intake (AI) has been established for boron, the average daily intake is highly variable, having been estimated at between 0.5 and 7 mg/day. The tolerable upper limit (UL) for boron is 20 mg/day for adult men and women. An analysis by USDA scientists suggests that a significant number of people do not consistently consume more than 1 mg/day of boron (Nielsen, 1998). Boron consumption of up to 20 mg/day is considered safe, but caution is warranted at higher intake levels because consumption of 50 mg or more has been linked to toxicity, loss of appetite, nausea, vomiting, skin rashes, lethargy, and diarrhea. Boron is found in relatively high levels in foods of plant origin, such as dried fruits, nuts, dark green leafy vegetables, applesauce, grape juice, and cooked dried beans and peas. Daily needs for boron probably fall somewhere between 1–20 mg but are thought to vary considerably based on stress levels, immune status, and intake of other bone-active minerals (Penland, 1998). Approximately 1 mg of boron is provided by the following foods: 1.5 oz of raisins or prunes, 2 oz of almonds or peanuts, and 4 oz of red wine.

REFERENCES

Beattie JH, Peace HS. The influence of a low-boron diet and boron supplementation on bone, major mineral and sex steroid metabolism in postmenopausal women. Br J Nutr 1993;69(3):871–884.

Benderdour M, Bui-Van T, Dicko A, Belleville F. In vivo and in vitro effects of boron and boronated compounds. J Trace Elem Med Bio 1998r;12(1):2–7.

Helliwell TR, Kelly SA, Walsh HP, Klenerman L, Haines J, Clark R, Roberts NB. Elemental analysis of femoral bone from patients with fractured neck of femur or osteoarthrosis. Bone 1996;18(2):151–157.

McCoy H, Kenney MA, Montgomery C, Irwin A, Williams L, Orrell R. Relation of boron to the composition and mechanical properties of bone. Environ Health Perspect 1994;102(suppl 7):49–53.

Meacham SL, Taper LJ, Volpe SL. Effect of boron supplementation on blood and urinary calcium, magnesium, and phosphorus, and urinary boron in athletic and sedentary women. Am J Clin Nutr 1995;61(2):341–345.

Meacham SL, Taper LJ, Volpe SL. Effects of boron supplementation on bone mineral density and dietary, blood, and urinary calcium, phosphorus, magnesium, and boron in female athletes. Environ Health Perspect 1994;102(suppl 7):79–82.

Naghii MR, Samman S. The role of boron in nutrition and metabolism. Prog Food Nutr Sci 1993;17(4):331–349.

Newnham RE. Essentiality of boron for healthy bones and joints. Environ Health Perspect 1994;102(suppl 7):83–5.

Nielsen FH. Biochemical and physiologic consequences of boron deprivation in humans. Environ Health Perspect 1994;102(suppl 7):59–63.

Nielsen FH. The justification for providing dietary guidance for the nutritional intake of boron. Biol Trace Elem Res 1998;66(1–3):319–330.

Nielsen FH, Hunt CD, Mullen LM, Hunt JR. Effect of dietary boron on mineral, estrogen, and testosterone metabolism in postmenopausal women. FASEB J 1987;1(5):394–397.

Penland JG. The importance of boron nutrition for brain and psychological function. Biol Trace Elem Res 1998;66(1–3):299–317.

Schaafsma A, de Vries PJ, Saris WH. Delay of natural bone loss by higher intakes of specific minerals and vitamins. Crit Rev Food Sci Nut 2001;41(4):225–249.

Sutherland B, Strong P, King JC. Determining human dietary requirements for boron. Biol Trace Elem Res 1998;66(1–3):193–204.

ADDITIONAL RESOURCES

Ferrando AA, Green NR. The effect of boron supplementation on lean body mass, plasma testosterone levels, and strength in male bodybuilders. Int J Sport Nutr 1993;3(2):140–149.

Green NR, Ferrando AA. Plasma boron and the effects of boron supplementation in males. Environ Health Perspect 1994;102(suppl 7):73–77.

Hunt CD, Herbel JL, Nielsen FH. Metabolic responses of postmenopausal women to supplemental dietary boron and aluminum during usual and low magnesium intake: boron, calcium, and magnesium absorption and retention and blood mineral concentrations. Am J Clin Nutr 1997;65(3):803–813.

Meacham SL, Hunt CD. Dietary boron intakes of selected populations in the United States. Biol Trace Elem Res 1998;66(1–3):65–78.

Naghii MR. The significance of dietary boron, with particular reference to athletes. Nutr Health 1999;13(1):31–37.

Nielsen FH. Studies on the relationship between boron and magnesium which possibly affects the formation and maintenance of bones. Magnes Trace Elem 1990;9(2):61–69.

Rainey CJ, Nyquist LA, Christensen RE, Strong PL, Culver BD, Coughlin JR. Daily boron intake from the American diet. J Am Diet Assoc 1999;99(3):335–340.

Samman S, Naghii MR, Lyons Wall PM, Verus AP. The nutritional and metabolic effects of boron in humans and animals. Biol Trace Elem Res 1998;66(1–3):227–235.

Volpe SL, Taper LJ, Meacham S. The relationship between boron and magnesium status and bone mineral density in the human: a review. Magnes Res 1993;6(3):291–296.

CALCIUM

Overall Rank

★★★★★ for bone health
★★★ for blood pressure control
★★★ for maintaining metabolic rate
★★★ for alleviating symptoms of premenstrual syndrome (PMS)
★★ for reducing the risk of colon cancer

OVERVIEW

Calcium is the most abundant mineral in the human body. The average adult skeleton contains about 2–3 lb of calcium, with 99% found in the bones and teeth. The remaining 1% of body calcium is found in the blood and within cells, where calcium helps with dozens of metabolic processes. This 1% of blood and cellular calcium is so tightly maintained within normal ranges that the body will draw on calcium stores in the bones, even at the expense of causing osteoporosis. Good dietary sources of calcium include all dairy products and several vegetables, like broccoli, bok choy, and kale. A cup of milk contains about 300 mg of calcium.

Because of the predominant role of calcium in bone health, it is covered in this chapter, but calcium is also an essential mineral for maintenance of blood pressure and nerve conduction. Therefore, dietary supplements containing calcium are frequently marketed for controlling blood pressure, reducing the risk of colon cancer, and alleviating certain symptoms of PMS.

COMMENTS

Calcium is cheap, widely available, and well tolerated as a supplement. Practically nobody consumes enough calcium in a "normal" daily diet, so calcium is one of the nutrients for which supplementation is highly recommended. When it comes to choosing a calcium supplement, a prudent approach is to select a product that combines calcium with other bone-specific nutrients such as vitamin D, vitamin K, and magnesium. The form of calcium, however, seems to be less important. Although a few studies suggest that one form of calcium may have superior intestinal absorption compared with another form, most comparison studies show no appreciable differences among the absorption rates of the various forms of calcium available as dietary supplements (milk, milk powder, carbonate, citrate, hydroxyapatite, and others).

SCIENTIFIC SUPPORT

The most obvious need for calcium is to help build and maintain strong bones, but calcium is also important for blood clotting, muscle contraction, nerve transmission, and maintenance of normal blood pressure. There is also some evidence that calcium supplements may be helpful in reducing the risk of colon cancer, regulating heart rhythms, and treating PMS.

For decades, we have known about the important role that calcium plays in achieving and maintaining strong bones and helping to prevent osteoporosis. Numerous studies have shown the skeletal benefit of using calcium supplements (generally, 500–1,000 mg/day) to increase bone mass in women from adolescence to old age (Martini and Wood, 2002; Stear et al., 2003). Not all studies, however, have found that an increase in calcium intake translates into a reduction in fracture risk (Feskanich et al., 2003), suggesting that vitamin D and vitamin K status may be as important as calcium intake for optimal absorption, transport, and skeletal assimilation of bone minerals.

The dietary source of calcium does not appear to be as important as the overall level or its combination with vitamins D and K. Martini and Wood (2002) have shown that the bioavailability of calcium and suppression of parathyroid hormone (PTH, a reliable index of calcium status) does not differ between calcium supplements provided as calcium citrate malate (in fortified orange juice), skim milk, or calcium carbonate.

Data from various nutrition questionnaires and surveys indicate that 50–70% of American men and women fail to consume the recommended amounts of calcium (Dawson-Hughes et al., 2002); thus, it is prudent for most Americans to consider a daily calcium supplement as one approach to increasing total calcium intake. Although calcium, when supplemented alone, has been shown to significantly improve bone density at various skeletal sites (Cleghorn et al., 2001), other studies suggest that the optimal bone-sparing effects of calcium are achieved in combination with vitamin D (Jensen et al., 2001). Such combined dosing is also likely to enhance the efficacy of estrogens and bisphosphonates, approximately doubling the increase in bone mass at various skeletal sites in supplemented versus nonsupplemented subjects (Nieves et al., 1998).

More recent research, much of it conducted over the past 5 years, has suggested a number of other beneficial health effects of getting adequate calcium in the diet. Among the more exciting research, scientists have recently shown that eating more calcium-rich foods reduces the risk of colon cancer in men and that taking daily calcium supplements can cut in half women's premenstrual symptoms (pain, bloating, mood swings, and food cravings). In other studies, researchers found that adequate calcium intake (along with vitamin D) can reduce blood pressure in women with mild hypertension and in black teenagers (two groups who rarely consume enough calcium). The hypertensive effects of a high-salt diet tend to be most pronounced among people whose diets are low in calcium. In addition, women who take calcium supplements during pregnancy tend to give birth to children with healthier blood pressure levels (lower than average for the first seven years of life), which may reduce the child's risk of developing high blood pressure later in life.

SAFETY/DOSAGE

Side effects from calcium supplements are rare, but nausea, diarrhea, constipation, or other gastrointestinal effects may be possible at extremely high intakes. The UL for calcium is 2,500 mg/day. Intakes above 1,500 mg/day have not been associated with any greater benefits than more moderate intakes in the RDA ranges of 1,000–1,300 mg/day for men and women.

The recommended dietary reference intake (DRI) for calcium are 1,300 mg for ages 9–18; 1,000 mg for adults aged 19–50; and 1,200 mg for adults over age 50. For postmenopausal women not taking hormone replacement therapy, 1,500 mg/day of calcium is recommended.

REFERENCES

Cleghorn DB, O'Loughlin PD, Schroeder BJ, Nordin BE. An open, crossover trial of calcium-fortified milk in prevention of early postmenopausal bone loss. Med J Aust 2001;175(5):242–245.

Dawson-Hughes B, Harris SS, Dallal GE, Lancaster DR, Zhou Q. Calcium supplement and bone medication use in a US Medicare health maintenance organization. Osteoporos Int 2002;13(8):657–662.

Feskanich D, Willett WC, Colditz GA. Calcium, vitamin D, milk consumption, and hip fractures: a prospective study among postmenopausal women. Am J Clin Nutr 2003;77(2):504–511.

Jensen LB, Kollerup G, Quaade F, Sorensen OH. Bone minerals changes in obese women during a moderate weight loss with and without calcium supplementation. J Bone Miner Res 2001;16(1):141–147.

Martini L, Wood RJ. Relative bioavailability of calcium-rich dietary sources in the elderly. Am J Clin Nutr 2002;76(6):1345–1350.

Nieves JW, Komar L, Cosman F, Lindsay R. Calcium potentiates the effect of estrogen and calcitonin on bone mass: review and analysis. Am J Clin Nutr 1998;67(1):18–24.

Stear SJ, Prentice A, Jones SC, Cole TJ. Effect of a calcium and exercise intervention on the bone mineral status of 16–18-y-old adolescent girls. Am J Clin Nutr 2003;77(4):985–992.

ADDITIONAL RESOURCES

Abrams SA. Bone turnover during lactation--can calcium supplementation make a difference? J Clin Endocrinol Metab 1998;83(4):1056–1058.

Dawson-Hughes B. Vitamin D and calcium: recommended intake for bone health. Osteoporos Int 1998;8(suppl 2):S30–S34.

Fardellone P, Brazier M, Kamel S, Gueris J, Graulet AM, Lienard J, Sebert JL. Biochemical effects of calcium supplementation in postmenopausal women: influence of dietary calcium intake. Am J Clin Nutr 1998;67(6):1273–1278.

Feit JM. Calcium and vitamin D supplements for elderly patients. J Fam Pract 1997;45(6):471–472.

Heaney RP. Calcium, dairy products and osteoporosis. J Am Coll Nutr 2000;19(2 suppl):83S–99S.

Heaney RP, McCarron DA, Dawson-Hughes B, Oparil S, Berga SL, Stern JS, Barr SI, Rosen CJ. Dietary changes favorably affect bone remodeling in older adults. J Am Diet Assoc 1999;99(10):1228–1233.

Howat PM, Crombie A, Brooks ER. Dietary/supplement intake and bone mineral density. J Am Diet Assoc 2001;101(5):520–521.

Lesser GT. Long-term prevention of bone loss. Ann Intern Med 2000;133(1):72–73.

Meunier PJ. Calcium, vitamin D and vitamin K in the prevention of fractures due to osteoporosis. Osteoporos Int 1999;9(suppl 2):S48–S52.

Need AG, Horowitz M, Morris HA, Nordin BE. Effects of three different calcium preparations on urinary calcium and hydroxyproline excretion in postmenopausal osteoporotic women. Eur J Clin Nutr 1991;45(7):357–361.

Recker RR, Davies KM, Dowd RM, Heaney RP. The effect of low-dose continuous estrogen and progesterone therapy with calcium and vitamin D on bone in elderly women. A randomized, controlled trial. Ann Intern Med 1999;130(11):897–904.

Ricci TA, Chowdhury HA, Heymsfield SB, Stahl T, Pierson RN Jr, Shapses SA. Calcium supplementation suppresses bone turnover during weight reduction in postmenopausal women. J Bone Miner Res 1998;13(6):1045–1050.

Riggs BL, O'Fallon WM, Muhs J, O'Connor MK, Kumar R, Melton LJ III. Long-term effects of calcium supplementation on serum parathyroid hormone level, bone turnover, and bone loss in elderly women. J Bone Miner Res 1998;13(2):168–174.

Scopacasa F, Horowitz M, Wishart JM, Need AG, Morris HA, Wittert G, Nordin BE. Calcium supplementation suppresses bone resorption in early postmenopausal women. Calcif Tissue Int 1998;62(1):8–12.

Storm D, Eslin R, Porter ES, Musgrave K, Vereault D, Patton C, Kessenich C, Mohan S, Chen T, Holick MF, Rosen CJ. Calcium supplementation prevents seasonal bone loss and changes in biochemical markers of bone turnover in elderly New England women: a randomized placebo-controlled trial. J Clin Endocrinol Metab 1998;83(11):3817–3825.

Magnesium

Overall Rank

★★★★★ for bone health
★★★ for blood pressure control
★★★ for alleviating PMS
★★★ for alleviating anxiety

OVERVIEW

Magnesium is a mineral that functions as a coenzyme for more than 300 biochemical reactions, including nerve and muscle function, regulation of body temperature, energy metabolism, DNA and RNA synthesis, and the formation of bones. Most of the body's magnesium (about 60%) is found in the bones. Food sources include green vegetables, artichokes, nuts, beans, whole grains, and shellfish. Dietary supplements containing magnesium are frequently claimed to help build bone, increase energy levels, promote heart health, and enhance protein synthesis (muscle building).

COMMENTS

Magnesium is needed as a cofactor for several enzymes to help convert carbohydrates, protein, and fat into energy. Magnesium supplements may play a role in maintaining energy metabolism, but they are not meant for "boosting" energy levels. Owing to the role of magnesium in conducting nerve impulses, numerous magnesium-based supplements have been promoted for support of heart function, and supplementation with magnesium indeed appears to help control blood pressure in many people.

Perhaps the most "solid" of the roles for magnesium supplements is its role in maintaining adequate intestinal calcium absorption. There is some controversy surrounding the "optimal" dosing of magnesium to enhance calcium absorption, but most of the research on magnesium for bone metabolism and blood pressure suggests that combinations of magnesium with calcium and potassium (as in fruits and vegetables) are most effective for modulating blood pressure, and combinations of magnesium with calcium and vitamin D are most effective for maintenance of bone mass. Therefore, it seems prudent to avoid supplementing the diet with magnesium on its own and to choose instead a combination approach, as evidenced by the studies outlined in the next section.

SCIENTIFIC SUPPORT

The scientific support for magnesium as an adjunct to calcium supplements is fairly well founded. Magnesium can help improve calcium absorption, or at least prevent the drop in calcium absorption seen with suboptimal magnesium levels, and may help maintain bone density in persons at risk for excessive bone loss. Although a handful of small studies have suggested a potential role for magnesium supplements in energy metabolism by showing increased exercise efficiency and power output in athletes (Brilla and Haley, 1992), other studies have failed to show a beneficial effect on exercise performance (Terblanche et al., 1992). In general, there is no overwhelming evidence to suggest any increases in muscular strength or elevated energy levels following magnesium supplementation (Schwenk and Costley, 2002).

Blood Pressure
Most of the data on magnesium as a dietary supplement focuses on blood pressure and bone metabolism. Evidence from large population studies, such as the Health Professionals Follow-up studies from Harvard's School of Public Health, have suggested that greater magnesium intake is significantly associated with a lower risk of hypertension. Large prospective intervention trials, such as the Dietary Approaches to Stopping Hypertension study, have also shown that high blood pressure can be significantly lowered by a diet high in magnesium, potassium, and calcium (and also low in sodium and fat). These findings may suggest why diets that are high in fruits and vegetables, which also tend to be rich sources of potassium and magnesium, are also consistently associated with lower blood pressure.

Anxiety
Magnesium supplements have been associated with a reduction in anxiety, perceived stress, and depression in a handful of studies. In one study of healthy males, a magnesium-containing multimineral product delivered consistent and statistically significant reductions in anxiety and perceived stress as well as subjective reports of less fatigue and better concentration (Carroll et al., 2000). In two studies of PMS, magnesium supplementation reduced anxiety-related PMS symptoms such as nervous tension, mood swings, irritability, and anxiety. In one study (De Souza et al., 2000), magnesium (200 mg as magnesium oxide) was combined with vitamin B_6 (50 mg), showing relief of PMS symptoms within the time frame of one or two menstrual cycles (Bendich, 2000; Walker et al., 1998).

Bone Metabolism

As with the evidence linking magnesium supplements to lower blood pressure, there exist both retrospective and population studies showing a higher bone mass in people historically consuming a high-magnesium diet, as well as prospective intervention studies showing that adding magnesium supplements to a marginal diet can improve bone mass. In one study with both cross-sectional and longitudinal design (Tucker et al., 1999), higher magnesium intake was associated with greater bone mass at several skeletal sites in men and women and was further associated with a slower decline in bone density over the course of 4 years in a group of elderly volunteers. A portion of the beneficial effect of magnesium on bone mass may be related to the "alkalizing" effect of magnesium on systemic pH, an effect that could reduce the resorption of calcium from skeletal stores for the same pH-balancing effect. In addition, when magnesium is consumed along with calcium, there is some evidence for a transient increase in calcium absorption (Spencer et al., 1994) that may or may not result in long-term enhancement of calcium status.

SAFETY/DOSAGE

The daily value (DV) for magnesium is 400 mg/day, but requirements may be elevated somewhat by stressors such as exercise and when taking calcium supplements for bone building or prevention of bone loss. In addition, a number of prescription medications can increase urinary loss of magnesium (some diuretics, some antibiotics, and some chemotherapy agents such as Cisplatin).

The RDA for magnesium is 400–420 mg/day for adult men and 310–320 mg/day for adult women. The Food and Nutrition Board has established a UL for magnesium supplements of 350 mg/day (above that obtained from food and water), and the Council for Responsible Nutrition has established a NOAEL (no observed adverse effect level) for magnesium of 700 mg/day (from all sources). Excessive magnesium intake can cause diarrhea and general gastrointestinal distress as well as interfere with calcium absorption and bone metabolism.

REFERENCES

Bendich A. The potential for dietary supplements to reduce premenstrual syndrome (PMS) symptoms. J Am Coll Nutr 2000;19(1):3–12.

Brilla LR, Haley TF. Effect of magnesium supplementation on strength training in humans. J Am Coll Nutr 1992;11(3):326–329.

Carroll D, Ring C, Suter M, Willemsen G. The effects of an oral multivitamin combination with calcium, magnesium, and zinc on psychological well-being in healthy young male volunteers: a double-blind placebo-controlled trial. Psychopharmacology (Berl) 2000;150(2):220–225.

De Souza MC, Walker AF, Robinson PA, Bolland K. A synergistic effect of a daily supplement for 1 month of 200 mg magnesium plus 50 mg vitamin B6 for the relief of anxiety-related premenstrual symptoms: a randomized, double-blind, crossover study. J Womens Health Gend Based Med 2000;9(2):131–139.

Schwenk TL, Costley CD. When food becomes a drug: nonanabolic nutritional supplement use in athletes. Am J Sports Med 2002;30(6):907–916.

Spencer H, Fuller H, Norris C, Williams D. Effect of magnesium on the intestinal absorption of calcium in man. J Am Coll Nutr 1994;13(5):485–492.

Terblanche S, Noakes TD, Dennis SC, Marais D, Eckert M. Failure of magnesium supplementation to influence marathon running performance or recovery in magnesium-replete subjects. Int J Sport Nutr 1992;2(2):154–164.

Tucker KL, Hannan MT, Chen H, Cupples LA, Wilson PW, Kiel DP. Potassium, magnesium, and fruit and vegetable intakes are associated with greater bone mineral density in elderly men and women. Am J Clin Nutr 1999;69(4):727–736.

Walker AF, De Souza MC, Vickers MF, Abeyasekera S, Collins ML, Trinca LA. Magnesium supplementation alleviates premenstrual symptoms of fluid retention. J Womens Health 1998;7(9):1157–1165.

ADDITIONAL RESOURCES

Altura BM, Altura BT. New perspectives on the role of magnesium in the pathophysiology of the cardiovascular system. Clinical aspects. Magnesium 1985;4(5–6):226–244.

Altura BM, Gebrewold A, Altura BT, Brautbar N. Magnesium depletion impairs myocardial carbohydrate and lipid metabolism and cardiac bioenergetics and raises myocardial calcium content in-vivo: relationship to etiology of cardiac diseases. Biochem Mol Biol Int 1996;40(6):1183–1190.

Bhandari N, Bahl R, Taneja S. Effect of micronutrient supplementation on linear growth of children. Br J Nutr 2001;85(suppl 2):S131–S137.

Chia RY, Hughes RS, Morgan MK. Magnesium: a useful adjunct in the prevention of cerebral vasospasm following aneurysmal subarachnoid haemorrhage. J Clin Neurosci 2002;9(3):279–281.

Dorup I, Skajaa K, Thybo NK. Oral magnesium supplementation restores the concentrations of magnesium, potassium and sodium-potassium pumps in skeletal muscle of patients receiving diuretic treatment. J Intern Med 1993;233(2):117–123.

Doyle L, Flynn A, Cashman K. The effect of magnesium supplementation on biochemical markers of bone metabolism or blood pressure in healthy young adult females. Eur J Clin Nutr 1999;53(4):255–261.

Hallfrisch J, Muller DC. Does diet provide adequate amounts of calcium, iron, magnesium, and zinc in a well-educated adult population? Exp Gerontol 1993;28(4–5):473–483.

Makrides M, Crowther CA. Magnesium supplementation in pregnancy. Cochrane Database Syst Rev 2001;(4):CD000937.

Mortensen L, Charles P. Bioavailability of calcium supplements and the effect of Vitamin D: comparisons between milk, calcium carbonate, and calcium carbonate plus vitamin D. Am J Clin Nutr 1996;63(3):354–357.

Vormann J, Worlitschek M, Goedecke T, Silver B. Supplementation with alkaline minerals reduces symptoms in patients with chronic low back pain. J Trace Elem Med Biol 2001;15(2–3):179–183.

Zive MM, Nicklas TA, Busch EC, Myers L, Berenson GS. Marginal vitamin and mineral intakes of young adults: the Bogalusa Heart Study. J Adolesc Health 1996;19(1):39–47.

VITAMIN D (CALCIFEROL, CHOLECALCIFEROL)

Overall Rank

★★★★★ for correcting nutrient deficiency
★★★★★ for bone health
  ★★ for anticancer effects

OVERVIEW

Although vitamin D is typically classified as a fat-soluble vitamin, it actually functions as a hormone in the body. Because it can be manufactured by the body (formed in the skin following exposure to the ultraviolet rays of the sun), vitamin D is not technically classified as an essential nutrient at all. In the skin, exposure to ultraviolet rays converts vitamin D precursors (compounds with structures similar to cholesterol) into an inactive form of vitamin D. This inactive form is then converted to the active form by enzymes located in the liver and kidneys. Regular sunlight exposure is the primary way that most of us get our vitamin D. Food sources of vitamin D include only a few, such as milk fortified with vitamin D (100 IU/cup), cod liver oil, and fatty fish such as salmon. Small amounts of vitamin D are also found in egg yolks and liver. Because of the role of vitamin D in stimulating calcium absorption, dietary supplements for bone health are the main supplement category.

COMMENTS

The primary effect of vitamin D is to maintain calcium levels in the blood. To do this, vitamin D promotes both the absorption of calcium from the intestines into the blood and the removal of calcium from the bones into the blood. Vitamin D also reduces calcium loss in the urine. In most cases, the increased calcium absorption results in an increase in bone density and bone strength, which can help reduce the risk of osteoporosis.

For most people, there is no reason to take more than the recommended AI level (200–600 IU) of vitamin D. During the winter months, however, synthesis of vitamin D in the skin is severely reduced because of reduced exposure to sunlight. In some parts of the country (northern latitudes such as Boston and Seattle), virtually no vitamin synthesis occurs in skin during the winter months (November through February). Therefore, vitamin D supplementation should be considered for people living in northern cities as well as for those who are not exposed to sunlight on a regular basis (Margiloff et al., 2001; Patel et al., 2001). In addition, older people should consider vitamin D supplements because with aging, skin loses its ability to adequately synthesize vitamin D and kidneys lose some of their ability to convert vitamin D precursors to their most active form. People who use sunblock frequently might also consider a vitamin D supplement because a sunblock with a sun protection factor (SPF) of 8 or greater can reduce the skin's ability to produce vitamin D.

SCIENTIFIC SUPPORT

It is well accepted that adequate vitamin D levels are crucial for healthy bone development, maintenance of bone density and bone strength, and prevention of osteoporosis. Vitamin D exists in several forms within the body, with both the liver and kidney helping to convert vitamin D into its most active hormone form (1,25OH-D3). Vitamin D deficiency results in rickets (in children) and osteomalacia (in adults), both of which are characterized by a reduced level of calcium being deposited in bones and a weakening of bone strength.

Several studies have clearly demonstrated that supplemental vitamin D intake (200–1,000 IU/day), usually combined with calcium, increases bone density and helps prevent osteoporosis (Feskanich et al., 2003). In one study, 240 healthy postmenopausal women consumed calcium (900 mg/day) and vitamin D (200 IU/day) for 2 years. Results showed a reduced loss of calcium in the urine and a highly significant increase of almost 2% in lumbar spine bone mineral density (Recker et al., 1999). Another study, also in postmenopausal women, gave supplements containing 1,000 mg of calcium (as calcium carbonate) and 500 IU of vitamin D and showed a positive effect on bone density (Baeksgaard et al., 1998), even though initial calcium and vitamin D status was adequate. It is interesting to note that although supplementation with calcium and vitamin D reduces bone loss and prevents fractures in elderly people, after discontinuing the supplements, bone turnover (loss) rates return to their original high levels, and the supplement-induced increases in bone mineral density are lost within 2 years (Dawson-Hughes et al., 2000), suggesting that supplementation needs to be continued for prolonged benefits.

As with calcium supplementation and with milk consumption, some controversy exists concerning the value of vitamin D supplementation in preventing osteoporotic fractures. In shorter supplementation trials, higher calcium intake, higher milk consumption, and higher vitamin D status were associated with reduced bone loss in postmenopausal women (Dawson-Hughes, 1998). Longer observation trials, however, do not generally find a lower risk of fractures associated with calcium intake or milk consumption, but a mediating factor may be vitamin D intake. Feskanich et al. (2003) assessed the relationship between postmenopausal hip fracture risk and intake of milk, calcium, and vitamin D, finding a significant relationship only between a higher vitamin D intake and lower risk of hip fractures. Supporting this finding are data from Deroisy et al. (2002) showing that a dietary supplement combining calcium (500 mg) plus vitamin D (200 IU) for 90 days was more effective than calcium alone in reducing hyperparathyroidism in a population of postmenopausal women. Other researchers (Reginster et al., 2002) have shown related effects on serum PTH with similar combinations of calcium (500–1,000 mg/day) and vitamin D (400–880 IU/day).

SAFETY/DOSAGE

In the United States, milk is fortified with 10 µg (400 IU) of vitamin D per quart, meaning that each 1-cup serving of milk provides about one fourth of the estimated daily need for vitamin D. Because there is not sufficient evidence to establish an RDA for vitamin D, an AI was established in 1998 to ensure maintenance of healthy blood levels of active vitamin D. Men and women have the same daily AI level of vitamin D within the following age ranges: 19–50 years, 5 µg or 200 IU; 51–69 years, 10 µg or 400 IU; and 70+ years, 15 µg or 600 IU.

Because vitamin D is a fat-soluble vitamin, it is stored in the body and has the potential to reach toxic levels if taken in high doses for prolonged periods. Getting too much vitamin D from food sources is unlikely unless high consumption of cod liver oil is routine. Prolonged sunlight exposure does not cause buildup of vitamin D as the body downregulates its production when levels are adequate. The Food and Nutrition Board considers an intake of 50 µg (2,000 IU) to be the UL for vitamin D in adults. Intakes over that amount can cause nausea, diarrhea, skin rash, headaches, muscle weakness, calcium deposits, and kidney stones.

The DV for vitamin D is 400 IU, and supplements at this level have been shown to be safe and effective in reducing calcium loss and maintaining bone density in postmenopausal women. Dietary supplements are not necessary in healthy, young individuals who are frequently exposed to moderate amounts of sunlight (15 minutes or so per day). In dietary supplements, vitamin D and calcium do not have to be taken together to be effective, but many calcium/vitamin D combinations are available and may be more convenient than taking separate tablets.

REFERENCES

Baeksgaard L, Andersen KP, Hyldstrup L. Calcium and vitamin D supplementation increases spinal BMD in healthy, postmenopausal women. Osteoporos Int 1998;8(3):255–260.

Dawson-Hughes B. Vitamin D and calcium: recommended intake for bone health. Osteoporos Int 1998;8(suppl 2):S30–S34.

Dawson-Hughes B, Harris SS, Krall EA, Dallal GE. Effect of withdrawal of calcium and vitamin D supplements on bone mass in elderly men and women. Am J Clin Nutr 2000;72(3):745–750.

Deroisy R, Collette J, Albert A, Jupsin I, Reginster JY. Administration of a supplement containing both calcium and vitamin D is more effective than calcium alone to reduce secondary hyperparathyroidism in postmenopausal women with low 25(OH)vitamin D circulating levels. Aging Clin Exp Res 2002;14(1):13–17.

Feskanich D, Willett WC, Colditz GA. Calcium, vitamin D, milk consumption, and hip fractures: a prospective study among postmenopausal women. Am J Clin Nutr 2003;77(2):504–511.

Margiloff L, Harris SS, Lee S, Lechan R, Dawson-Hughes B. Vitamin D status of an outpatient clinic population. Calcif Tissue Int 2001;69(5):263–267.

Patel R, Collins D, Bullock S, Swaminathan R, Blake GM, Fogelman I. The effect of season and vitamin D supplementation on bone mineral density in healthy women: a double-masked crossover study. Osteoporos Int 2001;12(4):319–325.

Recker RR, Davies KM, Dowd RM, Heaney RP. The effect of low-dose continuous estrogen and progesterone therapy with calcium and vitamin D on bone in elderly women. A randomized, controlled trial. Ann Intern Med 1999;130(11):897–904.

Reginster JY, Zegels B, Lejeune E, Micheletti MC, Kvsaz A, Seidel L, Sarlet N. Influence of daily regimen calcium and vitamin D supplementation on parathyroid hormone secretion. Calcif Tissue Int 2002;70(2):78–82.

ADDITIONAL RESOURCES

Davies PS, Bates CJ, Cole TJ, Prentice A, Clarke PC. Vitamin D: seasonal and regional differences in preschool children in Great Britain. Eur J Clin Nutr 1999;53(3):195–198.

Feit JM. Calcium and vitamin D supplements for elderly patients. J Fam Pract 1997;45(6):471–472.

Holzherr ML, Retallack RW, Gutteridge DH, Price RI, Faulkner DL, Wilson SG, Will RK, Stewart GO, Stuckey BG, Prince RL, Criddle RA, Kent GN, Bhagat CI, Dhaliwal SS, Jamrozik K. Calcium absorption in postmenopausal osteoporosis: benefit of HRT plus calcitriol, but not HRT alone, in both malabsorbers and normal absorbers. Osteoporos Int 2000;11(1):43–51.

Jensen LB, Kollerup G, Quaade F, Sorensen OH. Bone minerals changes in obese women during a moderate weight loss with and without calcium supplementation. J Bone Miner Res 2001;16(1):141–147.

Meunier PJ. Calcium, vitamin D and vitamin K in the prevention of fractures due to osteoporosis. Osteoporos Int 1999;9(suppl 2):S48–S52.

Outila TA, Lamberg-Allardt CJ. Ergocalciferol supplementation may positively affect lumbar spine bone mineral density of vegans. J Am Diet Assoc 2000;100(6):629.

Reid IR. The roles of calcium and vitamin D in the prevention of osteoporosis. Endocrinol Metab Clin North Am 1998;27(2):389–398.

VITAMIN K (PHYLLOQUINONE, MENAQUINONE)

Overall Rank

★★★★★ for correcting nutrient deficiency
★★★★ for bone health

OVERVIEW

Vitamin K is a fat-soluble vitamin required as a coenzyme during the synthesis of many proteins involved in blood clotting and bone formation. Good food sources include brussels sprouts, avocado, liver, and dark leafy greens (spinach, kale, broccoli, parsley). One cup of spinach provides enough vitamin K to meet the current AI levels (90 μg/day for adult women and 120 μg/day for adult men). No adverse effects have been associated with vitamin K consumption from food or supplements, but patients on anticoagulant therapy should monitor their vitamin K intake to ensure a consistent daily intake.

COMMENTS

Vitamin K is involved in both blood clotting (via prothrombin synthesis) and bone metabolism (via carboxylation of osteocalcin). Vitamin K is typically added in small amounts to most multivitamins and is frequently found as part of many bone formulas. As a dietary supplement for promoting bone health, vitamin K is needed as a cofactor in the production of osteocalcin, a key protein required for bone formation, and for the adequate deposition of calcium within the bone matrix. Vitamin K is required for full activity of the osteocalcin protein, and elderly subjects with low vitamin K intake have been shown to have inadequate carboxylated osteocalcin, suboptimal bone density, and increased risk of osteoporotic fractures.

SCIENTIFIC SUPPORT

Vitamin K's primary function is to regulate normal blood clotting (owing to its role in the synthesis of prothrombin). The newest DRI report from the National Academy of Sciences establishes an AI level of vitamin K at 90 µg/day for adult women and 120 µg/day for adult men. The vitamin K content of most foods is very low (<10 µg/100 g), and the bulk of dietary vitamin K intake is provided by a few leafy green vegetables (spinach, kale, parsley, broccoli) and vegetable oils (soybean, cottonseed, canola, olive). For the two types of naturally occurring vitamin K, absorption of phylloquinone from plant foods is poor and the small amounts of menaquinone produced by intestinal bacteria provide only a minor portion of daily requirements.

In bones, vitamin K mediates the λ carboxylation of glutamyl residues on several bone proteins, most notably, the bone formation protein osteocalcin. High serum concentrations of undercarboxylated osteocalcin and low serum concentrations of vitamin K are associated with lower bone mineral density and increased risk of hip fracture. Women with higher vitamin K intakes have a significantly lower relative risk of hip fracture (about 30% lower) than do women with lower vitamin K intake (less than 70 µg/day; Booth et al., 2003). In a similar study of 888 elderly men and women, those with the highest vitamin K intake (median of 254 µg/day) had a significantly lower adjusted relative risk (0.35) of hip fracture than did those with lower vitamin K intake (median of 56 µg/day; Booth et al., 2000). Feskanich et al. (1999) have shown that the risk of hip fracture in postmenopausal women is reduced by almost half for those women with the highest lettuce consumption. Those women who consumed one or more servings of lettuce per day were 45% less likely to have low bone density compared with women eating one or fewer servings of lettuce each week. Studies in postmenopausal women and older men have shown that an increased intake of vitamin K results in an increase in bone formation and osteocalcin levels and a slowing of bone loss (McKeown et al., 2002). Another study, conducted in female athletes, also showed that 1 month of vitamin K supplementation increased the body's ability to bind calcium in the bones and resulted in a 15–20% increase in bone formation and a 20–25% decrease in bone breakdown (Craciun et al., 1998). These findings suggest that low dietary intake of vitamin K may increase the risk of hip fracture in women.

SAFETY/DOSAGE

High intake of vitamin K from either foods or supplements is not recommended for patients taking anticoagulant medications such as warfarin (Coumadin). It is widely assumed that a dietary vitamin K–warfarin interaction exists, and patients taking the drug are instructed to consume a constant dietary intake of vitamin K (to avoid fluctuations in the activity of the blood-thinning medication). In most cases, a constant dietary intake of vitamin K from dietary supplements containing AI levels (90–120 µg/day) of vitamin K is the most acceptable practice for patients on warfarin. As with any fat-soluble vitamin, chronic consumption of doses above AI levels is not recommended because of concerns regarding buildup and toxicity.

REFERENCES

Booth SL, Broe KE, Gagnon DR, Tucker KL, Hannan MT, McLean RR, Dawson-Hughes B, Wilson PW, Cupples LA, Kiel DP. Vitamin K intake and bone mineral density in women and men. Am J Clin Nutr 2003;77(2):512–516.

Booth SL, Tucker KL, Chen H, Hannan MT, Gagnon DR, Cupples LA, Wilson PW, Ordovas J, Schaefer EJ, Dawson-Hughes B, Kiel DP. Dietary vitamin K intakes are associated with hip fracture but not with bone mineral density in elderly men and women. Am J Clin Nutr 2000;71(5):1201–1208.

Craciun AM, Wolf J, Knapen MH, Brouns F, Vermeer C. Improved bone metabolism in female elite athletes after vitamin K supplementation. Int J Sports Med 1998;19(7):479–484.

Feskanich D, Weber P, Willett WC, Rockett H, Booth SL, Colditz GA. Vitamin K intake and hip fractures in women: a prospective study. Am J Clin Nutr 1999;69(1):74–79.

McKeown NM, Jacques PF, Gundberg CM, Peterson JW, Tucker KL, Kiel DP, Wilson PW, Booth SL. Dietary and nondietary determinants of vitamin K biochemical measures in men and women. J Nutr 2002;132(6):1329–1334.

ADDITIONAL RESOURCES

Booth SL, O'Brien-Morse ME, Dallal GE, Davidson KW, Gundberg CM. Response of vitamin K status to different intakes and sources of phylloquinone-rich foods: comparison of younger and older adults. Am J Clin Nutr 1999;70(3):368–377.

Garber AK, Binkley NC, Krueger DC, Suttie JW. Comparison of phylloquinone bioavailability from food sources or a supplement in human subjects. J Nutr 1999;129(6):1201–1203.

Melhus H, Michaelsson K, Kindmark A, Bergstrom R, Holmberg L, Mallmin H, Wolk A, Ljunghall S. Excessive dietary intake of vitamin A is associated with reduced bone mineral density and increased risk for hip fracture. Ann Intern Med 1998;129(10):770–778.

Meunier PJ. Calcium, vitamin D and vitamin K in the prevention of fractures due to osteoporosis. Osteoporos Int 1999;9(suppl 2):S48–S52.

Reichel H. No effect of vitamin K1 supplementation on biochemical bone markers in haemodialysis patients. Nephrol Dial Transplant 1999;14(1):249–250.

CHAPTER 5

Joint Support Supplements

Boswellia (*Boswellia serrata*)
Cetyl Myristoleate
Chondroitin Sulfate
Devil's Claw (*Harpagophytum procumbens*)
Glucosamine
Green-Lipped Mussel (*Perna canaliculus*)

Hydrolyzed Collagen Protein (HCP, Gelatin)
MSM (Methylsulfonylmethane)
Sea Cucumber (*Stichopus japonicus*, Other Genera Depending on Location)

BOSWELLIA (*BOSWELLIA SERRATA*)

Overall Rank

★★★ for inflammatory diseases
★★ for joint pain and sports recovery

OVERVIEW

Boswellia, also known as frankincense, is known for its important role in ayurvedic medicine and more recently has been used and confirmed by science for its role in inflammatory conditions. Boswellia is thought to benefit inflammation because of its content of boswellic acids, which are known specific, noncompetitive, nonredox inhibitors of 5-lipoxygenase—the key enzyme that biosynthesizes leukotrienes. The leukotrienes are thought to promote inflammatory conditions of several chronic diseases (Ammon, 2002).

COMMENTS

Although boswellia is mostly used for inflammation, joint pain, and sports injuries, its clinical efficacy has focused in other more chronic inflammatory conditions; therefore, studies are needed in the area of inflammatory conditions caused by sports injuries and in other sources of joint pain. Overall, the theory and preclinical work with boswellia seem to support its use in inflammatory conditions, and clinical studies are just beginning to confirm this.

SCIENTIFIC SUPPORT

Anti-inflammatory

BRONCHIAL ASTHMA. Gupta et al. (1998) studied the treatment of bronchial asthma with boswellia in a double-blind, placebo-controlled study. In the boswellia group, 40 patients took 300 mg 3 times daily for 6 weeks; in the control group, 40 patients were treated with 300 mg of lactose 3 times daily for 6 weeks. Symptomatic parameters studied were dyspnea; rhonchi; number of attacks; increases in FEV subset 1, FVC, and PEFR; and decreases in eosinophilic count and ESR. In the treatment group, 70% of the patients showed disappearance of the symptomatic parameters and thus improvement in their condition; in the control group, 27% showed improvement.

COLITIS. Gupta et al. (2001) studied the treatment of 30 patients with chronic colitis and gave 20 patients a boswellia gum preparation (900 mg/day divided in three doses for 6 weeks), and 10 patients sulfasalazine (3 g/day divided in three doses for 6 weeks). They concluded that boswellia was an effective treatment with few side effects, because 14 of the 20 patients treated went into remission, and furthermore, 18 of the 20 patients showed improvement in one or more parameters of stool properties; histopathology and scanning electron microscopy; and hemoglobin, serum iron, calcium, phosphorus, proteins, total leukocytes, and eosinophils. In comparison, in the group taking sulfasalazine, 4 of 10 went into remission, and 6 of 10 showed improvement in one or more of the previously mentioned parameters. Because the inflammatory processes of colitis is associated with leukotrienes, boswellia was thought to act to counter the inflammatory symptoms by being a known non-redox, noncompetitive inhibitor of 5-lipoxygenase (which is responsible for the synthesis of leukotrienes). In a similar earlier study (Gupta et al., 1997), patients with ulcerative colitis grades 2 and 3 were given boswellia (350 mg 3 times daily for 6 weeks) and compared with patients taking sulfasalazine (1 g 3 times daily). The parameters studied were stool properties; histopathology and scan microscopy of rectal biopsies; and blood parameters, including hemoglobin, serum iron, calcium, phosphorus, proteins, total leukocytes, and eosinophils. Treatment with boswellia compared favorably with treatment with sulfasalazine: 82% of patients taking boswellia went into remission versus 75% of patients taking sulfasalazine.

CROHN DISEASE. Gerhardt et al. (2001) studied patients with Crohn disease, comparing those treated with boswellia (a boswellic acid preparation called H15) with those treated with mesalazine in a randomized, double-blind, parallel group comparison. The main parameter studied for outcome was the Crohn Disease Activity Index (CDAI) assessment from the start to the end of treatment. In the boswellia group of 44 patients, the CDAI was reduced by 90; in the mesalazine group of 39 patients, the CDAI was reduced by 53. These outcomes, however, were not statistically significantly different. The authors reported that the study confirmed that treatment with boswellia is not inferior to mesalazine treatment and when compared in terms of risk-benefit, boswellia is superior.

Edema and Leukoencephalopathy

In an uncontrolled clinical study, boswellia (phytotherapeutic agent H15) was given to patients who had either edema (from tumor progression) or leukoencephalopathy (caused by radiation treatment). The H15 preparation was given orally at 1,200 mg 3 times daily. Magnetic resonance imaging and clinical examinations were performed before treatment and at weeks 1 and 4 after treatment began. Two of the seven patients with edema and three of the five patients with leukoencephalopathy had reduced edema after treatment. All patients tolerated H15 well, with no side effects reported (Streffer et al., 2001).

Rheumatoid Arthritis and Osteoarthritis

In a multicenter, controlled clinical trial, 18 patients were given boswellia (H15, 3,600 mg/day) and 19 were given a placebo in addition to their previous therapy (with the ability to adjust amounts of nonsteroidal anti-inflammatory drugs [NSAIDs] whenever needed). The parameters studied at baseline and at 6 and 12 weeks into the study were the Ritchies Index for swelling and pain, ESR, CRP, pain on VAS, and NSAID dose. There were no differences in either subjective, clinical, or laboratory analysis of the parameters studied between the two groups (Sander et al., 1998).

Two promising clinical trials were conducted involving a formulation with boswellia in treatment of osteoarthritis. Because other substances were used in the mixtures tested, it is not known to what degree boswellia contributed to the efficacy of the studies (Kulkarni et al., 1991, 1992).

SAFETY/DOSAGE

The typical dosage of boswellia is about 450–1,200 mg/day, taken in three divided doses throughout the day. Standardized extracts are recommended to provide 30–60% boswellic acids. No reports of serious side effects are known, but some studies have mentioned mild and transitory gastrointestinal upset (Kimmatkar et al., 2003).

REFERENCES

Ammon HP. Boswellic acids (components of frankincense) as the active principle in treatment of chronic inflammatory diseases. Wien Med Wochenschr 2002;152(15–16):373–378.

Gerhardt H, Seifert F, Buvari P, Vogelsang H, Repges R. Therapy of active Crohn's disease with Boswellia serrata extract H15. Zeitschrift Fuer Gastroenterologie 2001;39(1):11–17.

Gupta I, Gupta V, Parihar A, Gupta S, Ludtke R, Safayhi H, Ammon HP. Effects of Boswellia serrata gum resin in patients with bronchial asthma: results of a double-blind, placebo-controlled, 6-week clinical study. Eur J Med Res 1998;3(11):511–514.

Gupta I, Parihar A, Malhotra P, Gupta S, Ludtke R, Safayhi H, Ammon HP. Effects of gum resin of Boswellia serrata in patients with chronic colitis. Planta Med 2001;67(5):391–395.

Gupta I, Parihar A, Malhotra P, Singh GB, Ludtke R, Safayhi H, Ammon HP. Effects of Boswellia serrata gum resin in patients with ulcerative colitis. Eur J Med Res 1997;2(1):37–43.

Kimmatkar N, Thawani V, Hingorani L, Khiyani R. Efficacy and tolerability of Boswellia serrata extract in treatment of osteoarthritis of knee—a randomized double blind placebo controlled trial. Phytomedicine 2003;10(1):3–7.

Kulkarni RR, Patki PS, Jog VP, Gandage SG, Patwardhan B. Efficacy of an Ayervedic formulation in rheumatoid arthritis, a double-blind placebo-controlled cross-over study. Indian J Pharmacol 1992;24(2):98–101.

Kulkarni RR, Patki PS, Jog VP, Gandage SG, Patwardhan B. Treatment of osteoarthritis with a herbomineral formulation: a double-blind, placebo-controlled, cross-over study. J Ethnopharmacol 1991;33(1–2):91–95.

Sander O, Herborn G, Rau R. Is H15 (resin extract of Boswellia serrata, "incense") a useful supplement to established drug therapy of chronic polyarthritis? Results of a double-blind pilot study. Z Rheumatol 1998;57(1):11–16.

Streffer JR, Bitzer M, Schabet M, Dichgans J, Weller M. Response of radiochemotherapy-associated cerebral edema to a phytotherapeutic agent, H15. Neurology 2001;56(9):1219–1221.

CETYL MYRISTOLEATE

Overall Rank

★★★ for joint pain

OVERVIEW

Cetyl myristoleate, or cis-9-cetyl myristoleate, is a combination of cetylated fatty acids (CFAs)—primarily, myristoleic acid (14:1)—and a long-chain alcohol molecule, cetyl alcohol. Cetyl myristoleate and other CFAs are naturally found in nuts, vegetables, and dairy products and may be especially high in the tissues of people who consume a diet rich in olive oil. Oral dosing with cetyl myristoleate in patients with osteoarthritis has shown a benefit in improving pain, stiffness, and mobility, yet the precise mechanism remains unclear. Studies suggest that cetyl myristoleate may serve as a general anti-inflammatory as well as a surfactant to lubricate joints (Diehl and May, 1994; Hesslink et al., 2002). Myristoleic acid, a component of cetyl myristoleate, has been shown to inhibit 5-lipoxygenase in tissue culture, suggesting general anti-inflammatory effects for the cetylated form of the fatty acid (Morelli et al., 2003).

COMMENTS

Cetyl myristoleate, also known as CMO, CM, and CM complex, appears to provide some anti-inflammatory benefits when supplemented to patients with osteoarthritis. Through its proposed mechanisms of action, which include inhibition of both 5-lipoxygenase (Bonnet et al., 1995; Iguchi et al., 2001) and 5-α-reductase (Liang and Liao, 1992), cetyl myristoleate may have clinical benefits as a general anti-inflammatory agent and as a potential regulator of androgen activity in various target tissues, such as the prostate gland and breast tissue. Because at this point cetyl myristoleate supplementation has been studied in humans only as a pain reliever in mild-to-moderate cases of osteoarthritis, it should be viewed as a general anti-inflammatory agent with specific utility in cases of arthritis.

SCIENTIFIC SUPPORT

Epidemiological and clinical research indicate that patients with both rheumatoid arthritis and osteoarthritis benefit from higher levels of dietary eicosapentaenoic acid and docosahexaenoic acid—whether consumed in the form of fatty fish (which are high in these ω-3 polyunsaturated fatty acids) or as dietary supplements of fish body oils (Kremer, 2000; Kremer et al., 1985, 1987). In addition, cetylated monounsaturated fatty acids have been shown to provide protection against arthritis in rats (Diehl and May, 1994) and increased knee range of motion and reduced pain in patients with osteoarthritis (Hesslink et al., 2002).

The process of inflammation in osteoarthritis involves the release of proinflammatory cytokines (e.g., interleukin 1β and tumor necrosis factor α). Various combinations of fatty acids have been proposed to reduce chronic inflammation by reducing cytokine expression (e.g., leukotriene B4 and interleukin 1; Curtis et al., 2000; Kremer, 2000) and reducing the activity of proteoglycan-degrading enzymes and their signaling (Heraud et al., 2000; Kremer, 1996). The proposed involvement of both chronic inflammation and androgen dysregulation in some forms of cancer, most notably cancers of the prostate and breast, suggest a potential role for fatty acids with demonstrated effect in modulating these events. Myristoleic acid has been identified as a putative active compound in extracts of saw palmetto (Serenoa repens, typically used for treatment of benign prostatic hyperplasia) with cytotoxic activity against isolated prostate cancer cells (Iguchi et al., 2001). Myristoleic acid has also been strongly positively correlated with total intake of conjugated linoleic acid (also a putative anticancer agent) and negatively correlated with breast cancer incidence (Simonsen et al., 1998).

Cetyl myristoleate was first identified in isolates from mice that were resistant to experimentally induced arthritis. Whether isolated or synthesized from myristoleic acid and cetyl alcohol, the resulting cetyl myristoleate protected rodents from induced arthritis while other fatty acids (cetyl oleate, cetyl myristate, and cetyl elaidate) were ineffective (Diehl and May, 1994). In humans, cetyl myristoleate in a complex of CFAs has been shown to reduce pain, improve knee function, and increase knee range of motion following oral supplementation for 68 days (Hesslink et al., 2002) and following topical application for 30 days (Kraemer et al., 2003; Ratamess et al., 2003).

SAFETY/DOSAGE

No adverse side effects are known for dietary supplements containing cetyl myristoleate, but a test-tube study has suggested a possible increase in glycolysis (Duan et al., 1997), and an animal study has shown an elevation of serum cholesterol levels (Smith et al., 1996). Whether or not these effects would be seen in human feeding studies is unknown, but one study using 2 g/day of CFAs for 2 months found no adverse effects in subjects with osteoarthritis (Hesslink et al., 2002). Cetyl myristoleate is known to be absorbed from the gastrointestinal tract (Gallaher et al., 2002; Islam et al., 2003) but may be less well absorbed across the skin compared with other fatty acids (Taguchi et al., 1999). In the most convincing study supporting the antipain benefits of cetyl myristoleate, patients with osteoarthritis received 2 g/day of cetylated fatty acids for a period of 2 months (Hesslink et al., 2002).

REFERENCES

Bonnet C, Bertin P, Cook-Moreau J, Chable-Rabinovitch H, Treves R, Rigaud M. Lipoxygenase products and expression of 5-lipoxygenase and 5-lipoxygenase-activating protein in human cultured synovial cells. Prostaglandins 1995;50(3):127–135.

Curtis CL, Hughes CE, Flannery CR, Little CB, Harwood JL, Caterson B. N-3 fatty acids specifically modulate catabolic factors involved with articular cartilage degradation. J Biol Chem 2000;275:721–724.

Diehl HW, May EL. Cetyl myristoleate isolated from Swiss albino mice: an apparent protective agent against adjuvant arthritis in rats. J Pharm Sci 1994;83(3):296–299.

Duan YJ, Murase S, Okuda J, Tamura A, Miwa I. Stimulatory effect of fatty acid treatment on glucose utilization in human erythrocytes. Biochim Biophys Acta 1997;1334(1):89–97.

Gallaher DD, Gallaher CM, Hesslink R Jr. Digestion and metabolism of cetylated fatty acids in rats. FASEB J 2002;16(4):A365.

Heraud F, Heraud A, Harmand MF. Apoptosis in normal and osteoarthritic human articular cartilage. Ann Rheum Dis 2000;59:959–965.

Hesslink R, Armstrong D, Nagendran MV, Sreevatsan S, Barathur R. Cetylated fatty acids improve knee function in patients with osteoarthritis. J Rheumatol 2002;29:1708–1712.

Iguchi K, Okumura N, Usui S, Sajiki H, Hirota K, Hirano K. Myristoleic acid, a cytotoxic component in the extract from Serenoa repens, induces apoptosis and necrosis in human prostatic LNCaP cells. Prostate 2001;47(1):59–65.

Islam A, Gallaher CM, Gallaher DD. Absorption and metabolism of a cetylated fatty acid. FASEB J 2003;17(4):A341.

Kraemer WJ, Ratamess NA, Anderson JA, Tiberio DP, Joyce ME, Messinger BN, French DN, Sharman MJ, Rubin MR, Gomez AL, Volek JS, Hesslink R Jr. The Effects of Cetylated Fatty Acid Cream on Pain, Range of Motion and Quality of Life of Patients with Osteoarthritis. San Francisco, CA: American College of Sports Medicine, 2003.

Kremer JM. Effects of modulation of inflammatory and immune parameters in patients with rheumatic and inflammatory disease receiving dietary supplementation of N-3 and N-6 fatty acids. Lipids 1996;31(suppl):S243–S247.

Kremer JM. N-3 fatty acid supplements in rheumatoid arthritis. Am J Clin Nutr 2000;71(suppl):349S–351S.

Kremer JM, Bigauoette J, Michalek AV, Timchalk MA, Lininger L, Rynes RI, Huyck C, Zieminski J, Bartholomew LE. Effects of manipulation of dietary fatty acids on clinical manifestations of rheumatoid arthritis. Lancet 1985;1:184–187.

Kremer JM, Jubiz W, Michalek A, Rynes RI, Bartholomew LE, Bigaouette J, Timchalk M, Beeler D, Lininger L. Fish-oil fatty acid supplementation in active rheumatoid arthritis. A double-blinded, controlled, crossover study. Ann Intern Med 1987;106:497–503.

Liang T, Liao S. Inhibition of steroid 5 alpha-reductase by specific aliphatic unsaturated fatty acids. Biochem J 1992;285(pt 2):557–562.

Ratamess NA, Kraemer WJ, Anderson JA, Tiberio DP, Joyce ME, Messinger BN, French DN, Sharman MJ, Rubin MR, Gomez AL, Volek JS, Hesslink R Jr. The Effects of a Cetylated Fatty Acid Cream on Functional Mobility and Performance in Patients with Osteoarthritis. San Francisco, CA: American College of Sports Medicine, 2003.

Simonsen NR, Fernandez-Crehuet Navajas J, Martin-Moreno JM, Strain JJ, Huttunen JK, Martin BC, Thamm M, Kardinaal AF, van't Veer P, Kok FJ, Kohlmeier L. Tissue stores of individual monounsaturated fatty acids and breast cancer: the EURAMIC study. European Community Multicenter Study on Antioxidants, Myocardial Infarction, and Breast Cancer. Am J Clin Nutr 1998;68(1):134–141.

Smith DR, Knabe DA, Cross HR, Smith SB. A diet containing myristoleic plus palmitoleic acids elevates plasma cholesterol in young growing swine. Lipids 1996;31(8):849–858.

Taguchi K, Fukushima S, Yamaoka Y, Takeuchi Y, Suzuki M. Enhancement of propylene glycol distribution in the skin by high purity cis-unsaturated fatty acids with different alkyl chain lengths having different double bond position. Biol Pharm Bull 1999;22(4):407–411.

ADDITIONAL RESOURCES

Barathur RR, Bookout JB, Sreevatsan S, Freedland ES, Hesslink RL Jr. A fatty acid ester (CMC) improves quality of life outcomes in osteoarthritis (OA) patients. FASEB J 2001;15(4):A265.

Hesslink RL, Sprouse S. The effects of a cetylated fatty acid complex on canine osteoarthritis. Presented at the 2nd International Symposium on Rehabilitation and Physical Therapy in Veterinary Medicine, Knoxville, TN, 2002.

Jiang J, Wolk A, Vessby B. Relation between the intake of milk fat and the occurrence of conjugated linoleic acid in human adipose tissue. Am J Clin Nutr 1999;70(1):21–27.

CHONDROITIN SULFATE

Overall Rank

★★★★ for joint health

OVERVIEW

Chondroitin sulfate falls into a category of compounds known as glycosaminoglycans—basically, long chains of specialized polysaccharides (sugars). In the body, chondroitin is used as a building block for larger structures known as proteoglycans, which are in turn used to form connective tissues such as cartilage. Chondroitin is related in structure and function to another sugar derivative, glucosamine, both of which are widely used as dietary supplements to nourish joint cartilage. Chondroitin sulfate is not found in the diet in appreciable amounts. The primary source is animal cartilage (such as the trachea of cows). Like glucosamine, chondroitin supplements are typically marketed to consumers with joint pain, whether or not true osteoarthritis exists.

COMMENTS

Now that a bit more is known about the effectiveness of chondroitin sulfate, it appears that the supplements can indeed result in a reduction in the pain associated with osteoarthritis (following about 2–4 months of treatment). Because the scientific data are also quite strong for the effectiveness of glucosamine in alleviating joint pain, it may be wise to select chondroitin supplements that include the effective dose of glucosamine (1,500 mg/day).

SCIENTIFIC SUPPORT

The theory behind the use of chondroitin sulfate to treat osteoarthritis involves two primary concepts. The first, and most basic, is that chondroitin sulfate simply provides the raw material that cartilage needs to repair itself. The second theory is that chondroitin sulfate may block the activity of enzymes that break down cartilage, thereby reducing inflammation and protecting cartilage from further damage. Both theories are interesting in light of the clinical findings that chondroitin supplementation can relieve much of the pain and stiffness associated with mild-to-moderate osteoarthritis in many parts of the body but that these supplements are only effective in osteoarthritis and have no pure pain-relieving effect in other conditions (Conrozier, 1998). For many years, critics of chondroitin sulfate use for treating arthritis argued that the large size of the chondroitin sulfate molecule would prevent it from being absorbed into the body. It is now known, however, that as much as 10–20% of the chondroitin sulfate is absorbed intact (and perhaps substantially more for the newer low-molecular-weight chondroitin), while the remaining percentage is likely digested and absorbed as its component parts (Conte et al., 1995; Ronca and Conte, 1993; Silvestro et al., 1994).

Until recently, the scientific evidence for the effectiveness of chondroitin sulfate in alleviating joint pain has been relatively weak. Several small studies have provided some evidence of a reduction in joint pain, but several other studies have found no clear benefits (McAlindon and Biggee, 2005). In studies of the combined use of glucosamine (typically, 1,500 mg/day) and chondroitin (typically, 1,200 mg/day), some authors have attributed the beneficial changes in pain or stiffness to glucosamine rather than to chondroitin or the combination (McAlindon et al., 2000; Richy et al., 2003). Separate groups of researchers have performed meta-analyses of all studies using chondroitin sulfate to treat osteoarthritis.

This type of statistical analysis gathers the evidence from the available research studies and looks at them together, allowing researchers to combine several small studies into one large analysis and providing scientists with more *power* (a statistical term) to determine whether an actual beneficial effect exists for a treatment. Both research groups found that over the course of approximately 4 months of treatment, chondroitin sulfate was significantly superior to placebo in relieving joint pain and that patients taking chondroitin sulfate showed improvements of at least 50% in measurements such as pain level, joint stiffness, and walking speed (McAlindon et al., 2000; Richy et al., 2003).

The pain-relieving effects of chondroitin have been compared favorably to NSAIDs such as naproxen and ibuprofen (Bucsi and Poor, 1998; Rovetta et al., 2002). Several studies demonstrate a significant reduction in the amount of over-the-counter pain relievers used in subjects taking chondroitin versus placebo (Nguyen et al., 2001). When examining the course of pain relief, several authors have found that NSAIDs offer a quicker onset of action but pain reappears following cessation of treatment, whereas chondroitin takes longer to become effective but the therapeutic response lasts up to 3 months following cessation of supplements (Morreale et al., 1996). In other studies, chondroitin sulfate appears to slow the progression of cartilage degradation in the knee joint—an effect measured by a stabilization of the medial femorotibial (knee) joint width (Conrozier, 1998; Uebelhart et al., 1998). Joints of the fingers appear to respond favorably to chondroitin, with supplements of either chondroitin sulfate or chondroitin polysulfate being shown to prevent the progression (but not the development) of erosive osteoarthritis (Rovetta et al., 2002; Verbruggen et al., 2002). Additionally, at least one report suggests that topically applied chondroitin has some benefits in alleviating joint pain in patients with osteoarthritis (Cohen et al., 2003), but it is unclear whether this effect is truly the result of the chondroitin or to other ingredients (e.g., camphor) in the topical preparation.

SAFETY/DOSAGE

Aside from some mild gastrointestinal complaints (heartburn and nausea), chondroitin sulfate has not been associated with any serious adverse side effects. The typical dosage recommendation for chondroitin supplementation is 1,200 mg/day, but effective doses studied have ranged from 800 to 1,600 mg/day (supplemented alone or in combination with glucosamine). Although the daily dose is frequently supplied in divided doses of 400 mg (taken 3 times a day) or 600 mg (taken 2 times a day), taking the entire 1,200 mg in one dose appears to be well tolerated and just as effective in alleviating joint pain (Bourgeois et al., 1998). Many dietary supplements combine chondroitin with glucosamine, but it is still not known whether this combination of ingredients is any better than either supplement on its own.

REFERENCES

Bourgeois P, Chales G, Dehais J, Delcambre B, Kuntz JL, Rozenberg S. Efficacy and tolerability of chondroitin sulfate 1200 mg/day vs chondroitin sulfate 3 x 400 mg/day vs placebo. Osteoarthritis Cartilage 1998;6(suppl A):25–30.

Bucsi L, Poor G. Efficacy and tolerability of oral chondroitin sulfate as a symptomatic slow-acting drug for osteoarthritis (SYSADOA) in the treatment of knee osteoarthritis. Osteoarthritis Cartilage 1998;6(suppl A):31–36.

Cohen M, Wolfe R, Mai T, Lewis D. A randomized, double blind, placebo controlled trial of a topical cream containing glucosamine sulfate, chondroitin sulfate, and camphor for osteoarthritis of the knee. J Rheumatol 2003;30(3):523–528.

Conrozier T. Anti-arthrosis treatments: efficacy and tolerance of chondroitin sulfates (CS 4&6). Presse Med 1998;27(36):1862–1865.

Conte A, Volpi N, Palmieri L, Bahous I, Ronca G. Biochemical and pharmacokinetic aspects of oral treatment with chondroitin sulfate. Arzneimittelforschung 1995;45(8):918–925.

McAlindon TE, Biggee BA. Nutritional factors and osteoarthritis: recent developments. Curr Opin Rheumato 2005;17(5):647–652.

McAlindon TE, LaValley MP, Gulin JP, Felson DT. Glucosamine and chondroitin for treatment of osteoarthritis: a systematic quality assessment and meta-analysis. JAMA 2000;283(11):1469–1475.

Morreale P, Manopulo R, Galati M, Boccanera L, Saponati G, Bocchi L. Comparison of the antiinflammatory efficacy of chondroitin sulfate and diclofenac sodium in patients with knee osteoarthritis. J Rheumatol 1996;23(8):1385–1391.

Nguyen P, Mohamed SE, Gardiner D, Salinas T. A randomized double-blind clinical trial of the effect of chondroitin sulfate and glucosamine hydrochloride on temporomandibular joint disorders: a pilot study. Cranio 2001;19(2):130–139.

Richy F, Bruyere O, Ethgen O, Cucherat M, Henrotin Y, Reginster JY. Structural and symptomatic efficacy of glucosamine and chondroitin in knee osteoarthritis: a comprehensive meta-analysis. Arch Intern Med 2003;163(13):1514–1522.

Ronca G, Conte A. Metabolic fate of partially depolymerized shark chondroitin sulfate in man. Int J Clin Pharmacol Res 1993;13(suppl):27–34.

Rovetta G, Monteforte P, Molfetta G, Balestra V. Chondroitin sulfate in erosive osteoarthritis of the hands. Int J Tissue React 2002;24(1):29–32.

Silvestro L, Lanzarotti E, Marchi E, Gori M, Pescador R, Ferro L, Milani MR, Da Col R, Coppini A. Human pharmacokinetics of glycosaminoglycans using deuterium-labeled and unlabeled substances: evidence for oral absorption. Semin Thromb Hemost 1994;20(3):281–292.

Uebelhart D, Thonar EJ, Delmas PD, Chantraine A, Vignon E. Effects of oral chondroitin sulfate on the progression of knee osteoarthritis: a pilot study. Osteoarthritis Cartilage 1998;6(suppl A):39–46.

Verbruggen G, Goemaere S, Veys EM. Systems to assess the progression of finger joint osteoarthritis and the effects of disease modifying osteoarthritis drugs. Clin Rheumatol 2002;21(3):231–243.

ADDITIONAL RESOURCES

Das A Jr, Hammad TA. Efficacy of a combination of FCHG49 glucosamine hydrochloride, TRH122 low molecular weight sodium chondroitin sulfate and manganese ascorbate in the management of knee osteoarthritis. Osteoarthritis Cartilage 2000;8(5):343–350.

Leffler CT, Philippi AF, Leffler SG, Mosure JC, Kim PD. Glucosamine, chondroitin, and manganese ascorbate for degenerative joint disease of the knee or low back: a randomized, double-blind, placebo-controlled pilot study. Mil Med 1999;164(2):85–91.

Mazieres B, Combe B, Phan Van A, Tondut J, Grynfeltt M. Chondroitin sulfate in osteoarthritis of the knee: a prospective, double blind, placebo controlled multicenter clinical study. J Rheumatol 2001;28(1):173–181.

McAlindon TE, LaValley MP, Gulin JP, Felson DT. Glucosamine and chondroitin for treatment of osteoarthritis: a systematic quality assessment and meta-analysis. JAMA 2000;283(11):1469–1475.

Towheed TE, Anastassiades TP. Glucosamine and chondroitin for treating symptoms of osteoarthritis: evidence is widely touted but incomplete. JAMA 2000;283(11):1483–1484.

DEVIL'S CLAW (*HARPAGOPHYTUM PROCUMBENS*)

Overall Rank

★★★★   for joint, low back, and arthritis pain

OVERVIEW

This herb's name definitely stimulates the imagination, but imagination may not be far from reality: devil's claw produces a hard fruit with large clawlike appendages that lie waiting for a passerby on which to grip and hitch a ride for dispersal, only to eventually work its way into or tear out of the skin of its host. It is native to South Africa (though unrelated "devil's claws" are found in North America) and traditional healers have used it to reduce pain and inflammation. Today, its anti-inflammatory attributes are being confirmed by science, and it is primarily used as an herb for the pain and inflammation of arthritis and back pain. The German Commission E has approved its claims for "degenerative disorders of the locomotor system" (Blumenthal et al., 1998).

COMMENTS

Early preclinical and clinical studies showed mixed results, indicating that perhaps only certain types of inflammatory disease benefit from devil's claw (Chrubasik et al., 2003). More recent clinical data, however, have indicated a benefit for back pain and osteoarthritis of the knee and hip (Chantre et al., 2000).

SCIENTIFIC SUPPORT

In a randomized, double-blind, double-placebo clinical study involving patients with exacerbated low back pain, Chrubasik et al. (2003) compared a devil's claw extract (Doloteffin) to the COX-2 inhibitor rofecoxib. Eighty-eight patients were split into two groups and given either devil's claw extract (60 mg/day) or rofecoxib (12.5 mg/day) for 6 weeks. Rescue medication of 400 mg/day of tramadol was allowed all participants. No significant differences between outcome measures were observed, but there was a trend toward greater pain reduction and fewer side effects from the devil's claw group.

A postmarketing survey was performed to assess the safety and efficacy of a proprietary devil's claw extract (Doloteffin) in 227 people suffering from back pain or osteoarthritis pain of the knee or hip. The parameters measured were several validated and unvalidated measures of pain and symptoms. The authors concluded that 50–70% of the participants bene-fited from the treatment with Doloteffin, and that both the generic and disease-specific outcomes improved in all groups. Few adverse effects were reported, with 10% found to be possibly caused by Doloteffin (Chrubasik et al., 2002a, 2000b).

Gobel et al. (2001) examined the effect of devil's claw extract (480 mg of Rivoltan 2 times a day or placebo for 4 weeks) in a randomized, double-blind, placebo-controlled study on people with slight to moder-ate muscular tension or slight muscular pain of the back, shoulder, and neck. The treatment group showed clear improvement in clinical global scores and in patient and physician subjective ratings. Highly significant results were found in the test measures of the visual analogue scale, pressure algometer test, muscle stiffness test, and muscular ischaemia test. The mechanism of action of the extract was reported to have an influence on sensory and vascular muscular response and to reduce muscle stiffness without affecting the central nervous system. No serious adverse effects were noted, and tolerability was good.

Patients suffering from nonradicular back pain were studied in an open, multicenter study of devil's claw extract (480 mg of Rivoltan 2 times a day for 8 weeks). Significant improvement of pain symptoms and mobility were found (using the multidimensional pain scale, Arhus back pain index, finger-floor distance, and Schober's sign). No serious side effects were found, and the authors reported that it appeared to be an excellent herbal alternative for chronic back pain, though further studies were needed (Laudahn and Walper, 2001).

A double-blind, randomized, multicenter, comparison study was per-formed on a 4-month treatment of Harpadol (six 435-mg capsules per day) versus diacerhein (100 mg/day) in 122 patients with knee and hip osteoarthritis. Although there were no significant differences between the two groups in efficacy, by the end of the study, patients in the devil's claw treatment group were using significantly less of other pain medications and had fewer reported adverse effects. The authors con-cluded that Harpadol is safer than and equally as effective as diacerhein (Chantre et al., 2000; Chrubasik et al., 2002a, 2002b). A similar study was performed to compare the efficacy of devil's claw extract versus diacerhein, and after 4 months of treatment, the same overall results were found. The devil's claw extract showed similar efficacy for knee and hip osteoarthritis and fewer side effects than diacerhein, and the need for other pain medications was reduced in the devil's claw group (Leblan et al., 2000).

In a randomized, double-blind study involving 197 patients with chronic back pain, two doses of devil's claw extract (WS 1531, 600 and 1,200 mg containing 50 and 100 mg of the marker compound harpagoside, respectively) were compared with a placebo over 4 weeks of treatment. Using the principal outcome measure of the number of patients free from pain without using the rescue medication (tramadol), the results were 3 for the placebo group, 6 for the 600-mg group, and

10 for the 1,200-mg group. Using analysis based on the Arhus back pain index, however, the 600-mg group showed more benefits. The only minor reported side effects were mild and infrequent gastrointestinal upset (Chrubasik et al., 1999).

SAFETY/DOSAGE

The typical dosage of devil's claw extract is between 600 and 6,000 mg/day (standardized between 1% and 3% of iridoid glycosides, often calculated as harpagoside), taken in divided doses. Only mild side effects of transitory gastrointestinal upset have been reported, if any. Because devil's claw extract is able to stimulate gastric acid secretion, it is not recommended for people with ulcers.

REFERENCES

Blumenthal M, Busse WR, Goldberg A, Gruenwald J, Hall T, Riggins CW, Rister RS, eds. The Complete German Commission E Monographs. Austin, TX: American Botanical Council, 1998.

Chantre P, Cappelaere A, Leblan D, Guedon D, Vandermander J, Fournie B. Efficacy and tolerance of Harpagophytum procumbens versus diacerhein in treatment of osteoarthritis. Phytomedicine 2000;7(3):177–183.

Chrubasik S, Junck H, Breitschwerdt H, Conradt C, Zappe H. Effectiveness of Harpagophytum extract WS 1531 in the treatment of exacerbation of low back pain: a randomized, placebo-controlled, double-blind study. Eur J Anaesthesiol 1999;16(2):118–129.

Chrubasik S, Model A, Black A, Pollak S. A randomized double-blind pilot study comparing Doloteffin and Vioxx in the treatment of low back pain. Rheumatology (Oxford) 2003;42(1):141–148.

Chrubasik S, Pollak S, Black A. Effectiveness of devil's claw for osteoarthritis. Rheumatology 2002a;41(11):1332–1333.

Chrubasik S, Thanner J, Kunzel O, Conradt C, Black A, Pollak S. Comparison of outcome measures during treatment with the proprietary Harpagophytum extract Doloteffin in patients with pain in the lower back, knee or hip. Phytomedicine 2002b;9(3):181–194.

Gobel H, Heinze A, Ingwersen M, Niederberger U, Gerber D. Effects of Harpagophytum procumbens LI 174 (devil's claw) on sensory, motor and vascular muscle agility in the treatment of unspecific back pain. Schmerz 2001;15(1):10–18.

Laudahn D, Walper A. Efficacy and tolerance of Harpagophytum extract LI 174 in patients with chronic non-radicular back pain. Phytother Res 2001;15(7):621–624.

Leblan D, Chantre P, Fournie B. Harpagophytum procumbens in the treatment of knee and hip osteoarthritis. Four-month results of a prospective, multicenter, double-blind trial versus diacerhein. Joint Bone Spine 2000;67(5):462–467.

GLUCOSAMINE

Overall Rank
★★★★★ for joint health

OVERVIEW

Glucosamine is an aminopolysaccharide (a combination of an amino acid—glutamine—and a sugar—glucose). Glucosamine is concentrated in joint cartilage where it is incorporated into longer chains known as glycosaminoglycans and finally into very large structures known as proteoglycans. The proteoglycans function to attract water into the joint space for lubrication of the cartilage during movement. Glucosamine is available in supplements as glucosamine sulfate, glucosamine hydrochloride, and N-acetylglucosamine. Chondroitin sulfate (also covered in this chapter) is often combined with glucosamine. These supplements are generally promoted with claims for protecting joints and joint cartilage from injury, alleviating the stiffness and pain of osteoarthritis, and reducing inflammation.

COMMENTS

Glucosamine supplements typically take 1–3 months to exert noticeable effects (reduced pain and stiffness) in people with mild-to-moderate degrees of osteoarthritis. Because arthritis pain is one of the most debilitating conditions, most people dealing with such pain would gladly invest a dollar or two per day in a supplement that relieved their discomfort and helped repair their damaged cartilage tissue. For people with existing chronic joint pain, glucosamine supplements (whether or not combined with chondroitin sulfate) are worth the modest dollar investment for the benefits they deliver.

SCIENTIFIC SUPPORT

The major principle behind glucosamine supplementation is that the glucosamine is delivered to the joint space and incorporated into proteoglycans of joint cartilage to maintain structure and repair damage. Glucosamine may also stimulate chondrocytes (cartilage cells) to begin producing healthy new cartilage matrix (both collagen and proteoglycans).

Numerous European studies and a handful of North American reports show a clear benefit of glucosamine supplements for relief of joint pain and stiffness associated with arthritis (Das and Hammad, 2000; McAlindon et al., 2000a; Muller-Fassbender et al., 1994). One Australian study has even suggested a pain-relieving effect in osteoarthritis of topically applied glucosamine/chondroitin (Cohen et al., 2003), but that effect may have been the result of camphor in the topical formulation. While glucosamine supplements have been reported to modify disease activity in studies of rheumatoid arthritis (Lard et al., 2001), the majority of glucosamine studies have examined osteoarthritis of mild-to-moderate severity. Most studies examine patients with osteoarthritis of the knee and hip, but examples of glucosamine's pain-relieving effects can be found in studies of osteoarthritis of the fingers and temporomandibular joint (Nguyen et al., 2001; Thie et al., 2001). Several studies have compared the pain-relieving effects of glucosamine (1,500 mg/day) to NSAIDs such as ibuprofen (1,200 mg/day). These studies generally find that although NSAIDs tend to exert their pain-relieving effects faster (within the first week of treatment; Muller-Fassbender et al., 1994), the difference between treatments lessens with time (similar benefits at 2–4 weeks), with fewer side effects reported among glucosamine users (6% versus 35% on ibuprofen). When followed posttreatment, glucosamine shows a carryover effect, whereby pain and use of pain relievers is reduced for 3–4 months following cessation of supplementation (Qiu et al., 1998; Thie et al., 2001).

Many of the existing studies have been criticized for lack of scientific control, short duration, and small size (Towheed et al., 2000), and indeed not all studies of glucosamine supplementation show benefits in terms of relief of pain or stiffness (Houpt et al., 1999; Rindone et al., 2000). Meta-analyses of several smaller studies, however, have supported the beneficial role of glucosamine supplements as a safe and effective approach to treating osteoarthritis (McAlindon et al., 2000a, 2000b; Towheed et al., 2000). In general, 1–3 months of glucosamine supplementation seems to be as effective as many analgesics and NSAIDs, like acetaminophen and ibuprofen, in reducing the joint pain of osteoarthritis. In perhaps the longest-duration trial to date (Reginster et al., 2001), 3 years of glucosamine supplementation (1,500 mg/day) improved pain scores (while symptoms with placebo worsened) and maintained radiographic joint space of the knee (while placebo users experienced significant losses). At least two studies have shown that glucosamine may even slow or stop the destruction of cartilage in the knee joints of people with osteoarthritis (Bruyere et al., 2003; Pavelka et al., 2002); this effect may be especially dramatic in patients with less severe radiographic knee damage in whom intervention is started early (Bruyere et al., 2003). In these studies, oral glucosamine supplements (1,500 mg/day for 3 years) were shown to virtually halt the progressive joint space narrowing observed in the placebo group, suggesting a retardation of osteoarthritis progression. Studies of glucosamine supplementation in more severe forms of osteoarthritis are less positive than studies of mild-to-moderate forms of the disease (Das and Hammad, 2000).

SAFETY/DOSAGE

Occasional symptoms of gastrointestinal discomfort have been noted, but no significant adverse effects are associated with glucosamine supplementation. Although no long-term safety studies have been conducted in humans, animal studies on glucosamine have found it to be nontoxic (Towheed et al., 2005). Diabetics have been cautioned about using glucosamine supplements, based on findings from several animal studies that have suggested an increase in blood sugar levels caused by glucosamine (Monauni et al., 2000). Most of the animal studies have used injections of glucosamine, and recent feeding studies in humans have shown no changes in plasma levels of glucose or insulin (Scroggie et al., 2003), insulin sensitivity (Pouwels et al., 2001), or glucose oxidation (Monauni et al., 2000), suggesting that glucosamine has no significant effect on blood sugar metabolism when used as directed.

No dose-response studies have been conducted with glucosamine supplements. Virtually all oral supplementation studies on glucosamine have used 1,500 mg/day, usually in 2–3 divided doses of 500–750 mg each, but some recent studies have used higher levels of glucosamine (2,000 mg/day; Braham et al., 2003) or higher levels combined with chondroitin and other ingredients (Das and Hammad, 2000). Although higher doses appear to be effective, there is no information to suggest that a higher dose works better or faster or that a lower dose is less effective.

Glucosamine is also routinely combined with chondroitin sulfate, but no information currently exists to suggest that such a combined formulation is superior to either agent consumed alone at the proper dosage. There appear to be few, if any, differences among the various forms of glucosamine (sulfate, hydrochloride, N-acetyl), and each form has been shown to reduce pain and stiffness in studies of mild-to-moderate osteoarthritis (Talent and Gracy, 1996).

REFERENCES

Braham R, Dawson B, Goodman C. The effect of glucosamine supplementation on people experiencing regular knee pain. Br J Sports Med 2003;37(1):45–49, discussion 49.

Bruyere O, Honore A, Ethgen O, Rovati LC, Giacovelli G, Henrotin YE, Seidel L, Reginster JY. Correlation between radiographic severity of knee osteoarthritis and future disease progression. Results from a 3-year prospective, placebo-controlled study evaluating the effect of glucosamine sulfate. Osteoarthritis Cartilage 2003;11(1):1–5.

Cohen M, Wolfe R, Mai T, Lewis D. A randomized, double blind, placebo controlled trial of a topical cream containing glucosamine sulfate, chondroitin sulfate, and camphor for osteoarthritis of the knee. J Rheumatol 2003;30(3):523–528.

Das A Jr, Hammad TA. Efficacy of a combination of FCHG49 glucosamine hydrochloride, TRH122 low molecular weight sodium chondroitin sulfate and manganese ascorbate in the management of knee osteoarthritis. Osteoarthritis Cartilage 2000;8(5):343–350.

Houpt JB, McMillan R, Wein C, Paget-Dellio SD. Effect of glucosamine hydrochloride in the treatment of pain of osteoarthritis of the knee. J Rheumatol 1999;26(11):2423–2430.

Lard LR, Visser H, Speyer I, vander Horst-Bruinsma IE, Zwinderman AH, Breedveld FC, Hazes JM. Early versus delayed treatment in patients with recent-onset rheumatoid arthritis: comparison of two cohorts who received different treatment strategies. Am J Med 2001;111(6):446–451.

McAlindon TE, LaValley MP, Felson DT. Efficacy of glucosamine and chondroitin for treatment of osteoarthritis. JAMA 2000a;284(10):1241.

McAlindon TE, LaValley MP, Gulin JP, Felson DT. Glucosamine and chondroitin for treatment of osteoarthritis: a systematic quality assessment and meta-analysis. JAMA 2000b;283(11):1469–1475.

Monauni T, Zenti MG, Cretti A, Daniels MC, Targher G, Caruso B, Caputo M, McClain D, Del Prato S, Giaccari A, Muggeo M, Bonora E, Bonadonna RC. Effects of glucosamine infusion on insulin secretion and insulin action in humans. Diabetes 2000;49(6):926–935.

Muller-Fassbender H, Bach GL, Haase W, Rovati LC, Setnikar I. Glucosamine sulfate compared with ibuprofen in osteoarthritis of the knee. Osteoarthritis Cartilage 1994;2(1):61–69.

Nguyen P, Mohamed SE, Gardiner D, Salinas T. A randomized double-blind clinical trial of the effect of chondroitin sulfate and glucosamine hydrochloride on temporomandibular joint disorders: a pilot study. Cranio 2001;19(2):130–139.

Pavelka K, Gatterova J, Olejarova M, Machacek S, Giacovelli G, Rovati LC. Glucosamine sulfate use and delay of progression of knee osteoarthritis: a 3-year, randomized, placebo-controlled, double-blind study. Arch Intern Med 2002;162(18):2113–2123.

Pouwels MJ, Jacobs JR, Span PN, Lutterman JA, Smits P, Tack CJ. Short-term glucosamine infusion does not affect insulin sensitivity in humans. J Clin Endocrinol Metab 2001;86(5):2099–2103.

Qiu GX, Gao SN, Giacovelli G, Rovati L, Setnikar I. Efficacy and safety of glucosamine sulfate versus ibuprofen in patients with knee osteoarthritis. Arzneimittelforschung 1998;48(5):469–474.

Reginster JY, Deroisy R, Rovati LC, Lee RL, Lejeune E, Bruyere O, Giacovelli G, Henrotin Y, Dacre JE, Gossett C. Long-term effects of glucosamine sulphate on osteoarthritis progression: a randomised, placebo-controlled clinical trial. Lancet 2001;357(9252):251–256.

Rindone JP, Hiller D, Collacott E, Nordhaugen N, Arriola G. Randomized, controlled trial of glucosamine for treating osteoarthritis of the knee. West J Med 2000;172(2):91–94.

Scroggie DA, Albright A, Harris MD. The effect of glucosamine-chondroitin supplementation on glycosylated hemoglobin levels in patients with type 2 diabetes mellitus: a placebo-controlled, double-blinded, randomized clinical trial. Arch Intern Med 2003;163(13):1587–1590.

Talent JM, Gracy RW. Pilot study of oral polymeric N-acetyl-D-glucosamine as a potential treatment for patients with osteoarthritis. Clin Ther 1996;18(6):1184–1190.

Thie NM, Prasad NG, Major PW. Evaluation of glucosamine sulfate compared to ibuprofen for the treatment of temporomandibular joint osteoarthritis: a randomized double blind controlled 3 month clinical trial. J Rheumatol 2001;28(6):1347–1355.

Towheed TE, Anastassiades TP. Glucosamine and chondroitin for treating symptoms of osteoarthritis: evidence is widely touted but incomplete. JAMA 2000;283(11):1483–1484.

Towheed TE, Maxwell L, Anastassiades TP, Shea B, Houpt J, Robinson V, Hochberg MC, Wells G. Glucosamine therapy for treating osteoarthritis. Cochrane Database Syst Rev 2005;(2):CD002946.

ADDITIONAL RESOURCES

Barclay TS, Tsourounis C, McCart GM. Glucosamine. Ann Pharmacother 1998;32(5):574–579.

da Camara CC, Dowless GV. Glucosamine sulfate for osteoarthritis. Ann Pharmacother 1998;32(5):580–587.

D'Ambrosio E, Casa B, Bompani R, Scali G, Scali M. Glucosamine sulphate: a controlled clinical investigation in arthrosis. Pharmatherapeutica 1981;2(8):504–508.

Deal CL, Moskowitz RW. Nutraceuticals as therapeutic agents in osteoarthritis. The role of glucosamine, chondroitin sulfate, and collagen hydrolysate. Rheum Dis Clin North Am 1999;25(2):379–395.

Delafuente JC. Glucosamine in the treatment of osteoarthritis. Rheum Dis Clin North Am 2000;26(1):1–11.

Denham AC, Newton WP. Are glucosamine and chondroitin effective in treating osteoarthritis? J Fam Pract 2000;49(6):571–572.

Donohoe M. Efficacy of glucosamine and chondroitin for treatment of osteoarthritis. JAMA 2000;284(10):1241, discussion 1242.

Hughes R, Carr A. A randomized, double-blind, placebo-controlled trial of glucosamine sulphate as an analgesic in osteoarthritis of the knee. Rheumatology (Oxford) 2002;41(3):279–284.

Leeb BF, Schweitzer H, Montag K, Smolen JS. A metaanalysis of chondroitin sulfate in the treatment of osteoarthritis. J Rheumatol 2000;27(1):205–211.

Leffler CT, Philippi AF, Leffler SG, Mosure JC, Kim PD. Glucosamine, chondroitin, and manganese ascorbate for degenerative joint disease of the knee or low back: a randomized, double-blind, placebo-controlled pilot study. Mil Med 1999;164(2):85–91.

Lopes Vaz A. Double-blind clinical evaluation of the relative efficacy of ibuprofen and glucosamine sulphate in the management of osteoarthrosis of the knee in out-patients. Curr Med Res Opin 1982;8(3):145–149.

Mautone G. Efficacy of glucosamine and chondroitin for treatment of osteoarthritis. JAMA 2000;284(10):1241, discussion 1242.

Noack W, Fischer M, Forster KK, Rovati LC, Setnikar I. Glucosamine sulfate in osteoarthritis of the knee. Osteoarthritis Cartilage 1994;2(1):51–59.

Pujalte JM, Llavore EP, Ylescupidez FR. Double-blind clinical evaluation of oral glucosamine sulphate in the basic treatment of osteoarthrosis. Curr Med Res Opin 1980;7(2):110–114.

Rubin BR, Talent JM, Kongtawelert P, Pertusi RM, Forman MD, Gracy RW. Oral polymeric N-acetyl-D-glucosamine and osteoarthritis. J Am Osteopath Assoc 2001;101(6):339–344.

GREEN-LIPPED MUSSEL (*PERNA CANALICULUS*)

Overall Rank

★★★ arthritis, joint pain and stiffness
★★ inflammatory conditions
★★ promoting postexercise recovery

OVERVIEW

Green-lipped mussel has been promoted as a dietary supplement for relieving arthritis and joint pain and stiffness and for rebuilding connective tissue, tendons, ligaments, and cartilage because it contains a large amount and diversity of glycosaminoglycans (see the "Chondroitin Sulfate" and "Glucosamine" sections of this chapter). It also contains a high amount of ω-3 fatty acids that may help to reduce or prevent inflammation by balancing eicosanoid production.

COMMENTS

Although a few studies in animals have shown promise for green-lipped mussel as an anti-inflammatory and for the pain and stiffness of arthritis, there have been few and conflicting studies for its use in humans. If indeed it is a good anti-inflammatory, it may also help to promote postexercise recovery, but there is no direct clinical evidence in athletes to support this. With its theorized mode of action, and the lack of clinical studies to directly support it, it may be wiser to use a more concentrated form with more clinical support of glycosaminoglycans, such as chondroitin and glucosamine sulfate.

SCIENTIFIC SUPPORT

Inflammatory Conditions and Asthma

A lipid extract of New Zealand green-lipped mussel was tested in patients with atopic asthma in a double-blind, placebo-controlled, randomized clinical trial. The treatment group received a lipid extract (Lyprinol, 50 mg of ω-3 fatty acids and olive oil); the placebo group received only

150 mg of olive oil. The treatment group was found to have significantly reduced daytime wheeze and exhaled hydrogen peroxide and an increase in morning peak expiratory flow with no side effects. Since asthma is a chronic inflammatory disease involving the mediation of leukotrienes, it was suggested that *Perna canaliculus* worked at least partially through the mechanism of inhibiting 5-lipooxygenase and cyclo-oxygenase (which is responsible for production of eicosanoids), as it was found to do in experimental studies (Emelyanov et al., 2002).

Rheumatoid and Osteoarthritis

In a randomized, placebo-controlled clinical study of green-lipped mussel extract for rheumatoid arthritis, 35 patients were given either Seatone (green-lipped mussel extract) or a placebo for 6 months. The treatment group showed no difference in any of the clinical or laboratory outcome measures, and the researchers concluded the extract was not effective for rheumatoid arthritis (Larkin et al., 1985).

Caughey et al. (1983) tested a freeze-dried extract of New Zealand green-lipped mussel for the treatment of rheumatoid arthritis in an early clinical study. Treatment with the green-lipped mussel extract was found to be beneficial for the pain and inflammation associated with arthritis.

Gibson et al. (1980) examined the effect of green-lipped mussel (three 350-mg capsules daily) or matched placebo in a double-blind, randomized, clinical study involving 66 patients with rheumatoid arthritis (28) and osteoarthritis (38). All patients were allowed to continue their previous medication of NSAIDs during the study. The outcome measures studied for rheumatoid arthritis were articular index of joint tenderness, morning stiffness, grip strength, pain (using a visual analog scale), functional index, and a timed walking test. The outcome measures studied for osteoarthritis were degree of morning stiffness, pain (by visual analog scale), functional index, timed walking test, and range of movement in hip and knee joints. Separate physician- and patient-assessed improvement measures were also recorded in all groups. At the end of the trial, green-lipped mussel was concluded to be an effective supplement or possible alternative to regular treatment of both rheumatoid and osteoarthritis. Green-lipped mussel treatment was able to reduce the amount of pain and stiffness, improve the patients' ability to cope with their conditions, and enhance general health with a low occurrence of side effects.

SAFETY/DOSAGE

Dosage recommendations vary widely for green-lipped mussel, from 500 to 3,000 mg/day in divided doses. No serious side effects have been reported, but green-lipped mussel may cause a problem with people prone to shellfish allergy. Additionally, people who have an aversion to the smell of fish may be repelled by this supplement!

REFERENCES

Caughey DE, Grigor RR, Caughey EB, Young P, Gow PJ, Stewart AW. Perna canaliculus in the treatment of rheumatoid arthritis. Eur J Rheumatol Inflamm 1983;6(2):197–200.

Emelyanov A, Fedoseev G, Krasnoschekova O, Abulimity A, Trendeleva T, Barnes PJ. Treatment of asthma with lipid extract of New Zealand green-lipped mussel: a randomised clinical trial. Eur Respir J 2002;20(3):596–600

Gibson RG, Gibson SL, Conway V, Chappell D. Perna canaliculus in the treatment of arthritis. Practitioner 1980;224(1347):955–960.

Larkin JG, Capell HA, Sturrock RD. Seatone in rheumatoid arthritis: a six-month placebo-controlled study. Ann Rheum Dis 1985;44(3):199–201.

HYDROLYZED COLLAGEN PROTEIN (HCP, GELATIN)

Overall Rank

★★★   for joint health
★★★   for wound healing

OVERVIEW

Hydrolyzed collagen protein (HCP, also known as gelatin) is the chief structural protein that makes up connective tissues in the body (skin, bones, cartilage, tendons, and ligaments). Hydrolyzed collagen is simply a modified form of the protein that has been broken down into smaller pieces by enzymes. The hydrolysis process disrupts the ability of collagen to form a gel and thus makes the protein easier to incorporate into dietary products and may ease the digestion and absorption of the amino acids by the intestine. HCP is often used as a general protein source in bodybuilding products because it is relatively inexpensive, but the use of HCP as a protein for muscle building is flawed because of the incomplete nature of the amino acid profile in gelatin. Because of the high composition of amino acids found in collagen protein, HCP has most recently been used to promote joint health, nourish cartilage and bones, and help athletes recover from exercise and sports-related injuries.

COMMENTS

As a joint support supplement, HCP is typically much less expensive compared with other popular joint supplements such as glucosamine and chondroitin, but the level and quality of the scientific evidence is also not nearly as strong. It may be, however, that because HCP and glucosamine/chondroitin products target different parts of the cartilage structure (collagen and proteoglycans, respectively), one ingredient or the other may work better for some people. Several products have recently been developed to include combinations of ingredients designed to work on different parts of the connective tissue matrix simultaneously.

SCIENTIFIC SUPPORT

HCP is not generally considered as good a source of "high-quality" protein as meat, poultry, fish, and concentrated or isolated protein powders comprised of soy, egg, or milk/whey proteins. On the one hand, HCP is a "poor" protein source because it is low in the sulfur-containing amino acids, such as cysteine and methionine. On the other hand, HCP is the richest dietary source of the primary amino acids that make up the collagen molecule—glycine, proline, hydroxyproline, lysine, and hydroxylysine. As a concentrated source of these collagen amino acids, HCP is thought to help nourish the collagen-containing tissues throughout the body—tissues such as cartilage, bones, tendons, ligaments, and skin.

HCP has been widely used in Europe as a dietary supplement and an alternative treatment for arthritis and osteoporosis. In several small German and Czech studies, dosages of 7–10 g/day of HCP for 1–3 months have been shown to decrease the pain and stiffness associated with arthritis (Adam et al., 1976, 1980; Beuker and Rosenfeld, 1995; Brown et al., 1998). In some studies, HCP was as effective as oral painkillers such as acetaminophen/paracetamol (Tylenol) (Deal and Moskowitz, 1999). In other studies, subjects were able to decrease or discontinue their use of analgesic medications while consuming HCP (Moskowitz, 2000). The only large multicenter study of HCP supplementation found no statistically significant differences for the total study group (all sites in the United States, Great Britain, and Germany) in total mean pain score, but a significant advantage of HCP over a placebo was found at the German sites (Moskowitz, 2000).

Although proponents of HCP consumption claim that it "rebuilds" cartilage, such claims are merely speculation (though probably correct) based on the body of scientific data showing pain reduction. At least one small German study has shown a suppression of bone breakdown in osteoporotic women (Adam et al., 1996). In addition, animal studies have demonstrated that orally administered HCP is better absorbed and incorporated into connective tissues than a comparable amount of labeled proline (Oesser et al., 1999), giving hope to athletes who routinely use HCP as a method for recovering from intense exercise training or sports injuries.

SAFETY/DOSAGE

Aside from the possibility of mild gastrointestinal upset with large doses (up to 10 g/dose), no serious adverse effects are known to exist for consumption of hydrolyzed collagen protein. Clinical studies suggest that at least 7–10 g/day over the course of 30–90 days is needed for reduction of pain in patients with moderate osteoarthritis. Athletes wishing to supplement with HCP as a dietary source of connective tissue building blocks may or may not be able to use a lower dose, but it is unknown whether lower doses would be as effective or if higher doses might even be more effective or work faster.

REFERENCES

Adam M, Musilova J, Deyl Z. Cartilage collagen in osteoarthrosis. Clin Chim Acta 1976;69(1):53–59.

Adam M, Musilova J, Krabcova M, Brettschneider I, Pesakova V, Deyl Z. Effect of cartilage bone marrow extract on the metabolism of collagen in osteoarthrotic cartilage. Pharmacology 1980;21(1):53–58.

Adam M, Spacek P, Hulejova H, Galianova A, Blahos J. Postmenopausal osteoporosis. Treatment with calcitonin and a diet rich in collagen proteins. Cas Lek Cesk 1996;135(3):74–78.

Beuker, F, Rosenfeld, J. The effect of regular gel hydrolysate on chronic-degenerative damage to the supporting and movement system. Int J Sportmed 1996; 1–88, Suppl.1.

Brown KE, Leong K, Huang CH, Dalal R, Green GD, Haimes HB, Jimenez PA, Bathon J. Gelatin/chondroitin 6-sulfate microspheres for the delivery of therapeutic proteins to the joint. Arthritis Rheum 1998;41(12):2185–2195.

Moskowitz RW. Role of collagen hydrolysate in bone and joint disease. Semin Arthritis Rheum 2000;30(2):87–99.

Oesser S, Adam M, Babel W, Seifert J. Oral administration of (14)C labeled gelatin hydrolysate leads to an accumulation of radioactivity in cartilage of mice (C57/BL). J Nutr 1999;129(10):1891–1895.

ADDITIONAL RESOURCES

Arborelius M Jr, Konttinen YT, Nordstrom DC, Solovieva SA. Gly-X-Y repeat sequences in the treatment of active rheumatoid arthritis. Rheumatol Int 1999;18(4):129–135.

Becvar R, Myllyla R, Krbec M, Cech O, Adam M. Changes in collagen biosynthesis in patients with hip joint replacement surgery and reoperation. Acta Chir Orthop Traumatol Cech 1991;58(3):178–184.

Deal CL, Moskowitz RW. Nutraceuticals as therapeutic agents in osteoarthritis. The role of glucosamine, chondroitin sulfate, and collagen hydrolysate. Rheum Dis Clin North Am 1999;25(2):379–395.

Krajickova J, Macek J, Medova N, Adam M. Excretion of proteoglycan degradation products in the urine in patients with rheumatoid arthritis and osteoarthrosis. Vnitr Lek 1987;33(2):129–133.

Schattenkirchner M. Treatment of arthrosis. Internist (Berl) 1990;31(1):82.

MSM (METHYLSULFONYLMETHANE)

Overall Rank

★★★★ as a sulfur supplement
★★ for treating athletic injuries
★★ for treating or preventing arthritis and joint pain
★★ for treating or preventing seasonal allergic rhinitis
★ for preventing cancer
★ for treating bladder disorders

OVERVIEW

MSM (methylsulfonylmethane), also called vitamin U, is a metabolite derived from the well-known solvent that also has anti-inflammatory and analgesic properties, dimethylsulfoxide (DMSO). The theory of the use of MSM is that it is able to supply the body with sulfur, which is involved in a number of metabolic pathways, notably those involved in skin, hair, nail, tendon, and cartilage health. When MSM is used as a dietary supplement, it is thought to improve arthritis and joint health and pain because it is supplying much-needed sulfur in connective tissues. Increases in serum sulfur have been attributed to some of the therapeutic effects of MSM as well as DMSO and glucosamine sulfate (Gessler et al., 1991; Parcell, 2002; Robb-Nicholson, 2002).

Other dietary sources of sulfur are usually high in protein, because sulfur is a component of protein. Good sources include eggs, meat, and fish, as well as sulfur-containing amino acids, such as methionine and cysteine (Parcell, 2002).

COMMENTS

Although MSM is widely used for joint health, most often in combination with glucosamine sulfate, glucosamine hydrochloride, and/or chondroitin sulfate, little clinical support exists for its efficacy. For people who suspect they are low in sulfur, consuming more foods containing sulfur may be as effective, and certainly cheaper.

SCIENTIFIC SUPPORT

Cancer Prevention

An investigational study was conducted on common mechanisms of action of aspirin and MSM in cancer prevention. To investigate this, the inhibition of cyclooxygenase (COX) and prostaglandin production was examined under differentiation-inducing conditions in mouse erythroleukemia cells. Both MSM and aspirin were found to induce differentiation by a COX-independent mechanism, and the authors suggested that another mechanism common to both agents may activate gene functions leading to differentiation (Ebisuzaki, 2003).

Seasonal Allergic Rhinitis

A clinical study was conducted to investigate whether MSM could help in the treatment of seasonal allergic rhinitis. The main outcome parameters tested were symptoms associated with seasonal allergic rhinitis (such as respiratory symptoms and energy levels) tested by a questionnaire and by inflammatory reactions measured by plasma IgE, C-reactive protein, and histamine. Additionally, the study investigated possible adverse reactions and tried to discover MSM's mechanism of action. The 55 participants were given 2,600 mg of MSM daily for 30 days. The study found that by day 7, upper respiratory symptoms were significantly improved from baseline; by day 14, energy levels were increased significantly; and by day 21, lower respiratory symptoms were significantly improved from baseline. All improvements were sustained until the end of the study. The authors concluded that the results of the study suggest that MSM may be helpful for improving seasonal allergic rhinitis symptoms but that a larger well-designed study is needed to determine its use. MSM was found to be very safe, and few side effects were found with supplementation (Barrager et al., 2002).

SAFETY/DOSAGE

MSM is typically used in the range of 2–5 g/day for the beginning or loading dose and 50–200 mg/day for maintenance. MSM is considered safe for use as a dietary supplement, and studies in animals have found that toxicity only occurs in extremely high doses (Horvath et al., 2002).

REFERENCES

Barrager E, Veltmann JR Jr, Schauss AG, Schiller RN. A multicentered, open-label trial on the safety and efficacy of methylsulfonylmethane in the treatment of seasonal allergic rhinitis. J Altern Complement Med 2002;8(2):167–173.

Ebisuzaki K. Aspirin and methylsulfonylmethane (MSM): a search for common mechanisms, with implications for cancer prevention. Anticancer Res 2003;23(1A):453–458.

Gessler NN, Bezzubov AA, Podlepa EV, Bykhovskii VI. Metabolism of S-methylmethionine (vitamin U) in animals. Prikl Biokhim Mikrobiol 1991;27(3):358–364.

Horvath K, Noker PE, Somfai-Relle S, Glavits R, Financsek I, Schauss AG. Toxicity of methylsulfonylmethane in rats. Food Chem Toxicol 2002;40(10):1459–1462.

Parcell S. Sulfur in human nutrition and applications in medicine. Altern Med Rev 2002;7(1):22–44.

Robb-Nicholson C. By the way, doctor. Is MSM as good as it sounds? Can you tell me anything about the dietary supplement MSM? I've heard it's supposed to relieve arthritis pain. Harv Womens Health Watch 2002;9(12):8.

SEA CUCUMBER (STICHOPUS JAPONICUS, OTHER GENERA DEPENDING ON LOCATION)

Overall Rank

★ for joint pain
★ for fibromyalgia

OVERVIEW

Also called *beche del mer*, sea cucumber is not a vegetable but an animal that lives on the sea floor and is related to the starfish. Because sea cucumber contains chondroitin, glycosaminoglycan, and other mucopolysaccharides, it has been recommended for use as a dietary supplement for joint pain.

COMMENTS

Concerns exist regarding the sustainability of the harvest of sea cucumbers for dietary supplements because they are slow growing and are harvested as a delicacy in Asia. Furthermore, scientific support for sea cucumber's use in arthritis and joint pain as a whole ingredient is lacking. It is probably better to stick to other supplements because of a possible lack of sustainable supply and a lack of clinical evidence for sea cucumber.

SCIENTIFIC SUPPORT

Joint Pain and Fibromyalgia
No clinical studies were found that examine the usefulness of sea cucumber alone in treating joint pain or stiffness. Overall, the scientific support for the use of sea cucumber for joint health and pain is lacking. One clinical study included sea cucumber in a formulation with cerasomal-cis-9-cetyl myristoleate and shark cartilage. The study design was open, with a 21-day treatment period. The self-reported symptoms of sleep disturbance, severity of pain, and fatigue were found to be reduced with the treatment (Edwards, 2001). It is not known to what degree sea cucumber added to the efficacy of the preparation.

Cardiovascular Effects
While investigating the antithrombotic action of glycosaminoglycan, Zhiguang et al. (2000) performed a clinical study on cardiovascular recovery patients treated with glycosaminoglycan from sea cucumber. Glycosaminoglycan was found to have anticoagulant activity, to alter fat metabolism, and to reduce blood viscosity. The authors concluded that it had promise as a new drug in antithrombotic therapy and that its effects were similar to dermatan sulfate in efficacy and mechanism.

SAFETY/DOSAGE

The typical dosage is about 500–2,000 mg/day, but sea cucumber is often formulated with other arthritis dietary supplements, so it is usually found in smaller dosages. Sea cucumber has the potential to cause an anticoagulant and blood-thinning effect at high doses. No side effects have been reported.

REFERENCES

Edwards AM. CMO (cerasomal-cis-9-cetyl myristoleate) in the treatment of fibromyalgia: an open pilot study. J Nutr Environ Med 2001;11(2):105–111.
Zhiguang L, Hongli W, Jiazeng L, Guangshen Z, Cunji G. Basic and clinical study on the antithrombotic mechanism of glycosaminoglycan extracted from sea cucumber. Chin Med J (Engl) 2000;113(8):706–711.

Brain and Mood Support Supplements

5-HTP (5-Hydroxy-Tryptophan)
Choline
Feverfew
Ginkgo biloba
Kava Kava (*Piper methysticum*)
Melatonin

Phosphatidylserine
SAMe (S-Adenosyl-L-Methionine)
St. John's Wort
Valerian
Vinpocetine (from *Vinca minor*)

5-HTP (5-HYDROXY-TRYPTOPHAN)

Overall Rank

★★★★ for alleviating depression
★★★ for weight loss
★★★ for treating fibromyalgia
★★ for treating insomnia and sleep disorders
★★ for preventing diabetes
★★ for alleviating chronic headache

OVERVIEW

5-HTP (5 hydroxy-tryptophan) is a naturally occurring substance in the human body that is also the rate-limiting step in the biochemical synthesis of serotonin. In this synthesis, L-tryptophan is converted to 5-HTP by the enzyme tryptophan hydrolase, and then serotonin is produced from 5-HTP. If the tryptophan hydrolase enzyme is inhibited, serotonin is not produced. Several factors might inhibit this enzyme, such as stress, vitamin B_6 deficiency, insufficient magnesium, and insulin resistance. No significant level of 5-HTP is in the diet, but dietary supplements of 5-HTP made from the African plant *Griffonia simplicifolia* are

149

available. Supplementation of 5-HTP bypasses any deficiency or dysfunction in this enzyme's metabolism of serotonin and therefore results in higher serotonin levels.

COMMENTS

Although the hypothesis that serotonin levels can be improved with the supplementation of 5-HTP is probable, the clinical evidence for its efficacy is poor, and more well-designed studies are needed to ascertain which conditions respond best to supplementation. Additionally, wider availability of 5-HTP supplements requires quality assurances that eosinophilia-myalgia syndrome (EMS)–type reactions will not occur (see the "Safety/Dosage" subsection of this section).

SCIENTIFIC SUPPORT

Depression
A meta-analysis of the literature published from 1966 to 2000 on the use of 5-HTP and L-tryptophan for unipolar depression found that of 108 studies, only 2 (one on 5-HTP) met the study criteria. The review analysis suggested that both 5-HTP and L-tryptophan are better than placebo in the treatment of depression. The authors concluded that although positive studies are numerous, they are of poor quality and better-designed research is needed to make clinical recommendations (Shaw et al., 2002a, 2002b).

An open comparison between 5-HTP and tranylcypromine was conducted in patients with major depression who were unsuccessfully treated by at least two other cyclic antidepressant drugs. The 5-HTP-treated group showed no improvement, whereas the tranylcypromine-treated group showed efficacy in 50% of the patients tested. Those that responded to the tranylcypromine had depression that was more endogenous and of shorter duration than those that did not respond to its treatment (Nolen et al., 1988).

A double-blind, placebo-controlled comparison was conducted on 5-HTP and clomipramine in anxiety patients. A 90-item symptoms checklist and the state scale of the Spielberger State-Trait Anxiety Inventory were used as assessment parameters. The study found that 5-HTP did not alter the associated depressive symptomatology and compared with a placebo, showed only a moderate reduction in all the rating scales, whereas clomipramine showed significant improvements in all the rating scales (Kahn et al., 1987).

Major depressive patients who were unsuccessfully treated by other reuptake inhibitors were enrolled in an open, controlled, crossover comparison between 5-HTP and tranylcypromine. After 4 weeks of treatment (in a crossover design), no responses were found in the 17 patients in the 5-HTP group, but 15 of the 26 patients in the tranylcypromine group responded. The authors concluded that 5-HTP was not a viable option for patients with major depression that had not responded to other reuptake inhibitors (Nolen et al., 1985).

Obesity

The influence of 5-HTP on obesity was studied in 20 obese patients in a double-blind, randomized, placebo-controlled study. Either a placebo or 900 mg/day of 5-HTP was given to the subjects for two consecutive 6-week periods, with no dietary restrictions prescribed for the first period and a 5,040-kJ/day diet prescribed for the second period. The treatment group showed a significant weight loss for both periods of 5-HTP treatment, along with reductions in carbohydrate intake and increases in early satiety (Cangiano et al., 1992).

In a double-blind, crossover study involving 19 obese women, 5-HTP (8 mg/kg daily) was administered to subjects with body mass indexes between 30 and 40 for 5 weeks. No changes in mood were observed with 5-HTP administration, but it did result in decreased food intake and weight loss (Ceci et al., 1989).

Fibromyalgia

Puttini and Caruso (1992) tested 5-HTP in fibromyalgia patients using an open 90-day study design. The clinical variables tested for fibromyalgia (tender points, anxiety, pain, quality of sleep, and fatigue) showed an overall improvement compared with baseline, with approximately 50% of patients showing a "good" or "fair" clinical improvement. About 30% of the subjects treated reported side effects, but only one patient withdrew from the study for that reason.

In an earlier study on 5-HTP for fibromyalgia, 50 patients were enrolled in a double-blind, placebo-controlled study design. The authors found that all clinical parameters significantly improved, noting only mild or transient side effects (Caruso et al., 1990).

Insomnia and Sleep Disorders

5-HTP was tested in a double-blind, placebo-controlled, crossover study of 48 students with recurring headaches and sleep disorders. The authors concluded that 5-HTP can reduce headaches and sleep disorders, especially frequent awakenings and parasomnias (De Giorgis et al., 1987).

Chronic Headache

Because previous studies on 5-HTP had been inconclusive, a double-blind crossover study involving 31 patients looked at the role of 5-HTP in mitigating chronic primary headache. In the treatment group, 5-HTP was administered in doses of 400 mg/day orally for 2 months. Treatment with 5-HTP resulted in a nonsignificant reduction in severity and frequency of headache, and mild and transient side effects occurring in 19% of the treatment group (De Benedittis and Massei, 1985).

In a study to characterize the clinical subgroup that responds best to 5-HTP treatment, 100 patients with chronic primary headache were given 300 mg/day. The clinical subgroup that responded best was identified as having major mood disturbances, minor frequency of anxiety, previous positive response to pizotifen treatment, longer disease occurrence, and higher frequency of associated symptoms (Bono et al., 1984).

Diabetes

Because diabetes mellitus is associated with low levels of serotonin in the brain, carbohydrate cravings, and overeating, the use of 5-HTP was clinically tested for its ability to normalize serotonin and eating behaviors in diabetic patients. In a double-blind, placebo-controlled, randomized study, 5-HTP was given to 25 overweight patients with diabetes mellitus in 750-mg/day doses or placebo for 2 weeks. Treatment with 5-HTP resulted in significant reductions of brain tryptophan, body weight, and daily energy intake compared with placebo (Cangiano et al., 1998).

SAFETY/DOSAGE

Generally, the initial dosage recommended for 5-HTP is 50 mg 3 times daily, and the dosage is increased to up to 900 mg/day until the desired effect is noted. Not enough clinical data are available to safely recommend 5-HTP treatment in pregnant or lactating women. Interactions may exist between 5-HTP and other antidepressant products, especially selective serotonin reuptake inhibitors.

The foremost concern regarding the use of 5-HTP is the possibility of people contracting EMS, similar to a 1983 episode in which a contaminated batch of L-tryptophan was linked to production methods involving bacterial fermentation followed by inadequate filtration. Because 5-HTP is produced by extraction from plant sources, however, such contamination is unlikely to occur. Nonetheless, two reported cases of EMS-like symptoms have been described in patients taking 5-HTP. One case in 1980 involved the use of very high doses (1,400 mg/day); the product itself was never tested for contamination. A second case involved a family (a mother and two children) who had been confirmed to have taken contaminated 5-HTP (Bono et al., 1994; Michelson et al., 1994).

Another concern regarding the use of 5-HTP is the possibility of developing heart valve disease. In 1997, the Food and Drug Administration (FDA) banned the sale of redux and fen-phen because of an "unacceptable risk" of developing heart valve disease. According to Michael Murray, there have been "no reports of heart valve disease or other problems related to serotonin syndrome in people who take 5-HTP by itself" (Puttini and Caruso, 1992).

REFERENCES

Bono G, Micieli G, Sances G, Calvani M, Nappi G. L-5HTP treatment in primary headaches: an attempt at clinical identification of responsive patients. Cephalalgia 1984;4(3):159–165.

Cangiano C, Ceci F, Cascino A, Del Ben M, Laviano A, Muscaritoli M, Antonucci F, Rossi-Fanelli F. Eating behavior and adherence to dietary prescriptions in obese adult subjects treated with 5-hydroxytryptophan. Am J Clin Nutr 1992;56(5):863–867.

Cangiano C, Laviano A, Del Ben M, Preziosa I, Angelico F, Cascino A, Rossi-Fanelli F. Effects of oral 5-hydroxy-tryptophan on energy intake and macronutrient selection in non-insulin dependent diabetic patients. Int J Obes Relat Metab Disord 1998;22(7):648–654.

Caruso I, Sarzi Puttini P, Cazzola M, Azzolini V. Double-blind study of 5-hydroxytryptophan versus placebo in the treatment of primary fibromyalgia syndrome. J Int Med Res 1990;18(3):201–209.

Ceci F, Cangiano C, Cairella M, Cascino A, Del Ben M, Muscaritoli M, Sibilia L, Rossi Fanelli F. The effects of oral 5-hydroxytryptophan administration on feeding behavior in obese adult female subjects. J Neural Transm 1989;76(2):109–117.

De Benedittis G, Massei R. Serotonin precursors in chronic primary headache. A double-blind cross-over study with L-5-hydroxytryptophan vs. placebo. J Neurosurg Sci 1985;29(3):239–248.

De Giorgis G, Miletto R, Iannuccelli M, Camuffo M, Scerni S. Headache in association with sleep disorders in children: a psychodiagnostic evaluation and controlled clinical study—L-5-HTP versus placebo. Drugs Exp Clin Res 1987;13(7):425–433.

Kahn RS, Westenberg HG, Verhoeven WM, Gispen-de Wied CC, Kamerbeek WD. Effect of a serotonin precursor and uptake inhibitor in anxiety disorders; a double-blind comparison of 5-hydroxytryptophan, clomipramine and placebo. Int Clin Psychopharmacol 1987;2(1):33–45.

Michelson D, Page SW, Casey R, Trucksess MW, Love LA, Milstein S, Wilson C, Massaquoi SG, Crofford LJ, Hallett M, et al. An eosinophilia-myalgia syndrome related disorder associated with exposure to L-5-hydroxytryptophan. J Rheumatol 1994;21(12):2261–2265.

Nolen WA, van de Putte JJ, Dijken WA, Kamp JS. L-5HTP in depression resistant to re-uptake inhibitors. An open comparative study with tranylcypromine. Br J Psychiatry 1985;147:16–22.

Nolen WA, van de Putte JJ, Dijken WA, Kamp JS, Blansjaar BA, Kramer HJ, Haffmans J. Treatment strategy in depression, part II: MAO inhibitors in depression resistant to cyclic antidepressants: two controlled crossover studies with tranylcypromine versus L-5-hydroxytryptophan and nomifensine. Acta Psychiatr Scand 1988;78(6):676–683.

Puttini PS, Caruso I. Primary fibromyalgia syndrome and 5-hydroxy-L-tryptophan: a 90-day open study. J Int Med Res 1992;20(2):182–189.

Shaw K, Turner J, Del Mar C. Are tryptophan and 5-hydroxytryptophan effective treatments for depression? A meta-analysis. Aust N Z J Psychiatry 2002a;36(4):488–491.

Shaw K, Turner J, Del Mar C. Tryptophan and 5-hydroxytryptophan for depression. Cochrane Database Syst Rev 2002b;(1):CD003198. Review.

ADDITIONAL RESOURCES

Murray M. 5-HTP: The Natural Way to Overcome Depression, Obesity, and Insomnia. New York: Bantam Books, 1998.

CHOLINE

Overall Rank

★★★★ for general nutritional support
★★★ for memory support
★ as a fat burner

OVERVIEW

Choline is an essential B vitamin that functions as a precursor for the neurotransmitter acetylcholine and as a building block for phospholipids in cellular membranes and lipoproteins and for the methyl donor betaine. It can be manufactured in the body (from the amino acid methionine), although whether it can be made in sufficient amounts for optimal health is a matter of some debate. Folic acid and vitamin B_{12} are also needed to process choline. Choline plays a role in liver function, cardiovascular health, and brain development (as an amine precursor for the neurotransmitter acetylcholine). In 1998, the Food and Nutrition Board (FNB) of the National Academy of Sciences established adequate intake (AI) levels for choline of 550 mg/day for men and 425 mg/day for women. In setting AI levels for choline, the FNB also noted that "there are few data to assess whether a dietary supply of choline is needed at all stages of the life cycle and it may be that choline requirement can be met by endogenous synthesis at some of these stages" (National Academy of Sciences, 1998). Nevertheless, numerous choline-based dietary supplements are marketed with claims for improving memory, protecting the cardiovascular system, preventing cancer, and delaying fatigue.

COMMENTS

Choline is found in the diet in milk, liver, eggs, peanuts, and soybeans, where it is available as free choline or is bound as esters such as phosphocholine, glycerophosphocholine, sphingomyelin, or phosphatidylcholine. Choline can also be found in various "brain support" supplements, including lecithin (phosphatidylcholine). Although adequate maternal choline intake has been shown to be important for fetal brain development during pregnancy, dietary sources of choline (eggs and peanuts) are the preferred method of increasing choline intake for pregnant women. Among endurance athletes, choline supplements may be warranted because intake of choline is presumed low (owing to reliance on a high-carbohydrate diet for energy) and loss of choline following exercise is greater. Although it is important to ensure an adequate daily intake of choline to support normal nerve function and cell membrane structure, it is unlikely that additional choline in supplement form will boost mental acuity or endurance exercise performance (common product claims).

SCIENTIFIC SUPPORT

Choline is required to make essential membrane phospholipids, as a precursor for the biosynthesis of the neurotransmitter acetylcholine, and as an important source of labile methyl groups in numerous methylation reactions throughout the body (Zeisel et al., 1991). The AI levels for choline (425–550 mg/day) are based on the prevention of liver damage as assessed by serum alanine aminotransferase levels. Healthy humans fed a choline-deficient diet develop impaired methylation capabilities and liver dysfunction within 3 weeks, suggesting that choline is an essential nutrient (Jacob et al., 1995; Zeisel et al., 1991). Choline participates in lipid (fat) transport in the body and may reduce accumulation of fat in the liver (Zeisel et al., 1991). As a dietary supplement and ergogenic aid, however, claims surrounding choline are mostly the result of its role as a component of acetylcholine (the neurotransmitter needed for conduction of nerve signals and brain function). Claims in this area typically involve mental performance, memory, and reaction time.

During pregnancy, the mother's choline intake may influence memory and brain development in the growing fetus. Studies on choline and lecithin supplementation clearly show an increase in blood choline levels following supplementation with 1–5 g of choline (or 5–15 g of lecithin). Despite the wide range of commercial products claiming choline as a memory aid, no studies support that role. Studies of choline supplementation for fat metabolism have shown that choline does not increase fat metabolism; moreover, choline appears to reduce serum and urinary carnitine levels—an effect that could be expected to reduce overall fat metabolism (Daily and Sachan, 1995; Hongu and Sachan, 2003).

Choline has also been studied in humans as an aid to endurance exercise. Because plasma choline levels are known to fall after strenuous exercise, it has been suggested that choline supplementation might delay fatigue and enhance performance by increasing the synthesis of acetylcholine for muscle contractions (Spector et al., 1995; Warber et al., 2000). Studies of choline supplementation in athletes, however, have been disappointing. In one study of soldiers, 8.425 g of choline citrate given before and midway through a 4-hour treadmill exercise increased plasma choline levels by 128% but had no significant effect on any performance measurement (Warber et al., 2000). In another study, trained cyclists were supplemented with 2.43 g of choline bitartrate 1 hour before either a brief supramaximal (150% maximum power) or prolonged submaximal (70% maximum power) exercise test. Choline supplementation increased plasma choline levels 37–52%, but no significant changes were noted for measures of fatigue or exercise performance for either test (Spector et al., 1995).

SAFETY/DOSAGE

The AI levels for choline are 550 mg/day for men and 425 mg/day for women. The upper limit (UL) for adults is 3.5 g/day. Choline has a high margin of safety as a dietary supplement, and consumers can select foods with higher choline by looking for FDA-approved nutrient content claims on products with preexisting or added choline, such as this: "Good source of choline. Contains 55 mg of choline per serving, which is 10% of the daily value for choline (550 mg)." No adverse effects of choline supplements have been noted at levels of 1–2 g, whereas doses closer to 3–5 g (above the UL of 3.5 g/day) may be associated with side effects such as diarrhea, nausea, and abdominal discomfort. Anecdotal reports have been made of "fishy body odor" in people consuming high daily doses of choline or lecithin.

REFERENCES

Daily JW III, Sachan DS. Choline supplementation alters carnitine homeostasis in humans and guinea pigs. J Nutr 1995;125(7):1938–1944.

Hongu N, Sachan DS. Carnitine and choline supplementation with exercise alter carnitine profiles, biochemical markers of fat metabolism and serum leptin concentration in healthy women. J Nutr 2003;133(1):84–89.

Jacob RA, Pianalto FS, Henning SM, Zhang JZ, Swendseid ME. In vivo methylation capacity is not impaired in healthy men during short-term dietary folate and methyl group restriction. J Nutr 1995;125(6):1495–1502.

National Academy of Science, Institute of Medicine, Food and Nutrition Board. Dietary Reference Intakes for Thiamin, Riboflavin, Niacin, Vitamin B6, Folate, Vitamin B12, Pantothenic Acid, Biotin, and Choline. Washington, DC: National Academy of Sciences, 1998.

Spector SA, Jackman MR, Sabounjian LA, Sakkas C, Landers DM, Willis WT. Effect of choline supplementation on fatigue in trained cyclists. Med Sci Sports Exerc 1995;27(5):668–673.

Warber JP, Patton JF, Tharion WJ, Zeisel SH, Mello RP, Kemnitz CP, Lieberman HR. The effects of choline supplementation on physical performance. Int J Sport Nutr Exerc Metab 2000;10(2):170–181.

Zeisel SH, Da Costa KA, Franklin PD, Alexander EA, Lamont JT, Sheard NF, Beiser A. Choline, an essential nutrient for humans. FASEB J 1991;5(7):2093–2098.

ADDITIONAL RESOURCES

Growdon JH, Wurtman RJ. Dietary influences on the synthesis of neurotransmitters in the brain. Nutr Rev 1979;37(5):129–136.

Hoeger WW, Harris C, Long EM, Hopkins DR. Four-week supplementation with a natural dietary compound produces favorable changes in body composition. Adv Ther 1998;15(5):305–314.

Leathwood PD, Schlosser B. Phosphatidylcholine, choline and cholinergic function. Int J Vitam Nutr Res Suppl 1986;29:49–67.

Wurtman RJ, Growdon JH. Dietary enhancement of CNS neurotransmitters. Hosp Pract 1978;13(3):71–77.

Zeisel SH. Choline: an important nutrient in brain development, liver function and carcinogenesis. J Am Coll Nutr 1992;11(5):473–481.

Zeisel SH, Blusztajn JK. Choline and human nutrition. Annu Rev Nutr 1994;14:269–296.

Zeisel SH, Growdon JH, Wurtman RJ, Magil SG, Logue M. Normal plasma choline responses to ingested lecithin. Neurology 1980;30(11):1226–1229.

Zhang AQ, Mitchell SC, Smith RL. Dietary precursors of trimethylamine in man: a pilot study. Food Chem Toxicol 1999;37(5):515–520.

FEVERFEW

Overall Rank

★★★★ for migraine prevention

OVERVIEW

Feverfew (*Tanacetum parthenium*) is a member of the daisy family. It has been used in traditional medicine as far back as the first century for inflammatory conditions and to prevent the occurrence of migraine headaches. Traditionally consumed as whole fresh or dried leaves or as a tea, feverfew is available in supplemental form as an encapsulated powder standardized for the potential active ingredient known as parthenolide. Although many feverfew extracts are standardized to parthenolide, the predominant sesquiterpene lactone, it is unknown whether parthenolide is necessary for the antimigraine effect for which feverfew supplements are so popular and effective. Feverfew extracts standardized for parthenolide, as well as extracts not standardized, have been shown effective for reducing the occurrence of migraine headaches and for reducing the severity and range of side effects of migraine episodes that do occur.

COMMENTS

Migraines can cause excruciating pain and often completely incapacitate the sufferer. Feverfew is relatively inexpensive and safe and has shown clear effects in reducing the number of migraine attacks in some people. Although some studies suggest that it is important to look for a supplement that is standardized to at least 0.2% parthenolide (Knight, 1995), this sesquiterpene lactone may be only one of several active constituents that deliver the antimigraine effects associated with feverfew.

SCIENTIFIC SUPPORT

Although feverfew's mechanism of action is not yet fully understood, researchers have suggested several possibilities. Biological and plant studies have revealed that the plant extracts of feverfew have been found to exhibit inhibitory effects on the release of 5-hydroxy-tryptamine (serotonin) from blood platelets and polymorphonuclear leukocytes; platelet aggregation and secretion; prostaglandin, thromboxane, and leukotriene production; antimicrobial activity; and an antithrombotic potential (Awang, 1997). The parthenolide in feverfew causes most of this activity. Specifically, parthenolide inhibits thromboxane B_2 and leukotriene B_4 in human leukocytes, producing an anti-inflammatory effect (Sumner et al., 1992). These properties also consist of inhibition of the enzyme phospholipase A_2, which facilitates the release of arachidonic acid from the phospholipid cellular membrane (Heptinstall, 1988). Parthenolide has also been shown to inhibit expression of inducible cyclo-oxygenase-2 and proinflammatory cytokines in macrophages and may interfere with contractile and relaxant mechanisms in blood vessels (Knight, 1995; Sumner et al., 1992).

Laboratory and clinical studies have shown an effect of feverfew leaves and extracts on inflammatory processes, including arachidonate metabolism and platelet function (Sumner et al., 1992). Feverfew extracts produce a clear inhibition of histamine release and reduce production of prostaglandins, which may explain some of the anti-inflammatory activities of feverfew (Knight, 1995). Parthenolide and related sesquiterpenes may interfere with serotonin release from platelets (which has been suggested as a primary cause of migraines), suggesting a mechanism by which feverfew functions to inhibit smooth muscle cell contraction and prevent migraines from occurring (Vogler et al., 1998).

Several clinical trials have assessed the use of feverfew preparations to prevent migraine headaches. A randomized, double-blind, placebo-controlled, crossover study evaluated the use of dried feverfew leaves in 72 patients who had experienced, over more than two years, classic or common migraine headaches, with at least one attack monthly (Murphy et al., 1988). After a 1-month, single-blind, placebo run-in phase, patients were randomized to placebo or feverfew groups. These patients received one capsule daily for 4 months and then were crossed over to the other treatment group. Results of the study illustrated that feverfew capsules (70–114 mg) decreased the number of attacks by 24% and decreased symptoms of nausea and vomiting compared with the placebo (Johnson et al., 1985).

A similar 4-month randomized, double-blind, placebo-controlled, crossover trial was conducted to assess the effectiveness of feverfew as a prophylactic therapy for migraines in 57 patients who had never taken feverfew before. Patients who attended an outpatient pain clinic were selected at random and divided into two groups that completed three phases of the study. Phase 1 was an open-label run-in phase in which both groups received 100 mg (two capsules) daily of encapsulated, dried, powdered feverfew leaves for 2 months. In phases 2 and 3, the study groups were randomized to receive 100 mg of feverfew/day or a matching placebo for 1 month and then cross over for another month. No washout period occurred between the crossover phases. Patients completed a questionnaire that included parameters such as the number of years suffering, frequency and duration of migraine attacks, pain intensity, and symptoms accompanying migraine attacks, such as nausea, vomiting, and sensitivity to light and noise. A numerical self-assessment pain scale was used, in which 0 represented no pain and 10 represented severe pain. The linked symptoms were estimated by the patients on a numerical analog scale in which 0 represented no pain and 4 represented severe pain. The results demonstrated a significant reduction in pain intensity, nausea, vomiting, and sensitivity to light and noise compared with the placebo. These results provide convincing evidence that feverfew may be used prophylactically for migraine attacks (Murphy et al., 1988, Pittler and Vogler, 2000).

Another randomized, double-blind, placebo-controlled trial evaluated 17 patients who chronically ate feverfew leaves for self-prophylaxis of migraines. Patients were randomized to receive either 50 mg/day of feverfew or a matching placebo. All patients were then instructed to take two capsules (25 mg each) every morning with food for six periods of 4 weeks. They were also instructed to treat acute migraine attacks with soluble aspirin or their usual drug. Patients recorded and graded various visual symptoms, nausea, vomiting, and headache on dietary cards provided for them. The results showed that the placebo group experienced a significant increase in the frequency and severity of headaches, nausea, and vomiting. Patients given feverfew, however, showed no change in the frequency or severity of headaches, suggesting that feverfew may be taken prophylactically to prevent attacks of migraines (Palevitch et al., 1997).

In subjects consuming 80 mg/day of feverfew for 1 month, 25% experienced a reduction in the number of migraine attacks and a clear reduction in the occurrence of the nausea and vomiting that often accompany migraine attacks (Palevitch et al., 1997). In another study, subjects consumed 100 mg/day of dried feverfew leaves (standardized to contain 0.2 mg of parthenolide) and showed reduced migraine intensity after 60 days (Prusinski et al., 1999).

SAFETY/DOSAGE

Several side effects have been noted in clinical studies, including mouth ulcers (when the leaves are chewed), gastrointestinal discomfort, and dry mouth (Johnson et al., 1985; Murphy et al., 1988). Women who are pregnant or lactating should avoid consuming feverfew, as should people with known sensitivities to other members of the same plant family, such as ragweed and chamomile. Long-term use may be associated with an anticoagulant effect, so feverfew should probably not be used in conjunction with other blood-thinning agents (Sriramarao and Rao, 1993).

Most studies have used dosages ranging from 25 mg to 125 mg of feverfew leaf per day, many with a parthenolide content of at least 0.2 mg (0.2–0.9%). Supplements should be taken prophylactically to prevent the occurrence of migraines, rather than in an attempt to relieve a migraine attack once it occurs. A period of 1–2 months of taking feverfew is recommended before achieving the therapeutic effect. Some alternative practitioners recommend an occasional break from treatment, but be aware that a "feverfew rebound" syndrome has been reported in which tension headaches follow the abrupt discontinuance of feverfew consumption (Vogler et al., 1998).

REFERENCES

Awang DV. Feverfew products. CMAJ 1997;157(5):510–511.

Heptinstall S. Feverfew—an ancient remedy for modern times? J R Soc Med 1988;81(7):373–374.

Johnson ES, Kadam NP, Hylands DM, Hylands PJ. Efficacy of feverfew as prophylactic treatment of migraine. BMJ 1985;291:569–573.

Knight DW. Feverfew: chemistry and biological activity. Nat Prod Rep 1995;12(3):271–276.

Murphy JJ, Heptinstall S, Mitchell JR. Randomised double-blind placebo-controlled trial of feverfew in migraine prevention. Lancet 1988;2(8604):189–192.

Palevitch D, Earon G, Carasso R. Feverfew (Tanacetum parthenium) as a prophylactic treatment for migraine: a double-blind placebo-controlled study. Phytother Res 1997;11:508–511.

Pittler MH, Vogler BK, Ernst E. Feverfew for preventing migraine. Cochrane Database Syst Rev 2000;(3):CD002286.

Prusinski A, Durko A, Niczyporuk-Turek A. Feverfew as a prophylactic treatment of migraine. Neurol Neurochir Pol 1999;33(suppl 5):89–95.

Sriramarao P, Rao PV. Allergenic cross-reactivity between Parthenium and ragweed pollen allergens. Int Arch Allergy Immunol 1993;100(1):79–85.

Sumner H, Salan U, Knight DW, Hoult JR. Inhibition of 5-lipoxygenase and cyclo-oxygenase in leukocytes by feverfew. Involvement of sesquiterpene lactones and other components. Biochem Pharmacol 1992;43(11):2313–2320.

Vogler BK, Pittler MH, Ernst E. Feverfew as a preventive treatment for migraine: a systematic review. Cephalalgia 1998;18(10):704–708.

ADDITIONAL RESOURCES

Williams CA, Harborne JB, Geiger H, Hoult JR. The flavonoids of Tanacetum parthenium and T. vulgare and their anti-inflammatory properties. Phytochemistry 1999;51(3):417–423.

Wong HC. Is feverfew a pharmacologic agent? CMAJ 1999;160(1):21–22.

GINKGO BILOBA

Overall Rank

★★★★★ for improving cognitive function (senile dementia)
★★★★ for improving systemic blood flow
★★★★ for intermittent claudication
★★ for asthma

OVERVIEW

Ginkgo biloba is often referred to as a "living fossil" because, at about 200 million years old, it is believed to be the world's oldest living species. The ginkgo tree has been used in Traditional Chinese Medicine (TCM) for more than 4,000 years. Various parts of the tree were reportedly used in the treatment of respiratory ailments, to improve circulation, as a digestive aid, as a tonic for memory loss in the elderly, and as a longevity elixir.

In Germany, ginkgo is a top-selling over-the-counter and prescription drug. Modern Ginkgo biloba extracts are produced from the leaves of cultivated trees and still enjoy a large audience for the treatment of various disorders. High-quality *Ginkgo biloba* extract is normally standardized to 24% ginkgo flavone glycosides and 6% terpene lactones, with modern-day usage as a dietary supplement for improving memory, reducing depression, reducing symptoms of senile dementia, and improving peripheral circulation (a benefit for mental function, heart health, and sexual function).

The two groups of phytochemicals to which *Ginkgo biloba* is normally standardized, ginkgo flavone glycosides and terpene lactones, are considered to be the primary active constituents. The flavone glycosides, which include quercetin, kaempherol, and isorhamnetin, are responsible for the antioxidant properties of *Ginkgo biloba* extract. The terpene lactones, which include ginkgolides A, B, and C as well as bilobalide, possess several activities, including neuroprotection, improvement of choline uptake in brain synapses, and inhibition of platelet activating factor (which reduces the tendency of the blood to clot).

COMMENTS

Ginkgo biloba is valuable for a broad array of health concerns related to problems with microcirculation, whether they be in the brain, legs or sex organs. Ginkgo's neuroprotective effects are also well established, and its benefits in improving mental function and memory in healthy subjects looks promising.

SCIENTIFIC SUPPORT

Laboratory and clinical studies have found a great deal of support for most claims made for the therapeutic use of *Ginkgo biloba* extract. The German Commission E approves ginkgo for effective therapy in cases of memory deficits, impaired concentration, depression, dizziness, tinnitus (ringing in the ears), or headache. The primary groups of dementias targeted for treatment with ginkgo are primary degenerative dementia, vascular dementia, and mixed forms of both. Ginkgo is also approved for use in the improvement of pain-free walking in patients diagnosed with intermittent claudication or peripheral arterial occlusive disease (both are conditions in which improved circulation helps relieve symptoms). Lastly, the Commission E recommends ginkgo for vertigo and tinnitus, which also may be caused by inadequate circulation (Blumenthal et al., 1998).

Various clinical studies have been conducted on the benefits of *Ginkgo biloba* extract, many in Germany but several in the United States. Major findings include enhanced oxygen use and improvement of tolerance to hypoxia, increased brain circulation, inhibition or prevention of brain damage following trauma and/or toxicity, neurotransmitter support, inhibition of age-related loss of choline receptors, stimulation of choline uptake in the hippocampus region of the brain, increased memory performance and learning capacity, improved systemic circulation (improvement of blood flow, particularly in microcirculation of capillaries), and general improvements in cardiovascular function (antioxidant effects and reduced activity of platelet activating factor).

One meta-analysis looked at more than 40 clinical studies investigating *Ginkgo biloba* extract for the treatment of cerebral insufficiency (which is associated with age-related mental decline or dementia). The resulting analysis concluded that *Ginkgo biloba* extract is effective in reducing all symptoms of cerebral insufficiency and impaired mental function (Pittler and Ernst, 2000).

In a placebo-controlled, double-blind, randomized study, 72 patients with cerebral insufficiency (lack of blood flow to the brain) were subjected to a computerized test of short-term memory. At the end of 6 weeks, the group receiving *Ginkgo biloba* extract exhibited a statistically significant improvement in short-term memory capacity, while the placebo group showed no significant increase (Le Bars et al., 2002).

Clinical evidence indicates that *Ginkgo biloba* extract may be useful in the treatment of certain types of depression—notably "resistant" depression. At least one study correlated a reduction of cerebral blood flow to depression in patients. In one placebo-controlled study, patients who continued to exhibit symptoms of depression after the use of antidepressants were given 240 mg/day of *Ginkgo biloba* extract. The patients receiving the extract experienced a significant reduction in depressive symptoms as well as an improvement in cognitive function (Kang et al., 2002). In an open clinical trial of 60 patients with erectile dysfunction, 50% of the patients regained potency and 25% showed improved arterial blood flow following 6 months of supplementation with 60 mg/day of *Ginkgo biloba* extract (Garg et al., 1995).

Whether *Ginkgo biloba* extract can improve cognitive function in healthy subjects has been questioned. Two studies of healthy volunteers measured brain activity using sensitive electroencephalography and found that dosages of 120–240 mg of *Ginkgo biloba* extract increase cognitive function (measured as alpha wave activity) within 30 minutes, with peak measures recorded 2–3 hours after consuming the supplements (Kunkel, 1993; Itil and Martorano, 1995). The enhancement in alpha wave activity was similar to that achieved through the use of drugs that improve cognitive function. Both studies concluded that *Ginkgo biloba* extract improves cognitive function in healthy subjects.

SAFETY/DOSAGE

Ginkgo biloba extract is, very rarely, associated with gastrointestinal upset, allergic skin reaction, and headache. *Ginkgo biloba* is not known to be toxic at high dosages, although its inhibition of platelet-activating factor could pose a concern to patients with blood-clotting problems or those taking anticoagulant medications.

Typical dosage recommendations for the treatment of microcirculation problems in the extremities, including vertigo, tinnitus, and intermittent claudication, are in the range of 120–180 mg/day. For treatment of dementia, mild depression, and improvement of cognitive abilities, higher doses (about 240 mg/day) are recommended. For best results, daily dosage is typically split into two or three doses. Extracts should be standardized to at least 24% ginkgo flavone glycosides and 6% terpene lactones, the type of extract that has been shown effective in virtually every clinical trial.

REFERENCES

Blumenthal M, Busse WR, Goldberg A, Gruenwald J, Hall T, Riggins CW, Rister RS, eds. The Complete German Commission E Monographs. Austin, TX: American Botanical Council, 1998.

Garg RK, Nag D, Agrawal A. A double blind placebo controlled trial of ginkgo biloba extract in acute cerebral ischaemia. J Assoc Physicians India 1995;43(11):760–763.

Itil T, Martorano D. Natural substances in psychiatry (Ginkgo biloba in dementia). Psychopharmacol Bull 1995;31(1):147–158.

Kang B, Lee S, Kim M, Cho M. A placebo-controlled, double-blind trial of Ginkgo biloba for antidepressant-induced sexual dysfunction. Hum Psychopharmacol Clin Exp 2002;17:279–284.

Kunkel H. EEG profile of three different extractions of Ginkgo biloba. Neuropsychobiology 1993;27(1):40–45.

Le Bars P, Velasco F.M., Ferguson J.M., Dessain E.C., Kieser M, Hoerr R. Influence of the severity of cognitive impairment on the effect of the Ginkgo biloba extract Egb 761 in Alzheimer's disease. Neuropsychobiology 2002;45:19–26.

Pittler M, Ernst E. Ginkgo biloba extract for the treatment of intermittent claudication: a meta-analysis of randomized trials. Am J Med 2000;108:276–281.

ADDITIONAL RESOURCES

Allard M. Treatment of the disorders of aging with Ginkgo biloba extract. From pharmacology to clinical medicine. Presse Med 1986;15(31):1540–1545.

Christen Y. Oxidative stress and Alzheimer disease. Am J Clin Nutr 2000;71(2):621S–629S.

Crews D, Mix J. A double-blind, placebo-controlled, randomized trial of Ginkgo biloba extract Egb 761 in a sample of cognitively intact older adults: neuropsychological findings. Hum Psychopharmacol Clin Exp 2002;17:267–277.

Deberdt W. Interaction between psychological and pharmacological treatment in cognitive impairment. Life Sci 1994;55(25–26):2057–2066.

Diamond BJ, Shiflett SC, Feiwel N, Matheis RJ, Noskin O, Richards JA, Schoenberger NE. Ginkgo biloba extract: mechanisms and clinical indications. Arch Phys Med Rehabil 2000;81(5):668–678.

Drew S, Davies E. Effectiveness of Ginkgo biloba in treating tinnitus: double blind, placebo controlled trial. BMJ 2001;322:1–6.

Hofferberth B. The effect of Ginkgo biloba extract on neurophysiological and psychometric measurement results in patients with psychotic organic brain syndrome. A double-blind study against placebo. Arzneimittelforschung 1989;39(8):918–922.

Itil TM, Eralp E, Ahmed I, Kunitz A, Itil KZ. The pharmacological effects of ginkgo biloba, a plant extract, on the brain of dementia patients in comparison with tacrine. Psychopharmacol Bull 1998;34(3):391–397.

Kidd PM. A review of nutrients and botanicals in the integrative management of cognitive dysfunction. Altern Med Rev 1999;4(3):144–161.

Kleijnen J, Knipschild P. Ginkgo biloba. Lancet 1992;340(8828):1136–1139.

Le Bars P, Kieser M, Kurt Z. A 26-week analysis of a double-blind, placebo-controlled trial of the Ginkgo biloba extract Egb 761 in dementia. Dement Geriatr Cogn Disord 2000;11:230–237.

Massoni G, Piovella C, Fratti L. Effects on microcirculation of Ginkgo-biloba in elderly people. G Gerontol 1972;20(5):444–450.

Moulton P, Boyko L, Fitzpatrick J, Petros T. The effect of Ginkgo biloba on memory in healthy male volunteers. Physiol Behav 2001;73:659–665.

Perry EK, Pickering AT, Wang WW, Houghton P, Perry NS. Medicinal plants and Alzheimer's disease: integrating ethnobotanical and contemporary scientific evidence. J Altern Complement Med 1998;4(4):419–428.

Pidoux B. Effects of Ginkgo biloba extract on functional brain activity.. An assessment of clinical and experimental studies. Presse Med 1986;15(31):1588–1591.

Pitchumoni SS, Doraiswamy PM. Current status of antioxidant therapy for Alzheimer's disease. J Am Geriatr Soc 1998;46(12):1566–1572.

Raabe A, Raabe M, Ihm P. Therapeutic follow-up using automatic perimetry in chronic cerebroretinal ischemia in elderly patients. Prospective double-blind study with graduated dose ginkgo biloba treatment. Klin Monatsbl Augenheilkd 1991;199(6):432–438.

Racagni G, Brunello N, Paoletti R. Neuromediator changes during cerebral aging. The effect of Ginkgo biloba extract. Presse Med 1986;15(31):1488–1490.

Solomon P, Adams F, Silver A, Zimmer J, DeVeaux R. Ginkgo for memory enhancement. JAMA 2002;288(7):835–840.

Taillandier J, Ammar A, Rabourdin JP, Ribeyre JP, Pichon J, Niddam S, Pierart H. Treatment of cerebral aging disorders with Ginkgo biloba extract. A longitudinal multicenter double-blind drug vs. placebo study. Presse Med 1986;15(31):1583–1587.

Warburton DM. Clinical psychopharmacology of Ginkgo biloba extract. Presse Med 1986;15(31):1595–1604.

KAVA KAVA (*PIPER METHYSTICUM*)

Overall Rank

 WARNING: Some contaminated kava supplements have been implicated in isolated cases of hepatotoxicity. Readers are referred to the "Safety/Dosage" subsection of this section for a discussion.

★★★★ for anxiety and stress
★★★ for insomnia
★★★ for reducing musculoskeletal pain
★★ for reducing menstrual discomfort and anxiety
★★ for benzodiazepine withdrawal
★★ for attention-deficit/hyperactivity disorder (ADHD)
★★ for headaches and migraines
★ as an aphrodisiac
★ as an analgesic
ZERO for treating or preventing upper respiratory infection (URI)
ZERO for treating or preventing urinary tract infections (UTI)

OVERVIEW

Kava kava (*Piper methysticum*) is a perennial shrub with a heart-shaped leaf. It was discovered by Captain Cook, who named the plant "intoxicating pepper." Ceremonially, kava kava had been used in the Pacific regions of Polynesia, Melanesia, and Micronesia as a beverage to induce relaxation and thus promote discussion and interaction. It was prepared by chewing the root, which became fermented in saliva, leaving a bitter, hot, numbing taste. Other preparations included pounding the root or grating it into a powder and using hot water to extract the kava. Currently, kava kava—also known more simply as kava—is prepared commercially by either ethanol or acetone, which yields 30–70% kava lactones, respectively. The active components of kava are referred to as kavapyrones and consist of kavain, dihydrokavain, methysticin, dihydromethysticin, yangonin, and desmethoxyyangonin.

Although only the anxiolytic properties of kava have been studied in humans to date, empirical data suggest usefulness in several other areas. In response to a report about alleged hepatotoxic reactions to kava use, worldwide controversy sprang up (FDA/CFSAN Consumer Advisory, 2002). As a result, kava was banned in many countries, and Merck, the manufacturer of two kava supplements, withdrew the supplements from the market (Abt and Hammerly, 2003; DerMarderosian, 2003).

The pharmacologic mechanism of action of kava is largely attributed to the kavapyrones kavain, dihydrokavain, methysticin, dihydromethysticin, and yangonin. Preliminary evidence indicates kava can inhibit the cytochrome P4503A4 enzyme and possibly others. In vitro, kava extract and kavapyrones, desmethoxyyangonin, and methysticin have been shown to be reversible inhibitors of monoamine oxidase B through competitive inhibition. In vitro, two kavapyrones have been shown to inhibit the uptake of noradrenaline in the cerebral cortex, suggesting antidepressant activity. The sedative effects of kava may be the result of an increased number of γ-aminobutyric acid (GABA)-binding sites or dopamine antagonism. The psychotropic actions of kava are thought to stem from the kavapyrones (+)-methysticin, and (+)-kavain, by noradrenaline uptake inhibition. Kava is also thought to inhibit inflammation by inhibiting COX-1 and COX-2.

COMMENTS

Reports linking liver toxicity to kava use have been widely debated, and their validity is still controversial. A systematic review of clinical trials and short-term postmarketing surveillance studies found that the adverse effects associated with kava use are rare, mild, and reversible. Although the data for short-term use of kava have found it to be safe, with only mild side effects, more studies on the side effects of long-term use would benefit our understanding of its use for longer periods (Stevinson et al., 2002).

SCIENTIFIC SUPPORT

A meta-analysis of randomized, double-blind, placebo-controlled studies of kava found that 11 trials with a total of 645 participants met the criteria for the analysis. The analysis of six of the trials found the Hamilton Anxiety Scale (HAMA) total score to show a significant improvement in symptoms, with few adverse effects (Pittler and Ernst, 2003).

An earlier meta-analysis by Pittler and Ernst (2000) found seven trials met the inclusion criteria. All seven trials suggested that kava extract was better than a placebo for anxiety; the meta-analysis of three of the trials suggested a significant lowering in the HAMA total score for anxiety for the use of kava over a placebo.

Lehrl (2004) tested the clinical efficacy of a kava extract (WS 1490) in sleep disturbances associated with anxiety disorders. In the multicenter, randomized, double-blind study, 61 patients received 200 mg of the extract or a placebo for 4 weeks. A significant increase in the quality of sleep and the recuperative effect after sleep was found for the group taking the kava extract. The HAMA also showed superior effects for kava, and significant effects were found in the self-ratings of well-being.

A double-blind, placebo-controlled study was conducted to obtain dosage range information on kava (WS 1490) in patients with nonpsychotic anxiety. The drug was well tolerated and had a safety profile with no drug-related adverse events or post-study withdrawal symptoms. The authors found that 150 mg of WS 1490 was an effective treatment for nonpsychotic anxiety syndromes (Geier and Konstantinowicz, 2004).

In an earlier randomized, placebo-controlled, double-blind study, kava was studied for its effect on climacteric-related symptomology. Patients received 300 mg of kava (WS 1490) 3 times daily or a placebo for 8 weeks. After only 1 week of treatment, the target variable—anxiety as measured by the HAMA—showed significant improvement. Over the study period, kava showed a high level of efficacy for neurovegetative and psychosomatic dysfunctions in the climacteric woman (Warnecke, 1991).

In a randomized, double-blind placebo-controlled study, kava was tested for its effect on anxiety syndrome. Kava (WS 1490, or Laitan) was given at the rate of 100 mg 3 times daily for 4 weeks, or a placebo was administered. After 4 weeks, the HAMA score was significantly improved, as was the Adjectives List Scale and the Clinical Global Impression Scale. No adverse effects were found (Kinzler et al., 1991).

In an 8-week, randomized, multicenter, double-blind, controlled study, 400 mg of kava (LI) was studied for generalized anxiety disorder. Kava or one of two reference drugs, buspirone (10 mg) or opipramol (100 mg) was given to 129 outpatients. Kava was found to be as effective as the reference drugs and well tolerated in the acute treatment of people suffering from generalized anxiety disorder (Boerner et al., 2003).

In a 5-week, randomized, placebo-controlled, double-blind study, kava was investigated for its use for treating nonpsychotic nervous anxiety, tension, and restlessness. Kava (WS 1490) was administered at the dosage of 50 mg/day, increasing to 300 mg/day in the first week as the pretreatment of benzodiazepines was tapered off over 2 weeks. The kava extract was found to be superior to the placebo according to the HAMA and a subjective well-being scale. The tolerance to kava was the same as to the placebo. The authors concluded that further symptom reduction is possible after a changeover from benzodiazepine treatment (Malsch and Keiser, 2001).

De Leo et al. (2001) studied the use of kava in combination with hormone replacement therapy in the treatment of menopausal anxiety. A significant reduction in the HAMA score was observed in four groups receiving hormone replacement therapy, with or without progestogens and with kava extract or placebo for 6 months. The groups with kava treatment had the more significant reductions in HAMA scores, and the authors concluded that kava accelerated the betterment of psychological symptoms with hormone therapy. An earlier study also investigated the use of kava with hormone replacement therapy and found significantly lower HAMA scores after 3 and 6 months of treatment in all four groups studied, although the groups treated with kava in combination with the hormone replacement showed the best improvements (De Leo et al., 2000).

In a study on anxiety of nonpsychotic origin (criteria of the *Diagnostic and Statistical Manual of Mental Disorders* [*DSM-III-R*]: agoraphobia, specific phobia, generalized anxiety disorder, and adjustment disorder with anxiety), kava (WS 1490) was tested in a multicenter, randomized, placebo-controlled, double-blind test design. Starting at week 8, the kava treatment group resulted in significant improvement in HAMA scores as well as other secondary outcomes. The authors concluded that this supported using WS 1490 instead of tricyclic antidepressants and benzodiazepines in anxiety disorders, with none of the side effects of conventional treatment (Volz and Kieser, 1997).

In a placebo-controlled, double-blind trial with 84 subjects, kavain improved memory and reaction time. In a similar study with 38 subjects, kavain showed equivalent activity to oxazepam (Lindenberg and Pitule-Schodel, 1990).

SAFETY/DOSAGE

For typical anxiolytic uses, 70% kava lactones (kavapyrones) is recommended. In capsule form, the recommended dosage is 300 mg (70 mg kava lactone) daily for 1 to 8 weeks. As a tincture, 30 drops with water 3 times daily is recommended. Dosage varies depending on the kava lactones present in the source. For the typical tea preparation, 2–4 g of kava root should be simmered in 150 mL of boiling water for 5–10 minutes and then strained (Abt and Hammerly, 2003; Brinker, 2002; Cupp, 2000).

Kava can adversely affect the liver, possibly leading to hepatitis, cirrhosis, and liver failure requiring a transplant. The use of kava for as little as 1–3 months has resulted in the need for liver transplants, and even death. Symptoms may resolve following discontinuation. Other adverse effects include gastrointestinal distress, headache, dizziness, drowsiness, enlarged pupils, disturbances of oculomotor equilibrium and accommodation, dry mouth, allergic skin reaction (rare), and extrapyramidal symptoms (oral and lingual reflexes, and head and trunk twisting movements). With chronic use at high doses (greater than 400 mg/day), endocrine and metabolic effects can result, including weight loss, reduced protein levels, puffy face, hematuria, increased red blood cell volume, decreased platelets and lymphocytes, and possible pulmonary hypertension. Chronic use of kava has also been associated with dermopathy (reddened eyes; dry, scaly, flaky skin; temporary yellow discoloration of the skin, hair, and nails). These effects usually resolve with discontinuation (Abt and Hammerly, 2003; Brinker, 2002; Cupp, 2000).

Many concerns have been expressed about the use of kava with alcohol. In reality, this effect varies with the type of extract. For example, 200 mg/kg of kava lipid-soluble extract (resin administered orally in mice) increased the hypnotic effect of ethanol, whereas kava extract (WS 1490, administered orally in humans) showed no negative additive effects (Lehrl, 2004). The risk of drowsiness and motor reflex depression is increased because of depression of the central nervous system. Pyrones in kava with pentobarbital increased sleeping time in mice (Abt and Hammerly, 2003; Brinker, 2002; Cupp, 2000).

Possible drug interactions include the following:

- Levodopa: The kavapyrone yangonin is a potent dopamine antagonist that decreases the efficacy of levodopa and worsens the symptoms of Parkinson disease.
- Benzodiazepines: In vitro, kavapyrones may indirectly increase the affinity of $GABA_A$-receptor binding sites with the use of alprazolam and may increase the number of GABA binding sites. Other studies report the possible interaction because of kava's inhibition of cytochrome P450 enzymes.
- Strychnine: Kavapyrones kavain, dihydrokavain, methysticin, and dihydromethysticin protect against strychnine poisoning more effectively than does mephenesin.
- Warfarin: Because of its interaction with the cytochrome P450 system, kava may increase warfarin's effects.
- Antiplatelets: May result in an increased risk of bleeding.
- Monoamine oxidase inhibitors: Additive effects.
- Hepatotoxic drugs: Include, but are not limited to, acarbose, amiodarone, atorvastatin, azathioprine, carbamazepine, gemfibrozil, itraconazole, methotrexate, valproic acid, zileuton.
- Hepatotoxic herbals: Include, but are not limited to, chaparral (*Larrea tridentate*), Russian comfrey (*Symphytum x uplandicum*), coltsfoot (*Tussilago farfara*), germander (*Teucrium chamaedrys*), jin bu huan, pennyroyal (*Mentha pulegium, Hedeoma pulegoides*), and petasites (*Petasites japonicus*). Additionally, androstenedione, coenzyme Q_{10} (in high doses), dehydroepiandrosterone, niacin, red yeast, skullcap, and valerian have been reported to adversely affect the liver with concomitant use.
- Sedative herbals: Include, but are not limited to, 5-HTP, calamus, calendula, California poppy, catnip, capsicum, celery, couch grass, elecampane, German chamomile, goldenseal, gotu kola, hops, Jamaican dogwood, lemon balm, melatonin, sage, St. John's wort, sassafras, skullcap, shepherd's purse, Siberian ginseng, stinging nettle, valerian, wild carrot, wild lettuce, ashwangandha root, and

yerba mansa; all may increase the risk of excessive drowsiness with concomitant use with kava (Abt and Hammerly, 2003; Brinker, 2002; Cupp, 2000).

Kava is contraindicated in pregnancy because pyrones may result in the loss of uterine tone. Pyrones may also be carried in breast milk. Kava resin and the pyrones dihydrokawain and dihydromethysticin may contribute to suicidal tendencies. Kava is associated with elevated liver transaminases with or without concomitant hepatic damage. Patients with Parkinson disease should not use kava because of its dopamine antagonism (Abt and Hammerly, 2003; Brinker, 2002; Cupp, 2000).

REFERENCES

Abt L, Hammerly M. AltMedDex System. Greenwood Village, CO: Micromedex, 2003.

Boerner RJ, Sommer H, Berger W, Kuhn U, Schmidt U, Mannel M. Kava-kava extract LI 150 is as effective as opipramol and buspirone in generalised anxiety disorder—an 8-week randomized, double-blind multi-centre clinical trial in 129 out-patients. Phytomedicine 2003;10(suppl 4):38–49.

Brinker F. Herb Contraindications and Drug Interactions. 3rd Ed. London: Pharmaceutical Press, 2002.

Cupp M, ed. Toxicology and Clinical Pharmacology of Herbal Products. Totowa, NJ: Humana Press, 2000.

De Leo V, la Marca A, Lanzetta D, Palazzi S, Torricelli M, Facchini C, Morgante G. Assessment of the association of kava-kava extract and hormone replacement therapy in the treatment of postmenopause anxiety. Minerva Ginecol 2000;52(6):263–267.

De Leo V, la Marca A, Morgante G, Lanzetta D, Florio P, Petraglia F. Evaluation of combining kava extract with hormone replacement therapy in the treatment of postmenopausal anxiety. Maturitas 2001;39(2):185–188.

DerMarderosian A. Review of Natural Products. St. Louis: Facts and Comparisons, 2003.

Food and Drug Administration/Center for Food Safety and Applied Nutrition (FDA/ CFSAN) Consumer Advisory. Kava-containing dietary supplements may be associated with severe liver injury. March 25, 2002. http://www.cfsan.fda.gov/~dms/ addskava.html. Accessed May 6, 2006.

Geier FP, Konstantinowicz T. Kava treatment in patients with anxiety. Phytother Res 2004;18(4):297–300.

Kinzler E, Kromer J, Lehmann E. Effect of a special kava extract in patients with anxiety-, tension-, and excitation states of non-psychotic genesis. Double blind study with placebos over 4 weeks. Arzneimittelforschung 1991;41(6):584–588.

Lehrl S. Clinical efficacy of kava extract WS 1490 in sleep disturbances associated with anxiety disorders. Results of a multicenter, randomized, placebo-controlled, double-blind clinical trial. J Affect Disord 2004;78(2):101–110.

Lindenberg D, Pitule-Schodel H. D,L-kavain in comparison with oxazepam in anxiety disorders. A double-blind study of clinical effectiveness. Fortschr Med 1990;108(2):49–50, 53–54.

Malsch U, Kieser M. Efficacy of kava-kava in the treatment of non-psychotic anxiety, following pretreatment with benzodiazepines. Psychopharmacology (Berl) 2001;157(3):277–283.

Pittler MH, Ernst E. Efficacy of kava extract for treating anxiety: systematic review and meta-analysis. J Clin Psychopharmacol 2000;20(1):84–89.

Pittler MH, Ernst E. Kava extract for treating anxiety. Cochrane Database Syst Rev 2003;(1):CD003383.

Stevinson C, Huntley A, Ernst E. A systematic review of the safety of kava extract in the treatment of anxiety. Drug Saf 2002;25(4):251–261.

Volz HP, Kieser M. Kava-kava extract WS 1490 versus placebo in anxiety disorders—a randomized placebo-controlled 25-week outpatient trial. Pharmacopsychiatry 1997;30(1):1–5.

Warnecke G. Psychosomatic dysfunctions in the female climacteric. Clinical effectiveness and tolerance of Kava Extract WS 1490. Fortschr Med 1991;109(4):119–122.

ADDITIONAL RESOURCES

Barnes J, Anderson LA, Phillipson JD. Herbal Medicines: A Guide for Healthcare Professionals. 2nd Ed. Chicago: Pharmaceutical Press, 2002.

Fetrow CW, Avila JR. Professionals Handbook of Complimentary and Alternative Medicine. 2nd Ed. Springhouse, PA: Springhouse, 2001.

Mills S, Bone K. Principles and Practice of Phytotherapy: Modern Herbal Medicine. New York: Harcourt, 2000.

MELATONIN

Overall Rank

★★★★ as a sleep aid
★★★★ for alleviating jet lag
★★★ as an antioxidant
★ for antiaging effects
★ for depression

OVERVIEW

Melatonin is a hormone produced by the pineal gland in the brain. It is synthesized from the amino acid tryptophan (tryptophan can also be converted into serotonin and the serotonin converted into melatonin). Melatonin levels are lowest during midday (and subsequent to sunlight exposure), and production peaks at night (typically, from 2:00 to 4:00 AM). In some animals, melatonin is necessary for regulation of light/dark cycle behaviors like sleeping and waking and sexual maturation. In animals, melatonin seems to help regulate seasonal behaviors (e.g., mating, molting, hibernation), which are related to daily light/dark cycles. In humans, melatonin helps regulate the "internal clock." The onset of darkness results in an increased production of melatonin in the brain, while the light of morning tells the brain to stop producing melatonin. Melatonin levels are 10 times higher at night than during the day.

Dietary supplements containing melatonin are generally used for promoting sleep, reducing insomnia, and reducing the symptoms of jet lag. Numerous claims for melatonin supplements exist for its preliminary effects as an antioxidant, anticancer adjunct, and antiaging agent. Interestingly, melatonin has been found in other herbal remedies, such as St. John's wort flower, green feverfew leaves, and skullcap. It may be obtained by extraction from the pineal glands of cattle or by chemical synthesis in the laboratory from 5-methoxyindole. The synthetic form is available from numerous manufacturers and is preferred over animal-derived supplements.

COMMENTS

Melatonin can be viewed as a relatively inexpensive and nonaddictive alternative to over-the-counter chemical sleep aids. It may be particularly useful as a short-term regulator of sleep/wake cycles in cases such as getting one's internal clock back on schedule after crossing several time zones (jet lag) and in cases of transient insomnia.

SCIENTIFIC SUPPORT

Melatonin is produced from tryptophan, which is converted to 5-hydroxytryptophan, then to serotonin, then to N-acetylserotonin, and finally to melatonin (Lewy et al., 1992). By altering membrane characteristics, melatonin is thought to increase the binding of GABA to its receptors, subsequently decreasing central nervous system activity (Sack et al., 1997). In addition, the hormone seems to have a role in the regulation of circadian rhythm, endocrine secretions, and sleep cycles (Sack et al., 1997). When melatonin is administered, it induces sleep and may lower alertness, body temperature, and blood pressure. Melatonin supplementation has been shown to lower core body temperature, produce acute hypnotic effects, and induce the onset of sleep in various subjects, including military pilots, jet-lagged travelers, elderly patients, and people with delayed-sleep disorder (Kato et al., 1998; Petri et al., 1993). Melatonin has also shown some benefit in helping to reset the internal clocks of shift workers who tend to have peak melatonin levels during the day (Kuhn et al., 1998).

As an antioxidant, melatonin has shown benefits in protecting cells against oxidative stress by scavenging hydroxyl radicals and preventing oxidative damage to DNA, lipids, and cellular proteins (DeFrance and Quera-Salva, 1998). Melatonin is also thought to play a role in the regulation of the human menstrual cycle, as evidenced by the finding that women with hypothalamic amenorrhea (lack of menstrual periods) have melatonin levels 3 times higher than normal (Lewy et al., 1992).

Numerous clinical trials have monitored the effectiveness of melatonin use for the treatment of insomnia (Kato et al., 1998; Kuhn et al., 1998; Petrie et al., 1993). Most of these trials have concluded that melatonin improves quality, onset, and duration of sleep (Jan and Espezel, 1995). In one randomized, double-blind, placebo-controlled trial, the effects of immediate-release melatonin and sustained-release melatonin were compared in patients with sleep-onset and sleep-maintenance insomnia. Although a significant improvement in sleep onset was noted in patients receiving 0.5 mg immediate-release melatonin, melatonin was not effective for the treatment of sleep-maintenance insomnia. The researchers concluded that melatonin would not be the ideal sleep medication for elderly patients, because the primary causes of insomnia in the elderly are related to sleep-maintenance issues (Hughes et al., 1998).

Numerous clinical studies have concluded that melatonin is effective in reducing symptoms of jet lag, such as daytime fatigue and unpleasant mood (Arendt and Deacon, 1997; Chase and Gidal, 1997; Jan et al., 1998). In most of these studies, the effectiveness of melatonin has been demonstrated at doses from 0.5 mg to 5 mg for jet lag symptoms.

SAFETY/DOSAGE

The interactions of melatonin with other supplements or drugs is unknown, but some studies suggest that melatonin can induce or deepen depression in susceptible people. Melatonin supplements may also be dangerous for people with cardiovascular risks, owing to the possibility of vasoconstriction and increased blood pressure. Studies of melatonin as a sleep aid or for relief of symptoms associated with jet lag have shown 0.5–5 mg to be effective, depending on the degree of sleep disturbance. High-dose melatonin supplements (about 50 mg) may disrupt female fertility and menstrual patterns and should be avoided except under the supervision of a reproductive physician.

REFERENCES

Arendt J, Deacon S. Treatment of circadian rhythm disorders—melatonin. Chronobiol Int 1997;14(2):185–204.

Chase JE, Gidal BE. Melatonin: therapeutic use in sleep disorders. Ann Pharmacother 1997;31(10):1218–1226.

Hughes RJ, Sack RL, Lewy AJ. The role of melatonin and circadian phase in age-related sleep-maintenance insomnia: assessment in a clinical trial of melatonin replacement. Sleep 1998;21:52–68.

Jan JE, Espezel H, Freeman RD, Fast DK. Melatonin treatment of chronic sleep disorders. J Child Neurol 1998;13(2):98.

Lewy AJ, Ahmed S, Jackson JM, Sack RL. Melatonin shifts human circadian rhythms according to a phase-response curve. Chronobiol Int 1992;9(5):380–392.

Sack RL, Hughes RJ, Edgar DM, Lewy AJ. Sleep-promoting effects of melatonin: at what dose, in whom, under what conditions, and by what mechanisms? Sleep 1997;20(10):908–915.

ADDITIONAL RESOURCES

Avery D, Lenz M, Landis C. Guidelines for prescribing melatonin. Ann Med 1998;30(1):122–130.

Defrance R, Quera-Salva MA. Therapeutic applications of melatonin and related compounds. Horm Res 1998;49(3–4):142–146.

Jan JE, Espezel H. Melatonin treatment of chronic sleep disorders. Dev Med Child Neurol 1995;37(3):279–280.

Kato M, Kajimura N, Sekimoto M, Watanabe T, Takahashi K. Melatonin treatment for rhythm disorder. Psychiatry Clin Neurosci 1998;52(2):262–263.

Kendler BS. Melatonin: media hype or therapeutic breakthrough? Nurse Pract 1997;22(2):66–67, 71–72, 77.

Kryger MH. Controversies in sleep medicine: melatonin. Sleep 1997;20(10):898.

Kuhn WF, Wellman A. The use of melatonin as a potential treatment for shiftwork sleep disorder. Acad Emerg Med 1998;5(8):842–843.

Petrie K, Conaglen JV, Thompson L, et al: Effect of melatonin on jet lag after a treatment for jet lag in international cabin crew. Biol Psychiatry 1993;33:526–530.

Sack RL, Lewy AJ, Hughes RJ. Use of melatonin for sleep and circadian rhythm disorders. Ann Med 1998;30(1):115–121.

Skene DJ, Lockley SW, Arendt J. Melatonin in circadian sleep disorders in the blind. Biol Signals Recept 1999;8(1–2):90–95.

Skene DJ, Lockley SW, Arendt J. Use of melatonin in the treatment of phase shift and sleep disorders. Adv Exp Med Biol 1999;467:79–84.

Spitzer RL, Terman M, Williams JB, Terman JS, Malt UF, Singer F, Lewy AJ. Jet lag: clinical features, validation of a new syndrome specific scale, and lack of response to melatonin in a randomized, double-blind trial. Amer J Psychiatr 1999;156:1392–1396.

Wurtman RJ, Zhdanova I. Improvement of sleep quality by melatonin. Lancet 1995;346:1491.

Zhdanova IV, Lynch HJ, Wurtman RJ. Melatonin: a sleep-promoting hormone. Sleep 1997;20(10):899–907.

PHOSPHATIDYLSERINE

Overall Rank

★★★★   for cognitive function
★★★   for anti-stress effects

OVERVIEW

Phosphatidylserine (PS) is an aminophospholipid—a molecule made up of two fatty acids and a phosphate group attached to a glycerol backbone (derived from the amino acid serine). PS is synthesized in the body and concentrated in cells of the brain, where it may be related to brain cell function and neurotransmitter metabolism. PS is also found in other cell membranes, such as muscle tissue and cells of the immune system, where it may play both a structural and functional role in muscle metabolism and immune system function. Dietary supplements of PS are most often promoted for their role in maintaining brain function, boosting memory, and improving cognitive ability, as well as for their role in modulating stress response and cortisol metabolism. Because of its effects on controlling stress hormones, PS is often found in supplements that target immune function, exercise recovery, and relaxation.

COMMENTS

Although not all studies are unanimous in their findings for a cognitive benefit of phosphatidylserine supplements, enough evidence exists to consider recommending PS for patients in the early stages of age-related cognitive decline, as well as for those who are under increased physical or emotional stress. In May 2003, the FDA reviewed the scientific evidence for PS as a dietary supplement for preventing cognitive dysfunction and dementia in the elderly. Although the FDA determined that there was a lack of "significant scientific agreement" (the standard by which it may award a health claim), the agency also determined that the evidence was appropriate to issue the following qualified health claim for PS: "Consumption of phosphatidylserine may reduce the risk of dementia [or cognitive dysfunction] in the elderly." In addition, all claims on products must also carry this qualification language: "Very limited and preliminary scientific research suggests that phosphatidylserine may reduce the risk of dementia [or cognitive dysfunction] in the elderly. FDA concludes that there is little scientific evidence supporting this claim" (Letter Updating..., 2004). A daily dose of PS is important because it is an expensive ingredient and many commercial products fail to provide clinically effective levels.

SCIENTIFIC SUPPORT

Phosphatidylserine, like other phospholipids, is a major constituent of cellular membranes. Maintenance of membrane integrity is crucial for proper function, but there is little direct evidence that PS supplements improve membrane integrity or cellular function. PS has, however, been linked to a suppression of cortisol secretion during periods of intense training (20–30%), an effect that may help enhance recovery and repair, particularly following intense exercise or injury (Monteleone et al., 1990).

Although not all studies have shown a benefit of PS in reducing symptoms of age-associated memory impairment (AAMI), there are several studies showing improvements in memory, learning, concentration, word recall, and mood in middle-aged and elderly subjects with dementia or age-related cognitive decline. Some of the differences in findings among studies may be related to the degree of cognitive decline in subjects enrolled. For example, one study of 120 elderly subjects with moderate levels of AAMI found no effect of 300 mg or 600 mg of PS daily for 12 weeks on measures of learning, memory, attention, or reaction time (Jorissen et al., 2001). Other studies of PS supplementation in elderly subjects with milder memory impairment (Crook et al., 1991; Engel et al., 1992) or mild depression (Maggioni et al., 1990) have shown significant improvements on global measurements of cognitive function and psychological testing. Likewise, PS has shown benefits on overall cognitive functioning in more severely affected subjects—those with moderate to severe senile dementia (Cenacchi et al., 1993; Delwaide et al., 1986) and Alzheimer disease (Crook et al., 1992; Heiss et al., 1994). Additionally, isolated reports exist concerning the use of PS to alleviate some symptoms associated with physical stress (Monteleone et al., 1992), Parkinson disease (Funfgeld et al., 1989), and thyroid hormone dysregulation (Masturzo et al., 1990).

Interestingly, PS could also be considered a general antistress nutrient, providing benefits for athletes subjected to the physical stress of exercise as well as for persons under chronic emotional stress from hectic lifestyles, job deadlines, and many of the other stresses of modern life. PS has been shown to reduce blood levels of cortisol, a hormone produced in response to stress (Monteleone et al., 1992). One of the effects of elevated cortisol production is accelerated amino acid catabolism, which could lead to muscle breakdown. Suppression of cortisol levels could theoretically maintain muscle mass during periods of increased stress and intense training, including during the "stress" of dieting for weight loss.

SAFETY/DOSAGE

There do not appear to be any significant side effects associated with dietary supplements containing phosphatidylserine, but owing to concerns about "mad cow disease," it is generally recommended that patients select PS supplements derived from soybeans rather than those forms extracted from cow brains (bovine cortex). Soy-derived PS supplements are known to be well tolerated up to doses of 600 mg/day (Jorissen et al., 2002). Although concentrated PS supplements are available in doses of 50–100 mg/day, they are very expensive. For brain and mental support, 300–400 mg/day of PS is recommended for 1–6 months (Cenacchi et al., 1993; Delwaide et al., 1986; Engel et al., 1992; Maggioni et al., 1990). Athletes may need as much as 800 mg/day to help modulate cortisol levels associated with exercise stress cortisol secretion and to promote muscle recovery.

REFERENCES

Cenacchi T, Bertoldin T, Farina C, Fiori MG, Crepaldi G. Cognitive decline in the elderly: a double-blind, placebo-controlled multicenter study on efficacy of phosphatidylserine administration. Aging (Milano) 1993;5(2):123–133.

Crook T, Petrie W, Wells C, Massari DC. Effects of phosphatidylserine in Alzheimer's disease. Psychopharmacol Bull 1992;28(1):61–66.

Crook T, Tinklenberg J, Yesavage J, Petrie W, Nunzi MG, Massari DC. Effects of phosphatidylserine in age-associated memory impairment. Neurology 1991;41(5):644–649.

Delwaide PJ, Gyselynck-Mambourg AM, Hurlet A, Ylieff M. Double-blind randomized controlled study of phosphatidylserine in senile demented patients. Acta Neurol Scand 1986;73(2):136–140.

Engel RR, Satzger W, Gunther W, Kathmann N, Bove D, Gerke S, Munch U, Hippius H. Double-blind cross-over study of phosphatidylserine vs. placebo in patients with early dementia of the Alzheimer type. Eur Neuropsychopharmacol 1992;2(2):149–155.

Funfgeld EW, Baggen M, Nedwidek P, Richstein B, Mistlberger G. Double-blind study with phosphatidylserine (PS) in parkinsonian patients with senile dementia of Alzheimer's type (SDAT). Prog Clin Biol Res 1989;317:1235–1246.

Heiss WD, Kessler J, Mielke R, Szelies B, Herholz K. Long-term effects of phosphatidylserine, pyritinol, and cognitive training in Alzheimer's disease. A neuropsychological, EEG, and PET investigation. Dementia 1994;5(2):88–98.

Jorissen BL, Brouns F, Van Boxtel MP, Ponds RW, Verhey FR, Jolles J, Riedel WJ. The influence of soy-derived phosphatidylserine on cognition in age-associated memory impairment. Nutr Neurosci 2001;4(2):121–134.

Jorissen BL, Brouns F, Van Boxtel MP, Riedel WJ. Safety of soy-derived phosphatidylserine in elderly people. Nutr Neurosci 2002;5(5):337–343.

Letter Updating the Phosphatidylserine and Cognitive Function and Dementia Qualified Health Claim. CFSAN/Office of Nutritional Products, Labeling, and Dietary Supplements, November 24, 2004. Accessed at: http://www.cfsan.fda.gov/~dms/ds-ltr39.html.

Maggioni M, Picotti GB, Bondiolotti GP, Panerai A, Cenacchi T, Nobile P, Brambilla F. Effects of phosphatidylserine therapy in geriatric patients with depressive disorders. Acta Psychiatr Scand 1990;81(3):265–270.

Masturzo P, Murialdo G, de Palma D, Filippi U, Balbi D, Bonura ML, Toffano G, Polleri A. TSH circadian secretions in aged men and effect of phosphatidylserine treatment. Chronobiologia 1990;17(4):267–267.

Monteleone P, Maj M, Beinat L, Natale M, Kemali D. Blunting by chronic phosphatidylserine administration of the stress-induced activation of the hypothalamo-pituitary-adrenal axis in healthy men. Eur J Clin Pharmacol 1992;42(4):385–388.

ADDITIONAL RESOURCES

Monteleone P, Beinat L, Tanzillo C, Maj M, Kemali D. Effects of phosphatidylserine on the neuroendocrine response to physical stress in humans. Neuroendocrinology 1990;52(3):243–248.

Rosadini G, Sannita WG, Nobili F, Cenacchi T. Phosphatidylserine: quantitative EEG effects in healthy volunteers. Neuropsychobiology 1990–1991;24(1):42–48.

SAME (S-ADENOSYL-L-METHIONINE)

Overall Rank

★★★★ for depression
★★★★ for liver disease
★★★ for osteoarthritis
★ for fibromyalgia

OVERVIEW

SAMe (S-adenosyl-L-methionine) is a substance naturally found in many of the body's tissues. It is made up of the amino acid methionine (a sulfur-containing amino acid) combined with adenosine. SAMe is used in several of the body's processes that require sulfur, especially methylation reactions. Many favorable clinical studies on SAMe indicate it has potential as a therapy for osteoarthritis, depression, and liver disease. SAMe's general mechanism of action as a supplement is as a methyl donor for methylation reactions in our body's natural processes. A deficiency of SAMe could be caused by a deficiency in the cofactors of its production, such as methionine, choline, and B vitamins. A defect in methylation may also cause a deficiency in SAMe. Overall, SAMe has been found to have anti-inflammatory, analgesic, and antidepressive effects.

One theory on depression and other neuropsychiatric disorders is that they are caused by a defect in biochemical methylation reactions. Low levels of folate (used in methylation reactions) and serotonin have been linked to lower levels of SAMe in depressed patients; in clinical studies, SAMe supplementation has been shown to have an antidepressant effect that may increase serotonin levels (Bressa, 1994; Fetrow and Avila, 2001).

The National Institute on Alcohol Abuse and Alcoholism and the Office of Dietary Supplements sponsored a conference examining the possible role of SAMe in treating alcoholic liver disease. Because oxidant stress is known to play a major role in the development of liver disease, and SAMe is involved in the manufacture of important liver antioxidant compounds (glutathione), SAMe is being studied for its role in the treatment of alcoholic liver disease. SAMe's potential for osteoarthritis is based on its ability to support a higher production of proteoglycans, a substance that makes up cartilage.

COMMENTS

SAMe seems to be a relatively safe and effective way of correcting our biochemical methylation reactions, which may lead to causes of depression, osteoarthritis, liver disease, and other conditions. More clinical studies are needed to understand the kinds of depression for which SAMe works best, its specific risks and therapeutic side effects, and its potential for other disease processes before it can be accepted as a treatment method for these and other conditions.

SCIENTIFIC SUPPORT

Depression

A review of the published literature (from 1966 to 2001) on SAMe found that most of the clinical evidence for its use has been conducted on various depressive disorders, osteoarthritis, and fibromyalgia, and sample sizes and the doses used varied widely (Fetrow and Avila, 2001). Several reviews and meta-analyses have been published, all concluding that SAMe was better than placebo in treating depression and equally as effective as the standard tricyclic antidepressants. The authors pointed out, however, that even though SAMe seems well tolerated, with most side effects being presented as gastrointestinal complaints, it may have the potential risk of psychiatric and cardiovascular adverse side effects. They concluded that until the side effects are more thoroughly researched, people should not be consuming it in an unmonitored fashion, and health care providers should be aware of the need for more research into the potential for adverse events (Bressa, 1994; Fetrow and Avila, 2001).

SAMe was tested in depressive patients and compared with imipramine in two multicenter studies. In one study (involving 143 patients over 6 weeks), 1,600 mg/day of SAMe was given orally, and in the second study (involving 138 patients over 4 weeks), 400 mg/day of SAMe was given intramuscularly. In both studies, the SAMe treatment was compared (in 138 patients over 6 weeks) to the effects of 150 mg of imipramine given orally each day in a double-blind manner. The assessment measures were the Hamilton Depression Rating Scale (HAM-D) and the Clinical Global Impression Scale at the endpoint. The authors stated that SAMe is the most important methyl donor in the central nervous system, and they concluded that both treatments of SAMe were as effective as 150 mg/day of imipramine orally and were associated with significantly fewer adverse events (Delle Chiaie et al., 2002).

In one pilot study involving 13 depressed patients with Parkinson disease, for which no other previously tried antidepressant agents were effective (and were with intolerable side effects), SAMe was administered in doses of 800 to 3,600 mg/day for 10 weeks. Ten of the 11 patients that completed the study showed at least a 50% improvement in the HAM-D score. One patient did not improve, and two dropped out because of increased anxiety. The only side effects noted in the others were mild nausea (in one patient) and mild and transient diarrhea (in two others). The authors concluded that this preliminary trial showed that SAMe is well tolerated and may be a safe alternative to current antidepressant agents used in Parkinson patients (Di Rocco et al., 2000).

In an open, multicenter study involving 195 patients, 400 mg of SAMe was given parenterally for 15 days. Depressive symptoms were found to decrease after days 7 and 15 of treatment, with no serious adverse events reported. The authors concluded that further double-blind studies are needed to confirm the findings that SAMe not only is a safe and effective antidepressant but also is fast-acting and may be a method for reducing the delay in antidepressant response (Fava et al., 1995).

The antidepressive effect of SAMe was compared with desipramine in a double-blind randomized clinical study involving 26 patients. In the SAMe group, 62% showed significant improvement compared with 50% in the desipramine group. Regardless of the treatment group, the plasma SAMe concentration was shown to have been significantly improved in all patients that showed a 50% decrease in their HAM-D assessment. The authors concluded that this latter finding showed that SAMe played a major role in regulating mood (Bell et al., 1994).

Another study examined the effect of SAMe in depressed post-menopausal women in a 30-day double-blind, placebo-controlled, ran-domized design. Eighty women who were diagnosed with *DSM-III-R* major depressive disorder or dysthymia 6–36 months subsequent to menopause (either natural or through hysterectomy) were given 1,600 mg/day of SAMe or a placebo. A significant improvement was found in depressive symptoms compared with placebo starting on day 10 of the study, and side effects were mild and transient (Salmaggi et al., 1993).

In an effort to study the effect of speeding up the onset of action of the antidepressant imipramine, SAMe was given to 40 patients in a double-blind manner alongside imipramine at 150 mg/day. SAMe was administered at 200 mg/day intramuscularly and was found to effectively increase the onset of the antidepressive action of imipramine (Berlanga et al., 1992).

In an earlier study, SAMe was administered both orally and intraven-ously, and levels of SAMe were found to significantly rise in the cerebro-spinal fluid, indicating that it crossed the blood-brain barrier. The authors also pointed out that SAMe levels were low in a group of Alzh-eimer patients and that this suggested a problem in methylation that the use of SAMe might treat (Bottiglieri et al., 1990).

Osteoarthritis

A meta-analysis of randomized, controlled, clinical trials was conducted on the use of SAMe compared with nonsteroidal anti-inflammatory drugs (NSAIDs) for osteoarthritis. SAMe was found to be as effective as NSAIDs in reducing pain and the functional limitations of osteoarthritis but without the side effects associated with NSAIDs (Soeken et al., 2002).

In another meta-analysis of the use of SAMe in osteoarthritis, all randomized clinical trials on SAMe and oxaceprol were reviewed for their efficacy in osteoarthritis. Assessments of clinical trials were based mostly on pain scores and pain and function scores. Because there were only a few trials that had a mixture of results, the authors cautioned that the results of the meta-analysis had to be interpreted very carefully. The authors concluded that overall, the evidence was insufficient to recommend using SAMe and oxaceprol for the treatment of osteoarthritis, but that the effect of the substances was comparable to that of NSAIDs (Witte et al., 2002).

SAMe was tested in a bicentric, randomized, double-blind, placebo-controlled study on its effectiveness for treatment on 81 patients with osteoarthritis. After a 7-day washout period, patients were administered either 400-mg boluses of SAMe intravenously for 5 days followed by 200 mg 3 times daily for 23 days or a matching placebo regimen. The major outcome measures were the Stanford Health Assessment Questionnaire disability and pain scales and supplemental visual analog scales for rest and walking pain. In one center, where the patients tended to have a milder baseline of osteoarthritis, the SAMe showed a significantly greater effect in reducing overall pain and resting pain than the placebo. In the other center, the baseline osteoarthritis was much more severe, and no difference was seen between treatment groups in outcome measures. The authors concluded that SAMe is beneficial to the treatment of osteoarthritis in some patients and that intravenous loading of SAMe may be a more effective strategy than beginning oral treatment (Bradley et al., 1994).

Fibromyalgia

In one study of SAMe for fibromyalgia, 34 patients in a double-blind, crossover trial were given 600 mg of SAMe intravenously or a placebo for 10 days. The primary outcome measure was the tender-point change between the treatment groups. No significant difference between the two was found, even though there was a trend toward the SAMe group showing significantly improved measures of perception of pain (Volkmann et al., 1997).

In another double-blind, placebo-controlled study on fibromyalgia treatment using SAMe, 800 mg/day of SAMe or a placebo was administered orally for 6 weeks. The measured outcome parameters that showed improvement compared with the placebo were clinical disease activity, subjective symptoms (visual analog scale) of pain experienced during the last week, fatigue, morning stiffness, and mood parameters (evaluated by the face scale). Parameters for which no improvement were found were tender-point score, isokinetic muscle strength, and mood evaluated by the Beck Depression Inventory. The authors noted no differences in side effects between the treatment and placebo groups and concluded that SAMe is beneficial to primary fibromyalgia (Jacobsen et al., 1991).

Liver Disease

A review of clinical and preclinical science on SAMe was undertaken to give relevance to new findings of the role of SAMe in liver growth, differentiation, and injury. Through genome sequence analysis, it was revealed that all organisms make SAMe, and a large percentage of all genes are SAMe-dependent methyltransferases. Because most methylation reactions and a large percentage of methionine metabolism occur in the liver, the authors contended that the liver is essential in the regulation of blood methionine. They added that SAMe is not only an intermediate in methionine catabolism but also a control switch that works intracellularly to regulate liver regeneration, differentiation, and protection (Mato et al., 2002).

A systematic review of the clinical studies on the use of SAMe in alcoholic liver disease first assessed the methodology of each one using the components of quality and the Jadad score. Although eight placebo-controlled randomized clinical trials were found, only one (involving 123 patients) used the adequate methodology and reported with clarity on mortality and liver transplantation. The authors found no significant effect of SAMe on mortality, liver-related mortality, liver transplantation, or liver complications, and therefore did not recommend SAMe for alcoholic liver disease outside clinical trials (Mato et al., 1999; Rambaldi and Gluud, 2001).

SAMe was tested in a randomized, placebo-controlled study involving 32 women with intrahepatic cholestasis of pregnancy. The study groups were divided into those who were treated with ursodeoxycholic acid, SAMe, both drugs, or a placebo. The authors found the combination treatment, administering both ursodeoxycholic acid and SAMe, to be significantly more effective than the placebo or than either drug alone (Nicastri et al., 1998).

In another study comparing SAMe treatment to ursodeoxycholic acid for intrahepatic cholestasis of pregnancy, 20 women were treated with either SAMe (1,000 mg/day intramuscularly) or ursodeoxycholic acid (450 mg/day) from the last trimester of pregnancy until time of delivery. Ursodeoxycholic acid was shown to be more effective than SAMe in treating pruritus and total bile acids and was recommended for further testing in this indication (Floreani et al., 1996). Earlier studies on the use of SAMe for intrahepatic cholestasis of pregnancy have likewise given mixed results (Frezza et al., 1990; Ribalta et al., 1991).

Parkinson Disease

See Di Rocco et al. (2000) and the discussion in the "Depression" subsection earlier in this section.

SAFETY/DOSAGE

Experimental studies have found that SAMe does not cause the same side effects as other nonsteroidal anti-inflammatory agents (e.g., aspirin), including gastric irritation, interference with blood-clotting mechanisms, or inhibition of prostaglandins. In clinical studies, the noted side effects of SAMe have been mostly mild and transient, especially gastrointestinal discomfort.

SAMe appears to be well absorbed through intravenous and intramuscular routes and through oral administration when an enteric-coated capsule is used. In clinical studies, the amounts taken ranged from 600 mg/day to 1,600 mg/day for osteoarthritis. For depression, higher amounts of SAMe are recommended, starting with a high dosage of 1,600 mg/day (divided into two or four doses daily) for 2–3 weeks, and then reducing the dosage to a maintenance level depending on the patient's depressive symptoms (such as 800 mg or 400 mg daily). Preclinical studies suggest that SAMe functions when folate and vitamin B_{12} levels are normal, not low (Grazi and Costa, 1999).

REFERENCES

Bell KM, Potkin SG, Carreon D, Plon L. S-adenosylmethionine blood levels in major depression: changes with drug treatment. Acta Neurol Scand Suppl 1994;154:15–18.

Berlanga C, Ortega-Soto HA, Ontiveros M, Senties H. Efficacy of S-adenosyl-L-methionine in speeding the onset of action of imipramine. Psychiatry Res 1992;44(3):257–262.

Bottiglieri T, Godfrey P, Flynn T, Carney MW, Toone BK, Reynolds EH. Cerebrospinal fluid S-adenosylmethionine in depression and dementia: effects of treatment with parenteral and oral S-adenosylmethionine. J Neurol Neurosurg Psychiatry 1990;53(12):1096–1098.

Bradley JD, Flusser D, Katz BP, Schumacher HR Jr, Brandt KD, Chambers MA, Zonay LJ. A randomized, double blind, placebo controlled trial of intravenous loading with S-adenosylmethionine (SAM) followed by oral SAM therapy in patients with knee osteoarthritis. J Rheumatol 1994;21(5):905–911.

Bressa GM. S-adenosyl-l-methionine (SAMe) as antidepressant: meta-analysis of clinical studies. Acta Neurol Scand Suppl 1994;154:7–14.

Delle Chiaie R, Pancheri P, Scapicchio P. Efficacy and tolerability of oral and intramuscular S-adenosyl-L-methionine 1,4-butanedisulfonate (SAMe) in the treatment of major depression: comparison with imipramine in 2 multicenter studies. Am J Clin Nutr 2002;76(5):1172S–1176S.

Di Rocco A, Rogers JD, Brown R, Werner P, Bottiglieri T. S-Adenosyl-Methionine improves depression in patients with Parkinson's disease in an open-label clinical trial. Mov Disord 2000;15(6):1225–1229.

Fava M, Giannelli A, Rapisarda V, Patralia A, Guaraldi GP. Rapidity of onset of the antidepressant effect of parenteral S-adenosyl-L-methionine. Psychiatry Res 1995;56(3):295–297.

Fetrow CW, Avila JR. Efficacy of the dietary supplement S-adenosyl-L-methionine. Ann Pharmacother 2001;35(11):1414–1425.

Floreani A, Paternoster D, Melis A, Grella PV. S-adenosylmethionine versus ursodeoxycholic acid in the treatment of intrahepatic cholestasis of pregnancy: preliminary results of a controlled trial. Eur J Obstet Gynecol Reprod Biol 1996;67(2):109–113.

Frezza M, Surrenti C, Manzillo G, Fiaccadori F, Bortolini M, Di Padova C. Oral S-adenosylmethionine in the symptomatic treatment of intrahepatic cholestasis. A double-blind, placebo-controlled study. Gastroenterology 1990;99(1):211–5.

Grazi S, Costa M. The European Arthritis and Depression Breakthrough: SAMe. Rocklin, CA: Prima Health, 1999.

Jacobsen S, Danneskiold-Samsoe B, Andersen RB. Oral S-adenosylmethionine in primary fibromyalgia. Double-blind clinical evaluation. Scand J Rheumatol 1991;20(4):294–302.

Mato JM, Camara J, Fernandez de Paz J, Caballeria L, Coll S, Caballero A, Garcia-Buey L, Beltran J, Benita V, Caballeria J, Sola R, Moreno-Otero R, Barrao F, Martin-Duce

A, Correa JA, Pares A, Barrao E, Garcia-Magaz I, Puerta JL, Moreno J, Boissard G, Ortiz P, Rodes J. S-adenosylmethionine in alcoholic liver cirrhosis: a randomized, placebo-controlled, double-blind, multicenter clinical trial J Hepatol 1999;30(6):1081–1089.

Mato JM, Corrales FJ, Lu SC, Avila MA. S-Adenosylmethionine: a control switch that regulates liver function. FASEB J 2002;16(1):15–26.

Nicastri PL, Diaferia A, Tartagni M, Loizzi P, Fanelli M. A randomised placebo-controlled trial of ursodeoxycholic acid and S-adenosylmethionine in the treatment of intrahepatic cholestasis of pregnancy. Br J Obstet Gynaecol 1998;105(11):1205–1207.

Rambaldi A, Gluud C. S-adenosyl-L-methionine for alcoholic liver diseases. Cochrane Database Syst Rev 2001;(4):CD002235.

Ribalta J, Reyes H, Gonzalez MC, Iglesias J, Arrese M, Poniachik J, Molina C, Segovia N. S-adenosyl-L-methionine in the treatment of patients with intrahepatic cholestasis of pregnancy: a randomized, double-blind, placebo-controlled study with negative results. Hepatology 1991;13(6):1084–1089.

Salmaggi P, Bressa GM, Nicchia G, Coniglio M, La Greca P, Le Grazie C. Double-blind, placebo-controlled study of S-adenosyl-L-methionine in depressed postmenopausal women. Psychother Psychosom 1993;59(1):34–40.

Soeken KL, Lee WL, Bausell RB, Agelli M, Berman BM. Safety and efficacy of S-adenosylmethionine (SAMe) for osteoarthritis. J Fam Pract 2002;51(5):425–430.

Volkmann H, Norregaard J, Jacobsen S, Danneskiold-Samsoe B, Knoke G, Nehrdich D. Double-blind, placebo-controlled cross-over study of intravenous S-adenosyl-L-methionine in patients with fibromyalgia. Scand J Rheumatol 1997;26(3):206–211.

Witte S, Lasek R, Victor N. Meta-analysis of the efficacy of adenosylmethionine and oxaceprol in the treatment of osteoarthritis. Orthopade 2002;31(11):1058–1065.

St. John's Wort

Overall Rank

★★★★★ for mild-to-moderate depression or anxiety

OVERVIEW

St. John's wort (*Hypericum perforatum*), also called Klamath weed, is a five-petaled yellow flower especially plentiful in northern California and southern Oregon. The "St. John's" name comes from the red color of the extract (from squeezed buds and flowers), which was associated with the blood of Saint John the Baptist, and the fact that the herb typically flowers around the time of the feast of Saint John. St. John's wort has been used for centuries for everything from protecting against "evil spirits" (depression) to wound healing. Its most common present-day use is as an antidepressant. The active ingredients in St. John's wort extract are unknown, but extracts standardized to contain naphthodianthrone compounds such as hypericin and pseudohypericin along with phloroglucinols such as hyperforin and adhyperforin are known to be effective in alleviating mild-to-moderate depressive symptoms.

As an antidepressant, St. John's wort has been shown to inhibit the enzyme catechol-O-methyltransferase, which degrades certain neurotransmitters, such as dopamine. It has also been shown to inhibit serotonin reuptake in the brain and to reduce expression of interleukin-6 and GABA uptake. Each of these actions can help alleviate depression by slowing the recycling of the neurotransmitters needed to maintain emotional balance. As an antiviral agent, St. John's wort has been reputed to inhibit replication of several viruses, including the herpes simplex virus, HIV, and the virus that causes mononucleosis, but its use as a dietary supplement for treating viral infections is generally not supported.

COMMENTS

St. John's wort appears to be helpful in about 50–60% of cases of mild-to-moderate depression, but as with prescription antidepressants, the full effect takes about 4–6 weeks to develop. It is important to note that St. John's wort should never be used for the treatment of severe depression (feelings of suicide, extreme inability to cope with daily life, severe anxiety, or extreme fatigue), as physician-directed drug therapy may mean the difference between life and death.

St. John's wort is sold in various forms, including tea, drops, tablets, and capsules. In tablet or capsule form, standardized St. John's wort extracts (300–900 mg/day) represent a relatively safe and effective dietary supplement for those with mild-to-moderate depression, anxiety, or seasonal affective disorder.

SCIENTIFIC SUPPORT

Several clinical studies have been conducted to determine the efficacy of St. John's wort for those with mild-to-moderate depression. In one review of 23 randomized trials (15 placebo-controlled and eight drug comparisons) including nearly 2,000 patients with mild-to-moderate depressive disorders, extracts of St. John's wort were nearly 3 times more effective than a placebo and were comparable to prescription antidepressants with fewer side effects (Gaster and Holroyd, 2000). Across the studies, fewer than 1% of participants taking St. John's wort dropped out compared with a drop-out rate of 3% taking prescription antidepressants. Perhaps the most encouraging results were that in contrast to the high percentage of side effects experienced by patients taking prescription antidepressants (52.8%), only 19.8% of those taking St. John's wort experienced any adverse effects (Linde et al., 1996).

Other well-controlled studies comparing the St. John's wort extract LI 160 (from Lichtwer Pharma) to prescription antidepressants such as fluoxetine (Prozac), sertraline (Zoloft), paroxetine (Paxil), imipramine, amitriptyline, and maprotiline have found St. John's wort to be comparable in effectiveness but superior to prescription drugs with regard to tolerability. Overall, more than a dozen double-blind, placebo-controlled (mostly small) studies have been conducted, with most supporting the case for the effectiveness of St. John's wort in alleviating mild-to-moderate depression (e.g., Hansgen et al., 1994; Harrer et al., 1994; Philipp et al., 1999).

In the one study that explored the use of St. John's wort as a retroviral agent for use in HIV-infected patients (Woelk et al., 1994), more than half the patients discontinued treatment early because of severe cutaneous phototoxicity (skin sensitivity to sunlight exposure). Among those who remained in the study, no significant changes in virologic markers were found. It should be noted that HIV-positive patients should *not* use St. John's wort without the specific advice and consultation of their personal physicians, because the herb has been shown to almost completely inactivate the effects of certain antiviral medications (e.g., indinavir and other protease inhibitors).

SAFETY/DOSAGE

St. John's wort is quite safe in terms of observed side effects, the most common of which are mild gastrointestinal upset, mild allergic reactions (skin rash), tiredness, and insomnia or restlessness. No published reports note serious adverse effects from taking the herb alone, and animal studies with large doses of St. John's wort have not shown any serious problems. The most commonly studied adverse effect of St. John's wort is its ability to cause photosensitivity, especially in fair-skinned people. This condition is reversible by discontinuing the herb. Thus, those using the supplement should take special care to avoid ultraviolet light, to frequently apply sunscreen, and to wear sunglasses (because of an increased risk of cataracts) when they must be outside. Other side effects, including gastrointestinal symptoms, dizziness, confusion, and tiredness, tend to be equivalent in incidence to placebo.

Scientific studies conducted in vitro have shown St. John's wort to be mutagenic and toxic to sperm, suggesting that it should not be taken by persons trying to become pregnant. On the other hand, St. John's wort has also been shown to interfere with the action of certain oral contraceptives (birth control pills). St. John's wort is not recommended for children or for women who are pregnant or lactating.

Although direct side effects from consuming St. John's wort appear to be quite rare, several recent reports have raised the possibility that the herb may interact with and decrease the effectiveness of various medications, including HIV drugs (protease inhibitors), immunosuppressants (such as cyclosporin for organ transplants), digoxin (for congestive heart failure), blood thinners (Coumadin, warfarin), chemotherapy drugs, (olanzapine, clozapine), and asthma medications (theophylline). Patients currently taking any of these or other prescription medications should not begin taking or discontinue taking St. John's wort without first consulting their personal physicians. Abrupt withdrawal of the herb could increase blood levels of various medications, which could be dangerous in certain cases.

The recommended dosage for St. John's wort is 900 mg/day (300 mg taken 3 times daily) of an extract of the flowers and leaves standardized to contain 0.3% hypericin in a complex of other natural compounds, or 3–5% hyperforin (the main constituent that is thought to inhibit neurotransmitter reuptake). Minimal treatment time is 4–6 weeks. St. John's wort is sold in the United States only as an herbal supplement, although it is marketed as a drug in Germany for the treatment of mild depression and anxiety.

REFERENCES

Gaster B, Holroyd J. St. John's wort for depression: a systematic review. Arch Intern Med 2000;160(2):152–156.

Hansgen KD, Vesper J, Ploch M. Multicenter double-blind study examining the antidepressant effectiveness of the hypericum extract LI 160. J Geriatr Psychiatry Neurol 1994;7(suppl 1):S15–S18.

Harrer G, Hubner WD, Podzuweit H. Effectiveness and tolerance of the hypericum extract LI 160 compared with maprotiline: a multicenter double-blind study. J Geriatr Psychiatry Neurol 1994;7(suppl 1):S24–S28.

Linde K, Ramirez G, Mulrow CD, Pauls A, Weidenhammer W, Melchart D. St. John's wort for depression—an overview and meta-analysis of randomised clinical trials. BMJ 1996;313(7052):253–258.

Philipp M, Kohnen R, Hiller KO. Hypericum extract versus imipramine or placebo in patients with moderate depression: randomised multicentre study of treatment for eight weeks. BMJ 1999;319(7224):1534–1538.

Woelk H, Burkard G, Grunwald J. Benefits and risks of the hypericum extract LI 160: drug monitoring study with 3250 patients. J Geriatr Psychiatry Neurol 1994;7(suppl 1):S34–S38.

ADDITIONAL RESOURCES

Cott JM, Fugh-Berman A. Is St. John's wort (Hypericum perforatum) an effective antidepressant? J Nerv Ment Dis 1998;186(8):500–501.

Firenzuoli F, Luigi G. Safety of Hypericum perforatum. J Altern Complement Med 1999;5(5):397–398.

Fugh-Berman A, Cott JM. Dietary supplements and natural products as psychotherapeutic agents. Psychosom Med 1999;61(5):712–728.

Holsboer-Trachsler E, Vanoni C. Clinical efficacy and tolerance of the hypericum special extract LI 160 in depressive disorders—a drug monitoring study. Schweiz Rundsch Med Prax 1999;88(37):1475–1480.

Hubner WD, Lande S, Podzuweit H. Hypericum treatment of mild depressions with somatic symptoms. J Geriatr Psychiatry Neurol 1994;7(suppl 1):S12–S14.

Jobst KA, McIntyre M, St. George D, Whitelegg M. Safety of St. John's wort. Lancet 2000;355(9203):575.

Johne A, Brockmoller J, Bauer S, Maurer A, Langheinrich M, Roots I. Pharmacokinetic interaction of digoxin with an herbal extract from St. John's wort (Hypericum perforatum). Clin Pharmacol Ther 1999;66(4):338–345.

Kasper S. Treatment of seasonal affective disorder (SAD) with hypericum extract. Pharmacopsychiatry 1997;30(suppl 2):89–93.

Laakmann G, Schule C, Baghai T, Kieser M. St. John's wort in mild to moderate depression: the relevance of hyperforin for the clinical efficacy. Pharmacopsychiatry 1998;31(suppl 1):54–59.

Martinez B, Kasper S, Ruhrmann S, Moller HJ. Hypericum in the treatment of seasonal affective disorders. J Geriatr Psychiatry Neurol 1994;7(suppl 1):S29–S33.

Miller AL. St. John's wort (Hypericum perforatum): clinical effects on depression and other conditions. Altern Med Rev 1998;3(1):18–26.

Sommer H, Harrer G. Placebo-controlled double-blind study examining the effectiveness of an hypericum preparation in 105 mildly depressed patients. J Geriatr Psychiatry Neurol 1994;7(suppl 1):S9–S11.

Stevinson C, Ernst E. Hypericum for depression. An update of the clinical evidence. Eur Neuropsychopharmacol 1999;9(6):501–505.

Volz HP, Laux P. Potential treatment for subthreshold and mild depression: a comparison of St. John's wort extracts and fluoxetine. Compr Psychiatry 2000;41(2 suppl 1):133–137.

Vorbach EU, Arnoldt KH, Hubner WD. Efficacy and tolerability of St. John's wort extract LI 160 versus imipramine in patients with severe depressive episodes according to ICD-10. Pharmacopsychiatry 1997;30(suppl 2):81–85.

Vorbach EU, Hubner WD, Arnoldt KH. Effectiveness and tolerance of the hypericum extract LI 160 in comparison with imipramine: randomized double-blind study with 135 outpatients. J Geriatr Psychiatry Neurol 1994;7(suppl 1):S19–S23.

Wheatley D. LI 160, an extract of St. John's wort, versus amitriptyline in mildly to moderately depressed outpatients—a controlled 6-week clinical trial. Pharmacopsychiatry 1997;30(suppl 2):77–80.

Williams JW Jr, Mulrow CD, Chiquette E, Noel PH, Aguilar C, Cornell J. A systematic review of newer pharmacotherapies for depression in adults: evidence report summary. Ann Intern Med 2000;132(9):743–756.

VALERIAN

Overall Rank

★★★★★ as a sleep aid
★★★★ for anxiety

OVERVIEW

Valerian (*Valeriana officinalis* or *Valerianae radix*) has been used as a medicinal antianxiety herb and sleep aid since the days of the Roman Empire. The dried roots of the plant are used in teas, tinctures, capsules, and tablets. The fresh root has no distinctive odor; however, over time, hydrolysis of compounds present in the volatile oil produce isovaleric acid, which has an offensive odor (akin to sweaty socks). Traditionally, valerian was used to treat migraine headache, anxiety, fatigue, and seizures, and many traditional Chinese remedies include valerian for treatment of numbness resulting from rheumatic conditions, colds, menstrual difficulties, bruises, and wounds. Currently, valerian may be used orally for the treatment of insomnia, restlessness, sleeping disorders with anxiety, mood disorders, muscle and joint pain, menstrual cramps, and menopausal symptoms. It is unclear which of the numerous compounds is the true "active," but the combination of compounds appears to work together in the brain to produce an overall effect similar to the action of prescription tranquilizers such as Valium and Halcion.

COMMENTS

As a mild tranquilizer and sleep aid, valerian may be an effective herb for dealing with temporary feelings of anxiety, nervousness, or insomnia. The effects of valerian are generally quite mild compared with prescription medications and synthetic over-the-counter products and generally do not result in "morning after hangover" effects that some sleep aids produce.

SCIENTIFIC SUPPORT

Valerian taken before bedtime appears to reduce the amount of time that it takes to fall asleep (sleep latency) (Donath et al., 2000; Schulz et al., 1994). It is unknown, however, whether the quality of the sleep is affected. Valerian is generally regarded as a mild tranquilizer and has been deemed safe by the German Commission E for treating "restlessness and sleeping disorders brought on by nervous conditions" (Donath et al., 2000). The medicinal portion of the plant is the root, and most of the pharmacological effects of valerian root have been attributed to valepotriate and volatile oil constituents—specifically, monoterpenes and sesquiterpenes. Multiple constituents, however, may be responsible for the root's therapeutic effects, rather than a single active compound. Valepotriate constituents are believed to have sedative, hypnotic, and spasmolytic effects, while the sesquiterpenes, valerenic acid, and kessyl glycol have been shown to cause sedation in animals (Houghton, 1999). Another mechanism of action is likely to involve valerenic acid's ability to inhibit the enzyme system responsible for the central catabolism of GABA, increasing GABA concentrations and decreasing central nervous system activity (Houghton, 1999).

Several studies have examined the effects of valerian on sleep. In one placebo-controlled crossover study with 128 participants, 400 mg of valerian extract (plus hops) reduced sleep latency and improved sleep quality compared with placebo (Leathwood et al., 1982). Analysis of the results suggested that valerian had an increased effect in participants who described themselves as "poor" or "irregular" sleepers. Another trial evaluated the effectiveness of 450–900 mg of valerian on healthy volunteers between the ages of 21 and 44 (Kuhlmann et al., 1999). Sleep quality was measured using a questionnaire, nighttime motor activity recordings, and spectral analysis of the sleep electroencephalogram. Both doses elicited mild hypnotic effects and improved sleep quality. Other studies of valerian supplementation have shown improvements in slow-wave (deeper-stage) sleep compared with placebo and equivalence of 600 mg of valerian with 10 mg of oxazepam for indices of overall sleep quality (Vonderheid-Guth et al., 2000). In terms of anxiolytic effects, several studies have shown 100–300 mg of valerian root extract to be more effective than a placebo and as effective as 20 mg of propranolol on measures of social stress, somatic arousal, anxiety, and emotional tension (Kohnen and Oswald, 1988).

SAFETY/DOSAGE

Occasional reports of headaches and mild nausea are documented, but habituation or dependency is unlikely when used as directed. Valerian should be avoided by pregnant and lactating women and should not be consumed by children. Patients currently taking sedative drugs or antidepressant medications should be advised by their personal physicians before taking valerian. Additionally, patients should not take valerian in conjunction with alcohol or other tranquilizers and should not consume valerian for more than 2 weeks.

Because the activity and strength of valerian preparations can vary significantly from one product to the next, patients should select a standardized product (0.5–1.0% valerenic acids) whenever possible and follow the directions on the particular product. As a general guideline, approximately 200–900 mg of a standardized extract can be taken 30–60 minutes before bed (as a sleep aid) or as needed as a mild tranquilizer.

REFERENCES

Donath F, Quispe S, Diefenbach K, Maurer A, Fietze I, Roots I. Critical evaluation of the effect of valerian extract on sleep structure and sleep quality. Pharmacopsychiatry 2000;33(2):47–53.

Houghton PJ. The scientific basis for the reputed activity of Valerian. J Pharm Pharmacol 1999;51(5):505–512.

Kohnen R, Oswald WD. The effects of valerian, propranolol, and their combination on activation, performance, and mood of healthy volunteers under social stress conditions. Pharmacopsychiatry 1988;21(6):447–448.

Kuhlmann J, Berger W, Podzuweit H, Schmidt U. The influence of valerian treatment on "reaction time, alertness and concentration" in volunteers. Pharmacopsychiatry 1999;32(6):235–241.

Leathwood PD, Chauffard F, Heck E, Munoz-Box R. Aqueous extract of valerian root (Valeriana officinalis L.) improves sleep quality in man. Pharmacol Biochem Behav 1982;17(1):65–71.

Vonderheid-Guth B, Todorova A, Brattstrom A, Dimpfel W. Pharmacodynamic effects of valerian and hops extract combination (Ze 91019) on the quantitative-topographical EEG in healthy volunteers. Eur J Med Res 2000;5(4):139–144.

ADDITIONAL RESOURCES

Assemi M. Herbs affecting the central nervous system: gingko, kava, St. John's wort, and valerian. Clin Obstet Gynecol 2001;44(4):824–835.

Balderer G, Borbely AA. Effect of valerian on human sleep. Psychopharmacology (Berl) 1985;87(4):406–409.

Cauffield JS, Forbes HJ. Dietary supplements used in the treatment of depression, anxiety, and sleep disorders. Lippincotts Prim Care Pract 1999;3(3):290–304.

Heiligenstein E, Guenther G. Over-the-counter psychotropics: a review of melatonin, St. John's wort, valerian, and kava-kava. J Am Coll Health 1998;46(6):271–276.

Kammerer E. Phytogenic sedatives-hypnotics—does a combination of valerian and hops have a value in the modern drug repertoire? Z Arztl Fortbild (Jena) 1993;87(5):401–406.

Kirkwood CK. Management of insomnia. J Am Pharm Assoc (Wash) 1999;39(5):688–696.

Leathwood PD, Chauffard F. Aqueous extract of valerian reduces latency to fall asleep in man. Planta Med 1985;(2):144–148.

Plushner SL. Valerian: Valeriana officinalis. Am J Health Syst Pharm 2000;57(4):328, 333, 335.

Schulz H, Stolz C, Muller J. The effect of valerian extract on sleep polygraphy in poor sleepers: a pilot study. Pharmacopsychiatry 1994;27(4):147–151.

Willey LB, Mady SP, Cobaugh DJ, Wax PM. Valerian overdose: a case report. Vet Hum Toxicol 1995;37(4):364–365.

Wong AH, Smith M, Boon HS. Herbal remedies in psychiatric practice. Arch Gen Psychiatry 1998;55(11):1033–1044.

VINPOCETINE (FROM *VINCA MINOR*)

Overall Rank

★★★★ for cerebrovascular disease
★★ as a memory enhancer
★★ for dementia

OVERVIEW

Vinpocetine is a derivative of the alkaloid vincamine (extracted from vinca minor) and is used in many countries in the treatment and prevention of stroke and vascular dementia. Although no single mechanism of action has been agreed on for vinpocetine, many activities are known to stem from its use, such as dilating blood vessels, enhancing circulation to the brain, improving oxygen utilization and reducing blood clotting, and inhibiting platelet aggregation. Vinpocetine works on altering the ischemic cascade in several areas, including depletion of adenosine triphosphate, activation of voltage-sensitive sodium and calcium channels, and release of glutamate and free radicals. The most important of these effects to neuroprotective activity of vinpocetine seems to be the interference of voltage-sensitive sodium channels and possibly its strong antioxidant activity (Hadjiev, 2003).

One main Hungarian company markets vinpocetine in Europe as a drug (Cavinton) for improving several types of cerebral insufficiency conditions and for improving cerebral metabolism. In studies involving vinpocetine's use in chronic stroke patients, positron emission tomography scans showed that it improves the brain metabolism and blood flow, especially around stroke-damaged areas (Gulyas et al., 2002; Szakall et al., 1998; Vas et al., 2002).

COMMENTS

There seems to be a good amount of preclinical science and little clinical science to back vinpocetine's use in cerebrovascular disorders. With its low toxicity and side effects, however, it shows excellent potential for the future in preventing and treating stroke. Its effects on memory in healthy people have some merit but need more clinical backing.

SCIENTIFIC SUPPORT

Cerebrovascular Disease

Hadjiev (2003) reviewed the actions of vinpocetine on the ischemic cascade and discussed how it may be a new therapeutic approach to treatment and prophylactic neuroprevention in patients with asymptomatic ischemic cerebrovascular disorders (AICVD) and cerebrovascular disease. A subclinical noninvasive diagnosis of AICVD has been recently introduced by the American Heart Association, and its treatment was identified as being important in prevention of ischemic stroke and cognitive decline. As a potential treatment to AICVD, the neuroprotective effects of vinpocetine were discussed.

Szapary et al. (2003) examined the high- and low-dose therapies of vinpocetine on rheological parameters in acute and chronic stroke patients. Although vinpocetine is used mainly in a preventative manner, this study sought to determine if it had value as a treatment for chronic disease. The authors concluded that after parenteral administration with low (30 mg/day) and high (70 mg/day) doses of vinpocetine, the high dose showed significant decreases in hematocrit, whole-blood and plasma viscosity, and red blood cell aggregation, indicating a beneficial role in the treatment of chronic cerebrovascular disease.

A pilot clinical study treated 30 patients with vinpocetine to determine the safety and feasibility of a full-scale clinical study. Patients were given either dextran alone or dextran in combination with vinpocetine; the study found that the two treatment groups were comparable in their major prognostic variables. The National Institutes of Health Stroke Scale score, however, was slightly improved in the vinpocetine group at follow-up of 3 months, and no significant side effects were seen. The authors concluded that a full-scale clinical study was warranted (Feigin et al., 2001).

A systematic review of the literature and researchers in the field (including drug companies) was conducted to determine if therapy with vinpocetine on stroke was effective. Only one trial was found to be of an unconfounded, randomized, placebo-controlled design. The authors concluded that no deaths or drug dependencies were found but that not enough studies had been conducted to determine the efficacy of vinpocetine in stroke patients (Bereczki and Fekete, 1999, 2000).

Because vinpocetine had been used for more than 20 years in the treatment of cognitive impairment caused by vascular diseases, and because many preclinical findings had suggested several important mechanisms of action, no consensus had been reached on its efficacy. Therefore, a search was conducted to review the existing literature worldwide to analyze unconfounded, double-blind studies pertaining to vinpocetine treatment of vascular dementia, Alzheimer dementia, and other dementias. The authors concluded that although the preclinical science done on vinpocetine was persuasive and few adverse effects were found, the clinical science was inconclusive and did not support clinical use. The authors called for more clinical work on well-defined types of cognitive impairment (Szatmari and Whitehouse, 2003).

Memory
In a randomized, double-blind, crossover study, 12 healthy females were given vinpocetine (in dosages of 10, 20, or 40 mg) or a placebo for 2 days

and assessed for psychopharmacological effects. Assessment parameters were measured on day 3, including Critical Flicker Fusion, Choice Reaction Time, Subjective Ratings of Drug Effects, and the Sternberg Memory Scanning Test. Significant improvements were found in memory as a function of the Sternberg test at the dosage level of 40 mg. The results suggested that vinpocetine has a specific effect on the serial comparison stage of the reaction process (Subhan and Hindmarch, 1985).

SAFETY/DOSAGE

To improve mild-to-moderate dementia in patients, 5–10 mg taken 2–3 times daily is the typical dosage recommendation; larger dosages, however, have been used clinically for acute treatment. Because vinpocetine is difficult to absorb in large quantities, dividing the daily doses as suggested above is recommended.

Side effects of vinpocetine are rare and transient (with discontinued use) at the recommended dosages. Typical side effects include gastrointestinal upset, low blood pressure, dry mouth, insomnia, headaches, and heart palpitations. Persons on anticoagulant therapy should not use vinpocetine because it may interfere with clotting. The safety or efficacy of vinpocetine for pregnant or lactating women is undocumented.

REFERENCES

Bereczki D, Fekete I. A systematic review of vinpocetine therapy in acute ischaemic stroke. Eur J Clin Pharmacol 1999;55(5):349–352.

Bereczki D, Fekete I. Vinpocetine for acute ischaemic stroke. Cochrane Database Syst Rev 2000;(2):CD000480.

Feigin VL, Doronin BM, Popova TF, Gribatcheva EV, Tchervov DV. Vinpocetine treatment in acute ischaemic stroke: a pilot single-blind randomized clinical trial. Eur J Neurol 2001;8(1):81–85.

Gulyas B, Halldin C, Sandell J, Karlsson P, Sovago J, Karpati E, Kiss B, Vas A, Cselenyi Z, Farde L. PET studies on the brain uptake and regional distribution of [11C]vinpocetine in human subjects. Acta Neurol Scand 2002;106(6):325–332.

Hadjiev D. Asymptomatic ischemic cerebrovascular disorders and neuroprotection with vinpocetine. Ideggyogy Sz 2003;56(5–6):166–172.

Subhan Z, Hindmarch I. Psychopharmacological effects of vinpocetine in normal healthy volunteers. Eur J Clin Pharmacol 1985;28(5):567–571.

Szakall S, Boros I, Balkay L, Emri M, Fekete I, Kerenyi L, Lehel S, Marian T, Molnar T, Varga J, Galuska L, Tron L, Bereczki D, Csiba L, Gulyas B. Cerebral effects of a single dose of intravenous vinpocetine in chronic stroke patients: a PET study. J Neuroimaging 1998;8(4):197–204.

Szapary L, Horvath B, Alexy T, Marton Z, Kesmarky G, Szots M, Nagy F, Czopf J, Toth K. Effect of vinpocetin on the hemorheologic parameters in patients with chronic cerebrovascular disease. Orv Hetil 2003;144(20):973–978.

Szatmari SZ, Whitehouse PJ. Vinpocetine for cognitive impairment and dementia. Cochrane Database Syst Rev 2003;(1):CD003119.

Vas A, Sovago J, Halldin C, Sandell J, Karlsson P, Karpati E, Kiss B, Cselenyi Z, Farde L, Gulyas B. Cerebral uptake and regional distribution of [11C]-vinpocetin after intravenous administration to healthy men: a PET study. Orv Hetil 2002;143(47):2631–2636.

CHAPTER 7

Heart Health Supplements

Alfalfa (*Medicago sativa*)
Arginine
B-Complex Vitamins (B$_6$, B$_{12}$, Folic Acid, Niacin)
Coenzyme Q$_{10}$ (CoQ$_{10}$)
Essential Fatty Acids (ω-3, ω-6, Fish Oil, Evening Primrose Oil, Borage Seed Oil, Flaxseed Oil)

Garlic
Hawthorn (*Crataegus oxyacantha* L.)
Red Yeast Rice
Soy

ALFALFA (*MEDICAGO SATIVA*)

Overall Rank

★★★ for cholesterol reduction
★★ for increasing energy levels
★★ for liver health and detoxification
★ for reducing the pain of arthritis
★ for reducing hot flashes associated with menopause

OVERVIEW

Because alfalfa has long been used as fodder for livestock and horses, much of what has been studied in the scientific literature is based on its use in animals. It has been revered as a food for horses that increases strength and speed, and this has contributed to its folkloric use as an herbal supplement for increasing energy, lowering cholesterol, detoxifying, relieving the pain of arthritis, and relieving the hot flashes associated with menopause.

Alfalfa truly is a nutritive food, with high levels of protein (up to 50%), B vitamins, and minerals. These characteristics may play a large part in explaining alfalfa's claims for energy and reduction of fatigue. Additionally, alfalfa contains saponins, which could explain some of its adaptogenic reputation; its antioxidants and alkalizing nature could explain its detoxification claims. The use of alfalfa for hot flashes and cancer may be explained by its high estrogenic activity.

COMMENTS

Clinical research to back up alfalfa's many claims is still lacking, but as a nutritive food, alfalfa's use in many kinds of wellness formulations may have some credence. In a study on the estrogenic activity of several legumes, alfalfa sprout extract was found to increase cell proliferation above levels found for estradiol; the authors concluded that it contains phytoestrogens with a high level of activity (Boue et al., 2003).

SCIENTIFIC SUPPORT

Supplementation of alfalfa seeds was clinically tested in patients with hyperlipoproteinemia (HLP) types 2A, 2B, and 4. All patients were given 40 g of alfalfa seeds 3 times daily with meals for 8 weeks. At the end of the 8-week period, patients with type 2 HLP showed a 17% lowering of total plasma cholesterol and an 18% decrease in the low density lipoprotein (LDL) levels. The largest decreases observed were 26% in total cholesterol and 30% in LDL. The authors concluded that alfalfa seeds may be used to normalize serum cholesterol levels in patients with type 2 HLP (Molgaard et al., 1987).

SAFETY/DOSAGE

Although the clinical study on alfalfa for lowering cholesterol used an extremely high dosage (120 g/day), typical dosages for alfalfa tend to range from 250–1,000 mg 2–3 times daily with meals. In this dosage range, there are no known side effects of alfalfa except a possible mild blood-thinning effect.

REFERENCES

Boue SM, Wiese TE, Nehls S, Burow ME, Elliott S, Carter-Wientjes CH, Shih BY, McLachlan JA, Cleveland TE. Evaluation of the estrogenic effects of legume extracts containing phytoestrogens. J Agric Food Chem 2003;51(8):2193–2199.

Molgaard J, von Schenck H, Olsson AG. Alfalfa seeds lower low density lipoprotein cholesterol and apolipoprotein B concentrations in patients with type II hyperlipoproteinemia. Atherosclerosis 1987;65(1–2):173–179.

ARGININE

Overall Rank
★★★★ for cardiovascular disease
★★★ for sexual dysfunction
★★★ for immune function
★★ for high cholesterol
★★ for high blood pressure

OVERVIEW

L-arginine is a substance that is produced in the body. It plays an essential role in the nitric oxide pathway—a pathway involved in the cascade reactions responsible for vasodilation. Thus, arginine supplements are associated with cardiovascular health, especially in conditions in which the nitric oxide pathway may not be working sufficiently. For example, there is evidence that in the development of arteriosclerosis, people with high cholesterol have an endothelium with a reduced ability to produce nitric oxide, and therefore their arteries cannot dilate effectively (Rasmusen et al., 1995). As a consequence, their blood cells have the ability to attach to inner vessels and cause blockages. L-arginine has also been shown to stimulate lymphocyte production and has therefore been studied in diets of surgery patients.

During the nitric oxide pathway, the nitric oxide synthase enzyme catalyzes the oxidation of arginine to citrulline and nitric oxide. The production of nitric oxide in turn causes vasodilation and is involved in the regulation of overall vasoresistance. Because the human body produces arginine, the substance has been classified as a nonessential nutrient for supplementation, although there is some question whether the amount is sufficient for maintaining health (Luiking et al., 2004).

COMMENTS

Due to the popularity of dietary supplements for improving sexual function and the known action of arginine on the nitric oxide pathway, numerous supplements now include arginine in combination with other herbs for sexual function and performance. Few studies have confirmed the benefits of these combinations or the single components (Ito et al., 2001; Polan et al., 2004; Stanislavov and Nikolova, 2003).

SCIENTIFIC SUPPORT

Cardiovascular Health

A meta-analysis of the use of L-arginine in the enteral or oral diets of stressed patients was conducted to help determine whether the diets were immune enhancing and beneficial. Although the review found the L-arginine "immune-enhancing" diets to be beneficial, the author contended that nothing proved that this effect was not confounded by other bioactive components, including ω-3 fatty acids, RNAs, and antioxidant vitamins. The author also pointed out that the L-arginine-supplemented enteral or oral diets could have a harmful effect in hemo-dynamically unstable patients, and in patients with multiple organ failure (Cynober, 2003).

A medical food called the Heart Bar is now sold that looks just like the numerous other sports and protein bars. The Heart Bar is intended to nutritionally support cardiovascular health, with its major active constituent being arginine. Its use is substantiated by numerous peer-reviewed clinical studies, and it is regulated specially as a "medical food" by the Food and Drug Administration (FDA). In a randomized, double-blind, placebo-controlled, crossover trial, 36 stable angina outpatients were tested for the electrocardiographic, vascular, and clinical effects of the Heart Bar. This medical food was found to improve vascular function, exercise capacity, and aspects of quality of life in patients with stable angina (Maxwell et al., 2002).

L-arginine was clinically studied in a single-blind, controlled, crossover, dietary intervention study for its effect on certain cardiovascular parameters, especially blood pressure. Six subjects were given isocaloric diets for one week, with constant measures of sodium in each diet (approximately 180 mmol/day). Each participant received three diets in random order: (1) control, (2) L-arginine enriched by natural foods, and (3) L-arginine given orally to supplement the control diet. Both arginine-rich diets (2 and 3) resulted in a blood pressure decrease. Diet 2 resulted in lower total serum cholesterol and triglyceride levels and higher high-density lipoprotein (HDL) cholesterol. Diet 3, and to a lesser extent diet 2, resulted in higher creatine clearance (slight) and a fall in fasting glucose. The authors concluded that increasing L-arginine in the diet lowers blood pressure and affects kidney function and carbohydrate metabolism (Siani et al., 2000).

Fujita et al. (2000) clinically tested the ability of L-arginine to affect coronary perfusion abnormality during exercise. Twelve patients with angina pectoris and normal coronary arteries underwent exercise thallium-201 scintigraphy, either with intravenous L-arginine or without (control). The administration of L-arginine was found to prolong exercise time and improve the severity score. In 7 of the 12 patients, the Tl-201 redistribution disappeared after L-arginine administration, and the percentage of serum L-citrulline and the percentage of epicardial coronary diameter increased in response to acetylcholine more than in the other patients who did not show a change in TI-201 redistribution. The authors concluded that exogenous L-arginine was able to improve myocardial perfusion during exercise in this subset of patients.

High Blood Pressure

To determine whether a deficient L-arginine–nitric oxide system is active in cortisol-induced hypertension, the effect of L-arginine uptake was studied. Eight healthy men were given hydrocortisone acetate (50 mg) orally every 6 hours for 24 hours after a 5-day fixed-salt diet. L-arginine levels appeared unaffected by cortisol treatment; therefore, no correlation was found between cortisol-induced hypertension and the L-arginine transport system (Chin-Dusting et al., 2003).

Immune Function

L-arginine was clinically tested in patients with advanced gastric cancer for its ability to stimulate lymphocyte production, because it had been shown to stimulate lymphocyte production in healthy persons. The patients received a dietary supplement of L-arginine (30 g/day for 7 days), and the lymphocyte counts and T-cell:B-cell ratio in the peripheral blood were tested. Although L-arginine did not show any significant side effects (except transient nausea in one patient) or impair liver function, it also did not stimulate lymphocyte function. The authors suggested that the immune systems of the cancer patients may have been intrinsically defective and therefore not able to be stimulated (Wu et al., 1993).

Li et al. (1993) tested the ability of L-arginine to decrease the incidence of sepsis after surgery in patients with obstructive jaundice. Since arginine had been known as a T-lymphocyte stimulator, the use of supplementation and the immunological status of patients with obstructive jaundice after surgery were studied. Arginine was found to significantly enhance immune function of patients with obstructive jaundice.

To study the immunomodulatory effect of arginine in surgery patients, 30 cancer patients took part in a randomized study; 16 were given L-arginine (25 g/day) while the other 14 were given isonitrogenous L-glycine (43 g/day) for 7 days after major surgery. Parameters measured were nitrogen balance (daily) and immune parameters before and after surgery on days 1, 4, and 7. T-lymphocyte response was significantly enhanced to concanavalin A in the L-arginine group compared with the glycine group. L-arginine was also found to increase the CD4 phenotype. L-arginine was found to be beneficial in modulating the immune system in surgery patients. This immune-modulating effect was found to be nontoxic and distinct in its mechanism from its moderate effect on nitrogen metabolism (Daly et al., 1988).

SAFETY/DOSAGE

The daily requirement of arginine supplementation has been calculated to be approximately 8 g/day (for a 70-kg person). Supplements in the range of 8–21 g/day have been used clinically in people with high cholesterol to restore the proper functioning of the vasodilatory pathways. Supplements in the range of 9–14 g/day have been used clinically to increase blood flow to the peripheries and improve conditions of myocardial ischemia and walking pain caused by claudication.

The average daily intake of arginine in the American diet has been calculated to be approximately 5 g/day. The primary dietary sources of this amino acid are meats and other high-protein foods (e.g., nuts, eggs).

REFERENCES

Chin-Dusting JP, Ahlers BA, Kaye DM, Kelly JJ, Whitworth JA. L-arginine transport in humans with cortisol-induced hypertension. Hypertension 2003;41(6):1336–1340.

Cynober L. Immune-enhancing diets for stressed patients with a special emphasis on arginine content: analysis of the analysis. Curr Opin Clin Nutr Metab Care 2003;6(2):189–193.

Daly JM, Reynolds J, Thom A, Kinsley L, Dietrick-Gallagher M, Shou J, Ruggieri B. Immune and metabolic effects of arginine in the surgical patient. Ann Surg 1988;208(4):512–523.

Fujita H, Yamabe H, Yokoyama M. Effect of L-arginine administration on myocardial thallium-201 perfusion during exercise in patients with angina pectoris and normal coronary angiograms. J Nucl Cardiol 2000;7(2):97–102.

Ito TY, Trant AS, Polan ML. A double-blind placebo-controlled study of ArginMax, a nutritional supplement for enhancement of female sexual function. J Sex Marital Ther 2001;27(5):541–549.

Li H, Xiong ST, Zhang SX, Liu SB, Luo Y. Immunological status of patients with obstructive jaundice and immunostimulatory effect of arginine. J Tongji Med Univ 1993;13(2):111–115.

Luiking YC, Poeze M, Dejong CH, Ramsay G, Deutz NE. Sepsis: an arginine deficiency state? Crit Care Med 2004;32(10):2135–2145. Review.

Maxwell AJ, Zapien MP, Pearce GL, MacCallum G, Stone PH. Randomized trial of a medical food for the dietary management of chronic, stable angina. J Am Coll Cardiol 2002;39(1):37–45.

Polan ML, Hochberg RB, Trant AS, Wuh HC. Estrogen bioassay of ginseng extract and ArginMax, a nutritional supplement for the enhancement of female sexual function. J Womens Health (Larchmt) 2004;13(4):427–430.

Rasmusen C, Cynober L, Couderc R. [Arginine and statins: relationship between the nitric oxide pathway and the atherosclerosis development] Ann Biol Clin (Paris) 2005;63(5):443–455.

Siani A, Pagano E, Iacone R, Iacoviello L, Scopacasa F, Strazzullo P. Blood pressure and metabolic changes during dietary L-arginine supplementation in humans. Am J Hypertens 2000;13(5 pt 1):547–551.

Stanislavov R, Nikolova V. Treatment of erectile dysfunction with pycnogenol and L-arginine. J Sex Marital Ther 2003;29(3):207–213.

Wu CW, Chi CW, Chiu CC, Wu HS, Liu WY, P'eng FK, Wang SR. Can daily dietary arginine supplement affect the function and subpopulation of lymphocytes in patients with advanced gastric cancer? Digestion 1993;54(2):118–124.

B-COMPLEX VITAMINS (B$_6$, B$_{12}$, FOLIC ACID, NIACIN)

Overall Rank

★★★★★ for folate to prevent neural tube defects during pregnancy
★★★★★ for B$_6$, B$_{12}$, and folate to control homocysteine levels for heart health
★★★★ for niacin to control cholesterol

OVERVIEW

Four B vitamins are considered here in one section because of their related benefits as dietary supplements for promoting cardiovascular health—folic acid, vitamin B_6, and vitamin B_{12} for their effects in reducing homocysteine levels, and niacin for reducing cholesterol levels.

Vitamin B_6 is a water-soluble vitamin. It is also known by the names pyridoxine, pyridoxamine, and pyridoxal. Vitamin B_6 performs functions as a cofactor for about 70 enzyme systems, most of which have something to do with amino acid and protein metabolism. Because vitamin B_6 is also involved in the synthesis of neurotransmitters in the brain and nerve cells, it is frequently recommended as a nutrient to support mental function (mood) and nerve conduction. Some athletic supplements include vitamin B_6 because of its role in the conversion of glycogen to glucose for energy in muscle tissue. Perhaps the best data supporting the value of B_6 supplements are in the area of heart health through reduced homocysteine levels. Food sources include poultry, fish, whole grains, and bananas.

The water-soluble vitamin B_{12} is also known as cobalamin because it contains cobalt. The B_{12} form most commonly used in dietary supplements is called cyanocobalamin. Vitamin B_{12} is only produced by bacteria, so it is only found in food products of animal origin and in some fermented vegetable products such as tempeh and miso (fermented soybeans). B_{12} functions in various metabolic processes, many of which are involved in transferring methyl groups between amino acids. Vitamin B_{12} works closely with another B vitamin, folic acid, in reactions involved with DNA synthesis, blood cell formation, nervous system maintenance, and heart health. B_{12} is also involved in the metabolism of proteins, fats, and carbohydrates because it is needed to produce succinyl coenzyme A, an intermediary in the Krebs cycle that generates adenosine triphosphate (ATP) for cellular energy. Like B_6, vitamin B_{12} has been shown to reduce elevated homocysteine levels and thus can be considered a valuable supplement for promoting heart health.

Folic acid is a B vitamin that plays an important role in the synthesis of DNA and RNA, the production of red blood cells, and the maintenance of the nervous system. Fruits and vegetables are the best dietary sources (folic acid derives its name from *foliage*), especially dark leafy greens, oranges and orange juice, beans, and peas. Because folic acid is known to reduce the risk of neural tube defects in developing fetuses, the FDA requires folate-enrichment of refined cereal grains. At fortification levels of folic acid intake, homocysteine is partially normalized, but further increases in dietary intake, whether from foods or supplements, provide additional significant reductions in homocysteine levels.

Niacin is a water-soluble B vitamin and the common name for two very different compounds: nicotinic acid and niacinamide. Like all B vitamins, niacin plays a role in many aspects of energy metabolism and nervous system function. One of the most common uses for supplemental niacin is cholesterol regulation (used at very high doses; see the "Scientific Support" subsection of this section). Rich dietary sources of niacin include many high-protein foods, such as meat, chicken, tuna and other fatty fish, peanuts, pork, and milk. The nicotinic acid form of niacin is effective, when used at high levels, for reducing cholesterol and triglyceride levels as well as enhancing circulation.

COMMENTS

The dosage levels of these B vitamins that have been associated with cardioprotective effects (reduced homocysteine and cholesterol levels) generally fall within the ranges of 2–12.5 mg/day for B_6, 50–800 μg/day for B_{12}, 400–1,000 μg/day for folate (though much higher milligram levels are also effective) for control of homocysteine levels, and 250–2,000 mg/day of niacin (a very high level that should be monitored by a physician) for cholesterol and triglyceride reduction.

Vitamins B_6 and B_{12} are found in high concentrations in most protein-rich foods. Because folic acid is destroyed during cooking, levels are typically highest in raw or lightly steamed vegetables. The chemical form of folic acid found in foods, monoglutamic acid (conjugated), however, is less well absorbed (40–60% less) than the synthetic form found in dietary supplements, polyglutamic acid (unconjugated). This suggests that supplemental forms of folic acid may even be warranted in high-risk persons in addition to a well-balanced intake of fruits and vegetables.

Like the other B vitamins discussed in this section, niacin is very inexpensive; therefore, its effectiveness in reducing cholesterol levels may be an affordable solution to reducing a known risk factor for cardiovascular disease. When monitored properly, niacin therapy can be almost as effective as the popular (and expensive) statin drugs for lowering cholesterol and triglyceride levels. It is important to note that although niacin is a B vitamin, high-dose niacin therapy should be considered drug therapy and not nutritional therapy.

SCIENTIFIC SUPPORT

Although various "structure/function" rationales could be assigned to the value of supplementation with B_6, B_{12}, and folate, the clearest and most dramatic effect of these nutrients is the reduction of hyperhomocysteinemia (and of niacin, hypercholesterolemia reduction) for prevention of heart disease. Thus, although some structure/function claims are mentioned here, the focus of this section is on the strongest data set—reduction of heart disease risk.

Vitamin B_6, like most of the B vitamins, is a cofactor in a wide variety of enzyme systems. As such, structure/function claims can be made for virtually any health condition. For example, because B_6 is needed to convert the amino acid tryptophan into niacin, a common B_6 claim relates to healthy cholesterol levels (because niacin can help lower cholesterol in some people). Vitamin B_6 also plays a role in prostaglandin synthesis; therefore, claims are often made for B_6 in regulating blood pressure, heart function, and pain levels (each of which is partially regulated by prostaglandins). Vitamin B_6 needs are increased in people consuming high-protein diets as well as in women taking oral contraceptives. Vitamin B_6 supplements (in conjunction with folic acid) have been shown to have a significant effect in reducing plasma levels of homocysteine (an amino acid metabolite linked to increased risk of atherosclerosis; see further discussion later in this subsection).

Vitamin B_6 is often recommended as a treatment for carpal tunnel syndrome (CTS). Most cases of CTS are caused by repetitive hand and wrist motions (such as typing), which causes inflammation and nerve compression in a region of the wrist known as the carpal tunnel. CTS is also known to occur in some women during pregnancy, in which case the nerve compression may be related to water retention and swelling rather than to repetitive motion. Vitamin B_6 is the most frequently recommended dietary supplement in cases of CTS (traditional treatments often include rest, splints, anti-inflammatory medications, and surgery). In some cases of CTS, approximately 100–300 mg of vitamin B_6 in divided doses has been shown to alleviate symptoms, although these results are not consistent and several studies have found no benefit of vitamin B_6 in treating CTS.

Vitamin B_{12} is an essential cofactor for methylation reactions in the body (including homocysteine metabolism), many in conjunction with folic acid. Therefore, B_{12} is involved in metabolic pathways related to brain function, joint health, and cardiovascular function. Absorption of B_{12} begins in the stomach, where it must combine with intrinsic factor, a compound synthesized by the stomach and required for proper absorption of vitamin B_{12} in the small intestine. A common cause of vitamin B_{12} deficiency in the elderly is an inadequate production of intrinsic factor and hydrochloric acid. Because B_{12} is stored in the liver, the symptoms of deficiency develop very slowly, typically not showing up for 5–10 years. Strict vegetarians (vegans), who consume only plant foods, are at the highest risk for developing B_{12} deficiency and should consider supplements. Elevated plasma homocysteine concentrations are considered to be a risk factor for vascular disease and birth defects such as neural tube defects. Studies have shown that plasma homocysteine can be lowered by intake of folic acid (400–800 µg) in combination with vitamin B_{12} (6 µg). This combination is significantly more effective in reducing homocysteine levels than is folic acid alone (Booth and Wang, 2000; Bunout et al., 2000).

Because folic acid has functions in DNA synthesis and nervous system maintenance, it has been linked to fetal growth and development. Clinical evidence clearly shows a beneficial effect of adequate folic acid intake in reducing the risk of brain and spinal cord birth defects. Owing to its role in red blood cell formation and homocysteine metabolism and because a deficiency of folic acid results in megaloblastic anemia, supplemental levels are often associated with maintenance of energy levels and heart health.

An adequate intake of folic acid is essential during pregnancy. Overwhelming evidence has shown that women given folic acid supplements during pregnancy have a lower incidence of delivering babies with neural tube defects such as spina bifida (American Academy of Pediatrics, 1999; Bailey, 2000). Oral contraceptives have been associated with lower folate levels in women who conceived soon after they stopped taking the pill (Shojania, 1982). Former contraceptive users and women who have previously delivered babies with neural tube defects may especially benefit from supplemental levels of folic acid in their diets.

The U.S. Department of Health recommends that pregnant women (and those trying to conceive) take a daily folic acid supplement of 400 μg (0.4 mg); the U.S. Public Health Service recommends that all women of childbearing age consume the same amount of folic acid each day to decrease the risk of bearing a child with a neural tube defect (American Academy of Pediatrics, 1999). Three strategies are available to women to achieve this goal: eat more foods with naturally occurring folic acid (fruits and vegetables), eat foods fortified with folic acid (such as breakfast cereals), or use dietary supplements.

Despite the wide-ranging public health benefits of adequate folic acid intake and the widespread public awareness of these benefits, as many as 68–87% of American women of childbearing age still have folic acid intakes below the recommended 400 μg/day. Elderly populations are also thought to be at increased risk for folate deficiencies, which might exacerbate their already high risk of heart disease, cancer, and neurological impairments. Several studies have suggested that folate supplementation should be considered in older people, especially those with elevated plasma total homocysteine levels and cardiovascular disease, as well as in people experiencing neuropsychiatric disorders (Brouwer et al., 1999; Loew et al., 1999). Because high-dose folate supplements can mask the symptoms of vitamin B_{12} deficiencies (which are also common in older people), folic acid supplements should be given in conjunction with B_{12}.

Niacin is involved in the proper functioning of more than 200 metabolic enzymes; thus, it plays a role in a wide range of bodily processes, including the synthesis of hormones and blood cells and the release of energy from fats, carbohydrates, and proteins. Virtually no difference is seen in overall metabolism between the various chemical forms of niacin as a nutrient (vitamin B_3) when it is consumed at low doses (20–40 mg). In the mid-1950s, however, high doses of niacin (as nicotinic acid) were found to lower cholesterol levels (although the exact mechanism of action is still not known) (Goldberg, 1998). The other form of niacin (nicotinamide or niacinamide) does not provide a cholesterol-lowering effect.

Niacin has been studied for its cardiovascular benefits in numerous clinical trials. The primary cardiovascular measures such as cholesterol and triglyceride levels, heart attacks, and strokes are all significantly reduced with niacin therapy (sometimes used alone and sometimes used with other drug therapy). Overall, the use of niacin (nicotinic acid but not niacinamide) to prevent or treat elevated blood lipids and reduce cardiovascular disease risk is well substantiated (O'Connor et al., 1997). In clinical trials, nicotinic acid has been shown to consistently lower total and LDL cholesterol by about 15–20% and triglycerides by 10–25%, while increasing levels of HDL cholesterol by 15–25% (O'Connor et al., 1997). The downside is that the amount of niacin needed to lower cholesterol levels tends to result in "niacin intolerance" in 15–40% of people who try it; they may experience unpleasant skin flushing (similar to hot flashes) as well as the serious risk of liver damage (see the "Safety/Dosage" subsection of this section).

Niacin supplements are available in regular and slow-release forms. The slow-release forms of nicotinic acid are intended for prolonged release of niacin during its 6–8 hour transit time in the intestines, but are also associated with greater toxicity. Safe doses are only about half of normal-release forms of niacin (Capuzzi et al., 1998; Guyton et al., 2000; Morgan et al., 1998).

Folate, B_6, and B_{12} are often used in combination therapy to reduce serum levels of homocysteine (an amino acid produced during methionine metabolism). Plasma levels of homocysteine have been recognized in dozens of studies as an important cardiovascular risk factor that predicts adverse cardiac events in patients with established coronary atherosclerosis (Righetti et al., 2003) and influences the restenosis rate after percutaneous coronary intervention (Schnyder et al., 2002). A 5-μmol/L increase in total homocysteine level is associated with an increase of approximately 70% in the relative risk of cardiovascular disease in adults (Chait et al., 1999). When folic acid is supplemented alone at 5–15 mg/day for 1 year, no difference is seen in the degree of homocysteine reduction at different levels of folic acid within this range (Righetti et al., 2003), and much lower levels of folic acid (100–600 μg/day for 4 weeks) have resulted in significant reductions in plasma total homocysteine levels in several studies (Brouwer et al., 1999; Riddell et al., 2000; Silaste et al., 2003; Venn et al., 2002). Even in the face of folate enrichment of cereal grain products (at 140 μg per 100 g of flour), which would be expected to increase the baseline folic acid intake of the population, dietary supplementation with additional folate (2.5 g/day) for 12 weeks has been shown to further increase folic acid status and reduce total homocysteine levels in patients with coronary artery disease (Bostom et al., 2002). Much lower levels of folic acid supplementation (400 μg/day), when combined with B_{12} (500 μg/day) and B_6 (12.5 mg/day) for 3 months, reduced homocysteine levels by 15% in patients with documented coronary artery disease (Lobo et al., 1999).

In one study by Malinow et al. (1998), 75 men and women with coronary artery disease were studied to determine the effect of folate-fortified foods on plasma homocysteine levels. Results showed that cereal fortified with 127 μg/day of folate (approximately the level resulting from the FDA's policy on enrichment of cereal grains) increased plasma folic acid by 31% but reduced homocysteine by less then 4%. Cereals providing folic acid at 499 μg and 665 μg daily increased plasma folic acid levels by 65% and 106%, respectively, and decreased plasma total homocysteine levels by 11% and 14%, respectively (Malinow et al., 1998). These results suggest that higher levels of folic acid fortification than currently recommended by the FDA may be needed to control homocysteine levels. A similar study by Riddell et al. (2000) used forti-fied breakfast cereal or folic acid supplements to bring total daily folic acid intake to 600 µg/day. The authors found that a 21–24% drop in total homocysteine was negatively correlated to serum folate values. The increase in serum folate levels and the resulting reduction in total homocysteine tend to be more dramatic for supplements and fortified foods and more modest for nonenriched folate-containing foods (Riddell et al., 2000; Venn et al., 2002). Dietary interventions to encourage higher intakes of folate-rich foods are effective in increasing serum folate by approximately 11–14% and reducing total homocysteine levels by approximately 10–13% within 5–10 weeks (Chait et al., 1999; Silaste et al., 2003).

Like folic acid, vitamin B_{12} is an essential cofactor in methionine metabolism and an important coenzyme in various methylation reactions. In folate- and B_{12}-replete subjects, vitamin B_6 supplementation (pyridoxine at 1.6 mg/day for 12 weeks) has been shown to reduce plasma total homocysteine levels by an additional 7.5% (McKinley et al., 2001) and should thus be included in a cocktail of vitamins for reducing elevated plasma homocysteine levels.

Studies of therapies consisting of various combinations of folate, B_6, and B_{12} for reducing plasma total homocysteine levels have been nearly unanimous in their findings of significantly reducing elevated homocysteine levels while leaving other aspects of cardiovascular risk largely unchanged (Hirsch et al., 2002). In patients with established coronary artery disease, therapy with folate, B_6, and B_{12} for 6 months has been shown to significantly reduce homocysteine and to reduce the incidence of fatal and nonfatal myocardial infarctions (Schnyder et al., 2002).

Lipid-lowering therapy with fibrates is known to increase homocysteine levels by up to 40% (Dierkes et al., 2001a, 2001b)—an effect that could counteract the cardioprotective effect of lipid lowering. By combining fenofibrate treatment with daily folic acid (650 µg), B_{12} (50 µg), and B_6 (5 mg) for 6 weeks, the increase in homocysteine levels was cut by nearly half, from more than 47% with no vitamins to only 25% with vitamin supplementation. In most hemodialysis patients and patients with end-stage renal disease, levels of B vitamins are depleted and homocysteine levels are elevated (Dierkes et al., 2001a, 2001b; Henning et al., 2001; Tremblay et al., 2000). In these patients, supplementation with folate, B_6, and B_{12} through either an oral or intravenous route is effective in improving B-vitamin status and reducing hyperhomocysteinemia by 30–50% within 4 weeks to 6 months (Dierkes et al., 2001a, 2001b; Henning et al., 2001, Tremblay et al., 2000). Metformin therapy in diabetic patients is also known to reduce serum levels of vitamin B_{12} and folic acid by 8–17% and increase total homocysteine levels by nearly 15% (Carlsen et al., 1997), suggesting that homocysteine-lowering therapy with B-vitamin supplements may be beneficial in some diabetic patients.

SAFETY/DOSAGE

As water-soluble vitamins, all B vitamins are generally considered quite safe as dietary supplements. For B_6, excessive intakes (2–6 g acutely or 500 mg chronically) are associated with sensory neuropathy (loss of feeling in the extremities), which may or may not be reversible. The recommended dietary allowance (RDA) for vitamin B_6 is less than 2 mg/day—an amount contained in virtually all multivitamin supplements. Pregnant and lactating women should not take more than 100 mg of vitamin B_6 per day.

There are no confirmed reports of toxic side effects associated with vitamin B_{12} supplements, even at the very high injected doses commonly used to restore cognitive function in older patients suffering from B_{12} deficiency. Oral intakes as high as 3,000 μg per day are considered nontoxic (Wyn and Wyn, 1998). The daily value (DV) for vitamin B_{12} is 6 μg, with a lower RDA set at 2.4 μg.

Extremely high intakes of folic acid (1–5 mg/day) have been associated with masking the signs and symptoms of pernicious anemia (vitamin B_{12} deficiency) and should be avoided. The DV (and RDA) for folic acid is 400 μg, an amount that all women of childbearing age should consume each day. As with the other B vitamins, dietary needs for folic acid may be somewhat elevated during times of stress and during pregnancy and lactation. In older people, a daily folate supplement of 500 μg may be warranted, but it should not replace the need for a diet rich in fruit and vegetables.

The DV for niacin is only 20 mg and the RDA is only 14–16 mg (see Table 7.1), and the body can convert the amino acid tryptophan into niacin. Nonetheless, a "cholesterol-lowering" dose of niacin (as nicotinic acid, *not* niacinamide or nicotinamide) is typically in the range of 250–2,000 mg/day. Dosing is usually started at the low end (250 mg/day), with increasing doses of 250 mg each week or two until blood lipid levels start to normalize (or side effects develop). Side effects are usually minimized by increasing the dosage slowly to the common therapeutic range of 1,000–2,000 mg/day and should be divided into two or three separate doses of no more than 500–750 mg/dose. With high doses of niacin used for controlling cholesterol levels (anything above 100 mg/day), nicotinic acid can cause skin flushing and itching of the skin as well as headaches and hypotension. In some cases, the skin flushing and itching side effects can be reduced somewhat by combined use with aspirin (which also has the beneficial cardiovascular effect of reduced blood clotting). The niacinamide form of niacin does not cause these side effects, but it is not effective in reducing cholesterol levels, so it is seldom taken in such high doses.

The slow-release versions of niacin supplements for controlling blood lipids have the potential for causing liver damage (even at "lower" doses of 500 mg/day); therefore, blood tests to monitor for liver damage are recommended, and high-dose niacin supplementation should only be undertaken on the advice and guidance of a physician. The inositol

Table 7.1. B-Complex Dosage Ranges

Nutrient	RDA/AI	UL	THyc dose	NOAEL	LOAEL
Pyridoxine (vitamin B$_6$)	1.3–1.5 mg (F); 1.3–1.7 mg (M)	100 mg	2.0–12.5 mg	200 mg	500 mg
Cobalamin (vitamin B$_{12}$)	2.4 µg	Unknown	50–800 µg	3,000 µg	Unknown
Folic acid	400 µg	1,000 µg	400–1,000 µg (cholesterol reduction)	1,000 µg	Unknown
Niacin	14 mg (F); 16 mg (M)	35 mg	250–2,000 mg (cholesterol reduction)	Nicotinic acid = 500 mg (250 mg SR) Nicotinamide = 1,500 mg	Nicotinic acid = 1,000 mg (500 mg SR) Nicotinamide = 3,000 mg

AI = adequate intake; LOAEL = lowest observed adverse effect level—the lowest level at which the Council for Responsible Nutrition has determined that adverse effects are observed; NOAEL = no observed adverse effect level—level at which the Council for Responsible Nutrition has determined no adverse effects are likely to be observed; RDA = recommended dietary allowance; SR = slow-release; tHyc dose = dosage range showing positive effect in reducing total plasma homocysteine levels; UL = upper limit.

hexaniacinate (Niacinol) form of niacin may be less likely to cause liver damage compared with timed-release forms. Anybody with liver disease, including those who consume more than two drinks of alcohol daily, should not take high-dose niacin except on specific medical advice. All niacin therapy (at doses exceeding 100 mg/day) should be supervised and monitored by a physician.

REFERENCES

American Academy of Pediatrics, Committee on Genetics. Folic acid for the prevention of neural tube defects. Pediatrics 1999;104(2 pt 1):325–327.

Bostom AG, Jacques PF, Liaugaudas G, Rogers G, Rosenberg IH, Selhub J. Total homocysteine lowering treatment among coronary artery disease patients in the era of folic acid-fortified cereal grain flour. Arterioscler Thromb Vasc Biol 2002;22(3):488–491.

Booth GL, Wang EE. Preventive health care, 2000 update: screening and management of hyperhomocysteinemia for the prevention of coronary artery disease events. The Canadian Task Force on Preventive Health Care. CMAJ 2000;163(1):21–29.

Brouwer IA, van Dusseldorp M, Thomas CM, Duran M, Hautvast JG, Eskes TK, Steegers-Theunissen RP. Low-dose folic acid supplementation decreases plasma homocysteine concentrations: a randomized trial. Am J Clin Nutr 1999;69(1):99–104.

Bunout D, Garrido A, Suazo M, Kauffman R, Venegas P, de la Maza P, Petermann M, Hirsch S. Effects of supplementation with folic acid and antioxidant vitamins on homocysteine levels and LDL oxidation in coronary patients. Nutrition 2000;16(2):107–110.

Capuzzi DM, Guyton JR, Morgan JM, Goldberg AC, Kreisberg RA, Brusco OA, Brody J. Efficacy and safety of an extended-release niacin (Niaspan): a long-term study. Am J Cardiol 1998;82(12A):74U–81U.

Carlsen SM, Folling I, Grill V, Bjerve KS, Schneede J, Refsum H. Metformin increases total serum homocysteine levels in non-diabetic male patients with coronary heart disease. Scand J Clin Lab Invest 1997;57(6):521–527.

Chait A, Malinow MR, Nevin DN, Morris CD, Eastgard RL, Kris-Etherton P, Pi-Sunyer FX, Oparil S, Resnick LM, Stern JS, Haynes RB, Hatton DC, Metz JA, Clark S, McMahon M, Holcomb S, Reusser ME, Snyder GW, McCarron DA. Increased dietary micronutrients decrease serum homocysteine concentrations in patients at high risk of cardiovascular disease. Am J Clin Nutr 1999;70(5):881–887.

Dierkes J, Domrose U, Bosselmann KP, Neumann KH, Luley C. Homocysteine lowering effect of different multivitamin preparations in patients with end-stage renal disease. J Ren Nutr 2001a;11(2):67–72.

Dierkes J, Westphal S, Kunstmann S, Banditt P, Lossner A, Luley C. Vitamin supplementation can markedly reduce the homocysteine elevation induced by fenofibrate. Atherosclerosis 2001b;158(1):161–164.

Goldberg AC. Clinical trial experience with extended-release niacin (Niaspan): dose-escalation study. Am J Cardiol 1998;82(12A):35U–38U.

Guyton JR, Capuzzi DM. Treatment of hyperlipidemia with combined niacin-statin regimens. Am J Cardiol 1998;82(12A):82U–84U.

Henning BF, Zidek W, Riezler R, Graefe U, Tepel M. Homocyst(e)ine metabolism in hemodialysis patients treated with vitamins B_6, B_{12} and folate. Res Exp Med (Berl) 2001;200(3):155–168.

Hirsch S, Pia De la Maza M, Yanez P, Glasinovic A, Petermann M, Barrera G, Gattas V, Escobar E, Bunout D. Hyperhomocysteinemia and endothelial function in young subjects: effects of vitamin supplementation. Clin Cardiol 2002;25(11):495–501.

Lobo A, Naso A, Arheart K, Kruger WD, Abou-Ghazala T, Alsous F, Nahlawi M, Gupta A, Moustapha A, van Lente F, Jacobsen DW, Robinson K. Reduction of homocysteine levels in coronary artery disease by low-dose folic acid combined with vitamins B_6 and B_{12}. Am J Cardiol 1999;83(6):821–825.

Loew D, Wanitschke R, Schroedter A. Studies on vitamin B_{12} status in the elderly—prophylactic and therapeutic consequences. Int J Vitam Nutr Res 1999;69(3):228–233.

Malinow MR, Duell PB, Hess DL, Anderson PH, Kruger WD, Phillipson BE, Gluckman RA, Block PC, Upson BM. Reduction of plasma homocyst(e)ine levels by breakfast cereal fortified with folic acid in patients with coronary heart disease. N Engl J Med 1998;338(15):1009–1015.

McKinley MC, McNulty H, McPartlin J, Strain JJ, Pentieva K, Ward M, Weir DG, Scott JM. Low-dose vitamin B-6 effectively lowers fasting plasma homocysteine in healthy elderly persons who are folate and riboflavin replete. Am J Clin Nutr 2001;73(4):759–764.

Morgan JM, Capuzzi DM, Guyton JR. A new extended-release niacin (Niaspan): efficacy, tolerability, and safety in hypercholesterolemic patients. Am J Cardiol 1998;82(12A):29U–34U.

O'Connor PJ, Rush WA, Trence DL. Relative effectiveness of niacin and lovastatin for treatment of dyslipidemias in a health maintenance organization. J Fam Pract 1997;44(5):462–467.

Riddell LJ, Chisholm A, Williams S, Mann JI. Dietary strategies for lowering homocysteine concentrations. Am J Clin Nutr 2000;71(6):1448–1454.

Righetti M, Ferrario GM, Milani S, Serbelloni P, La Rosa L, Uccellini M, Sessa A. Effects of folic acid treatment on homocysteine levels and vascular disease in hemodialysis patients. Med Sci Monit 2003;9(4):PI19–PI24.

Schnyder G, Roffi M, Flammer Y, Pin R, Hess OM. Effect of homocysteine-lowering therapy with folic acid, vitamin B_{12}, and vitamin B_6 on clinical outcome after percutaneous coronary intervention: the Swiss heart study: a randomized controlled trial. JAMA 2002;288(8):973–979.

Shojania AM. Oral contraceptives: effect of folate and vitamin B_{12} metabolism. Can Med Assoc J 1982 1;126(3):244–247.

Silaste ML, Rantala M, Alfthan G, Aro A, Kesaniemi YA. Plasma homocysteine concentration is decreased by dietary intervention. Br J Nutr 2003;89(3):295–301.

Tremblay R, Bonnardeaux A, Geadah D, Busque L, Lebrun M, Ouimet D, Leblanc M. Hyperhomocysteinemia in hemodialysis patients: effects of 12-month supplementation with hydrosoluble vitamins. Kidney Int 2000;58(2):851–858.

Venn BJ, Mann JI, Williams SM, Riddell LJ, Chisholm A, Harper MJ, Aitken W, Rossaak JI. Assessment of three levels of folic acid on serum folate and plasma homocysteine: a randomised placebo-controlled double-blind dietary intervention trial. Eur J Clin Nutr 2002;56(8):748–754.

Wynn M, Wynn A. The danger of B_{12} deficiency in the elderly. Nutr Health 1998;12(4):215–226.

ADDITIONAL RESOURCES

Baik HW, Russell RM. Vitamin B_{12} deficiency in the elderly. Annu Rev Nutr 1999;19:357–377.

Bailey LB. New standard for dietary folate intake in pregnant women. Am J Clin Nutr 2000;71(5 suppl):1304S–1307S.

Carmody BJ, Arora S, Avena R, Cosby K, Sidawy AN. Folic acid inhibits homocysteine-induced proliferation of human arterial smooth muscle cells. J Vasc Surg 1999;30(6):1121–1128.

Chandna SM, Tattersall JE, Nevett G, Tew CJ, O'Sullivan J, Greenwood RN, Farrington K. Low serum vitamin B_{12} levels in chronic high-flux haemodialysis patients. Nephron 1997;75(3):259–263.

Elkin AC, Higham J. Folic acid supplements are more effective than increased dietary folate intake in elevating serum folate levels. BJOG 2000;107(2):285–289.

Ellis JM, McCully KS. Prevention of myocardial infarction by vitamin B_6. Res Commun Mol Pathol Pharmacol 1995;89(2):208–220.

Fanapour PC, Yug B, Kochar MS. Hyperhomocysteinemia: an additional cardiovascular risk factor. WMJ 1999;98(8):51–54.

Fenech M, Aitken C, Rinaldi J. Folate, vitamin B_{12}, homocysteine status and DNA damage in young Australian adults. Carcinogenesis 1998;19(7):1163–1171.

Folsom AR, Nieto FJ, McGovern PG, Tsai MY, Malinow MR, Eckfeldt JH, Hess DL, Davis CE. Prospective study of coronary heart disease incidence in relation to fasting total homocysteine, related genetic polymorphisms, and B vitamins: the Atherosclerosis Risk in Communities (ARIC) study. Circulation 1998;98(3):204–210.

Ford ES, Ballew C. Dietary folate intake in US adults: findings from the third National Health and Nutrition Examination Survey. Ethn Dis 1998;8(3):299–305.

Gardner SF, Marx MA, White LM, Granberry MC, Skelton DR, Fonseca VA. Combination of low-dose niacin and pravastatin improves the lipid profile in diabetic patients without compromising glycemic control. Ann Pharmacother 1997;31(6):677–682.

Gupta A, Moustapha A, Jacobsen DW, Goormastic M, Tuzcu EM, Hobbs R, Young J, James K, McCarthy P, van Lente F, Green R, Robinson K. High homocysteine, low folate, and low vitamin B_6 concentrations: prevalent risk factors for vascular disease in heart transplant recipients. Transplantation 1998;65(4):544–550.

Guyton JR, Blazing MA, Hagar J, Kashyap ML, Knopp RH, McKenney JM, Nash DT, Nash SD. Extended-release niacin vs gemfibrozil for the treatment of low levels of high-density lipoprotein cholesterol. Niaspan-Gemfibrozil Study Group. Arch Intern Med 2000;160(8):1177–1184.

Guyton JR, Goldberg AC, Kreisberg RA, Sprecher DL, Superko HR, O'Connor CM. Effectiveness of once-nightly dosing of extended-release niacin alone and in combination for hypercholesterolemia. Am J Cardiol 1998;82(6):737–743.

Lewis CJ, Crane NT, Wilson DB, Yetley EA. Estimated folate intakes: data updated to reflect food fortification, increased bioavailability, and dietary supplement use. Am J Clin Nutr 1999;70(2):198–207.

Littell JT. Relationship of dietary folate and vitamin B_6 with coronary heart disease in women. JAMA 1998;280(5):418–419.

Liu S, Stampfer MJ, Hu FB, Giovannucci E, Rimm E, Manson JE, Hennekens CH, Willett WC. Whole-grain consumption and risk of coronary heart disease: results from the Nurses' Health Study. Am J Clin Nutr 1999;70(3):412–419.

Murua AL, Quintana I, Janson J, Batista M, Camera MI, Kordich LC. Plasmatic homocysteine response to vitamin supplementation in elderly people. Thromb Res 2000;100(6):495–500.

Newman PE. Can reduced folic acid and vitamin B_{12} levels cause deficient DNA methylation producing mutations which initiate atherosclerosis? Med Hypotheses 1999 Nov;53(5):421–424.

Nilsson-Ehle H. Age-related changes in cobalamin (vitamin B_{12}) handling. Implications for therapy. Drugs Aging 1998;12(4):277–292.

Novy MA. Are strict vegetarians at risk of vitamin B_{12} deficiency? Cleve Clin J Med 2000;67(2):87–88.

Omenn GS, Beresford SA, Motulsky AG. Preventing coronary heart disease: B vitamins and homocysteine. Circulation 1998;97(5):421–424.

Philipp CS, Cisar LA, Saidi P, Kostis JB. Effect of niacin supplementation on fibrinogen levels in patients with peripheral vascular disease. Am J Cardiol 1998;82(5):697–699, A9.

Rimm EB, Willett WC, Hu FB, Sampson L, Colditz GA, Manson JE, Hennekens C, Stampfer MJ. Folate and vitamin B_6 from diet and supplements in relation to risk of coronary heart disease among women. JAMA 1998;279(5):359–364.

Selhub J, Jacques PF, Bostom AG, D'Agostino RB, Wilson PW, Belanger AJ, O'Leary DH, Wolf PA, Rush D, Schaefer EJ, Rosenberg IH. Relationship between plasma homocysteine, vitamin status and extracranial carotid-artery stenosis in the Framingham Study population. J Nutr 1996;126(4 suppl):1258S–1265S.

Selhub J, Jacques PF, Bostom AG, D'Agostino RB, Wilson PW, Belanger AJ, O'Leary DH, Wolf PA, Schaefer EJ, Rosenberg IH. Association between plasma homocysteine concentrations and extracranial carotid-artery stenosis. N Engl J Med 1995;332(5):286–291.

Selhub J, Jacques PF, Wilson PW, Rush D, Rosenberg IH. Vitamin status and intake as primary determinants of homocysteinemia in an elderly population. JAMA 1993;270(22):2693–2698.

Simon J, Racek J, Rosolova H. Homocysteine, a less well-known risk factor in cardiac and vascular diseases. Cas Lek Cesk 1996;135(9):263–265.

Suitor CW, Bailey LB. Food folate vs synthetic folic acid: a comparison. J Am Diet Assoc 1999;99(3):285.

Vermaak WJ, Barnard HC, Potgieter GM, Theron HD. Vitamin B_6 and coronary artery disease. Epidemiological observations and case studies. Atherosclerosis 1987;63(2–3):235–238.

Willems HP, den Heijer M, Bos GM. Homocysteine and venous thrombosis: outline of a vitamin intervention trial. Semin Thromb Hemost 2000;26(3):297–304.

Willett WC. A prospective study of folate intake and the risk of breast cancer. JAMA 1999;281(17):1632–1637.

Zeitlin A, Frishman WH, Chang CJ. The association of vitamin B_{12} and folate blood levels with mortality and cardiovascular morbidity incidence in the old: the Bronx Aging Study. Am J Ther 1997;4(7–8):275–281.

COENZYME Q_{10} (COQ$_{10}$)

Overall Rank

★★★★ for heart patients, especially in conjunction with statins
★★★★ as an antioxidant
★★ for endurance performance
★★ for energy and chronic fatigue

OVERVIEW

Coenzyme Q_{10} (CoQ$_{10}$) is found in the mitochondria of all cells and is particularly enriched in tissues of the heart, liver, kidney, and pancreas. CoQ$_{10}$ functions as part of the cellular system that generates energy from oxygen (in the form of ATP) for bodily processes and can act as an antioxidant to help prevent cellular damage from free radicals created during exercise and during the generation of energy. Dietary supplements containing CoQ$_{10}$ (often suspended in soybean oil or some other oil base for better absorption) are generally marketed with claims of increasing energy and endurance levels, supporting heart function, reducing blood pressure, and improving overall heart strength.

Because CoQ$_{10}$ plays a role in the respiratory chain as an electron/proton carrier, it functions in the production of ATP in the mitochondria of the cell. CoQ$_{10}$ has also been shown to exhibit activity as a free radical scavenger and antioxidant. The theory of CoQ$_{10}$ supplementation posits that consumption of CoQ$_{10}$ increases tissue and mitochondrial CoQ$_{10}$ levels and supports ATP production as well as serving an antioxidant function.

COMMENTS

For athletes, the data do not consistently support the use of supplemental CoQ$_{10}$ as an ergogenic performance aid. As a general "energetic" dietary supplement for reducing fatigue and alleviating the symptoms of chronic fatigue syndrome, the effectiveness of CoQ$_{10}$ supplementation is largely unsupported. As an antioxidant, especially in combination with other antioxidants such as vitamins C and E, CoQ$_{10}$ appears to be beneficial. For heart patients, CoQ$_{10}$ appears to be especially indicated, particularly in those who may be taking cholesterol-lowering medications (3-hydroxy-3-methylglutaryl coenzyme A [HMG-CoA] reductase inhibitors in the class of statin medications, including lovastatin [Mevacor], simvastatin [Zocor], pravastatin [Pravachol], and fluvastatin [Lescol]).

SCIENTIFIC SUPPORT

Because CoQ_{10} levels peak around age 20 and decline thereafter, it seems logical that supplemental CoQ_{10} would be beneficial in older adults. The antioxidant effects of CoQ_{10} are well established. Many studies have shown that CoQ_{10} reduces the initiation and propagation of lipid peroxidation (free-radical damage) in cell membranes and in lipoprotein fractions (Taggart et al., 1996). Additionally, combined supplementation of CoQ_{10} and vitamin E produces a synergistic antioxidant effect on lipoproteins and "spares" the vitamin E (Kucharska et al., 1996).

In heart disease, CoQ_{10} has shown benefits in patients with heart failure, with 50 mg/day for 4 weeks resulting in improvements in dyspnea, heart rate, blood pressure, and ankle edema (Hofman-Bang et al., 1995). In most studies of heart failure, a significant reduction in hospitalizations and episodes of pulmonary edema and cardiac asthma are generally observed (Khatta et al., 2000). Cardiac patients supplemented with CoQ_{10} before heart surgery tend to recover sooner and maintain blood and tissue levels of CoQ_{10} better than patients not receiving supplements. In a one study, 144 patients suffering from acute mitral incompetence benefited from 28 days of CoQ_{10} at 120 mg/day compared with placebo by decreasing incidence of angina, arrhythmias, and poor left ventricular function (Soja et al., 1997a, 1997b). A handful of studies have suggested reductions in systolic and diastolic blood pressure of 7–10 mm Hg after 8–10 weeks of CoQ_{10} supplementation (Sacher et al., 1997; Singh et al., 1998).

In addition, patients taking cholesterol-lowering medications (HMG-CoA reductase inhibitors, known as statin drugs) may benefit from CoQ_{10} supplements because these medications can reduce blood levels of CoQ_{10} (Langsjoen and Langsjoen, 1999). In several studies, CoQ_{10} levels have been shown to be significantly reduced with simvastatin and related statin medications, resulting in an accompanying reduction in ejection fraction response to exercise, myocardial reserve, and myocardial contractile function (Kontush et al., 1997; Langsjoen and Langsjoen, 1999). CoQ_{10} was approved in 1974 in Japan for the treatment of congestive heart failure, and at least one formulation (UbiQGel), has received FDA orphan drug status for treating mitochondrial disorders (Greenberg and Frishman, 1990).

The one area in which data are most conflicting is for CoQ_{10} as an ergogenic aid for athletic performance. Because of its role in ATP synthesis, supplemental CoQ_{10} would be expected to support the process of cellular energy production. Research in this area has been conflicting, however, with some studies showing a benefit and others showing no effect (Weston et al., 1997).

SAFETY/DOSAGE

CoQ_{10} has a good safety profile, and daily doses of 50–100 mg are well tolerated. Reported side effects are rare but tend to be various forms of epigastric distress (heartburn, nausea, stomachache), which can be prevented by consuming the supplement with a meal. Intakes of 100–200 mg/day have been studied with no apparent adverse side effects, but muscle damage has been noted in at least one study in which 120 mg/day were administered over 20 days, perhaps because of a prooxidant effect and free-radical damage in the muscle (Kucharska et al., 1998).

Smoking is known to deplete CoQ_{10} levels in blood and tissues. Several medications can reduce blood and tissue levels of CoQ_{10}, including drugs for controlling cholesterol (statins, including a theoretical reduction in CoQ_{10} levels with use of red yeast rice supplements, which contain natural lovastatin); blood pressure (β blockers, by inhibiting CoQ_{10}-dependent enzymes); and blood sugar (some oral hypoglycemic agents); therefore, CoQ_{10} supplements may be warranted in patients taking these medications. HMG-CoA reductase inhibitors can reduce CoQ_{10} concentrations by approximately 32–47% by blocking the synthesis of mevalonic acid, a precursor of CoQ_{10}.

REFERENCES

Greenberg S, Frishman WH. Co-enzyme Q_{10}: a new drug for cardiovascular disease. J Clin Pharmacol 1990;30(7):596–608.

Hofman-Bang C, Rehnqvist N, Swedberg K, Wiklund I, Astrom H. Coenzyme Q_{10} as an adjunctive in the treatment of chronic congestive heart failure. The Q_{10} Study Group. J Card Fail 1995;1(2):101–107.

Khatta M, Alexander BS, Krichten CM, Fisher ML, Freudenberger R, Robinson SW, Gottlieb SS. The effect of coenzyme Q_{10} in patients with congestive heart failure. Ann Intern Med 2000;132(8):636–640.

Kontush A, Reich A, Baum K, Spranger T, Finckh B, Kohlschutter A, Beisiegel U. Plasma ubiquinol-10 is decreased in patients with hyperlipidaemia. Atherosclerosis 1997;129(1):119–126.

Kucharska J, Gvozdjakova A, Mizera S, Braunova Z, Schreinerova Z, Schramekova E, Pechan I, Fabian J. Participation of coenzyme Q_{10} in the rejection development of the transplanted heart: a clinical study. Physiol Res 1998;47(6):399–404.

Kucharska J, Gvozdjakova A, Mizera S, Margitfalvi P, Schreinerova Z, Schramekova E, Solcanska K, Notova P, Pechan I, Fabian J. Coenzyme Q_{10} and alpha-tocopherol in patients after heart transplantation. Bratisl Lek Listy 1996;97(10):603–606.

Langsjoen PH, Langsjoen AM. Overview of the use of CoQ_{10} in cardiovascular disease. Biofactors 1999;9(2–4):273–284.

Sacher HL, Sacher ML, Landau SW, Kersten R, Dooley F, Sacher A, Sacher M, Dietrick K, Ichkhan K. The clinical and hemodynamic effects of coenzyme Q_{10} in congestive cardiomyopathy. Am J Ther 1997;4(2–3):66–72.

Singh RB, Wander GS, Rastogi A, Shukla PK, Mittal A, Sharma JP, Mehrotra SK, Kapoor R, Chopra RK. Randomized, double-blind placebo-controlled trial of coenzyme Q_{10} in patients with acute myocardial infarction. Cardiovasc Drugs Ther 1998;12(4):347–353.

Soja AM, Mortensen SA. Treatment of chronic cardiac insufficiency with coenzyme Q_{10}, results of meta-analysis in controlled clinical trials. Ugeskr Laeger 1997a;159(49):7302–7308.

Soja AM, Mortensen SA. Treatment of congestive heart failure with coenzyme Q_{10} illuminated by meta-analyses of clinical trials. Mol Aspects Med 1997b;18(suppl):S159–S168.

Taggart DP, Jenkins M, Hooper J, Hadjinikolas L, Kemp M, Hue D, Bennett G. Effects of short-term supplementation with coenzyme Q_{10} on myocardial protection during cardiac operations. Ann Thorac Surg 1996;61(3):829–833.

Weston SB, Zhou S, Weatherby RP, Robson SJ. Does exogenous coenzyme Q_{10} affect aerobic capacity in endurance athletes? Int J Sport Nutr 1997;7(3):197–206.

ADDITIONAL RESOURCES

Gvozdjakova A, Kucharska J, Mizera S, Braunova Z, Schreinerova Z, Schramekova E, Pechan I, Fabian J. Coenzyme Q_{10} depletion and mitochondrial energy disturbances in rejection development in patients after heart transplantation. Biofactors 1999;9(2–4):301–306.

Langsjoen PH, Langsjoen A, Willis R, Folkers K. Treatment of hypertrophic cardiomyopathy with coenzyme Q_{10}. Mol Aspects Med 1997;18(suppl):S145–S151.

Mortensen SA. Coenzyme Q_{10} as an adjunctive therapy in patients with congestive heart failure. J Am Coll Cardiol 2000;36(1):304–305.

Munkholm H, Hansen HH, Rasmussen K. Coenzyme Q_{10} treatment in serious heart failure. Biofactors 1999;9(2–4):285–289.

Overvad K, Diamant B, Holm L, Holmer G, Mortensen SA, Stender S. Coenzyme Q_{10} in health and disease. Eur J Clin Nutr 1999;53(10):764–770.

Sinatra ST. Coenzyme Q_{10}: a vital therapeutic nutrient for the heart with special application in congestive heart failure. Conn Med 1997;61(11):707–711.

Sinatra ST. Refractory congestive heart failure successfully managed with high dose coenzyme Q_{10} administration. Mol Aspects Med 1997;18(suppl):S299–S305.

ESSENTIAL FATTY ACIDS (ω-3, ω-6, FISH OIL, EVENING PRIMROSE OIL, BORAGE SEED OIL, FLAXSEED OIL)

Overall Rank

★★★★★   for correcting essential fatty acid deficiency
★★★★★   for general heart health
★★★★   for controlling inflammation

OVERVIEW

The term *essential fatty acids* refers to two fatty acids, linoleic acid and linolenic acid, that our bodies cannot synthesize. These fatty acids, like the essential vitamins and minerals, must be consumed in the diet. These essential fatty acids are needed for the production of prostaglandins and eicosanoids, which help regulate blood clotting, blood pressure, heart rate, immune response, and a wide variety of other biological processes.

Linoleic acid is a polyunsaturated fatty acid with 18 carbon atoms and two double bonds. It is considered an ω-6 or n-6 fatty acid because the first of its double bonds occurs at the sixth carbon from the ω end. It is also referred to as C18:2n6, meaning 18 carbons and two double bonds, with the first double bond at the n-6 position. Linoleic acid is found in vegetable and nut oils such as sunflower, safflower, corn, soy, and peanut oil. Most Americans get adequate levels of these ω-6 oils in their diets because of a high consumption of margarines, salad dressings, and mayonnaise with vegetable oil bases.

Linolenic acid, or α-linolenic acid, is also an 18-carbon polyunsaturated fatty acid, but it is classified as an ω-3 or n-3 fatty acid because its first double bond (of three) is at the third carbon from the ω end. It is also known as C18:3n3, meaning 18 carbons and three double bonds, with the first double bond at the n-3 position. Three major types of ω-3 fatty acids are consumed in foods and utilized by the body: α-linolenic acid (ALA), eicosapentaenoic acid (EPA), and docosahexaenoic acid (DHA). ALA can be converted into EPA and DHA in the body. Good dietary sources of ALA are flaxseed oil (51% linolenic acid), canola oil (9%), and walnuts (7%), as well as margarine derived from canola oil. For example, a tablespoon of canola oil or canola oil margarine provides about 1 g of linolenic acid.

ω-3 fatty acids are generally found to reduce inflammation and thus to have a positive impact on heart disease, arthritis, and inflammatory conditions such as allergies, asthma, inflammatory bowel disease, and others. The existing data for the health benefits of ω-3 fatty acids are particularly strong for a reduced risk of heart disease (Marckmann and Gronbaek, 1999; Meydani, 2000).

COMMENTS

Over the last century, modern diets have come to rely heavily on fats derived from high-n-6 vegetable oils (sunflower, safflower, corn), bringing the ratio of n-6 to n-3 fatty acids from an estimated Paleolithic ratio of 1:1 to the modern-day range of 20–30:1. This unbalanced intake of high n-6 fatty acids and low n-3 fatty acids sets the stage for increases in blood viscosity, vasoconstriction, and generalized inflammation involving everything from heart health to pain levels.

Fatty acids of the n-3 variety, however, have opposing biological effects to the n-6 fatty acids, meaning that a higher intake of n-3 oils can deliver anti-inflammatory, antithrombotic, and vasodilatory effects that can lead to benefits in terms of heart disease, hypertension, diabetes, and a wide variety of inflammatory conditions such as rheumatoid arthritis and ulcerative colitis.

The most common supplemental sources of essential fatty acids are fish oils—good sources of the ω-3 fatty acids. Other oils, such as those made from flaxseed, borage seed, and evening primrose, are rich sources of essential fatty acids but typically do not provide the high levels of concentrated EPA and DHA found in many fish oil supplements. The highest quality fish oil supplements should provide 18–30% EPA and 12–20% DHA. Supplements with higher EPA and DHA contents are better but also more expensive.

Although γ-linoleic acid (GLA) supplements are widely available as extracts of evening primrose and borage seed, their claims of reducing menopausal hot flashes, symptoms of premenstrual syndrome (breast tenderness and irritability), and inflammatory conditions such as eczema, asthma, allergies, and rheumatoid arthritis are generally not well supported by objective scientific literature. The data in this area are mixed, and the response to GLA supplementation may be individual, based on initial GLA levels.

The best evidence for a beneficial health effect of essential fatty acid supplementation exists for the use of fish oil supplements (EPA and DHA) in reducing cardiovascular disease risk, prompting the FDA to issue a qualified health claim for ω-3 supplements indicating, "The scientific evidence about whether ω-3 fatty acids may reduce the risk of coronary heart disease (CHD) is suggestive, but not conclusive. Studies in the general population have looked at diets containing fish and it is not known whether diets or ω-3 fatty acids in fish may have a possible effect on a reduced risk of CHD. It is not known what effect ω-3 fatty acids may or may not have on risk of CHD in the general population" (FDA Announces..., 2004). Such language is permitted on foods or supplements provided that the product does not recommend a daily intake exceeding 3 g/day of EPA and DHA (which, for most standard fish oil supplements, would be in the range of 9–10 g/day of fish oil).

SCIENTIFIC SUPPORT

In the body, linoleic acid (n-6) is metabolized in the body to γ-linoleic acid and then to arachidonic acid, a precursor to specific "bad" eicosanoids that can promote vasoconstriction and elevated blood pressure. Although GLA is a fatty acid of the n-6 variety, when taken as a dietary supplement (typically from evening primrose oil, borage seed oil, and black currant seed oil), it may be converted largely to dihomo-γ-linoleic acid (DGLA), which is known to compete with arachidonic acid (typically found in egg yolks and meat) for conversion into pro-inflammatory eicosanoids. Therefore, GLA (via DGLA) is a potential anti-inflammatory fatty acid in conditions such as dermatitis (Thijs et al., 2000, van Gool et al., 2003), periodontics (Rosenstein et al., 2003), rheumatoid arthritis (Leventhal et al., 1993), and inflammatory respiratory disorders (Gadek et al., 1999).

Despite the potential anti-inflammatory effect of GLA, the scientific evidence supporting the anti-inflammatory effects of ω-3 fatty acids is much stronger (Blommers et al., 2002; Hederos and Berg, 1996; Henz et al., 1999). For example, linolenic acid (n-3) is metabolized in the body to EPA and DHA. EPA serves as the precursor to prostaglandin E3, which may have vasodilatory properties on blood vessels—effects that can counteract the vasoconstriction caused by n-6 fatty acids (Honstra et al., 1990, Kurlandsky et al., 1994).

Other studies have shown that consumption of linolenic acid and other n-3 fatty acids offers protection against heart disease and heart attacks (Leaf et al., 1998; Oomen et al., 2000). This is thought to be mediated through the synthesis of EPA and DHA. Fish oils contain large amounts of both, and most studies have used various concentrations of fish oil supplements to demonstrate the health benefits of these essential fatty acids. For example, 1 g of menhaden oil (a common fish source) provides about 300 mg of essential fatty acids. EPA is known to induce an antithrombotic (clot-preventing) effect through its inhibition of platelet cyclooxygenase (which converts arachidonic acid to thromboxane A2) and the "less sticky" platelets that result. Fish oil and its high content of EPA and DHA may also protect against heart disease through an anti-inflammatory effect (by reducing cytokine production and/or increasing nitric oxide production in the endothelium) (O'Keefe and Harris, 2000).

Flaxseed, a rich plant source of ω-3 fatty acids, has been shown to lower both systolic and diastolic blood pressure (1–2 tablespoons daily). Epidemiological studies have shown that subjects with high intakes of linolenic acid (n-3) have a 50% reduced risk of heart disease, which may be partly a result of the beneficial effects of n-3 on blood pressure, cholesterol levels, blood clotting, and heart rhythm. ω-3 fatty acids are known to reduce thromboxane activity, which could explain their benefits in reducing platelet aggregation (blood clotting), blood vessel constriction, and various inflammatory conditions such as dermatitis (Bjorneboe et al., 1989) and rheumatoid arthritis (Cleland et al., 1988).

Some evidence exists that ω-3 fatty acids from fish oil and flaxseed may help improve insulin sensitivity, modulate lipid metabolism, and combat both mild depression and attention-deficit/hyperactivity disorder (ADHD) (Hamazaki et al., 1996). Although the data are far from clear, it is known that ω-3 fatty acids are concentrated in the brain and that children and adults suffering from depression and/or ADHD typically show suboptimal blood levels of essential fatty acids. In addition, population studies suggest that a high consumption of fish (rich in ω-3 fatty acids) may be related to a lower risk of depression, including postpartum depression. Mothers pass large amounts of essential fatty acids to their babies during the last 3 months of fetal brain development and through breast milk—so much that new mothers have only half the normal blood levels of ω-3 fatty acids, and nursing mothers may have even lower levels (Holman et al., 1991).

Several scientific studies suggest that diets high in ω-3 oils may protect against the development of heart disease, ADHD, arthritis, colitis, and other inflammatory diseases (Hawkes et al., 2002, Volker et al., 2000), and that ω-3 fatty acids can reduce triglyceride levels in the blood as well as reduce blood pressure (Kestin et al., 1990). The effects of ω-3 fatty acids on cholesterol levels, however, are inconsistent and may require excessive doses of fish oil to be effective. In rare instances, high doses of fish oil supplements may even increase serum cholesterol levels in genetically predisposed persons.

A major heart protective effect of ω-3 oil is its effect in reducing the "stickiness" of platelets in the blood, thus reducing the likelihood of the formation of blood clots. Regular consumption of diets high in fish is clearly linked to a reduced incidence of heart attacks. In some studies, it even appears that the real importance is not how much fish you eat but that you eat it at all. In other words, eating fish once a week appears to be just as effective as eating it 3 or 4 times each week.

The strongest data supporting a heart health benefit of ω-3 fatty acid consumption come from intervention trials with CHD as the endpoint.

These studies, ranging in length from 1.0 to 3.5 years and in size from 223 people in one study location to 11,324 people in 172 separate centers, have reported significant reductions in CHD risk with increased consumption of ω-3 fatty acids, predominantly EPA and DHA at approximately 800–900 mg/day (Burr et al., 2000; Marchioli and Valagussa, 2000; Singh et al., 1997; von Schacky et al., 2000). Although some of these studies reported an increase in LDL levels, others reported a decrease in LDL and most reported no change. In particular, the longest (3.5 years) and largest (*n* = 11,324) trial found no change in LDL cholesterol, while also reporting a 15% decrease in relative risk of CHD (Marchioli and Valagussa, 2000). In prospective studies of fish intake (as opposed to intake of fish oil supplements), a strong decreased risk of CHD with increasing consumption of fish may be related to the drop in serum triglyceride levels associated with increasing ω-3 fatty acid intake (Albert et al., 1998, Guallar et al., 1995, Layne et al., 1996, Morris et al., 1995).

SAFETY/DOSAGE

No serious adverse side effects should be expected from regular consumption of essential fatty acid supplements or ω-3 oils, whether from fish oil or other common oil supplements. The FDA considers fish oil to be generally recognized as safe, but because of the tendency of n-3 fatty acids to reduce platelet aggregation (i.e., to "thin" the blood), increased bleeding times can occur in some people (Lund et al., 1999), and doses of EPA and DHA above 3 g/day should be avoided (9–10 g of most standard fish oils providing 30% ω-3 fatty acids). Other potential safety concerns of high-dose ω-3 consumption (since discounted) have included increased oxidation of cell membranes rich in ω-3 fatty acids, increased blood levels of LDL cholesterol, and reduced glycemic control among diabetics (Pedersen et al., 2003, Ramirez-Tortosa et al., 1999, Wander and Du, 2000).

ALA is found in flaxseeds, flaxseed oil, canola oil, soybeans, and soybean oil. The best dietary sources of EPA and DHA are cold-water fish such as trout, tuna, salmon, mackerel, herring, and sardines, which all contain about 1–2 g of n-3 oils per 3–4-oz serving. The Food and Nutrition Board of the National Academy of Sciences has established an adequate intake (AI) of total n-6 fatty acids (primarily linoleic acid) of 11–17 g/day and total n-3 fatty acids (primarily ALA) of 1.1–1.6 g/day for adults (an approximate 10:1 ratio of n-6 to n-3 fatty acids). A 4-oz portion of salmon may contain 900 mg of ω-3 fatty acids, while a 4-oz portion of Atlantic mackerel provides 2.6 g of EPA and DHA.

Supplements of linoleic acid (n-6) are typically not needed, whereas linolenic acid (n-3) supplements (2–4 g/day) and/or concentrated EPA and DHA supplements (400–1,000 mg/day) are recommended to support cardiovascular health. According to the International Society for the Study of Fatty Acids and Lipids, total EPA and DHA intake should be a minimum of 220 mg/day of each and should approach about 1 g/day, about evenly split between the two (Proceedings of the 5th Congress..., 2003). Pregnant and lactating women are advised to increase their DHA intake somewhat so they consume at least 300 mg of DHA daily to ensure adequate brain development in their growing babies. When using flaxseed oil as a concentrated source of essential fatty acids, a typical dose is 1–2 tablespoons per day or up to 3,000 mg/day from capsules as a dietary source of ALA. Diabetics may lose the ability to convert ALA to EPA and DHA and thus may need to supplement with fish oil.

GLA supplement recommendations are in the range of 1,000–15,000 mg/day or up to 3,000 mg of evening primrose oil. Levels of GLA above 3,000 mg/day may lead to higher conversion to ALA rather than to the blocking effect of DGLA.

REFERENCES

Albert CM, Hennekens CH, O'Donnell CJ, Ajani UA, Carey VJ, Willett WC, Ruskin JN, Manson JE. Fish consumption and risk of sudden cardiac death. JAMA 1998;279(1):23–28.

Burr ML. Lessons from the story of n-3 fatty acids. Am J Clin Nutr 2000;71(1 Suppl):397S–398S.

Bjorneboe A, Soyland E, Bjorneboe GE, Rajka G, Drevon CA. Effect of n-3 fatty acid supplement to patients with atopic dermatitis. J Intern Med Suppl 1989;225(731):233–236.

Blommers J, de Lange-De Klerk ES, Kuik DJ, Bezemer PD, Meijer S. Evening primrose oil and fish oil for severe chronic astalgia: a randomized, double-blind, controlled trial. Am J Obstet Gynecol 2002;187(5):1389–1394.

Cleland LG, French JK, Betts WH, Murphy GA, Elliott MJ. Clinical and biochemical effects of dietary fish oil supplements in rheumatoid arthritis. J Rheumatol 1988;15(10):1471–1475.

FDA Announces Qualified Health Claims for Omega-3 Fatty Acids. FDA News. September 8, 2004. Accessed at: http://www.cfsan.fda.gov/~lrd/fpqhco3.html.

Gadek JE, DeMichele SJ, Karlstad MD, Pacht ER, Donahoe M, Albertson TE, Van Hoozen C, Wennberg AK, Nelson JL, Noursalehi M. Effect of enteral feeding with eicosapentaenoic acid, gamma-linolenic acid, and antioxidants in patients with acute respiratory distress syndrome. Enteral Nutrition in ARDS Study Group. Crit Care Med 1999;27(8):1409–1420.

Guallar E, Hennekens CH, Sacks FM, Willett WC, Stampfer MJ. A prospective study of plasma fish oil levels and incidence of myocardial infarction in U.S. male physicians. J Am Coll Cardiol 1995;25(2):387–394.

Hamazaki TS, Sawazaki S, Itomura M, Asaoka E, Nagao Y, Nishimura N, Yazawa K, Kuwamori T, Kobayashi M. The effect of docosahexaenoic acid on aggression in young adults. J Clin Invest 1996;97(4):1129–1134.

Hawkes JS, Bryan DL, Makrides M, Neumann MA, Gibson RA. A randomized trial of supplementation with docosahexaenoic acid-rich tuna oil and its effects on the human milk cytokines interleukin 1 beta, interleukin 6, and tumor necrosis factor alpha. Am J Clin Nutr 2002;75(4):754–760.

Hederos CA, Berg A. Epogam evening primrose oil treatment in atopic dermatitis and asthma. Arch Dis Child 1996;75(6):494–497.

Henz BM, Jablonska S, van de Kerkhof PC, Stingl G, Blaszczyk M, Vandervalk PG, Veenhuizen R, Muggli R, Raederstorff D. Double-blind, multicentre analysis of the efficacy of borage oil in patients with atopic eczema. Br J Dermatol 1999;140(4):685–688.

Holman RT, Johnson SB, Ogburn PL. Deficiency of essential fatty acids and membrane fluidity during pregnancy and lactation. Proc Natl Acad Sci 1991;88:4835–4839.

Honstra G, van Houwelingen AC, Kivits GA, Fischer S, Uedelhoven W. Influence of dietary fish on eicosanoid metabolism in man. Prostaglandins 1990;40(3):311–329.

Kestin M, Clifton P, Belling GB, Nestel PJ. n-3 fatty acids of marine origin lower systolic blood pressure and triglycerides but raise LDL cholesterol compared with n-3 and n-6 fatty acids from plants. Am J Clin Nutr 1990;51(6):1028–1034.

Kurlandsky LE, Bennink MR, Webb PM, Ulrich PJ, Baer LJ. The absorption and effect of dietary supplementation with omega-3 fatty acids on serum leukotriene B4 in patients with cystic fibrosis. Pediatr Pulmonol 1994;18(4):211–217.

Layne KS, Goh YK, Jumpsen JA, Ryan EA, Chow P, Clandinin MT. Normal subjects consuming physiological levels of 18:3(n-3) and 20:5(n-3) from flaxseed or fish oils have characteristic differences in plasma lipid and lipoprotein fatty acid levels. J Nutr 1996;126(9):2130–2140.

Leaf A, Kang JX, Xiao YF, Billman GE. Dietary n-3 fatty acids in the prevention of cardiac arrhythmias. Curr Opin Clin Nutr Metab Care 1998;1(2):225–228.

Leventhal LJ, Boyce EG, Zurier RB. Treatment of rheumatoid arthritis with gammalinolenic acid. Ann Intern Med 1993;119(9):867–873.

Lund EK, Harvey LJ, Ladha S, Clark DC, Johnson IT. Effects of dietary fish oil supplementation on the phospholipid composition and fluidity of cell membranes from human volunteers. Ann Nutr Metab 1999;43(5):290–300.

Marchioli R, Valagussa F. The results of the GISSI-Prevenzione trial in the general framework of secondary prevention. Eur Heart J 2000;21(12):949–952.

Marckmann P, Gronbaek M. Fish consumption and coronary heart disease mortality. A systematic review of prospective cohort studies. Eur J Clin Nutr 1999;53(8):585–590.

Meydani M. Omega-3 fatty acids alter soluble markers of endothelial function in coronary heart disease patients. Nutr Rev 2000;58(2 pt 1):56–59.

Morris MC, Manson JE, Rosner B, Buring JE, Willett WC, Hennekens CH. Fish consumption and cardiovascular disease in the physicians' health study: a prospective study. Am J Epidemiol 1995;142(2):166–175.

O'Keefe JH Jr, Harris WS. From Inuit to implementation: omega-3 fatty acids come of age. Mayo Clin Proc 2000;75(6):607–614.

Oomen CM, Feskens EJ, Rasanen L, Fidanza F, Nissinen AM, Menotti A, Kok FJ, Kromhout D. Fish consumption and coronary heart disease mortality in Finland, Italy, and the Netherlands. Am J Epidemiol 2000;151(10):999–1006.

Pedersen H, Petersen M, Major-Pedersen A, Jensen T, Nielsen NS, Lauridsen ST, Marckmann P. Influence of fish oil supplementation on in vivo and in vitro oxidation resistance of low-density lipoprotein in type 2 diabetes. Eur J Clin Nutr 2003;57(5):713–720.

Proceedings of the 5th Congress of the International Society for the Study of Fatty Acids and Lipids (ISSFAL). May 7-11, 2002. Montreal, Canada. Lipids 2003;38(4):297–496.

Ramirez-Tortosa C, Lopez-Pedrosa JM, Suarez A, Ros E, Mataix J, Gil A. Olive oil- and fish oil-enriched diets modify plasma lipids and susceptibility of LDL to oxidative modification in free-living male patients with peripheral vascular disease: the Spanish Nutrition Study. Br J Nutr 1999;82(1):31–39.

Rosenstein ED, Kushner LJ, Kramer N, Kazandjian G. Pilot study of dietary fatty acid supplementation in the treatment of adult periodontitis. Prostaglandins Leukot Essent Fatty Acids 2003;68(3):213–218.

Simopoulos AP. Evolutionary aspects of omega-3 fatty acids in the food supply. Prostaglandins Leukot Essent Fatty Acids 1999;60(5–6):421–429.

Singh RB, Niaz MA, Sharma JP, Kumar R, Rastogi V, Moshiri M. Randomized, double-blind, placebo-controlled trial of fish oil and mustard oil in patients with suspected acute myocardial infarction: the Indian experiment of infarct survival--4. Cardiovasc Drugs Ther 1997;11(3):485–491.

Siscovick DS, Raghunathan T, King I, Weinmann S, Bovbjerg VE, Kushi L, Cobb LA, Copass MK, Psaty BM, Lemaitre R, Retzlaff B, Knopp RH. Dietary intake of long-chain n-3 polyunsaturated fatty acids and the risk of primary cardiac arrest. Am J Clin Nutr 2000;71(1 suppl):208S–212S.

Thijs C, Houwelingen A, Poorterman I, Mordant A, van den Brandt P. Essential fatty acids in breast milk of atopic mothers: comparison with non-atopic mothers, and effect of borage oil supplementation. Eur J Clin Nutr 2000;54(3):234–238.

van Gool CJ, Thijs C, Henquet CJ, van Houwelingen AC, Dagnelie PC, Schrander J, Menheere PP, van den Brandt PA. Gamma-linolenic acid supplementation for prophylaxis of atopic dermatitis—a randomized controlled trial in infants at high familial risk. Am J Clin Nutr 2003;77(4):943–951.

Volker D, Fitzgerald P, Major G, Garg M. Efficacy of fish oil concentrate in the treatment of rheumatoid arthritis. J Rheumatol 2000;27(10):2343–2346.

von Schacky C. N-3 fatty acids and the prevention of coronary atherosclerosis. Am J Clin Nutr 2000;71(1 suppl):224S–227S.

Wander RC, Du SH. Oxidation of plasma proteins is not increased after supplementation with eicosapentaenoic and docosahexaenoic acids. Am J Clin Nutr 2000;72(3):731–737.

ADDITIONAL RESOURCES

Appel LJ, Miller ER III, Seidler AJ, Whelton PK. Does supplementation of diet with fish oil reduce blood pressure? A meta-analysis of controlled clinical trials. Arch Intern Med 1993;153:1429–1438.

Bierenbaum ML, Reichstein R, Watkins TR. Reducing atherogenic risk in hyperlipemic humans with flax seed supplementation: a preliminary report. J Am Coll Nutr 1993;12(5):501–504.

Charnock JS. Omega-3 polyunsaturated fatty acids and ventricular fibrillation: the possible involvement of eicosanoids. Prostaglandins Leukot Essent Fatty Acids 1999;61(4):243–247.

Chenoy R, Hussain S, Tayob Y, O'Brien PM, Moss MY, Morse PF. Effect of oral gamolenic acid from evening primrose oil on menopausal flushing. BMJ 1994;308(6927):501–503.

Christensen JH, Christensen MS, Dyerberg J, Schmidt EB. Heart rate variability and fatty acid content of blood cell membranes: a dose-response study with n-3 fatty acids. Am J Clin Nutr 1999;70(3):331–337.

Connor WE. Importance of n-3 fatty acids in health and disease. Am J Clin Nutr 2000;71(1 suppl):171S–175S.

de Deckere EA, Korver O, Verschuren PM, Katan MB. Health aspects of fish and n-3 polyunsaturated fatty acids from plant and marine origin. Eur J Clin Nutr 1998;52(10):749–753.

de Lorgeril M, Renaud S, Mamelle N, Salen P, Martin JL, Monjaud I, Guidollet J, Touboul P, Delaye J. Mediterranean alpha-linolenic acid-rich diet in secondary prevention of coronary heart disease. Lancet 1994;343:1454–1459.

Demke DM, Peters GR, Linet OI, Metzler CM, Klott KA. Effects of a fish oil concentrate in patients with hypercholesterolemia. Atherosclerosis 1988;70(1–2):73–80.

Edwards R, Peet M, Shay J, Horrobin D. Omega-3 polyunsaturated fatty acids in the diet and in the red blood cell membranes of depressed patients. J Affect Disord 1998;48:149–155.

Gibney MJ, Hunter B. The effects of short- and long-term supplementation with fish oil on the incorporation of n-3 polyunsaturated fatty acids into cells of the immune system in healthy volunteers. Eur J Clin Nutr 1993;47(4):255–259.

Goh YK, Jumpsen JA, Ryan EA, Clandinin MT. Effect of omega 3 fatty acid on plasma lipids, cholesterol and lipoprotein fatty acid content in NIDDM patients. Diabetologia 1997;40(1):45–52.

Greenfield SM, Green AT, Teare JP, Jenkins AP, Punchard NA, Ainley CC, Thompson RP. A randomized controlled study of evening primrose oil and fish oil in ulcerative colitis. Aliment Pharmacol Ther 1993;7(2):159–166.

Horrocks LA, Yeo YK. Health benefits of docosahexaenoic acid. Pharmacol Res 1999;40(3):211–225.

Hu FB, Stampfer MJ, Manson JE, Rimm EB, Wolk A, Colditz GA, Hennekens CH, Willett WC. Dietary intake of alpha-linolenic acid and risk of fatal ischemic heart disease among women. Am J Clin Nutr 1999;69(5):890–897.

Hutchins AM, Martini MC, Olson BA, Thomas W, Slavin JL. Flaxseed consumption influences endogenous hormone concentrations in postmenopausal women. Nutr Cancer 2001;39(1):58–65.

Khoo SK, Munro C, Battistutta D. Evening primrose oil and treatment of premenstrual syndrome. Med J Aust 1990;153(4):189–192.

Kremer JM, Lawrence DA, Petrillo GF, Litts LL, Mullaly PM, Rynes RI, Stocker RP, Parhami N, Greenstein NS, Fuchs BR, et al. Effects of high-dose fish oil on rheumatoid arthritis after stopping nonsteroidal anti-inflammatory drugs. Clinical and immune correlates. Arthritis and Rheumatism 1995;38(8):1107–1114.

Lucas EA, Wild RD, Hammond LJ, Khalil DA, Juma S, Daggy BP, Stoecker BJ, Arjmandi BH. Flaxseed improves lipid profile without altering biomarkers of bone metabolism in postmenopausal women. J Clin Endocrinol Metab 2002;87(4):1527–1532.

Miller M. Current perspectives on the management of hypertriglyceridemia. Am Heart J 2000;140(2):232–240.

Oliwiecki S, Burton JL. Evening primrose oil and marine oil in the treatment of psoriasis. Clin Exp Dermatol 1994;19(2):127–129.

Olsen SF, Secher NJ. A possible preventive effect of low-dose fish oil on early delivery and pre-eclampsia: indications from a 50-year-old controlled trial. Br J Nutr 1990;64(3):599–609.

Pullman-Mooar S, Laposata M, Lem D, Holman RT, Leventhal LJ, DeMarco D, Zurier RB. Alteration of the cellular fatty acid profile and the production of eicosanoids in human monocytes by gamma-linolenic acid. Arthritis Rheum 1990;33(10):1526–1533.

Schmidt EB, Dyerberg J. n-3 fatty acids and coronary heart disease—the urgent need of clinical trials. Lipids 1999;34(suppl):S303–S305.

Shapiro JA , Koepsell TD, Voigt LF, Dugowson CE, Kestin M, Nelson JL. Diet and rheumatoid arthritis in women: a possible protective effect of fish consumption. Epidemiology 1996;7(3):256–263.

Simopoulos AP. Essential fatty acids in health and chronic disease. Am J Clin Nutr 1999;70(3 suppl):560S–569S.

Singer P. Effects of dietary oleic, linoleic and alpha-linolenic acids on blood pressure, serum lipids, lipoproteins and the formation of eicosanoid precursors in patients with mild essential hypertension. J Hum Hypertens 1990;4:227–233.

Singleton CB, Walker BD, Campbell TJ. N-3 polyunsaturated fatty acids and cardiac mortality. Aust N Z J Med 2000;30(2):246–251.

Stark KD, Park EJ, Maines VA, Holub BJ. Effect of a fish-oil concentrate on serum lipids in postmenopausal women receiving and not receiving hormone replacement therapy in a placebo-controlled, double-blind trial. Am J Clin Nutr 2000;72(2):389–394.

Stenius-Aarniala B, Aro A, Hakulinen A, Ahola I, Seppala E, Vapaatalo H. Evening primrose oil and fish oil are ineffective as supplementary treatment of bronchial asthma. Ann Allergy 1989;62(6):534–537.

Veale DJ, Torley HI, Richards IM, O'Dowd A, Fitzsimons C, Belch JJ, Sturrock RD. A double-blind placebo controlled trial of Efamol Marine on skin and joint symptoms of psoriatic arthritis. Br J Rheumatol 1994;33(10):954–958.

Whitaker DK, Cilliers J, de Beer C. Evening primrose oil (Epogam) in the treatment of chronic hand dermatitis: disappointing therapeutic results. Dermatology 1996;193(2):115–120.

GARLIC

Overall Rank

★★★★ for blood pressure control
★★★ for cholesterol control

OVERVIEW

Garlic has been used for centuries for its reported benefits in promoting heart health and preventing infection. For more than 5,000 years, humans have been cultivating garlic for use as a spice and a medicine, and records document its medicinal use by Egyptian pharaohs, Chinese emperors, and soldiers from the Middle Ages to World War II; among the latter, garlic juice was known as "Russian penicillin" for its antibiotic effects in wound healing.

Modern-day use of garlic as a dietary supplement generally centers around promotion of heart health by reducing serum lipid levels (total cholesterol, LDL, triglycerides), lowering blood pressure, and inhibiting blood clotting. The cardioprotective benefits associated with garlic are generally attributed to the various sulfur compounds that can be isolated from the raw clove. These compounds, which include alliin, allicin, S-allyl-cysteine, and S-methyl-cysteine, are found in varying concentrations in garlic, chives, leeks, shallots, and onions, but the chemical composition may vary considerably depending on processing methods and are generally highest in garlic compared with other plants in the allium family. The chemical responsible for the pungent smell of garlic, allicin, is produced from alliin (an odorless amino acid derivative) through the action of alliinase and is thought to contribute to many of the health effects associated with garlic supplements.

COMMENTS

A major concern with all garlic supplements is the total level of sulfur-containing compounds or the total allicin potential of commercial products. Raw garlic is more potent than cooked garlic, and fresh garlic is more potent than old garlic. Deodorized and aged garlic supplements typically contain only a fraction of the alliin found in fresh garlic. Because alliin is converted to the active allicin form (the source of garlic's unique odor) in the body, and because the precise mechanism by which garlic helps lower cholesterol is unknown, it is prudent to select a product with high allicin potential. General considerations for dosing are that each milligram of alliin yields approximately 50% of that amount as allicin; thus, 500 mg of a garlic extract standardized to 1% alliin would yield approximately 2,500 µg allicin (compared with a clove of fresh garlic, approximately 4 g, with 1% alliin yielding about 20,000 µg allicin). Owing to differences in strength and preparations of various commercial garlic supplements, consumers should pay attention to the allicin potential of a particular product.

SCIENTIFIC SUPPORT

Garlic is mostly used for its antihyperlipidemic and antihypertensive effects. It also has been reported to possess antibacterial, antiviral, and antifungal effects, but these are generally confined to topical applications. In patients with hyperlipidemia, garlic might lower cholesterol levels by acting as a mild HMG-CoA reductase inhibitor. Garlic is thought to protect vascular endothelial cells from injury by reducing oxidative stress and inhibiting LDL oxidation. Garlic has also been shown to have antithrombotic activity by increasing fibrinolytic activity and decreasing platelet aggregation. For hypertension, garlic is thought to reduce blood pressure by causing smooth cell relaxation and vasodilation by activating production of nitric oxide.

The health benefits of garlic supplements are controversial. Although quite a large number of studies appear to indicate a beneficial cardiovascular effect of garlic supplements, the most well-controlled studies generally suggest a lack of any beneficial effects (Arora et al., 1981; Buck et al., 1979) or suggest benefits only at high doses (Breithaupt-Grogler et al., 1997; Fogarty, 1993). For example, in a study of children with elevated blood cholesterol and triglycerides, 8 weeks of garlic supplementation (900 mg/day) produced no significant effect on total cholesterol, triglycerides, LDL, or HDL (Jepson et al., 2000). It is possible that these children, who had severe cases of familial hyperlipidemia, did not respond to the garlic supplements because their medical conditions were too advanced for treatment with a mild approach such as dietary supplementation. In support of this "noneffect," however, a multicenter study carried out over 12 weeks (also using 900 mg/day) showed no significant lipid or lipoprotein changes following garlic supplementation (Jepson et al., 2000). The FDA has gone so far as to issue a ruling to prohibit claims on dietary supplements promoting a relationship between garlic, decreased serum cholesterol, and the risk in adults of cardiovascular disease.

The lack of effects in the above-mentioned studies may have been the results of the dose used, with 900 mg/day being too low. Larger doses of garlic (4–10 g/day) have been more consistently associated with beneficial effects. For example, in a study of 30 patients with coronary artery disease (Simons et al., 1995), garlic supplements (4 capsules per day equivalent to 4 g of raw garlic) showed a significant reduction in serum cholesterol and triglyceride levels as well as an inhibition of platelet aggregation (reduced blood clotting). Further supporting the cardiovascular benefits in humans is a well-controlled study that compared the effect of aged garlic extract on blood lipids in a group of 41 men with moderately elevated cholesterol levels. Each subject received about 7 g of garlic extract per day over the course of 6 months. The major findings were a reduction in total serum cholesterol of approximately 7%, a drop in LDL of 4–5%, a 5.5% decrease in systolic blood pressure, and a modest reduction of diastolic blood pressure. The study concluded that "dietary supplementation with aged garlic extract has beneficial effects on the lipid profile and blood pressure of moderately hypercholesterolemic subjects," but this dose of garlic would certainly pose numerous practical issues such as compliance (Chutani and Bordia 1981).

SAFETY/DOSAGE

Adverse side effects associated with garlic supplements are rare. Occasionally, mild gastrointestinal symptoms such as heartburn and nausea may occur with high intakes. In some cases, high doses of garlic may potentiate the antithrombotic (blood-thinning) effects of anti-inflammatory medications such as aspirin and dietary supplements such as vitamin E and fish oil. The German Commission E monographs recommend a dose of 4 g/day of fresh garlic to lower blood lipids (Blumenthal et al., 1998). That amount of garlic would be equivalent to approximately 18,000 µg (18 mg) of alliin (9 mg of allicin) and 500 µg of S-allyl-cysteine.

REFERENCES

Arora RC, Arora S, Gupta RK. The long-term use of garlic in ischemic heart disease—an appraisal. Atherosclerosis 1981;40(2):175–179.

Blumenthal M, Busse WR, Goldberg A, Gruenwald J, Hall T, Riggins CW, Rister RS, eds. The Complete German Commission E Monographs. Austin, TX: American Botanical Council, 1998.

Breithaupt-Grogler K, Ling M, Boudoulas H, Belz GG. Protective effect of chronic garlic intake on elastic properties of aorta in the elderly. Circulation 1997;96(8):2649–2655.

Buck C, Simpson H, Willan A. Ischaemic heart-disease and garlic. Lancet 1979;2(8133):104–105.

Chutani SK, Bordia A. The effect of fried versus raw garlic on fibrinolytic activity in man. Atherosclerosis 1981;38(3–4):417–421.

Fogarty M. Garlic's potential role in reducing heart disease. Br J Clin Pract 1993;47(2):64–65.

Jepson RG, Kleijnen J, Leng GC. Garlic for peripheral arterial occlusive disease. Cochrane Database Syst Rev 2000;(2):CD000095.

Simons LA, Balasubramaniam S, von Konigsmark M, Parfitt A, Simons J, Peters W. On the effect of garlic on plasma lipids and lipoproteins in mild hypercholesterolaemia. Atherosclerosis 1995;113(2):219–225.

ADDITIONAL RESOURCES

Randerson K. Cardiology update. Garlic and the healthy heart. Nurs Stand 1993;7(30):51.

HAWTHORN (*CRATAEGUS OXYACANTHA* L.)

Overall Rank

★★★★ for cardiovascular health
★★★★ as an antioxidant
★★★ for high blood pressure
★★★ for arteriosclerosis

OVERVIEW

Hawthorn is an English shrub that has a long history of medicinal use in herbal medicine, including cardiovascular disorders, digestive complaints, dyspnea, and kidney stones. Today, hawthorn is a popular phytomedicine in Europe for use in cardiovascular disorders. With its ability to increase the integrity of the blood vessel walls, hawthorne can improve coronary blood flow and oxygen utilization and possesses positive inotropic activity. The cardiovascular effects of hawthorn are thought to be the result of these activities and primarily the result of the flavonoid group of compounds present in hawthorn. Clinical trials conducted on congestive heart failure (functional class 2) patients have shown good results, including positive implications on changing blood lipids (Rigelsky and Sweet, 2002).

COMMENTS

In Europe, hawthorn is widely used alone as a phytotherapy as well as in combination with digitalis for congestive heart failure. As clinical evidence continues to mount in favor of the use of hawthorn as a cardioprotectant, its popularity in the United States is also increasing.

SCIENTIFIC SUPPORT

Blood Pressure Reduction

Hawthorn extract was tested singly and in combination with magnesium supplements and compared with a placebo for its ability to lower blood pressure. Thirty-six mildly hypertensive people were involved in the study and randomly assigned to undergo a 10-week supplementation regimen of either 600 mg of magnesium, 500 mg of hawthorn extract, a combination of the two, or a placebo. A decline in systolic and diastolic blood pressure was found in all treatment groups, with no differences found among the groups. Factorial contrast analysis in analysis of variance found a reduction in resting diastolic blood pressure at the end of treatment in 19 of the subjects given hawthorn extract, along with a trend in the reduction of anxiety in that group. The authors noted the low dose of hawthorn extract used in the study and thought the results prompted further study for hawthorn (Walker et al., 2002).

Cardiovascular Disease

Pittler et al. (2003) conducted a meta-analysis of studies using hawthorn to treat chronic heart failure. Various database searches were performed, and experts and commercial manufacturers in the field were asked to contribute published and unpublished studies. Inclusion criteria of randomized, double-blind, placebo-controlled studies with hawthorn used alone in therapy resulted in 13 trials. Eight of those trials, which involved 632 patients, met the meta-analysis criteria. Improvement of outcome measures of workload and pressure heart rate were found in the hawthorn groups. Symptoms that showed improvement from hawthorn treatment included dyspnea and fatigue. Infrequent, mild, and transient side effects of nausea, dizziness, and cardiac and gastrointestinal complaints were found. The authors concluded that hawthorn extract proved to be a beneficial adjunct therapy for New York Heart Association (NYHA) class 2 cardiac disease.

Hawthorn extract (standardized extract of the fresh berries of *Crataegus oxyacantha* and *C. monogyna*) was tested in a placebo-controlled, randomized, parallel multicenter clinical study in patients with NYHA class 2 cardiac failure. The 143 participants were given either hawthorn extract (30 drops 3 times daily) or a placebo for 8 weeks. Primary outcome measurements were changes in exercise tolerance (bicycle exercise tolerance testing), and secondarily, blood pressure–heart rate product (BHP). In the hawthorn treatment group, a significant improvement was found, with dyspnea and fatigue not occurring until a significantly higher wattage of bicycle output had been reached. The authors concluded that NYHA class 2 patients undergoing long-term hawthorn therapy could expect improvement in their conditions (Degenring et al., 2003).

Hawthorn extract (Rob 10) was tested on exercise tolerance and quality of life in 88 patients in a placebo-controlled, randomized, double-blind, clinical study. Patients were given 25 drops 3 times daily of the hawthorn extract or placebo for 3 months. Treatment with hawthorn resulted in a significant increase in exercise time, and beneficially affected the quality of life assessment—the assessments of dyspnea. The authors concluded that hawthorn extract was able to be used safely and efficaciously in patients with NYHA class 2 congestive heart failure (Rietbrock et al., 2001).

Hawthorn extract (WS 1442 standardized to 18.72% oligomeric procyanidines) was tested in 40 NYHA class 2 patients in a randomized, placebo-controlled, double-blind, clinical study. Patients were treated with either hawthorn extract (1 capsule 3 times daily) or placebo for 12 weeks. The primary outcome in this study was the effect on exercise tolerance; as a secondary outcome, BHP was calculated. The treatment group produced a borderline significant improvement in exercise tolerance and a significant improvement in BHP. Administration of hawthorn extract was found to be safe, well tolerated, and effective for NYHA class 2 heart failure (Zapfe jun, 2001).

A standardized hawthorn extract (WS 1442) was tested in a multicenter utilization observational study. Hawthorn (Crataegutt novo 450, 1 tablet 2 times daily) was administered to 1,011 patients with NYHA class 2 cardiac insufficiency over 24 weeks. Hawthorn extract administration resulted in a significant improvement in the clinical symptoms of NYHA class 2 heart failure, including reduced exercise tolerance, fatigue, palpitation, and exercise dyspnea. Additionally, ankle edema and nocturia were reduced by 83% in half of the patients with those symptoms before treatment. Overall findings included increased exercise tolerance, reductions in blood pressure and BHP, stabilization in heart rate, improvement in measures of myocardial perfusion, and overall assessments of improvement by the patient and the physician from hawthorn treatment. The authors concluded that hawthorn extract is an efficient, well-tolerated, and easily regulated therapeutic alternative for NYHA class 2 patients (Tauchert et al., 1999).

Leuchtgens (1993) studied hawthorn extract (WS 1442) in NYHA class 2 cardiac insufficiency patients in a placebo-controlled, randomized, double-blind study. Hawthorn (1 capsule 2 times daily) or a placebo was administered for 8 weeks; the BHP and a subjective assessment of improvement were used as primary outcomes, and exercise tolerance, change in heart rate, and arterial blood pressure were used as secondary outcomes. Hawthorn treatment produced a statistically significant improvement in the measures of BHP, subjective assessments of improvement, and heart rate. Both groups produced a mild reduction in systolic and diastolic blood pressure, and no adverse reactions were observed.

SAFETY/DOSAGE

Generally, the recommended dosage level for hawthorn is 160–900 mg of a water-ethanol extract (equivalent to 30–169 mg of epicatechin or 3.5–19.8 mg of flavonoids) 2–3 times daily (Rigelsky and Sweet, 2002).

Side effects of hawthorn are usually mild and transitory but may include a mild rash, headache, sweating, dizziness, palpitations, sleepiness, agitation, and gastrointestinal upset. Drug interactions may occur with other vasodilators, and hawthorn is thought to potentially potentiate or interact with other drugs used for heart failure, hypertension, angina, and arrhythmias (Rigelsky and Sweet, 2002). A randomized, crossover, clinical study to determine the potential interaction with drugs that are P-glycoprotein substrates, such as digoxin, concluded that in the dosages studied (450 mg 2 times daily of an extract of hawthorn leaves and flowers and 0.25 mg of digoxin), the two medications could be coadministered safely (Tankanow et al., 2003).

REFERENCES

Degenring FH, Suter A, Weber M, Saller R. A randomised double blind placebo controlled clinical trial of a standardised extract of fresh crataegus berries (Crataegisan) in the treatment of patients with congestive heart failure NYHA II. Phytomedicine 2003;10(5):363–369.

Leuchtgens H. Crataegus Special Extract WS 1442 in NYHA II heart failure. A placebo controlled randomized double-blind study. Fortschr Med 1993;111(20–21):352–354.

Pittler MH, Schmidt K, Ernst E. Hawthorn extract for treating chronic heart failure: meta-analysis of randomized trials. Am J Med 2003;114(8):665–674.

Rigelsky JM, Sweet BV. Hawthorn: pharmacology and therapeutic uses. Am J Health Syst Pharm 2002;59(5):417–422.

Rietbrock N, Hamel M, Hempel B, Mitrovic V, Schmidt T, Wolf GK. Actions of standardized extracts of crataegus berries on exercise tolerance and quality of life in patients with congestive heart failure. Arzneimittelforschung 2001;51(10):793–798.

Tankanow R, Tamer HR, Streetman DS, Smith SG, Welton JL, Annesley T, Aaronson KD, Bleske BE. Interaction study between digoxin and a preparation of hawthorn (Crataegus oxyacantha). J Clin Pharmacol 2003;43(6):637–642.

Tauchert M, Gildor A, Lipinski J. High-dose crataegus extract WS 1442 in the treatment of NYHA stage II heart failure. Herz 1999;24(6):465–474, discussion 475.

Walker AF, Marakis G, Morris AP, Robinson PA. Promising hypotensive effect of hawthorn extract: a randomized double-blind pilot study of mild, essential hypertension. Phytother Res 2002;16(1):48–54.

Zapfe jun G. Clinical efficacy of crataegus extract WS 1442 in congestive heart failure NYHA class II. Phytomedicine 2001;8(4):262–266.

RED YEAST RICE

Overall Rank

 WARNING: Banned for sale as a dietary supplement in the United States.

★★★★★ for cholesterol control

OVERVIEW

Red yeast rice is a traditional Chinese "spice" used to flavor and color food such as Peking duck. The red yeast (*Monascus purpureus*) is grown on white rice and then fermented, creating the product known as red yeast rice. The yeast is then inactivated and the rice–yeast mixture is powdered. In Traditional Chinese Medicine (TCM), red yeast rice is used for healthy blood and to strengthen the heart; modern dietary supplements use red yeast rice to lower cholesterol levels. In many Asian countries, total daily consumption of red yeast rice from foods ranges from 10–50 g/day, while Western use as a dietary supplement is more in the range of 1–3 g/day.

The modern-day use of red yeast rice as a dietary supplement is for reducing cholesterol levels. Although the FDA has banned the sale of red yeast rice as a dietary supplement (considering it an unapproved drug because of the presence of naturally occurring lovastatin), many products containing red yeast rice remain on the market.

Red yeast rice contains many naturally occurring compounds known as monacolins, which are known to inhibit the activity of an enzyme in the liver (HMG-CoA reductase) that is needed to produce cholesterol. Red yeast rice also contains a mix of sterols (sitosterol, campesterol, and stigmasterol), isoflavones, and unsaturated fatty acids, which are thought to contribute to the cholesterol- and lipid-lowering effects of the monacolins. Of the dozen or so monacolins found in red yeast rice, one of them, monacolin K, is also known as lovastatin and is synthesized and marketed under the brand name Mevacor for reducing elevated cholesterol and triglyceride levels.

Although the precise mechanism of action for red yeast rice is not completely understood, the activity of the monacolins in reducing cholesterol synthesis does not appear to be sufficient to account for the entire effect observed in studies of red yeast rice supplementation. For example, the dose of total monacolins reported in clinical trials of red yeast rice supplementation is 9.6–13.5 mg/day, while the recommended dose of lovastatin is 20 mg, suggesting that the cholesterol-lowering effects of red yeast rice may be owing to the combined actions of monacolins and other constituents, such as sterols and fatty acids (possibly by simultaneously reducing cholesterol synthesis and absorption while promoting cholesterol excretion).

COMMENTS

Historically, red yeast rice was used in China to make rice wine and preserve food. As a medicinal agent, TCM practitioners use red yeast rice to promote blood circulation and as a general aid to heart health. As a dietary supplement, red yeast rice has been promoted as an alternative to cholesterol-lowering medications. In May 1998, however, the FDA declared red yeast rice dietary supplements to be unapproved drugs under the terms of the Federal Food, Drug, and Cosmetic Act; in March 2001, a federal appeals court supported the FDA's position that red yeast rice products should be removed from the market (though many products containing red yeast rice are still on the U.S. market).

As a natural approach to controlling moderately elevated cholesterol levels (between 200–240 mg/dL), red yeast rice supplements appear to be a safe and effective addition to a prudent diet-and-exercise regimen. For people with cholesterol levels well below 200 mg/dL, red yeast rice supplements probably do not justify the cost ($1.00 to $1.50 per day), while patients with cholesterol levels above 240 mg/dL should consult with their personal physicians to discuss the appropriateness of prescription medications for lowering cholesterol levels.

SCIENTIFIC SUPPORT

Red yeast rice contains HMG-CoA reductase inhibitors, primarily lovastatin, and large amounts of unsaturated fatty acids, including monounsaturated fatty acids and diene, triene, tetraene, and pentaene fatty acids. Red yeast rice contains monacolin K (lovastatin, mevinolin), an HMG-CoA reductase inhibitor that may contribute to its cholesterol-lowering effects.

Animal studies (mostly in rabbits) have clearly shown that consumption of red yeast rice reduces total and LDL cholesterol levels by 40–60% and triglyceride levels by 50–60%. The animal studies have also shown that red yeast rice can inhibit the formation of atherosclerotic plaques (Li et al., 1998). Several human studies have also shown the benefits of red yeast rice in reducing elevated cholesterol and correcting dyslipidemia. In one study of subjects with elevated cholesterol levels (average 230 mg/dL), supplementation of 1.2 g of red yeast rice per day (13.5 mg total monacolins) for 8 weeks reduced total cholesterol by 23%, LDL by 31%, and triglycerides by 34%, and elevated HDL by 20% (Keithley et al., 2002). In another study, subjects with elevated cholesterol were given red yeast rice (10–13 mg total monacolins) and showed a 20–36% reduction in cholesterol and triglyceride levels (Heber et al., 1999). One study used a combination of diet (American Heart Association Step 1 Diet) and red yeast rice supplements and found that a 2-month course of the supplements (2.4 g/day containing 9.6 mg total monacolins) reduced total cholesterol by 16%, LDL by 21%, and total triglyceride levels by 25%, while increasing HDL levels by 15% (Rippe et al., 1999). Discontinuation of red yeast rice supplements following the treatment led to a rapid return of serum lipids to prestudy levels despite adherence of the subjects to the American Heart Association Step 1 Diet.

SAFETY/DOSAGE

In both animal and human studies, red yeast rice appears to be quite safe as a dietary supplement. No serious side effects have been reported in human trials, though mild gastrointestinal symptoms are possible. It is important to note that some potentially serious adverse side effects have been noted for prescription statin medications (muscle pain and damage with flulike symptoms). Although such side effects have not been noted in published studies on red yeast rice, some supplement manufacturers err on the side of caution and post warning labels on their products to alert consumers to the possibility. Because of the likely mechanism of action of monacolins in the liver, the recommended amount should not be exceeded (see the next paragraph), nor should red yeast rice be taken by pregnant or lactating women or patients with liver disease.

Doses of 1.2–2.4 g/day of red yeast rice (9.6–13.5 mg of total monacolins) have been used to effectively reduce elevated cholesterol and triglyceride levels in several clinical trials. Because HMG-CoA reductase inhibitors, including the naturally occurring lovastatin and other monocolins found in red yeast rice, may cause liver damage and myopathy, levels of cholesterol (every 4–8 weeks), liver function (every 6 weeks for 3 months and then every 6 months), and creatine phosphokinase (every 8 weeks or in presence of muscle pain or weakness) should be obtained on a routine basis. Also, because of the well-described reduction of CoQ_{10} levels in patients taking HMG-CoA reductase inhibitors (statins), those taking red yeast rice supplements may also benefit from a daily supplement of CoQ_{10}.

REFERENCES

Heber D, Yip I, Ashely JM, Elashoff DA, Elashoff RM, Go VL. Cholesterol-lowering effects of a proprietary Chinese red-yeast-rice dietary supplement. Am J Clin Nutr 1999;69(2):231–236.

Keithley JK, Swanson B, Sha BE, Zeller JM, Kessler HA, Smith KY. A pilot study of the safety and efficacy of cholestin in treating HIV-related dyslipidemia. Nutrition 2002;18:201–204.

Li CL, Zhu Y, Wang Y, et al. Monascus purpureus-fermented rice (red yeast rice): a natural food product that lowers blood cholesterol in animal models of hypercholesterolemia. Nutr Res 1998;18:71–81.

Rippe J, Bonovich K, Colfer H, et al. A multicenter, self-controlled study of cholestin in subjects with elevated cholesterol. Presented at the 39th Annual Conference on Cardiovascular Disease Epidemiology and Prevention. Orlando, FL, March 25, 1999.

ADDITIONAL RESOURCES

Havel R. Dietary supplement or drug? The case of cholestin. Am J Clin Nutr 1999;69:175–176.

Heber D. Dietary supplement or drugs? The case for cholestin. Am J Clin Nutr 1999;70:106–108.

Heber D. Reply to EG Bliznakov. Am J Clin Nutr 2000;71:153–154.

Qin S, Zhang W, Qi P, et al. Elderly patients with primary hyperlipidemia benefited from treatment with a Monascus purpureus rice preparation: a placebo-control, double-blind clinical trial. Presented at the 39th Annual Conference on Cardiovascular Disease Epidemiology and Prevention, Orlando, FL, March 25, 1999.

Wang J, Lu Z, Chi J et al. Multicenter clinical trial of serum lipid-lowering effects of a Monascus purpureus (red yeast) rice preparation from traditional Chinese medicine. Curr Ther Res 1997;58(12):964–978.

Soy

Overall Rank

★★★★★ for cardiovascular disease
★★★★ for menopausal symptoms
★★★ for osteoporosis
★★★ for cancer prevention

OVERVIEW

The term *soy* is used to refer to many products derived from the soybean. In terms of health and wellness, the two most important dietary supplements derived from soybeans are isolated or concentrated soy proteins and soy extracts containing high amounts of compounds called isoflavones. Isoflavones have been associated with many beneficial health effects, ranging from protection from cancer and osteoporosis to a reduction in hot flashes and other symptoms of menopause. Soy protein, which may or may not contain a high level of isoflavones (depending on how it is processed) has been associated with a reduction in serum cholesterol and triglyceride levels and may protect against the development of coronary heart disease. Soy products are generally marketed with claims for their benefits in reducing cholesterol and triglyceride levels, reducing the risk of heart disease, suppressing menopausal symptoms such as hot flashes, and slowing bone breakdown during menopause.

COMMENTS

Depending on the method of processing, many soy foods have a relatively high content of chemical compounds called isoflavones, which possess weak estrogen-like effects and relatively powerful antioxidant properties. Under conditions of high estrogen exposure, which may promote certain cancers, the isoflavone compounds tend to block the adverse effects of estrogen and may prevent the growth of cancer cells. Under conditions of low estrogen exposure, such as during menopause, the isoflavones tend to act as weak estrogens, providing just enough estrogen-like effects to help alleviate some of the symptoms associated with menopause, such as hot flashes, headaches, and mood swings. In terms of heart disease risk, both isoflavones and concentrated soy proteins provide benefits through antioxidant effects (from the isoflavones) and cholesterol lowering (from the soy proteins).

As a high-quality protein source, soy-based protein powders provide an excellent amino acid profile along with the added benefits of heart health, cancer protection, bone maintenance, and in postmenopausal women, relief from menopausal symptoms. For women who cannot or choose not to undergo hormone replacement therapy following menopause, isoflavone supplements may provide an effective alternative to treating some of the symptoms associated with menopause, including hot flashes, night sweats, headaches, vaginal dryness, and mood swings.

SCIENTIFIC SUPPORT

Protein

In general, soybeans, like most legumes, have a high protein content (35–40% for whole soybeans). After processing, protein powders composed of soy concentrate provide about 70% protein, while the even more purified protein source, soy isolate, may contain close to 90% protein. As a protein source, soy tends to be somewhat low in the sulfur-containing amino acids such as cysteine and methionine. This has led to the perception that soy protein is a less desirable source of dietary protein than foods with higher sulfur content, such as meat, milk, and eggs. When the digestibility of the protein is taken into account, however, isolated soy protein scores on a par with egg white and milk proteins, and no differences have been noted in either the increase in muscle strength or the muscle cross-sectional area in men fed protein from beef or soy protein while performing resistance exercise for 12 weeks (Haub et al., 2002). Consumption of soy foods and soy proteins has been associated with beneficial health effects for heart disease, osteoporosis, cancer, and menopausal symptoms. It is still unclear, however, whether these effects stem from the displacement of animal protein with vegetable protein or from the combination of soy protein and the phytonutrients known as isoflavones.

Isoflavones

Soy is the richest dietary source of isoflavones. Typical soy foods like tofu contain approximately 40–100 mg of isoflavones per ounce. Soy milk provides about 100–150 mg of isoflavones per 8-oz glass. The isoflavones function as phytoestrogens in the body, where they possess weak estrogen-like effects. The two primary isoflavones found in soy are daidzein and genistein, both of which have been associated with the health benefits previously mentioned. The chemical structure of isoflavones is similar enough to that of estrogen that they can bind to the estrogen receptor on cells, yet it is different enough that they only perform very weak estrogen-like effects.

Among the various soy-based protein powders on the market, the isoflavone content can vary significantly, from almost zero for products extracted using alcohol to certified levels of 2–5 mg per gram of protein. In many Asian countries, where the incidence of heart disease, cancer, and menopausal symptoms is low, the daily isoflavone intake is estimated at an average of 50–100 mg/day. In contrast, the average Western intake is less than 5 mg/day.

Heart Protection

Results from several studies show the cholesterol-lowering benefits of including soy protein in the diet, and the American Heart Association supports the use of soy protein as a reliable method of reducing serum cholesterol and LDL levels (Jenkins et al., 2003). Reductions of 20–30% in total cholesterol, LDL, triglycerides, and C-reactive protein, with no lowering of HDL cholesterol levels, have been shown with soy protein intakes of 25–50 g/day, typically taken in 2–4 divided doses throughout the day (Jenkins et al., 2003). Cross-sectional studies of typical soy isoflavone intakes have shown positive correlations between total isoflavone intake and HDL cholesterol levels and inverse associations of isoflavones with insulin levels, both of which may be associated with a lower overall risk of coronary vascular disease in postmenopausal women (Goodman-Gruen and Kritz-Silverstein 2001).

Findings from several studies have prompted the FDA to approve a health claim for the prevention of coronary heart disease through a higher consumption of soy protein (permitted on products with at least 6.25 g of soy protein per serving). Such intakes have also been shown to improve arterial elasticity and vasodilatory function and reduce the susceptibility of the LDL particles to become oxidized (Nestel et al., 1997; Steinberg et al., 2003; Wiseman et al., 2000) to a similar degree as hormone replacement therapy in postmenopausal women (Chiechi et al., 2002). In some studies, soy protein added to the diet has reduced cholesterol as significantly as HMG-CoA reductase inhibitors such as lovastatin (Jenkins et al., 2003). Soy protein feeding (30–50 g/day of isolated soy protein) for 4–16 weeks has also been shown to protect blood vessels by reducing plasma total homocysteine levels (Tonstad et al., 2002) and overall exposure to inflammatory cytokines (Jenkins et al., 2002).

Cancer Risk

Epidemiological studies have suggested that Asian diets may provide protection from several cancers, including those of the breast, prostate gland, and colon. As mentioned earlier, the action of isoflavones as weak estrogens allows them to bind to estrogen receptors and block some of the detrimental effects of estrogen, such as promotion of cancer cell growth (Kumar et al., 2002). Tamoxifen, a prescription drug for treating breast cancer, is thought to act as an antiestrogen by binding to the estrogen receptor and "blocking" the growth-promoting effects of estrogen in cancer cells. Women using tamoxifen have a lower incidence of breast cancer and a 30–40% reduction in breast cancer cell growth rate. The isoflavones in soy are chemically similar to tamoxifen and therefore may also reduce the risk of hormone-dependent cancers through the same estrogen-blocking mechanism.

Dietary supplementation with 40 mg/day of isoflavones over a 12-week period resulted in a reduction of serum levels of estradiol and estrone and a lengthening of the menstrual cycle by 3.52 days—effects that may suggest a potential to reduce the risk of breast cancer (Kumar et al., 2002). Studies of the effects of isoflavone supplementation on breast tissue and endometrial epithelial cell proliferation have shown no effects in postmenopausal women at doses of 45 mg/day for 14 days (Hargreaves et al., 1999) or 120 mg/day for 93 days (Duncan et al., 1999), whereas other studies have suggested a stimulation of breast tissue proliferation following 14 days of 45-mg isoflavone supplementation in women with malignant or benign breast disease (McMichael-Phillips et al., 1998).

Bone Health

Soy protein consumption has been shown to reduce bone breakdown and slow calcium loss in animal models of osteoporosis, suggesting a possible beneficial role in preventing osteoporosis in humans. A diet high in soy protein has been shown to improve bone density in perimenopausal and postmenopausal women in both cross-sectional studies (Kritz-Silverstein and Goodman-Gruen, 2002) and after 3–6 months of intervention (Alekel et al., 2000; Anderson et al., 2002; Dalais et al., 1998), but no significant effect on bone density was noted following consumption of soy protein or isolated soy isoflavones (90 mg/day) in normally menstruating young (21–25 years of age) women even after 12 months (Anderson et al., 2002). Healthy men (59 years of age) supplemented with 40 g of soy protein for 3 months showed a higher level of serum insulin–like growth factor 1, which is associated with higher bone mass, although short-term changes in markers of bone formation and resorption did not change (Khalil et al., 2002).

It is also interesting to note that soy protein seems to cause a reduced loss of calcium from the body compared to other dietary sources of protein, which may promote calcium loss and bone breakdown when consumed at high levels. Ipriflavone, a synthetic isoflavone drug prescribed in Europe and available in the United States as a dietary supplement, may be metabolized in the body into daidzein and has potent effects on reducing bone resorption in postmenopausal women.

SAFETY/DOSAGE

Dietary consumption of soy-based protein concentrate or soy isolate is not associated with any significant side effects, aside from the mild gastrointestinal issues (bloating, flatulence) associated with any high-protein diet. High doses of concentrated isoflavone extracts are probably safe at levels up to about 200 mg/day (the maximum estimated amount contained in the average Japanese diet). Since the long-term effects of isolated isoflavone supplements are unknown and the potential for proestrogenic effects may exist for megadose isoflavone consumption, it is prudent to keep total isoflavone intake close to the levels found in dietary amounts.

- As a protein supplement: as needed. Typical protein recommendations are 1–2 g/day of protein per kilogram of body weight.
- For heart health: 25–50 g/day of soy protein isolate is effective in reducing cholesterol and triglyceride levels and in preventing the development of coronary heart disease (FDA-approved health claim).
- For menopausal symptoms: 25–50 mg/day of isoflavones is effective in alleviating some of the symptoms associated with menopause (e.g., hot flashes). Do not exceed more than 200 mg/day.

REFERENCES

Alekel DL, Germain AS, Peterson CT, Hanson KB, Stewart JW, Toda T. Isoflavone-rich soy protein isolate attenuates bone loss in the lumbar spine of perimenopausal women. Am J Clin Nutr 2000;72(3):844–852.

Anderson JJ, Chen X, Boass A, Symons M, Kohlmeier M, Renner JB, Garner SC. Soy isoflavones: no effects on bone mineral content and bone mineral density in healthy, menstruating young adult women after one year. J Am Coll Nutr 2002;21(5):388–393.

Chiechi LM, Secreto G, Vimercati A, Greco P, Venturelli E, Pansini F, Fanelli M, Loizzi P, Selvaggi L. The effects of a soy rich diet on serum lipids: the Menfis randomized trial. Maturitas 2002;41(2):97–104.

Dalais FS, Rice GE, Wahlqvist ML, Grehan M, Murkies AL, Medley G, Ayton R, Strauss BJ. Effects of dietary phytoestrogens in postmenopausal women. Climacteric 1998;1(2):124–129.

Duncan AM, Underhill KE, Xu X, Lavalleur J, Phipps WR, Kurzer MS. Modest hormonal effects of soy isoflavones in postmenopausal women. J Clin Endocrinol Metab 1999;84(10):3479–3484.

Goodman-Gruen D, Kritz-Silverstein D. Usual dietary isoflavone intake is associated with cardiovascular disease risk factors in postmenopausal women. J Nutr 2001;131(4):1202–1206.

Hargreaves DF, Potten CS, Harding C, Shaw LE, Morton MS, Roberts SA, Howell A, Bundred NJ. Two-week dietary soy supplementation has an estrogenic effect on normal premenopausal breast. J Clin Endocrinol Metab 1999;84(11):4017–4024.

Haub MD, Wells AM, Tarnopolsky MA, Campbell WW. Effect of protein source on resistive-training-induced changes in body composition and muscle size in older men. Am J Clin Nutr 2002;76(3):511–517.

Jenkins DJ, Kendall CW, Connelly PW, Jackson CJ, Parker T, Faulkner D, Vidgen E. Effects of high- and low-isoflavone (phytoestrogen) soy foods on inflammatory biomarkers and proinflammatory cytokines in middle-aged men and women. Metabolism 2002;51(7):919–924.

Jenkins DJ, Kendall CW, Marchie A, Faulkner DA, Wong JM, de Souza R, Emam A, Parker TL, Vidgen E, Lapsley KG, Trautwein EA, Josse RG, Leiter LA, Connelly PW. Effects of a dietary portfolio of cholesterol-lowering foods vs lovastatin on serum lipids and C-reactive protein. JAMA 2003;290(4):502–510.

Khalil DA, Lucas EA, Juma S, Smith BJ, Payton ME, Arjmandi BH. Soy protein supplementation increases serum insulin-like growth factor-I in young and old men but does not affect markers of bone metabolism. J Nutr 2002;132(9):2605–2608.

Kritz-Silverstein D, Goodman-Gruen DL. Usual dietary isoflavone intake, bone mineral density, and bone metabolism in postmenopausal women. J Womens Health Gend Based Med 2002;11(1):69–78.

Kumar NB, Cantor A, Allen K, Riccardi D, Cox CE. The specific role of isoflavones on estrogen metabolism in premenopausal women. Cancer 2002;94(4):1166–1174.

McMichael-Phillips DF, Harding C, Morton M, Roberts SA, Howell A, Potten CS, Bundred NJ. Effects of soy-protein supplementation on epithelial proliferation in the histologically normal human breast. Am J Clin Nutr 1998;68(6 suppl):1431S–1435S.

Nestel PJ, Yamashita T, Sasahara T, Pomeroy S, Dart A, Komesaroff P, Owen A, Abbey M. Soy isoflavones improve systemic arterial compliance but not plasma lipids in menopausal and perimenopausal women. Arterioscler Thromb Vasc Biol 1997;17(12):3392–3398.

Steinberg FM, Guthrie NL, Villablanca AC, Kumar K, Murray MJ. Soy protein with isoflavones has favorable effects on endothelial function that are independent of lipid and antioxidant effects in healthy postmenopausal women. Am J Clin Nutr 2003;78(1):123–130.

Tonstad S, Smerud K, Hoie L. A comparison of the effects of 2 doses of soy protein or casein on serum lipids, serum lipoproteins, and plasma total homocysteine in hypercholesterolemic subjects. Am J Clin Nutr 2002;76(1):78–84.

Wiseman H, O'Reilly JD, Adlercreutz H, Mallet AI, Bowey EA, Rowland IR, Sanders TA. Isoflavone phytoestrogens consumed in soy decrease F(2)-isoprostane concentrations and increase resistance of low-density lipoprotein to oxidation in humans. Am J Clin Nutr 2000;72(2):395–400.

ADDITIONAL RESOURCES

Adlercreutz H. Epidemiology of phytoestrogens. Baillieres Clin Endocrinol Metab 1998;12(4):605–623.

Clarkson TB, Anthony MS. Phytoestrogens and coronary heart disease. Baillieres Clin Endocrinol Metab 1998;12(4):589–604.

Dwyer J. Overview: dietary approaches for reducing cardiovascular disease risks. J Nutr 1995;125(3 suppl):656S–665S.

Figtree GA, Griffiths H, Lu YQ, Webb CM, MacLeod K, Collins P. Plant-derived estrogens relax coronary arteries in vitro by a calcium antagonistic mechanism. J Am Coll Cardiol 2000;35(7):1977–1985.

Gooderham MH, Adlercreutz H, Ojala ST, Wahala K, Holub BJ. A soy protein isolate rich in genistein and daidzein and its effects on plasma isoflavones concentrations, platelet aggregation, blood lipids and fatty acid composition of plasma phospholipid in normal men. J Nutr 1996;126(8):2000–2006.

Jacques H, Laurin D, Moorjani S, Steinke FH, Gagne C, Brun D, Lupien PJ. Influence of diets containing cow's milk or soy protein beverage on plasma lipids in children with familial hypercholesterolemia. J Am Coll Nutr 1992;11(suppl):69S–73S.

Knight DC, Eden JA. A review of the clinical effects of phytoestrogens. Obstet Gynecol 1996;87(5 pt 2):897–904.

Krauss RM, Chait A, Stone NJ. Soy protein and serum lipids. N Engl J Med 1995;333(25):1715–1716.

Maskarinec G, Robbins C, Riola B, Kane-Sample L, Franke AA, Murphy S. Three measures show high compliance in a soy intervention among premenopausal women. J Am Diet Assoc 2003;103(7):861–866.

Merz-Demlow BE, Duncan AM, Wangen KE, Xu X, Carr TP, Phipps WR, Kurzer MS. Soy isoflavones improve plasma lipids in normocholesterolemic, premenopausal women. Am J Clin Nutr 2000;71(6):1462–1469.

Messina M. Modern applications for an ancient bean: soybeans and the prevention and treatment of chronic disease. J Nutr 1995;125(3 suppl):567S–569S.

Mitchell JH, Collins AR. Effects of a soy milk supplement on plasma cholesterol levels and oxidative DNA damage in men—a pilot study. Eur J Nutr 1999;38(3):143–148.

Persky VW, Turyk ME, Wang L, Freels S, Chatterton R Jr, Barnes S, Erdman J Jr, Sepkovic DW, Bradlow HL, Potter S. Effect of soy protein on endogenous hormones in postmenopausal women. Am J Clin Nutr 2002;75(1):145–153.

Singh RB, Dubnov G, Niaz MA, Ghosh S, Singh R, Rastogi SS, Manor O, Pella D, Berry EM. Effect of an Indo-Mediterranean diet on progression of coronary artery disease in high risk patients (Indo-Mediterranean Diet Heart Study): a randomised single-blind trial. Lancet 2002;360(9344):1455–1461.

Tham DM, Gardner CD, Haskell WL. Clinical review 97: Potential health benefits of dietary phytoestrogens: a review of the clinical, epidemiological, and mechanistic evidence. J Clin Endocrinol Metab 1998;83(7):2223–2235.

Tikkanen MJ, Adlercreutz H. Dietary soy-derived isoflavone phytoestrogens. Could they have a role in coronary heart disease prevention? Biochem Pharmacol 2000;60(1):1–5.

Wilson TA, Behr SR, Nicolosi RJ. Addition of guar gum and soy protein increases the efficacy of the American Heart Association (AHA) step I cholesterol-lowering diet without reducing high density lipoprotein cholesterol levels in non-human primates. J Nutr 1998;128(9):1429–1433.

Wong WW, Smith EO, Stuff JE, Hachey DL, Heird WC, Pownell HJ. Cholesterol-lowering effect of soy protein in normocholesterolemic and hypercholesterolemic men. Am J Clin Nutr 1998;68(6 suppl):1385S–1389S.

Immune Support Supplements

Astragalus
Cat's Claw (*Uncaria tomentosa*)
Colostrum
Echinacea (*Echinacea angustifolia, E. pallida, E. purpurea*)
Glutamine

Goldenseal (*Hydrastis canadensis*)
Perilla Seed Oil (*Perilla frutescens*)
Shark Cartilage and Bovine Cartilage (Tracheal)
Vitamin A
Zinc

ASTRAGALUS

Overall Rank

★★★ for stimulating the immune system
★★★ for promoting resistance to stress (adaptogenic effect)
★★ for cancer protection

OVERVIEW

Astragalus is an herb used in Traditional Chinese Medicine (TCM) for its immune-enhancing properties, but is also recommended in TCM for "deficiency of chi" (life force), which might include symptoms such as lack of energy and fatigue. Similar to echinacea, astragalus exhibits immune-enhancing effects from the polysaccharides contained in the root. Modern medical practitioners have recently become involved in researching astragalus in reducing the side effects of chemotherapy, treating upper respiratory infections, promoting cardiovascular health, increasing hepatoprotection, and treating male infertility.

COMMENTS

Astragalus has been used as an herbal tonic for centuries in TCM and in Native American folk medicine. As a tonic, astragalus is primarily used throughout the cold and flu season as a "prevention" herb—a different use than the more popular echinacea, which is best used for early-stage cold treatment. Most of what is known about astragalus, however, comes from test-tube and animal experiments, which show that astragalus can help fight bacteria and viruses by enhancing various aspects of the body's normal immune response (enhanced function of specific immune system cells, such as T cells, lymphocytes, and neutrophils). In TCM, astragalus is often combined with other tonic herbs, such as ginseng, cordyceps, or ashwagandha, to keep the immune system "humming" during periods of high stress.

The scientific evidence for the ability of astragalus to enhance the immune system and improve cardiovascular disease and cancer comes from human, animal, and in vitro studies. Some of these studies show significant beneficial results for astragalus, although insufficient and unreliable data exist in the uses for this herb. Unless a patient has an autoimmune disease or is taking immune-suppressant medications, this herb is an option for treatment and/or symptom relief for various conditions.

SCIENTIFIC SUPPORT

The astragalus root is the part that contains the important saponin and polysaccharide constituents. These saponins have diuretic effects as well as anti-inflammatory and antihypertensive activity. Because of the various elements contained in the plant (amino acids, coumarins, flavanoids, isoflavanoids, polysaccharides, and trace minerals), it is unclear which agents provide which activities.

Several chemical constituents of astragalus have been identified as potential active compounds, including saponins, flavonoids, polysaccharides, and glycosides. Astragalus is often combined with other adaptogenic herbs, such as ginseng, and promoted as a guard against various internal and external stressors. The combination of astragalus with echinacea is often seen for protection against common infections of the mucous membranes (cold and flu).

Most of the scientific data on astragalus come from Chinese clinical evidence, in which astragalus appears to stimulate the immune system in patients with infections. At least one clinical trial in the United States has shown astragalus to boost T-cell levels close to normal in some cancer patients, suggesting the possibility of a synergistic effect of astragalus with chemotherapy. In animal studies, astragalus extracts have been shown effective in preventing infection of mice by influenza virus, possibly by increasing the phagocytotic activity of the white blood cells of the immune system.

In several Chinese studies (Duan and Wang, 2002; Zou et al., 2003), cancer patients have responded favorably to astragalus preparations (higher remission rate), probably owing to an inhibition of chemotherapy-induced immune suppression (lesser decrease of white blood cell count and higher IgG and IgM levels). Numerous animal studies have indicated astragalus also possesses broad antioxidant and hepatoprotective effects, likely the result of the presence of various saponin and flavonoid compounds (Chu et al., 1988; Sinclair, 1998; Zhao et al., 1990). As a general supporter of immune system function, astragalus has been studied in rodent models and in humans with a generally beneficial, if modest, effect on maintaining immune system function during chemotherapy and radiotherapy (Cha et al., 1994; Niu et al., 2001).

SAFETY/DOSAGE

When used as recommended, astragalus has no known side effects, but gastrointestinal distress and diarrhea are possible at high intakes. Astragalus is available as a single-ingredient supplement, but it may be even more effective in lower doses (100–200 mg/day) when combined with other immune-stimulating herbs and nutrients. Approximately 500 mg/day is recommended for stimulation of the immune system and to provide resistance to the effects of stress. Divided doses of 250 mg/day of a standardized (for saponins and flavonoids) root extract are preferred. Astragalus should be used with caution in autoimmune disease owing to the herb's immunostimulating properties. Patients should discontinue astragalus prior to surgery because the herb may increase the risk of bleeding.

REFERENCES

Cha RJ, Zeng DW, Chang QS. Non-surgical treatment of small cell lung cancer with chemo-radio-immunotherapy and traditional Chinese medicine. Zhonghua Nei Ke Za Zhi 1994;462–466.

Chu DT, Wong WL, Mavligit GM. Immunotherapy with Chinese medicinal herbs. II. Reversal of cyclophosphamide-induced immune suppression by administration of fractionated Astragalus membranaceus in vivo. J Clin Lab Immunol 1988;25(3):125–129.

Duan P, Wang ZM. Clinical study on effect of astragalus in efficacy enhancing and toxicity reducing of chemotherapy in patients of malignant tumor. Zhongguo Zhong Xi Yi Jie He Za Zhi 2002;22:515–517.

Niu HR, Lai ZH, Yuan L. Observation on effect of supplementary treatments by astragalus injection in treating senile pulmonary tuberculosis patients. Zhongguo Zhong Xi Yi Jie He Za Zhi 2001;21:346–350.

Sinclair S. Chinese herbs: a clinical review of Astragalus, Ligusticum, and Schizandrae. Altern Med Rev 1998;3(5):338–344.

Zhao KS, Mancini C, Doria G. Enhancement of the immune response in mice by Astragalus membranaceus extracts. Immunopharmacology 1990;20(3):225–233.

Zou YH, Liu XM. Effect of astragalus injection combined with chemotherapy on quality of life in patients with advanced non-small cell lung cancer. Zhongguo Zhong Xi Yi Jie He Za Zhi 2003;23(10):733–735.

ADDITIONAL RESOURCES

Chu DT, Lepe-Zuniga J, Wong WL, LaPushin R, Mavligit GM. Fractionated extract of Astragalus membranaceus, a Chinese medicinal herb, potentiates LAK cell cytotoxicity generated by a low dose of recombinant interleukin-2. J Clin Lab Immunol 1988;26(4):183–187.

Li SQ, Yuan RX, Gao H. Clinical observation on the treatment of ischemic heart disease with astragalus membranaceus. Zhongguo Zhong Xi Yi Jie He Za Zhi 1995;15:77–80.

Liu ZG, Xiong ZM, Yu XY. Effect of astragalus injection on immune function in patients with congestive heart failure. Zhongguo Zhong Xi Yi Jie He Za Zhi 2003;23:351–353.

Luo HM, Dai RH, Li Y. Nuclear cardiology study on effective ingredients of Astragalus membranaceus in treating heart failure. Zhongguo Zhong Xi Yi Jie He Za Zhi 1995;15:707–709.

Rittenhouse JR, Lui PD, Lau BH. Chinese medicinal herbs reverse macrophage suppression induced by urological tumors. J Urol 1991;146(2):486–490.

Sun Y, Hersh EM, Talpaz M, Lee SL, Wong W, Loo TL, Mavligit GM. Immune restoration and/or augmentation of local graft versus host reaction by traditional Chinese medicinal herbs. Cancer 1983;52(1):70–73.

Zhang JG, Gao DS, Wei GH. Clinical study on effect of Astragalus injection on left ventricular remodeling and left ventricular function in patients with acute myocardial infarction. Zhongguo Zhong Xi Yi Jie He Za Zhi 2002;22:346–348.

Zhang ZL, Wen QZ, Liu CX. Hepatoprotective effects of astragalus root. J Ethnopharmacol 1990;30:146–149.

Zhou ZL, Yu P, Lin D. Study on effect of astragalus injection in treating congestive heart failure. Zhongguo Zhong Xi Yi Jie He Za Zhi 2001;21:747–749.

CAT'S CLAW (*UNCARIA TOMENTOSA*)

Overall Rank

★★★★ for immune modulation
★★★ as an anti-inflammatory
★★★ for treating infections
★★★ for osteoarthritis
★★ as an antioxidant
★★ for cancer treatment

OVERVIEW

Although cat's claw (or *uña de gato*) is generally thought of as only coming from the rainforests of Peru, it is also found in the rainforests of surrounding countries such as Brazil and Bolivia. It has a number of traditional medicine uses, along with current uses such as immune system stimulation and modulation. It is known to possess antioxidant and anti-inflammatory activities and has been used for illnesses such as cancer, AIDS, colds and flu, yeast infections, intestinal and gastric ulcers, osteoarthritis, and rheumatoid arthritis.

COMMENTS

A lively debate exists about which chemotype or species (containing either pentacyclic or tetracyclic oxindole alkaloids) of cat's claw is the "best." A preclinical study by Sandoval et al. (2002) using in vitro methods concluded that although both species show antioxidant and anti-inflammatory effects, the presence of oxindole or pentacyclic alkaloids did not influence these activities. The authors further concluded that *Uncaria guianensis* is more potent than *Uncaria tomentosa* in these activities. Saventaro (manufactured by an Austrian company, Immodal Pharmaka) is the brand name of a cat's claw extract that contains the pentacyclic oxindole alkaloids (POAs).

Another debate centers on which part of the plant is the most efficacious. Although many references have been made to the traditional use of the root bark, the stem bark is more popular today, mostly because of its availability and higher sustainability of harvest.

Animal studies on a proprietary extract of cat's claw called C-Med 100 have found that it has the ability to increase spleen cell numbers dose dependently; the effect was not caused by an increasing proliferation rate but rather by the cells' survival rate. Thus, the authors noted the possible use of this extract for patients with leukopenia (Akesson et al., 2003).

SCIENTIFIC SUPPORT

Rheumatoid Arthritis

An extract of the pentacyclic chemotype of *U. tomentosa* was studied in 40 rheumatoid arthritis patients (also taking sulfasalazine or hydroxychloroquine) for its safety and efficacy. The study design was a 52-week two-phase study, with the first phase consisting of 24 weeks of double-blind, placebo-controlled study and the second phase consisting of 28 weeks with all patients taking the cat's claw treatment. In the first phase of the study, the treatment group showed a statistically significant reduction in the number of painful joints compared with the placebo group. In the second phase, treatment resulted in a reduction in the number of painful and swollen joints and in the Ritchie Index compared with the posttreatment values. Minor side effects were observed, and the treatment was concluded to be relatively safe and of modest benefit (Mur et al., 2002).

Osteoarthritis

Cat's claw was studied for its effect in patients with osteoarthritis of the knee, its safety, and its in vitro antioxidant and anti-inflammatory actions. In 45 patients with osteoarthritis of the knee, freeze-dried *U. guianensis* was given to 30 patients and placebo to 15, and hematological parameters were studied. No negative effects were found on the blood or liver, and no side effects were experienced compared with placebo. Symptoms that were significantly reduced by treatment were pain associated with activity and medical and patient assessment scores. No changes were found in knee pain at rest or at night and in knee circumference. In vitro studies of antioxidant (using the DPPH free-radical scavenging method) and anti-inflammatory (measuring tumor necrosis factor α [TNF-α] and prostaglandin E2 [PGE2] production) activity showed both species to be equally efficacious. Because of the dosages studied, it was hypothesized that anti-inflammatory activity may result from the ability to inhibit TNF-α rather than PGE2 (Piscoya et al., 2001).

The proprietary cat's claw extract called C-MED 100 (manufactured by CampaMed) was studied for its ability to affect the response to 23 valent pneumococcal vaccine. C-MED 100 had been found in earlier preclinical studies to produce immune-stimulating and anti-inflammatory effects. C-MED 100 was concluded to enhance the immune response through observed lymphocyte/neutrophil ratios of peripheral blood and the reduction of decline in antibody titer responses to the pneumococcal vaccination at 5 months. No negative side effects were found either through medical examination, clinical chemistry, or blood cell analysis (Lamm et al., 2001).

Anticancer

In a preliminary study, a decoction of *U. tomentosa* bark was given to a smoker for 15 days and found to decrease the mutagenicity induced by *Salmonella typhimurium* TA98 and TA100 through urine analysis. Fractions of the plant extract were tested in vitro and found to have no mutagenic effect in strains of *S. typhimurium* but rather to protect against the photomutagenic effects of 8-mehoxy-psoralen and UV-A. The study confirmed earlier reports of the antimutagenic activity of cat's claw but not of its purported mutagenic effects (Rizzi et al., 1993).

SAFETY/DOSAGE

Generally, dosages range from 20–60 mg/day for a week and then 20 mg/day as a maintenance dose. Saventaro is standardized to contain a minimum of 260 µg POAs in every 20-mg dose. C-MED-100 is manufactured to eliminate the indole alkaloids (< 0.05%) and other high-molecular-weight compounds such as tannins and to contain 8% or more carboxyl alkyl esters. The recommended dose of this product is 350 mg/day (McKenna et al., 2002).

Cat's claw is generally regarded as safe, but its use is not recommended during pregnancy or lactation because it has not been fully evaluated. Initial and temporary gastrointestinal side effects are sometimes experienced, such as gas, bloating, nausea, and diarrhea.

REFERENCES

Akesson C, Pero RW, Ivars F. C-Med 100, a hot water extract of Uncaria tomentosa, prolongs lymphocyte survival in vivo. Phytomedicine 2003;10(1):23–33.

Lamm S, Sheng Y, Pero RW. Persistent response to pneumococcal vaccine in individuals supplemented with a novel water soluble extract of Uncaria tomentosa, C-Med-100. Phytomedicine 2001;8(4):267–274.

McKenna D, Jones K, Hughes K, Humphrey S. Botanical Medicines: The Desk Reference for Major Herbal Supplements. 2nd Ed. Binghamton, NY: Haworth Press, 2002.

Mur E, Hartig F, Eibl G, Schirmer M. Randomized double blind trial of an extract from the pentacyclic alkaloid-chemotype of Uncaria tomentosa for the treatment of rheumatoid arthritis. J Rheumatol 2002;29(4):678–681.

Piscoya J, Rodriguez Z, Bustamante SA, Okuhama NN, Miller MJ, Sandoval M. Efficacy and safety of freeze-dried cat's claw in osteoarthritis of the knee: mechanisms of action of the species Uncaria guianensis. Inflamm Res 2001;50(9):442–448.

Rizzi R, Re F, Bianchi A, De Feo V, de Simone F, Bianchi L, Stivala LA. Mutagenic and antimutagenic activities of Uncaria tomentosa and its extracts. J Ethnopharmacol 1993;38(1):63–77.

Sandoval M, Okuhama NN, Zhang XJ, Condezo LA, Lao J, Angeles' FM, Musah RA, Bobrowski P, Miller MJ. Anti-inflammatory and antioxidant activities of cat's claw (Uncaria tomentosa and Uncaria guianensis) are independent of their alkaloid content. Phytomedicine 2002;9(4):325–337.

COLOSTRUM

Overall Rank

★★★★ for boosting gastrointestinal immunity
★★★ for boosting systemic immune function

OVERVIEW

Colostrum is the clear or cloudy "premilk" that female mammals secrete after giving birth and before producing milk. Colostrum for dietary supplements is usually derived from bovine sources and contains various immunoglobulins (also called antibodies) and antimicrobial factors (i.e., lactoferrin, lactoperoxidase, lysozyme) as well as insulin-like growth factors such as IGF-I and IGF-II. The concentration of IGF-I in bovine colostrum is 200–2,000 μg/L, whereas normal milk contains less than 10 μg/L. In normal, healthy adults, IGF-I occurs at a concentration of approximately 200 μg/L in serum. In terms of immunoglobulins, colostrum generally provides concentrations of IgG, IgM, and IgA that are 100-fold higher than in normal milk. The most prevalent claims for dietary supplements containing colostrum are in the area of generalized immune function as well as the specific areas of diarrhea prevention and treatment, overall gastrointestinal support, and improved recovery from intense exercise.

COMMENTS

The amino acid sequences of human and bovine IGF-I are identical. The increase in serum IGF-I observed in several human studies is most likely a result of an enhanced stimulation of endogenous IGF-I synthesis rather than a direct absorption of the growth factor from the adult gastrointestinal tract. It is likely that the natural target of colostrum-derived growth factors is the gastrointestinal tract, whereby the increased growth and turnover of the intestine provides for a healthier gut and an increased uptake of dietary components that may enhance growth, immune competence, and athletic performance generally.

SCIENTIFIC SUPPORT

Bovine colostrum contains the same disease-resistance factors (immuno-globins) found in human breast milk and unpasteurized cow's milk. Among the many immune factors that may be effective against various viruses, bacteria, yeast, and other invaders are immunoglobins (IgA, IgG, IgM), lactoferrin, lactalbumin, glycoproteins, cytokines (such as interleukin 1, interleukin 6, and interferon Y) and various polypeptides, growth factors, vitamins, and minerals. The antibodies present in colostrum are thought to combine with disease-causing microorganisms in the gastrointestinal tract. By adhering to pathogens, colostrum antibodies may be able to reduce the adhesive properties of bacteria and decrease their ability to attach to the intestinal wall (which could prevent their entrance into the body). It is unlikely that the "full" antimicrobial benefits of colostrum can be realized unless the user happens to be a baby cow, because the immunoglobulins are largely digested in the adult gut and cannot be absorbed intact (Mero et al., 2002). It may be possible, however, for partially digested immunoglobulin fragments to retain a small portion of their functional properties and deliver these immune benefits on absorption.

Numerous studies have been conducted in adults and children to show the benefits of ingesting colostrum in neutralizing the activity of several strains of bacteria and parasites that cause diarrhea (Ashraf et al., 2001; Bolke et al., 2002; Huppertz et al., 1999; Mitra et al., 1995; Nord et al., 1990; Okhuysen et al., 1998; Plettenberg et al., 1993; Rump et al., 1992; Sarker et al., 2001; Tacket et al., 1988; Tawfeek et al., 2003). Both the prophylactic and treatment effects of colostrum feeding against bacterial and parasitic infections of the gastrointestinal tract may be the result of the direct antimicrobial effects of colostrum-derived immune factors and/or a generalized stabilization of gut barrier function (Bolke et al., 2002; Playford et al., 2001). In studies of chronic gastritis, symptoms were improved and inflammation was reduced, but there was no evidence that colostrum was directly effective against *Helicobacter pylori* (the bacteria that causes stomach ulcers).

In terms of sports performance, several studies have investigated athletes who consumed colostrum (up to 60 g/day) compared with a placebo or whey protein. These studies found variable effects on IGF-I levels. In terms of overall athletic performance and exercise recovery, they found no differences in plasma IGF-1 concentrations in either group during the study period but they did find that the colostrum group ran further and did more work than the placebo group (equal to a 2% increase in performance; Antonio et al., 2001; Brinkworth et al., 2002; Buckley et al., 2002, 2003; Coombes et al., 2002; Hofman et al., 2002). One study examined rowing performance in a group of elite female rowers. Eight rowers completed a 9-week training program while consuming either colostrum (60 g/day) or whey protein. By week 9, rowers consuming colostrum had greater increases in the distance covered and work done compared to the whey protein group (Brinkworth et al., 2002).

Additional studies on bovine colostrum consumption suggest that it can also deliver some generalized anti-inflammatory benefits (Bolke et al., 2002; Playford et al., 2001) and help prevent and treat the gastric injury associated with nonsteroidal anti-inflammatory drugs. Such effects may also be of value for the treatment of ulcerative conditions of the bowel, such as colitis and irritable bowel syndrome (Khan et al., 2002).

Taken together, the available evidence for bovine colostrum is supportive of its benefits as an effective immune-supporting supplement, particularly when interactions with pathogens in the intestinal tract are possible. It is unlikely, however, that colostrum would provide immune benefits against airborne pathogens and upper respiratory tract infections such as cold and influenza or against pollen-related allergic responses (Leiferman et al., 1975).

SAFETY/DOSAGE

No adverse side effects are expected up to doses of 60 g/day, but people with milk allergies should avoid bovine colostrum. Doses of 10 g and up have been used in most human studies; it is unknown if lower doses provide any meaningful immune or gastrointestinal benefits. Many capsule-form products provide no more than 1 g of colostrum per serving, but powder forms may deliver levels associated with clinical effectiveness (10 g and higher).

REFERENCES

Antonio J, Sanders MS, Van Gammeren D. The effects of bovine colostrum supplementation on body composition and exercise performance in active men and women. Nutrition 2001;17(3):243–247.

Ashraf H, Mahalanabis D, Mitra AK, Tzipori S, Fuchs GJ. Hyperimmune bovine colostrum in the treatment of shigellosis in children: a double-blind, randomized, controlled trial. Acta Paediatr 2001;90(12):1373–1378.

Bolke E, Jehle PM, Hausmann F, Daubler A, Wiedeck H, Steinbach G, Storck M, Orth K. Preoperative oral application of immunoglobulin-enriched colostrum milk and mediator response during abdominal surgery. Shock 2002;17(1):9–12.

Brinkworth GD, Buckley JD, Bourdon PC, Gulbin JP, David A. Oral bovine colostrum supplementation enhances buffer capacity but not rowing performance in elite female rowers. Int J Sport Nutr Exerc Metab 2002;12(3):349–365.

Buckley JD, Abbott MJ, Brinkworth GD, Whyte PB. Bovine colostrum supplementation during endurance running training improves recovery, but not performance. J Sci Med Sport 2002;5(2):65–79.

Buckley JD, Brinkworth GD, Abbott MJ. Effect of bovine colostrum on anaerobic exercise performance and plasma insulin-like growth factor I. J Sports Sci 2003;21(7):577–588.

Coombes JS, Conacher M, Austen SK, Marshall PA. Dose effects of oral bovine colostrum on physical work capacity in cyclists. Med Sci Sports Exerc 2002;34(7):1184–1188.

Hofman Z, Smeets R, Verlaan G, Lugt R, Verstappen PA. The effect of bovine colostrum supplementation on exercise performance in elite field hockey players. Int J Sport Nutr Exerc Metab 2002;12(4):461–469.

Huppertz HI, Rutkowski S, Busch DH, Eisebit R, Lissner R, Karch H. Bovine colostrum ameliorates diarrhea in infection with diarrheagenic Escherichia coli, shiga toxin-producing E. coli, and E. coli expressing intimin and hemolysin. J Pediatr Gastroenterol Nutr 1999;29(4):452–456.

Khan Z, Macdonald C, Wicks AC, Holt MP, Floyd D, Ghosh S, Wright NA, Playford RJ. Use of the "nutriceutical", bovine colostrum, for the treatment of distal colitis: results from an initial study. Aliment Pharmacol Ther 2002;16(11):1917–1922.

Leiferman KM, Yunginger JW, Larson JB, Gleich GJ. The effect of immune milk as a treatment for ragweed pollinosis. Ann Allergy 1975;35(6):367–371.

Mero A, Kahkonen J, Nykanen T, Parviainen T, Jokinen I, Takala T, Nikula T, Rasi S, Leppaluoto J. IGF-I, IgA, and IgG responses to bovine colostrum supplementation during training. J Appl Physiol 2002;93(2):732–739.

Mitra AK, Mahalanabis D, Ashraf H, Unicomb L, Eeckels R, Tzipori S. Hyperimmune cow colostrum reduces diarrhoea due to rotavirus: a double-blind, controlled clinical trial. Acta Paediatr 1995;84(9):996–1001.

Nord J, Ma P, DiJohn D, Tzipori S, Tacket CO. Treatment with bovine hyperimmune colostrum of cryptosporidial diarrhea in AIDS patients. AIDS 1990;4(6):581–584.

Okhuysen PC, Chappell CL, Crabb J, Valdez LM, Douglass ET, DuPont HL. Prophylactic effect of bovine anti-Cryptosporidium hyperimmune colostrum immunoglobulin in healthy volunteers challenged with Cryptosporidium parvum. Clin Infect Dis 1998;26(6):1324–1329.

Playford RJ, MacDonald CE, Calnan DP, Floyd DN, Podas T, Johnson W, Wicks AC, Bashir O, Marchbank T. Co-administration of the health food supplement, bovine colostrum, reduces the acute non-steroidal anti-inflammatory drug-induced increase in intestinal permeability. Clin Sci (Lond) 2001;100(6):627–633.

Plettenberg A, Stoehr A, Stellbrink HJ, Albrecht H, Meigel W. A preparation from bovine colostrum in the treatment of HIV-positive patients with chronic diarrhea. Clin Investig 1993;71(1):42–45.

Rump JA, Arndt R, Arnold A, Bendick C, Dichtelmuller H, Franke M, Helm EB, Jager H, Kampmann B, Kolb P, et al. Treatment of diarrhoea in human immunodeficiency virus-infected patients with immunoglobulins from bovine colostrum. Clin Investig 1992;70(7):588–594.

Sarker SA, Casswall TH, Juneja LR, Hoq E, Hossain I, Fuchs GJ, Hammarstrom L. Randomized, placebo-controlled, clinical trial of hyperimmunized chicken egg yolk immunoglobulin in children with rotavirus diarrhea. J Pediatr Gastroenterol Nutr 2001;32(1):19–25.

Tacket CO, Losonsky G, Link H, Hoang Y, Guesry P, Hilpert H, Levine MM. Protection by milk immunoglobulin concentrate against oral challenge with enterotoxigenic Escherichia coli. N Engl J Med 1988;318(19):1240–1243.

Tawfeek HI, Najim NH, Al-Mashikhi S. Efficacy of an infant formula containing anti-Escherichia coli colostral antibodies from hyperimmunized cows in preventing diarrhea in infants and children: a field trial. Int J Infect Dis 2003;7(2):120–128.

ADDITIONAL RESOURCES

Casswall TH, Sarker SA, Albert MJ, Fuchs GJ, Bergstrom M, Bjorck L, Hammarstrom L. Treatment of Helicobacter pylori infection in infants in rural Bangladesh with oral immunoglobulins from hyperimmune bovine colostrum. Aliment Pharmacol Ther 1998;12(6):563–568.

Davidson GP, Whyte PB, Daniels E, Franklin K, Nunan H, McCloud PI, Moore AG, Moore DJ. Passive immunisation of children with bovine colostrum containing antibodies to human rotavirus. Lancet 1989;2(8665):709–712.

Ebina T, Sato A, Umezu K, Ishida N, Ohyama A, Oizumi A, Aikawa K, Katagiri S, Katsushima N, Imai A, et al. Prevention of rotavirus infection by oral administration of cow colostrum containing antihumanrotavirus antibody. Med Microbiol Immunol (Berl) 1985;174(4):177–185.

Greenberg PD, Cello JP. Treatment of severe diarrhea caused by Cryptosporidium parvum with oral bovine immunoglobulins concentrate in patients with AIDS. J Acquir Immune Defic Syndr Hum Retrovirol 1996;13:348–354.

He F, Tuomola E, Arvilommi H, Salminen S. Modulation of human humoral immune response through orally administered bovine colostrum. FEMS Immunol Med Microbiol 2001;31(2):93–96.

McClead RE Jr, Butler T, Rabbani GH. Orally administered bovine colostral anti-cholera toxin antibodies: results of two clinical trials. Am J Med 1988;85(6):811–816.

Mero A, Miikkulainen H, Riski J, Pakkanen R, Aalto J, Takala T. Effects of bovine colostrum supplementation on serum IGF-I, IgG, hormone, and saliva IgA during training. J Appl Physiol 1997;83(4):1144–1151.

Playford RJ, Floyd DN, Macdonald CE, Calnan DP, Adenekan RO, Johnson W, Goodlad RA, Marchbank T. Bovine colostrum is a health food supplement which prevents NSAID induced gut damage. Gut 1999;44(5):653–658.

Sarker SA, Casswall TH, Mahalanabis D, Alam NH, Albert MJ, Brussow H, Fuchs GJ, Hammerstrom L. Successful treatment of rotavirus diarrhea in children with immunoglobulin from immunized bovine colostrum. Pediatr Infect Dis J 1998;17(12):1149–1154.

Tacket CO, Binion SB, Bostwick E, Losonsky G, Roy MJ, Edelman R. Efficacy of bovine milk immunoglobulins concentrate in preventing illness after Shigella flexneri challenge. Amer J Trop Med Hyg 1992;47(3):276–283.

Takahashi N, Eisenhuth G, Lee I, Schachtele C, Laible N, Binion S. Nonspecific antibacterial factors in milk from cows immunized with human oral bacterial pathogens. J Dairy Sci 1992;75(7):1810–1820.

Warny M, Fatimi A, Bostwick EF, Laine DC, Lebel F, LaMont JT, Pothoulakis C, Kelly CP. Bovine immunoglobulin concentrate-clostridium difficile retains C difficile toxin neutralising activity after passage through the human stomach and small intestine. Gut 1999;44(2):212–217.

ECHINACEA (*ECHINACEA ANGUSTIFOLIA, E. PALLIDA, E. PURPUREA*)

Overall Rank

★★★★★ for prophylaxis and treatment of cold and flu symptoms
★★★★★ to increase resistance to colds, influenza, and other infections (oral formulations)
★★★ for wounds and inflammatory skin conditions (topical formulations)
★★★ for vaginal candidiasis
★★ for urinary tract infections
★★ for genital herpes (herpes simplex virus types 1 and 2)
★★ as an antimicrobial

OVERVIEW

Echinacea is native to the United States and a small region of southern Canada. Although there are nine species of echinacea (*Echinacea angustifolia, E. dicksoni, E. dubia, E. gloruisa, E. pallida, E. paradoxa, E. purpurea, E. simulate,* and *E. angustifolia*), only three are normally harvested for medicinal purposes (*E. angustifolia, E. pallida,* and *E. purpurea*). Echinacea was originally used in North America by Native Americans for therapeutic uses such as blood purification and treatment of snake bites, infections, and malignancy. In the late 1800s, a Nebraska physician, H. C. F. Meyer, learned of the plant being used by Native Americans and proposed its uses to a pharmaceutical manufacturer, Lloyd Brothers of Cincinnati. The physician expounded on the uses of echinacea, proposing that it could be used for rheumatism, streptococcal erysipelas, stomach upset, migraines, pain, sores, wounds, eczema, sore eyes, snake bites, gangrene, typhoid, diphtheria, rabies, hemorrhoids, dizziness, herbal poisoning, tumors, syphilis, malaria, and bee stings. At that time, it began to be marketed as an anti-infective (Blumenthal et al., 2000; Cupp, 2000; Rotblatt and Ziment, 2002).

Today, echinacea is mostly used as an immune modulator to help the body fight or prevent infections, such as the common cold, flu, and chronic infections like upper respiratory and lower urinary tract infections. In addition, a few studies have supported its use for chronic candidiasis. The active components of echinacea are phenolic compounds, terpenoid compounds, nitrogenous compounds like alkylamides and alkaloids, and carbohydrates like polysaccharides. Polysaccharide components have been proven to activate macrophages (stimulation of phagocytosis), increase leukocyte mobility, and increase cellular respiration that may lead to the attack of tumor cells (increased tumor necrosis factor) and microorganisms (Blumenthal et al., 2000; Cupp, 2000; Rotblatt and Ziment, 2002).

COMMENTS

Echinacea is a good example of an herb that proves there is no such thing as a generic herbal medicine. The quality of echinacea in studies has definitely had some influence on the confounding results of studies. Because echinacea comes in several pharmacologically important compounds, researchers should be careful to characterize the nature of their preparation. Likewise, consumers and health care professionals should be aware of the potential of buying a poor-quality product.

SCIENTIFIC SUPPORT

Common Cold and Flu

A randomized, double-blind, placebo-controlled study examined the efficacy of a standardized preparation of *E. purpurea* (100 mg of freeze-dried pressed juice from the aerial portion of the plant administered 3 times daily) on the severity and duration of the common cold. Of the 180 patients enrolled and given the active or placebo treatment, no statistical differences were found between groups in the total symptom scores or mean individual scores, nor was there a difference noted in the times to resolution of symptoms (Yale and Liu, 2004).

In another randomized, double-blind, placebo-controlled study, echinacea was again studied to elucidate its effects on the common cold. The authors theorized that much of the inconclusive nature of the studies to date resulted from the utilization of poorly standardized products devoid of active components. Therefore, they used a preparation (Echinilin) that was standardized to alkylamides (0.25 mg/mL), cichoric acid (2.5 mg/mL), and polysaccharides (25 mg/mL). The 282 healthy subjects were given either echinacea or a placebo to take at the onset of the first symptom related to a cold, consuming 10 doses on day 1 and 4 doses on the subsequent 7 days. The total daily symptom scores were 23.1% lower in the echinacea group than in the placebo, and the response rate was greater in the echinacea group throughout the study (Goel et al., 2004).

A randomized, double-blind, placebo-controlled, community-based trial was conducted to determine the efficacy of dried, encapsulated, whole-plant echinacea as early treatment for the common cold. The study concluded that compared with placebo, unrefined echinacea provided no detectable benefit or harm for participants who had the common cold. The study was designed with a power of 80% requiring 150 participants; 148 participants were enrolled (Barrett et al., 2002).

Researchers used a randomized, double-blind, placebo-controlled study to determine the efficacy of an echinacea compound herbal tea preparation given at early onset of cold or flu symptoms. The study concluded that treatment with the echinacea herbal tea was effective for relieving symptoms in a shorter time than the placebo. The placebo used was a different herbal tea that was marketed to promote healthy digestion and should not have improved or worsened the common cold or flu symptoms (Lindenmuth and Lindenmuth, 2000).

Researchers of an another randomized, placebo-controlled, double-blind study wanted to determine the effect of fluid extract (Madaus AG, 4 mL twice daily for 8 weeks) of E. purpurea on the incidence and severity of colds and respiratory infections. The study concluded that treatment with fluid extract of E. purpurea did not significantly decrease the incidence, duration, or severity of colds and respiratory infections compared with a placebo when tested in 109 participants (Grimm and Muller, 1999).

Four types of echinacea preparations were studied in 246 people who easily caught colds. The treatment groups were given (1) an E. purpurea crude extract consisting of 5% root and 95% above-ground parts (Echinaforce, 6.78 mg/tablet, 2 tablets 3 times daily); (2) the same extract at a higher dosage (48.27 mg/tablet, 2 tablets 3 times daily); (3) an unspecified crude extract of the root (E. purpurea, 29.60 mg/tablet, 2 tablets 3 times daily); or (4) a placebo. The participants were instructed to start taking their medications as soon as they felt a cold coming on until it was finished (not to exceed 7 days). The placebo and treatment 3 produced similar results, whereas treatments 1 and 2 produced an improvement of cold symptoms by 62.7% and 64.0%, respectively. The physicians found echinacea preparations to be 70% effective, and the patients judged them to be 80% effective. The authors concluded that echinacea is an effective and low-risk alternative for treating the symptoms of the common cold (Brinkeborn et al., 1999).

The expressed juice of the aerial parts of E. purpurea (Echinagard) was examined in a placebo-controlled study of 120 patients who presented with the first signs of the common cold. There was a highly significant decrease in the median time required before the patients improved in the treatment group versus placebo (zero versus 5 days); in patients determined to have developed "real colds," the difference between the treatment and placebo groups was 4 days versus 8 days, respectively (Hoheisel et al., 1997).

An herbal formulation containing *E. purpurea* root extract (25 mL), vitamin C (100 mg), fennel seed extract (10.3 mg), eucalyptus leaf extract (12.3 mg), and rosemary leaf extract (20.1 mg) was studied in 32 patients against the common cold. The other herbs in the formulation were added to provide expectorant and antiseptic properties. The groups were given 4 tablets of either the placebo or the herbal formulation for 44 days and evaluated based on the amount of discharge of the thin nasal mucus they produced and the number of tissues they used. The results of the groups were significantly different: the placebo group used a mean number of 1,168 tissues and recovered in 4.37 ± 1.57 days; the treatment group used 882 tissues and recovered in 3.37 ± 1.25 days (Scaglione and Lund, 1995).

The expressed juice of *E. purpurea* (4 mL of Echinacin twice daily for 8 weeks) versus a placebo was studied in 108 patients who had frequent cold infections. The patients who received the echinacea treatment took a longer time until contracting the cold: 40 days for the treatment group versus 25 days for the placebo. Also, 35.2% of the patients who received the treatment remained without infections versus 25.9% of those who received the placebo. The placebo group contracted infections that were more severe and showed evidence of a weakened immune system (Schöneberger, 1992).

General Immune Function

A systematic review of the trials in which echinacea was used as an immunomodulator (26 total) concluded that it is an effective immuno-modulator, although the authors also noted that the studies were not high quality, and recommended better-designed clinical trials to ascertain the doses for specific conditions and preparations (Melchart et al., 1994).

A study of the immunological changes produced by an extract of *E. purpurea* in 12 men found a 120% increased rate of granulocytic phagocytosis. This was compared with a placebo group, which showed only a 30% increase over the same period. After cessation of treatment, phagocytosis decreased to normal levels in 3 days. No changes were found in the immunoglobulin and leukocyte levels or in the erythrocyte sedimentation rate (Jurcic et al., 1989).

Exercise-induced immunosuppression was studied in 42 male tri-athletes. Three groups treated with *E. purpurea* extract, magnesium sup-plement, or a placebo were formed and followed as the athletes under-went regular competitive sprint training. The magnesium- and placebo-treated groups had similar results, but the echinacea group exhibited significantly enhanced exercise-induced decrease in levels of soluble IL-2 receptor (sIL-2R), significantly greater exercise-induced levels of urine

IL-6, and significantly greater exercise-induced increases in cortisol concentrations. The authors noted that the most common reported cytokine responses to strenuous exercise were increases in the release of IL-6 and sIL-2R and of IL-6 in the acute phase response to injury or infection. The absence of a significant decrease of natural killer cells in the echinacea groups suggested a countereffect of cortisol on these cells (Berg et al., 1998).

SAFETY/DOSAGE

Because many types of echinacea preparations are available and several immunologically active compounds are in echinacea, dosage recommendations vary. In the United States, commercial extracts are typically standardized to the echinacosides and 4-sesquiterpene esters; it has been suggested, however, that the caffeic acid derivatives (such as echinacoside and cichoric acid) and the polysaccharides, glycoproteins, alkylamides, and polyacetylenes make better standards. Some of the typical dosage recommendations are as follows (McKenna et al., 2002):

- Dried root or tea: 1–2 g 3 times daily
- Freeze-dried plant: 325–650 mg 3 times daily
- Juice of aerial portions stabilized in 22% ethanol: 2–3 mL 3 times daily
- Tincture (1:5): 3–4 mL 3 times daily
- Fluid extract (1:1): 1–2 mL 3 times daily
- Solid dry extract (6.5:1 or 3.5% echinacoside): 100–250 mg 3 times daily

Chronic use of echinacea is discouraged by some sources because it is believed to lose its ability to boost the immune system when needed during long-term use (Chua, 2003). When used at the recommended doses, side effects from taking echinacea are rare, and little or no toxicity is associated with its use. The LD_{50} (semilethal dose) of fresh-pressed *E. purpurea* juice in mice is 50 mL/kg, administered intravenously; and the polysaccharides of the aerial portions of the plant produced an LD_{50} of 1,000–2,500 mg/kg administered intraperitoneally to mice. Long-term administration of the fresh-pressed juice also produced no toxic effects at many times the human dose; and no significant acute or subacute toxicity was found from oral administration of up to 15 g/kg and 8 g/kg, respectively (McKenna et al., 2002).

Echinacea may interfere with drugs that have immunosuppressant effects, such as cyclosporine and corticosteroids. In vitro studies showed inhibition of 3A4 enzyme activity of the cytochrome P450 system, suggesting possible interactions with lovastatin, ketoconazole, fexofenadine, and triazolam. Patients taking metronidazole or disulfiram should avoid echinacea because of the varying alcohol contents of the herb. The use of acetaminophen, amiodarone, methotrexate, or ketoconazole with echinacea might increase the risk of hepatotoxicity (Abebe, 2002).

REFERENCES

Abebe W. Herbal medication: potential for adverse interactions with analgesic drugs. J Clin Pharm Ther 2002;27:391–401.

Barrett BP, Brown RL, Locken K, Maberry R, Bobula JA, D'Alessio D. Treatment of the common cold with unrefined echinacea: a randomized, double-blind, placebo-controlled trial. Ann Intern Med 2002;137:939–946.

Berg A, Northoff H, Konig D, et al. Influence of Echinacin (EC31) treatment on the exercise-induced immune response in athletes. J Clin Res 1998;1:367–380.

Blumenthal M, Goldberg A, Brinckmann J, Foster S, eds. Herbal Medicine: Expanded Commission E Monographs. Massachusetts: Integrative Medicine Communications, 2000.

Brinkeborn RM, Shah DV, Degenring FH. Echinaforce and other echinacea fresh plant preparations in the treatment of the common cold. A randomized, placebo-controlled, double-blind clinical trial. Phytomedicine 1999;6:1–5.

Chua D. Chronic use of echinacea should be discouraged. Am Fam Physician 2003;68(4):617.

Cupp MJ, ed. Toxicology and Clinical Pharmacology of Herbal Products. Totowa, NJ: Humana Press, 2000.

Goel V, Lovlin R, Barton R, Lyon MR, Bauer R, Lee TD, Basu TK. Efficacy of a standardized echinacea preparation (Echinilin) for the treatment of the common cold: a randomized, double-blind, placebo-controlled trial. J Clin Pharm Ther 2004;29(1):75–83.

Grimm W, Muller H. A randomized controlled trial of the effect of fluid extract of echinacea purpurea on the incidence and severity of colds and respiratory infections. Am J Med 1999;106:138–143.

Hoheisel O, Sandberg M, Dertram S, et al. Echinagard treatment shortens the course of the common cold: a double-blind, placebo-controlled clinical trial. European Journal of Clinical Research 1997;9:261–268.

Jurcic K, Melchart D, Holzmann M, et al. Two studies on the stimulation of the phagocytosis of granulocytes by drug preparations containing extracts of echinacea in healthy volunteers. Zeitschrift für Phytotherapie 1989;10:67–70.

Lindenmuth GF, Lindenmuth EB. The efficacy of echinacea compound herbal tea preparation on the severity and duration of upper respiratory and flu symptoms: a randomized, double-blind placebo-controlled study. J Altern Complement Med 2000;6(4):327–334.

McKenna D, Jones K, Hughes K, Humphrey S. Botanical Medicines: The Desk Reference for Major Herbal Supplements. 2nd Ed. Binghamton, NY: Haworth Press, 2002.

Melchart D, Linde K, Worku F, et al. Immunomodulation with echinacea—a systematic review of controlled clinical trials. Phytomedicine 1994;1:245–254.

Rotblatt M, Ziment I. Evidenced-Based Herbal Medicine. Philadelphia: Hanley and Belfus, 2002.

Scaglione F, Lund B. Efficacy in the treatment of the common cold of a preparation containing an Echinacea extract. Int J Immunother 1995;11:163–166.

Schöneberger D. The influence of immunostimulating effects of pressed juice from Echinacea purpurea on the course and severity of colds. Results of a double-blind study. Forum Immunologie 1992;8:2–12.

Yale SH, Liu K. Echinacea purpurea therapy for the treatment of the common cold: a randomized, double-blind, placebo-controlled clinical trial. Arch Intern Med 2004;164(11):1237–1241.

GLUTAMINE

Overall Rank

★★★★ to promote tissue repair
★★★★ to reduce muscle catabolism
★★★★ to prevent infections and boost immune system function

OVERVIEW

Glutamine is the most abundant amino acid in the body, comprising approximately half of the free amino acids in the blood and muscle. As a nonessential amino acid, glutamine can be produced in the body by conversion from another amino acid—glutamic acid (primarily by the skeletal muscle and liver). Glutamine has two main functions in the body: as a precursor in the synthesis of other amino acids and to convert into glucose for energy. Cells of the immune system, the small intestine, and the kidney are the major consumers of glutamine, making "immune boosting" and "immune maintenance" claims for glutamine supplements quite common. In addition, and peripherally related to the control of immune response and inflammation, are claims for glutamine supplements in maintaining muscle mass, reducing postexercise catabolism (muscle tissue breakdown), and accelerating recovery from intense exercise.

Intense exercise training results in a well-described drop in plasma glutamine levels. Chronically low glutamine levels have been implicated as a possible contributing factor in athletic overtraining syndrome as well as the transient immunosuppression and increased risk of infections that typically affect competitive athletes during intense training and competition. Under conditions of metabolic stress, the body's need for glutamine may become conditionally essential, meaning that the body cannot produce adequate levels and a dietary source is required to prevent catabolism of skeletal muscle, the primary source of stored glutamine in the body.

COMMENTS

Glutamine supplements are relatively inexpensive compared with other amino acid supplements. For people exposed to heightened levels of stress, such as those recovering from injury, surgery, or intense exercise, glutamine supplements represent an economical way to promote tissue repair, reduce muscle catabolism, and help prevent infections.

SCIENTIFIC SUPPORT

A significant body of scientific literature exists to support the beneficial effects of glutamine supplementation in maintaining muscle mass and immune system function in critically ill patients and in those recovering from extensive burns and major surgery (Carli et al., 1990). When plasma glutamine levels fall, skeletal muscles may enter a state of catabolism in which muscle protein is degraded to provide free glutamine for the rest of the body. Because skeletal muscle is the major source of glutamine (other than the diet), prolonged deficits in plasma glutamine can lead to a significant loss of skeletal muscle protein and muscle mass. Postsurgical deposition of collagen (a marker for wound healing) can be enhanced by amino acid supplementation containing 14 g of glutamine (Williams et al., 2002), but a lower dose of mixed amino acids containing glutamine (2.9 g) provides no change in athletic performance or on adaptations to cycling training (Vukovich et al., 1997).

In recent years, several studies have been conducted on glutamine supplementation in athletes, and a strong rationale exists for the efficacy of glutamine supplements in athletic populations. For example, glutamine's role in immune system support has been shown to prevent infections following intense bouts of physical activity (which tend to reduce plasma glutamine levels) (Castell and Newsholme, 1997; Smith and Norris, 2000). Glutamine supplements have also been shown to play a role in counteracting the catabolic (muscle-wasting) effects of stress hormones such as cortisol, which are typically elevated by strenuous exercise. Under conditions of stress-induced protein wasting in adults and children, including burns, surgery, and some forms of cancer, glutamine supplementation is associated with reduced protein (muscle tissue) breakdown (des Robert et al., 2002), enhanced lymphocyte function (Yoshida et al., 2001), reduced gut permeability (Klimberg et al., 1992; van Acker et al., 2000; Yoshida et al., 1998, 2001), and reduced infections (Barbosa et al., 1999; Burke et al., 1989; O'Riordain et al., 1996). Although glutamine supplementation has shown benefits in maintaining immune system function and enhancing tumoricidal effectiveness in rodents during chemotherapy and radiotherapy in various types of cancer (Klimberg et al., 1992), glutamine is also described as an essential factor for tumor growth (Medina, 2001; Souba, 1993).

The function of glutamine in stimulating glycogen synthase, the enzyme that controls the synthesis and storage of glycogen fuel storage in muscles and liver, may provide a mechanism by which glutamine supplements promote enhanced fuel stores. Glutamine is also thought to increase cell volume and may stimulate the activity of enzymes in the liver and muscles involved in glycogen storage as well as those involved in anabolic activities such as protein synthesis. Glutamine supplements have also been hypothesized to increase levels of growth hormone, which may be expected to help stimulate protein synthesis and encourage gains in muscle mass and strength, but reliable evidence for this effect has not been demonstrated by clinical studies.

SAFETY/DOSAGE

Glutamine supplements are well tolerated at levels up to at least 20 g/day, and intakes of as much as 40 g/day should induce no significant adverse effects other than mild gastrointestinal discomfort. As with any isolated amino acid supplement, consumption in divided doses throughout the day should increase total body stores without posing significant absorption issues. For the immune system support and anticatabolic actions that are of interest to most athletes, recommended doses range from 1–10 g/day.

REFERENCES

Barbosa E, Moreira EA, Goes JE, Faintuch J. Pilot study with a glutamine-supplemented enteral formula in critically ill infants. Rev Hosp Clin Fac Med Sao Paulo 1999;54(1):21–24.

Burke DJ, Alverdy JC, Aoys E, Moss GS. Glutamine-supplemented total parenteral nutrition improves gut immune function. Arch Surg 1989;124(12):1396–1399.

Carli F, Webster J, Ramachandra V, Pearson M, Read M, Ford GC, McArthur S, Preedy VR, Halliday D. Aspects of protein metabolism after elective surgery in patients receiving constant nutritional support. Clin Sci (Colch) 1990;78(6):621–628.

Castell LM, Newsholme EA. The effects of oral glutamine supplementation on athletes after prolonged, exhaustive exercise. Nutrition 1997;13(7–8):738–742.

des Robert C, Le Bacquer O, Piloquet H, Roze JC, Darmaun D. Acute effects of intravenous glutamine supplementation on protein metabolism in very low birth weight infants: a stable isotope study. Pediatr Res 2002;51(1):87–93.

Klimberg VS, Nwokedi E, Hutchins LF, Pappas AA, Lang NP, Broadwater JR, Read RC, Westbrook KC. Glutamine facilitates chemotherapy while reducing toxicity. JPEN 1992;16(6 suppl):83S–87S.

Medina MA. Glutamine and cancer. J Nutr 2001;131(9 suppl):2539S-2542S.

O'Riordain MG, De Beaux A, Fearon KC. Effect of glutamine on immune function in the surgical patient. Nutrition 1996;12(11–12 suppl):S82–S84.

Smith DJ, Norris SR. Changes in glutamine and glutamate concentrations for tracking training tolerance. Med Sci Sports Exerc 2000;32(3):684–689.

Souba WW. Glutamine and cancer. Ann Surg 1993;218(6):715–728.

van Acker BA, Hulsewe KW, Wagenmakers AJ, von Meyenfeldt MF, Soeters PB. Response of glutamine metabolism to glutamine-supplemented parenteral nutrition. Am J Clin Nutr 2000;72(3):790–795.

Vukovich MD, Sharp RL, Kesl LD, Schaulis DL, King DS. Effects of a low-dose amino acid supplement on adaptations to cycling training in untrained individuals. Int J Sport Nutr 1997;7(4):298–309.

Williams JZ, Abumrad N, Barbul A. Effect of a specialized amino acid mixture on human collagen deposition. Ann Surg 2002;236(3):369–374.

Yoshida S, Kaibara A, Ishibashi N, Shirouzu K. Glutamine supplementation in cancer patients. Nutrition 2001;17(9):766–768.

Yoshida S, Matsui M, Shirouzu Y, Fujita H, Yamana H, Shirouzu K. Effects of glutamine supplements and radiochemotherapy on systemic immune and gut barrier function in patients with advanced esophageal cancer. Ann Surg 1998;227(4):485–491.

ADDITIONAL RESOURCES

Alvestrand A, Bergstrom J, Furst P, Germanis G, Widstam U. Effect of essential amino acid supplementation on muscle and plasma free amino acids in chronic uremia. Kidney Int 1978;14(4):323–329.

Calder PC, Yaqoob P. Glutamine and the immune system. Amino Acids 1999;17(3):227–241.

Newsholme EA, Calder PC. The proposed role of glutamine in some cells of the immune system and speculative consequences for the whole animal. Nutrition 1997;13(7–8):728–730.

Walsh NP, Blannin AK, Robson PJ, Gleeson M. Glutamine, exercise and immune function. Links and possible mechanisms. Sports Med 1998;26(3):177–191.

Young LS, Bye R, Scheltinga M, Ziegler TR, Jacobs DO, Wilmore DW. Patients receiving glutamine-supplemented intravenous feedings report an improvement in mood. JPEN 1993;17(5):422–427.

GOLDENSEAL (*HYDRASTIS CANADENSIS*)

Overall Rank

★★★ for diarrhea (as a source of berberine)
★★★ for immune system support (as a source of berberine)
★★★ as an antimicrobial (as a source of berberine)

OVERVIEW

Many people consider the main active constituent in goldenseal to be berberine, and most of the clinical studies have been done on the single compound. Berberine is an alkaloid that also comes from several other plants, including *Coptis chinensis* (goldenthread), *Berberis aquifolium* (Oregon grape), *B. vulgaris* (barberry), and *B. aristata* (tree turmeric), which has a long history in folk medicine for diarrhea. Because goldenseal has had an endangered status, many herb companies have substituted it with other berberine-containing plants in formulas. Most commonly, goldenseal is used in immune support formulas (usually along with echinacea) or for its antioxidant, anticancer effects or for urinary tract infections.

Although goldenseal has a long history in the traditional medicine of Native Americans and later with the settlers, no clinical studies have been performed with the single herb in humans. Animal and in vitro studies have been done on goldenseal, however, and both preclinical and clinical data exist on berberine. Preclinical animal models have shown goldenseal root to be immunostimulatory and to decrease an enzyme involved with tumor growth in colon cancer (Lin et al., 1999). Preliminary studies have found berberine to be of possible value for diarrhea and liver cirrhosis (Choudhry et al, 1972; Gupte, 1975; Watanabe et al, 1982).

COMMENTS

Goldenseal is often piggy-backed with echinacea in immune-support formulas, but little clinical evidence yet confirms this use.

SCIENTIFIC SUPPORT

In a randomized controlled study, the effect of berberine sulfate was tested in 165 adults with acute diarrhea caused by either *Escherichia coli* or *Vibrio cholerae*. At the dosage of 400 mg of berberine sulfate, patients with *E. coli* experienced a significant reduction in mean stool volume during three consecutive 8-hour periods after treatment. At 24 hours past treatment, a significant number of *E. coli* patients treated with berberine sulfate were cured of their diarrhea compared with those in the control group. In the cholera group, patients receiving 1,200 mg of berberine sulfate showed only slight decreases in stool volume, and patients receiving berberine sulfate plus tetracycline did not show a significant difference in stool volume compared with the tetracycline-only group (Rabbani et al., 1987).

Khin-Maung-U et al. (1985) studied the effect of berberine, tetracycline, and the combination of berberine and tetracycline in 400 adult patients with diarrhea. In the 185 patients that suffered from diarrhea induced by cholera, the frequency and volume of diarrheal stools was significantly reduced in both treatment groups involving tetracycline, but not in the berberine-only group. Factorial design equations were able to show a 1-L reduction of diarrheal stools and a reduction of cyclic adenosine monophosphate concentrations in the berberine groups. In the 215 patients with noncholera diarrhea, neither tetracycline nor berberine showed benefit over placebo.

SAFETY/DOSAGE

Goldenseal is generally thought to be safe but should not be used during pregnancy or lactation. Goldenseal is contraindicated for people with high blood pressure or other cardiovascular diseases.

Berberine is considered safe at goldenseal's recommended dosages; however, it is contraindicated for pregnancy and may interfere with vitamin B metabolism. The LD_{50} in rats for berberine is greater than 1,000 mg/kg of body weight, indicating a low toxicity. Topical application of berberine may cause photosensitivity (Inbaraj et al., 2001; Kowalewski et al., 1975).

The typical dosage of goldenseal is 4–6 g/day of the powdered root or 250–500 mg of the extracted root (usually standardized to 5% berberine content) 3 times daily (McKenna et al., 2002).

REFERENCES
Choudhry VP, Sabir M, Bhide VN. Berberine in giardiasis. Indian Pediatr 1972;9(3):143–146.
Gupte S. Use of berberine in treatment of giardiasis. Am J Dis Child 1975;129(7):866.
Inbaraj JJ, Kukielczak BM, Bilski P, Sandvik SL, Chignell CF. Photochemistry and photocytotoxicity of alkaloids from goldenseal (Hydrastis canadensis L.), part I: berberine. Chem Res Toxicol 2001;14(11):1529–1534.
Khin-Maung-U, Myo-Khin, Nyunt-Nyunt-Wai, Aye-Kyaw, Tin-U. Clinical trial of berberine in acute watery diarrhoea. Br Med J (Clin Res Ed) 1985;291(6509):1601–1605.
Kowalewski Z, Mrozikiewicz A, Bobkiewicz T, Drost K, Hladon B. Toxicity of berberine sulfate. Acta Pol Pharm 1975;32(1):113–120.
Lin JG, Chung JG, Wu LT, Chen GW, Chang HL, Wang TF. Effects of berberine on arylamine N-acetyltransferase activity in human colon tumor cells. Am J Chin Med 1999;27(2):265–275.
McKenna D, Jones K, Hughes K, Humphrey S. Botanical Medicines: The Desk Reference for Major Herbal Supplements. 2nd Ed. Binghamton, NY: Haworth Press, 2002.

Rabbani GH, Butler T, Knight J, Sanyal SC, Alam K. Randomized controlled trial of berberine sulfate therapy for diarrhea due to enterotoxigenic Escherichia coli and Vibrio cholerae. J Infect Dis 1987;155(5):979–984.

Watanabe A, Obata T, Nagashima H. Berberine therapy of hypertyraminemia in patients with liver cirrhosis. Acta Med Okayama 1982;36(4):277–281.

PERILLA SEED OIL (*PERILLA FRUTESCENS*)

Overall Rank

★★★ for asthma and allergy
★★★ for inflammatory conditions
★★★ for cardiovascular health
  ★★ for immune function

OVERVIEW

Perilla, or shiso (also called beefsteak), is a popular vegetable in Asia that looks like a large-leafed basil. Because its seed oil is used in various foods in Asia, it has a long track record of safety in humans. In Asia it is also used for lung health and as a traditional treatment for coughs, cold, and flu. Perilla seed oil is high in ω-3 fatty acids, especially α-linolenic acid. The ω-3 fatty acids have been well tested as anti-inflammatory compounds that are useful for many inflammatory conditions, and are known to reduce the production of many allergic mediators when supplemented to the diet. In addition to essential fatty acids, perilla contains several pharmacologically active phenolic compounds, such as rosmarinic acid, apigenin, luteolin, chrysoleriol, quercetin, and catechin (Makino et al., 2003; Nakazawa et al., 2003; Takeda et al., 2002; Ueda et al., 2002).

COMMENTS

Few human studies yet exist on the therapeutic value of perilla seed oil, but many studies have been done on some of its chemical constituents, such as the ω-3 fatty acids and rosmarinic acid. Because of its traditional use in foods, interesting mixture of phenolic compounds, promising animal studies, and low cost, perilla may be an excellent alternative to fish oil supplementation.

SCIENTIFIC SUPPORT

Asthma and Allergies

Perilla seed oil, as a source of α-linolenic acid, was tested in asthma patients for the clinical features that accompanied leukotriene inhibition, including its effect on ventilatory parameters and lipid metabolism. The participants were divided into two groups. Group A comprised those who showed significantly suppressed leucocyte generation of leukotriene C_4 (LTC_4) by 4 weeks of perilla seed supplementation. Group B comprised those who showed no leukotriene inhibition but rather a significant increase in production after the same treatment. Analysis of the ventilatory clinical features and lipid metabolism in the groups prior to supplementation showed significant differences between the groups, and the groups responded differently to perilla seed oil supplementation. It was concluded that supplementation of perilla seed oil suppresses generation of LTC_4 in certain asthma patients and that its ability to do so is related to clinical features such as respiratory function and lipid metabolism (Okamoto et al., 2000a).

Okamoto et al. (2000b) studied the effects of perilla seed oil on bronchial asthma compared with the effects of corn oil on pulmonary function and the generation of leukotriene B_4 (LTB_4) and LTC_4 by leucocytes. Perilla seed oil is rich in the ω-3 fatty acids, whereas corn oil is rich in ω-6 fatty acids. Each group consisted of seven subjects, and supplementation of the respective oil proceeded for 4 weeks. Significant differences in pulmonary function and leukotriene production were found between the groups, and it was concluded that perilla seed oil is beneficial for the treatment of asthma because it suppresses LTB_4 and LTC_4 generation by leucocytes and improves pulmonary function.

In a small study involving five asthma patients, supplementation with perilla seed oil was reported to be helpful for asthma. After 2 weeks of supplementation, asthma symptoms and morning and evening mean and peak flow rates were improved significantly. Additionally, the generation of LTB_4 and LTC_4 by leukocytes was significantly reduced with supplementation (Kozo et al., 1997).

Cardiovascular Health

The effect of the long-term intake of perilla oil as a source of ω-3 fatty acid was compared with that of an ω-6 source, soybean oil, on the risk factors of coronary heart disease and serum levels of fatty acids. Twenty older Japanese subjects were given soybean oil for at least 6 months as a baseline period, put on a perilla oil diet for 10 months as the intervention period, and then returned to the soybean diet as the washout period. The changes in the ratio of ω-6 to ω-3 were 4:1 for the soybean oil treatment and 1:1 for the perilla oil treatment. At 3 months into the treatment period with perilla oil, the α-linolenic acid in the serum increased from 0.8% to 1.6%, and the eicosapentaenoic acid and docosahexaenoic acid increased from 2.5% to 3.6% and from 5.3% to 6.4% respectively after 10 months of treatment, and returned to baseline in the washout period. The concentration of the oxidized low-density lipoprotein did not change significantly. It was concluded that in elderly subjects the levels of α-linolenic acid, eicosapentaenoic acid, and docosahexaenoic acid could be increased significantly through dietary change without any adverse effects (Ezaki et al., 1999).

Bioavailability

In a study on the bioavailability of enteric-coated perilla seed oil (Entrox), 12 healthy volunteers were given enteric-coated or noncoated capsules containing 6 g of a perilla seed formulation. The perilla seed formulation was α-linolenic acid rich and was given in a single dose followed by a 3-week washout period. There were no difference in the pharmacokinetics of the two formulations; however, the levels of plasma α-linolenic acid measured within 24 hours were significantly higher for the enteric-coated treatment group (Kurowska et al., 2003).

SAFETY/DOSAGE

Although perilla has undergone few clinical studies in humans and most of the feeding studies have been done in animals, perilla seed oil has long been used as a food among Asian people with no associated safety problems. About 6 g/day of perilla seed oil would contribute about 3 g of α-linolenic acid to the diet. Contact dermatitis develops in about 20–50% of the long-term workers with perilla culture, which is thought to be caused by the 1-perillaldehyde and perillalcohol content of shiso oil (Okazaki et al., 1982).

REFERENCES

Ezaki O, Takahashi M, Shigematsu T, Shimamura K, Kimura J, Ezaki H, Gotoh T. Long-term effects of dietary alpha-linolenic acid from perilla oil on serum fatty acids composition and on the risk factors of coronary heart disease in Japanese elderly subjects. J Nutr Sci Vitaminol (Tokyo) 1999;45(6):759–772.

Kozo A., Fumihiro M, Takashi M, Yasuhiro H, Satoshi Y, Hirofumi T, Yoshiro T, Takao T. A pilot study: Effects of dietary supplementation with alpha-linolenic acid-enriched perilla seed oil on bronchial asthma. Allergology International 1997;46(3):181–185.

Kurowska EM, Dresser GK, Deutsch L, Vachon D, Khalil W. Bioavailability of omega-3 essential fatty acids from perilla seed oil. Prostaglandins Leukot Essentl Fatty Acids 2003;68(3):207–212.

Makino T, Furuta Y, Wakushima H, Fujii H, Saito K, Kano Y. Anti-allergic effect of Perilla frutescens and its active constituents. Phytother Res 2003;17(3):240–243.

Nakazawa T, Yasuda T, Ueda J, Ohsawa K. Antidepressant-like effects of apigenin and 2,4,5-trimethoxycinnamic acid from Perilla frutescens in the Forced Swimming Test. Biol Pharm Bull 2003;26(4):474–80.

Okamoto M, Mitsunobu F, Ashida K, Mifune T, Hosaki Y, Tsugeno H, Harada S, Tanizaki Y. Effects of dietary supplementation with n-3 fatty acids compared with n-6 fatty acids on bronchial asthma. Intern Med 2000a;39(2):107–111.

Okamoto M, Mitsunobu F, Ashida K, Mifune T, Hosaki Y, Tsugeno H, Harada S, Tanizaki Y, Kataoka M, Niiya K, Harada M. Effects of perilla seed oil supplementation on leukotriene generation by leucocytes in patients with asthma associated with lipometabolism. Int Arch Allergy Immunol 2000b;122(2):137–142.

Okazaki N, Matunaka M, Kondo M, Okamoto K. Contact dermatitis due to beefsteak plant Perilla-frutescens-var-acuta. Hifu 1982;24(2):250–256.

Takeda H, Tsuji M, Miyamoto J, Matsumiya T. Rosmarinic acid and caffeic acid reduce the defensive freezing behavior of mice exposed to conditioned fear stress. Psychopharmacology (Berl) 2002;164(2):233–235.

Ueda H, Yamazaki C, Yamazaki M. Luteolin as an anti-inflammatory and anti-allergic constituent of Perilla frutescens. Biol Pharm Bull 2002;25(9):1197–1202.

SHARK CARTILAGE AND BOVINE CARTILAGE (TRACHEAL)

Overall Rank

★ for anticancer effects (antiangiogenesis)

OVERVIEW

Shark cartilage extracts typically come from the fins, while cartilage from the trachea of cows is used in bovine cartilage supplements. The cartilage is pulverized, powdered, and packed into capsules with various claims made for preventing or treating cancer, promoting wound healing, and relieving the pain and stiffness of arthritis.

Cartilage consumption has been linked to the healing of connective tissue injuries since the middle part of the century (much as hydrolyzed collagen protein, glucosamine, and chondroitin are today). In the early 1980s, cartilage extracts became a popular alternative treatment for reducing the pain and stiffness associated with arthritis (although gelatin, SAMe, and glucosamine all appear to be more effective in this regard). Today, the most common use of cartilage supplements is as a cancer treatment. In theory, cartilage supplements inhibit tumor growth by inhibiting angiogenesis (growth of new blood vessels) and "choking off" the blood supply that the tumor needs to survive and grow. This popular, but unproven, theory generated a wave of media attention in the 1980s following publication of a popular pseudoscientific book misleadingly titled *Why Sharks Don't Get Cancer* (they actually do).

COMMENTS

At this time, cartilage extracts do not appear to provide significant value as a dietary supplement. As research into this area progresses, perhaps new findings will provide evidence of cartilage extracts in preventing angiogenesis in cancer patients. Currently, an experimental new drug derived from shark cartilage, Neovastat, is under investigation as an antitumor agent. Until then, other supplements have proven benefits in joint health and wound healing (hydrolyzed collagen protein, SAMe, glucosamine, and chondroitin) and cancer prevention (green tea and soy isoflavones).

SCIENTIFIC SUPPORT

Cancer tumors generally need new blood vessels to grow. Some researchers have theorized that cartilage, which does not have blood vessels,
might be a cancer preventive. Shark cartilage is known to harbor certain
compounds that seem to slow the creation of the new blood vessels
needed for tumors to grow and spread. Several processes are thought to
be involved. First, shark cartilage interferes with a group of enzymes
known as matrix metalloproteases, which are thought to be secreted by
tumors to break down surrounding tissue and allow the tumors to
spread. Vascular endothelial growth factor activity (which promotes the
formation of new blood vessels) is low in shark cartilage. Some rodent
studies using injected shark cartilage extracts have shown promising
initial results (Horsman et al., 1998), but when shark cartilage is taken
by mouth, not enough of the active ingredients may be absorbed from
the gastrointestinal tract to be effective. Controlled studies of either
oral or injected products in patients with advanced cancer treated with
conventional drugs, however, did not demonstrate effectiveness from
shark cartilage in producing complete or partial responses (Miller et al.,
1998). No studies involving patients with less advanced or previously
untreated cancer have been published, but clinical research is ongoing.

Although there is certainly no shortage of testimonials for "miracle"
cartilage products that "cure" cancer, the scientific evidence for such
effects is lacking. Despite shark and bovine cartilage supplements being
touted as cancer cures, careful scientific study in people with advanced
tumors have shown these claims to be wildly optimistic at best and
completely bogus in many cases (Blackadar, 1993; Ernst, 1998; Simone
and Simone, 1998). It is interesting to note, however, that for all the
outlandish and unsubstantiated claims for shark cartilage to "cure" cancer, a growing number of laboratory and early-stage clinical studies
(Davis et al., 1997) indicate that shark cartilage does indeed contain
compounds able to inhibit tumor angiogenesis (growth of new blood
vessels to feed the tumor). This means that something in cartilage prevents the growth of new blood vessels toward tumors, thereby restricting
tumor growth. The inhibitor is probably not a typical protein but may
be a heat-stable form of proteoglycans (long chains of sugars and amino
acids). Whatever this factor is, much more of it is in shark cartilage than
in cartilage from mammalian sources (such as cows). A major problem
with the shark cartilage theory of tumor prevention, however, is the lack
of clinical proof that this antiangiogenesis factor could even get into the
body when consumed as a dietary supplement.

Some studies, however, suggest that oral administration of liquid
cartilage extract delivers an antiangiogenic effect in humans similar to
that previously observed in lab animals and test-tube studies (Berbari
et al., 1999). In one study, 29 healthy males received either a placebo
or a liquid shark cartilage extract (7–21 mL) each day for 3–4 weeks
(Berbari et al., 1999). Midway through the supplementation period (day
12), a special sponge was inserted subcutaneously (under the skin of

each subject's arm) and removed on day 23. Researchers then counted the number of cells that had grown into the sponge as an indirect measurement of angiogenesis. Results from the study found that cell density was significantly lower in subjects who had received the liquid cartilage extract compared with the placebo. These results are the first to show that the antiangiogenic component of cartilage extracts is bioavailable in humans by oral administration and that oral intake of such extracts can actually reduce blood vessel growth in the body. The next step will be to conduct controlled clinical trials in cancer patients to see whether cartilage extracts can indeed "choke off" cancerous tumors (as those under way for the experimental drug Neovastat are attempting to do) and live up to the claims made for many supplements currently on the market (Batist et al., 2002).

SAFETY/DOSAGE

Although no specific safety studies have been conducted on cartilage extracts, the doses commonly suggested are not expected to cause any significant side effects (or dramatic benefits). In some isolated cases, bovine tracheal cartilage has been associated with contamination by thyroid tissue (the trachea is located adjacent to the thyroid gland) and could potentially lead to thyroid hormone toxicity. For patients choosing to supplement with cartilage extracts, typical dosage suggestions are likely to be in the range of 250–1,000 mg/day, although significant differences may exist among products.

REFERENCES

Batist G, Patenaude F, Champagne P, Croteau D, Levinton C, Hariton C, Escudier B, Dupont E. Neovastat (AE-941) in refractory renal cell carcinoma patients: report of a phase II trial with two dose levels. Ann Oncol 2002;13(8):1259–1263.

Berbari P, Thibodeau A, Germain L, Saint-Cyr M, Gaudreau P, Elkhouri S, Dupont E, Garrel DR, El-Khouri S. Antiangiogenic effects of the oral administration of liquid cartilage extract in humans. J Surg Res 1999;87(1):108–113.

Blackadar CB. Skeptics of oral administration of shark cartilage. J Natl Cancer Inst 1993;85(23):1961–1962.

Davis PF, He Y, Furneaux RH, Johnston PS, Ruger BM, Slim GC. Inhibition of angiogenesis by oral ingestion of powdered shark cartilage in a rat model. Microvasc Res 1997;54(2):178–182.

Ernst E. Shark cartilage for cancer? Lancet 1998;351(9098):298.

Horsman MR, Alsner J, Overgaard J. The effect of shark cartilage extracts on the growth and metastatic spread of the SCCVII carcinoma. Acta Oncol 1998;37(5):441–445.

Miller DR, Anderson GT, Stark JJ, Granick JL, Richardson D. Phase I/II trial of the safety and efficacy of shark cartilage in the treatment of advanced cancer. J Clin Oncol 1998;16(11):3649–3655.

Simone CB, Simone NL, Simone CB 2nd. Shark cartilage for cancer. Lancet 1998;351(9113):1440.

ADDITIONAL RESOURCES

Chen JS, Chang CM, Wu JC, Wang SM. Shark cartilage extract interferes with cell adhesion and induces reorganization of focal adhesions in cultured endothelial cells. J Cell Biochem 2000;78(3):417–428.

Dupont E, Savard PE, Jourdain C, Juneau C, Thibodeau A, Ross N, Marenus K, Maes DH, Pelletier G, Sauder DN. Antiangiogenic properties of a novel shark cartilage extract: potential role in the treatment of psoriasis. J Cutan Med Surg 1998;2(3):146–152.

Lee A, Langer R. Shark cartilage contains inhibitors of tumor angiogenesis. Science 1983;221(4616):1185–1187.

Liang JH, Wong KP. The characterization of angiogenesis inhibitor from shark cartilage. Adv Exp Med Biol 2000;476:209–223.

McGuire TR, Kazakoff PW, Hoie EB, Fienhold MA. Antiproliferative activity of shark cartilage with and without tumor necrosis factor-alpha in human umbilical vein endothelium. Pharmacotherapy 1996;16(2):237–244.

Oikawa T, Ashino-Fuse H, Shimamura M, Koide U, Iwaguchi T. A novel angiogenic inhibitor derived from Japanese shark cartilage (I). Extraction and estimation of inhibitory activities toward tumor and embryonic angiogenesis. Cancer Lett 1990;51(3):181–186.

Sauder DN, Dekoven J, Champagne P, Croteau D, Dupont E. Neovastat (AE-941), an inhibitor of angiogenesis: Randomized phase I/II clinical trial results in patients with plaque psoriasis. J Am Acad Dermatol 2002;47(4):535–541.

Sheu JR, Fu CC, Tsai ML, Chung WJ. Effect of U-995, a potent shark cartilage-derived angiogenesis inhibitor, on anti-angiogenesis and anti-tumor activities. Anticancer Res 1998;18(6A):4435–4441.

VITAMIN A

Overall Rank

★★★★★ for correcting vitamin A deficiency
★★★ for supporting immune function
★★★ for eye health

OVERVIEW

Vitamin A is a fat-soluble vitamin that is part of a family of compounds including retinol, retinal, and β carotene. Also known as provitamin A, β carotene can be converted into vitamin A when additional levels are required. Food sources of vitamin A include organ meats like liver and kidney, egg yolks, butter, cod liver oil, and fortified dairy products like milk and some margarines. For comparative purposes, one serving (3 oz) of beef liver contains approximately 30,000 IU of vitamin A, 1 cup of fortified milk contains 500 IU, and an egg contains 250–300 IU. For β carotene, an average carrot provides about 20,000 IU of vitamin A and one-half cup of spinach or sweet potato provides approximately 7,000 IU.

Vitamin A is involved in myriad metabolic reactions in the body. As a dietary supplement, however, the most prevalent claims are for promoting skin health, eyesight, and general immune function, with occasional claims made for antiaging and anticancer effects.

COMMENTS

Retinol, the most usable form of vitamin A, is often referred to as "preformed" vitamin A and is found in dietary supplements in various stabilized forms. β Carotene is a provitamin A carotenoid that is more efficiently converted into retinol than are other carotenoids. The most prudent approach to vitamin A and carotenoid supplementation, however, may be a combined approach that delivers small supplemental amounts of preformed vitamin A along with mixed carotenoids (versus purely β carotene at high doses).

SCIENTIFIC SUPPORT

Vitamin A is needed by all the body's tissues for general growth and repair processes and is especially important for bone formation, healthy skin and hair, night vision, and function of the immune system. Because of these myriad functions, the health claims associated with vitamin A are numerous.

Vitamin A may help boost immune system function and resistance to infection and the clinical and laboratory evidence to support such supplement claims is quite extensive. Vitamin A supplements have been suggested for the treatment and prevention of HIV infection, even though some in vitro data suggest that vitamin A may actually activate HIV (Humphrey et al., 1999; Nduati et al., 1995). Studies of vitamin A supplementation in HIV-positive patients (up to a single oral dose of 300,000 IU) showed no differences in any lymphocyte subset or activation marker or any change in viral load at any time during an 8-week follow-up period, suggesting no benefit or adverse effect of vitamin A supplements on immune parameters in HIV-positive patients (Humphrey et al., 1999).

In elderly Italian subjects, vitamin A supplementation (800 μg/day of retinol palmitate) has been shown to reduce T-cell numbers, suggesting a compromised cell-mediated immune function (Fortes et al., 1998). By contrast, in populations of healthy men (van Poppel et al., 1993), children with vitamin A deficiencies (Semba et al., 1992), lung cancer patients (Micksche et al., 1977), and older English patients (Penn at el., 1991), vitamin A (or β carotene) supplementation resulted in a significant increase in cell-mediated immunity, including the absolute number of T cells, T4 subsets, T4:T8 ratio, and lymphocyte proliferation responses.

Low plasma retinol concentrations indicate depleted levels of vitamin A, which can result not only from an inadequate intake of vitamin A but also from a deficiency in protein, calories, and zinc (all needed for the synthesis of retinol-binding protein, which is needed for the mobilization of vitamin A from liver stores to the general circulation).

The "immune" angle for vitamin A and its derivatives follows from its role in cell differentiation and maintenance of the surface linings of eyes and respiratory, urinary, and intestinal tracts as well as skin and mucous membranes throughout the body (thwarting bacterial infection). Vitamin A is also known to have wide-ranging effects on the general functioning of immune system cells, including lymphocytes.

SAFETY/DOSAGE

As a fat-soluble vitamin, vitamin A can be stored in the body and levels can build up over time. Possible toxicity can result with high-dose supplementation (50,000 IU/day) leading to vomiting, headaches, joint pain, skin irritation, gastrointestinal distress, and hair loss. Extreme caution should be exercised during pregnancy, as high doses of vitamin A have been associated with birth defects. A maximum intake of 5,000 IU of vitamin A is suggested during pregnancy.

Vegetarians who do not consume eggs and dairy foods often need greater amounts of provitamin A carotenoids to meet their need for vitamin A. Vegans may especially benefit from a daily supplement containing a blend of provitamin A carotenoids and preformed vitamin A.

The recommended dietary allowance (RDA) for vitamin A is listed in units referred to as retinol activity equivalents (RAEs) to account for differences in the activities of retinol and provitamin carotenoids such as β carotene. On dietary supplement labels, however, the daily value (DV) is used for all nutrients, with the value for vitamin A set at 5,000 IU for adults, although the RAEs for vitamin A are 2,330 IU (700 µg RAEs) for adult women and 3,000 IU (900 µg RAEs) for adult men. Based on the most recent evidence for the long-term effects of high vitamin A intake on bone health (see next paragraph), it is prudent to keep total vitamin A intake from foods, fortification, and supplements to less than 300 IU of preformed vitamin A daily. Although there is no established DV for β carotene, a daily intake of 5–20 mg would roughly approach those levels achieved by a diet high in fruits and vegetables; the Institute of Medicine suggests that a daily consumption of 3–6 mg of β carotene will maintain plasma β carotene levels in the range associated with a lower risk of chronic diseases.

Much has been made in the general media about the osteoporosis risk associated with higher-than-average vitamin A intakes. These stories are based on research studies that note the highest incidence of osteoporosis occurs in northern Europe—a population with a high vitamin A intake (Melhus et al., 1998). What the researchers further note (but many of the media reports fail to mention) is that this population has a reduced biosynthesis of vitamin D associated with lower levels of sun exposure. More recent studies of the effect of vitamin A intake on vitamin D metabolism and bone health have suggested that a high vitamin A intake may impair the ability of vitamin D to promote intestinal calcium absorption (Crandall, 2004). At very high levels (retinol intake at more than 1,500–3,000 µg/day, or 2–3 times the recommended amount for adults), studies have shown a reduced bone mineral density and an increased risk of hip fracture compared with lower intakes of vitamin A (500–1,250 μg/day). There does not seem to be any evidence of an association between β carotene intake and increased risk of osteoporosis or between recommended intakes of preformed vitamin A and osteoporosis (Feskanich et al., 2002). The upper limit (UL) for vitamin A is the same for men, women, and pregnant women: 3,000 μg RAEs, or 10,000 IU).

β Carotene as an antioxidant is covered in more detail in Chapter 9. Although some large clinical trials have associated β carotene supplements with a greater incidence of lung cancer and death in current heavy smokers, other large studies have found no adverse effects from up to 25–50 mg/day of β carotene in otherwise healthy subjects.

REFERENCES

Crandall C. Vitamin A intake and osteoporosis: a clinical review. J Womens Health 2004;13(8):939–953.

Feskanich D, Singh V, Willett WC, Colditz GA. Vitamin A intake and hip fractures among postmenopausal women. JAMA 2002;287(1):47–54.

Fortes C, Forastiere F, Agabiti N, Fano V, Pacifici R, Virgili F, Piras G, Guidi L, Bartoloni C, Tricerri A, Zuccaro P, Ebrahim S, Perucci CA. The effect of zinc and vitamin A supplementation on immune response in an older population. J Am Geriatr Soc 1998;46(1):19–26.

Humphrey JH, Quinn T, Fine D, Lederman H, Yamini-Roodsari S, Wu LS, Moeller S, Ruff AJ. Short-term effects of large-dose vitamin A supplementation on viral load and immune response in HIV-infected women. J Acquir Immune Defic Syndr Hum Retrovirol 1999;20(1):44–51.

Melhus H, Michaelsson K, Kindmark A, Bergstrom R, Holmberg L, Mallmin H, Wolk A, Ljunghall S. Excessive dietary intake of vitamin A is associated with reduced bone mineral density and increased risk for hip fracture. Ann Intern Med 1998;129(10):770–778.

Micksche M, Cerni C, Kokron O, Titscher R, Wrba H. Stimulation of immune response in lung cancer patients by vitamin A therapy. Oncology 1977;34(5):234–238.

Nduati RW, John GC, Richardson BA, Overbaugh J, Welch M, Ndinya-Achola J, Moses S, Holmes K, Onyango F, Kreiss JK. Human immunodeficiency virus type 1-infected cells in breast milk: association with immunosuppression and vitamin A deficiency. J Infect Dis 1995;172(6):1461–1468.

Penn ND, Purkins L, Kelleher J, Heatley RV, Mascie-Taylor BH, Belfield PW. The effect of dietary supplementation with vitamins A, C and E on cell-mediated immune function in elderly long-stay patients: a randomized controlled trial. Age Ageing 1991;20(3):169–74.

Semba RD, Muhilal, Scott AL, Natadisastra G, Wirasasmita S, Mele L, Ridwan E, West KP Jr, Sommer A. Depressed immune response to tetanus in children with vitamin A deficiency. J Nutr 1992;122(1):101–107.

van Poppel G, Spanhaak S, Ockhuizen T. Effect of beta-carotene on immunological indexes in healthy male smokers. Am J Clin Nutr 1993;57(3):402–407.

ADDITIONAL RESOURCES

Allende LM, Corell A, Madrono A, Gongora R, Rodriguez-Gallego C, Lopez-Goyanes A, Rosal M, Arnaiz-Villena A. Retinol (vitamin A) is a cofactor in CD3-induced human T-lymphocyte activation. Immunology 1997;90(3):388–396.

Daudu PA, Kelley DS, Taylor PC, Burri BJ, Wu MM. Effect of a low beta-carotene diet on the immune functions of adult women. Am J Clin Nutr 1994;60(6):969–972.

Molina EL, Patel JA. A to Z: vitamin A and zinc, the miracle duo. Indian J Pediatr 1996;63(4):427–431.

Ravaglia G, Forti P, Maioli F, Bastagli L, Facchini A, Mariani E, Savarino L, Sassi S, Cucinotta D, Lenaz G. Effect of micronutrient status on natural killer cell immune function in healthy free-living subjects aged >/=90 y. Am J Clin Nutr 2000;71(2):590–598.

Rosales FJ, Kjolhede C. A single 210-mumol oral dose of retinol does not enhance the immune response in children with measles. J Nutr 1994;124(9):1604–1614.

Rumore MM. Vitamin A as an immunomodulating agent. Clin Pharm 1993;12(7):506–514.

Schmidt K. Antioxidant vitamins and beta-carotene: effects on immunocompetence. Am J Clin Nutr 1991;53(1 suppl):383S–385S.

Semba RD. The role of vitamin A and related retinoids in immune function. Nutr Rev 1998;56(1 pt 2):S38–S48.

Semba RD. Vitamin A, immunity, and infection. Clin Infect Dis 1994;19(3):489–499.

Semba RD. Vitamin A and immunity to viral, bacterial and protozoan infections. Proc Nutr Soc 1999;58(3):719–727.

West CE, Rombout JH, van der Zijpp AJ, Sijtsma SR. Vitamin A and immune function. Proc Nutr Soc 1991;50(2):251–262.

ZINC

Overall Rank

★★★★★ for correcting zinc deficiency
★★★★ for support of immune function
★★★★ for treating colds (lozenge form)
★★★★ as a general antioxidant
★★★ for enhancing testosterone and sexual performance

OVERVIEW

Zinc is an essential trace mineral that functions as part of about 300 enzymes. As such, zinc plays a role in numerous biochemical pathways and physiological processes. More than 90% of the body's zinc is stored in the bones (30%) and muscles (60%), but zinc is also found widely distributed in small amounts in virtually all body tissues. The richest dietary sources of zinc are seafood (especially oysters), meat, fish, eggs, and poultry. Because of the varied roles of zinc in the body, claims for zinc-containing dietary supplements are numerous, including those for improved wound healing, general immune system support (including reduced severity and length of colds and upper respiratory tract infections), and support of various aspects of men's health (supporting a healthy prostate gland, preventing benign prostatic hyperplasia, and increasing fertility through enhanced sperm production.

COMMENTS

Zinc lozenges have become one of the most popular natural approaches to treating the common cold. The scientific evidence generally supports this use for short periods (1–2 weeks) (Eby, 1997). Zinc lozenges appear to reduce cold symptoms, such as sore throats, hoarseness, and coughing, and may even be able to shorten the duration of colds by a full day or so. Like vitamin C, zinc is an essential nutrient for optimal functioning of the immune system; both possess significant antiviral activity when consumed at elevated levels for short periods. It also appears, however, that some forms of zinc lozenges may be more effective than others, depending on the total amount of ionized zinc that the lozenge actually releases into the mouth and throat. At least one study has shown that lozenges containing zinc gluconate plus citric acid, sorbitol, or mannitol may not deliver high enough levels of ionized zinc, whereas lozenges containing glycine (an amino acid) appeared to deliver a higher quantity of ionized zinc (Eby et al., 1984).

SCIENTIFIC SUPPORT

Because zinc is an essential part of nearly 300 biochemical pathways, structure/function claims can be made for the nutrient's role in various processes, including digestion, wound healing, energy production, growth, cellular repair, collagen synthesis, bone strength, cognitive function, carbohydrate metabolism (glucose utilization and insulin production), and reproductive function. Even mild zinc deficiency has been associated with depressed immunity, decreased sperm count, and impaired memory. Perhaps the most popular claim for zinc is for its role in immunity: zinc delivered in lozenge form may interfere with the replication of the common cold virus (rhinovirus).

Zinc deficiency is common in developing countries and in some older and athletic populations (Bogden et al., 1990; Bunker et al., 1994; Johnson and Porter, 1997; Mahalanabis et al., 2002; Penny et al., 1999; Sazawal et al., 1998; Singh et al., 1994). In these populations, zinc supplementation at dosages of 10–25 mg/day improves most markers of immune function and duration of illness (diarrhea and upper respiratory tract infections).

Evidence exists to support the use of zinc lozenges in reducing the duration and severity of colds. Although concentrated zinc lozenges can help kill cold viruses in the mouth and throat, it is important to begin using them as soon as possible following the onset of cold symptoms (ideally, within the first 24–48 hours). Test-tube studies have shown that zinc can block the cold virus from replicating—an effect that could help the body's natural immune defenses "get a jump" on killing the viruses (Garland and Hagmeyer, 1998). Most studies of the effect of zinc lozenges (typically, zinc gluconate or zinc acetate) on the common cold have shown that subjects in the supplement group tend to have fewer "symptomatic" days (on average, 2–3 fewer sick days) compared with subjects receiving a placebo (measured in terms of coughing, sore throat, nasal congestion, and headache) (McElroy and Miller, 2002).

Occasionally, high-dose zinc supplements are recommended for diabetic patients, who commonly suffer from increased loss of zinc and reduced body stores of zinc. High doses of zinc have been shown to mimic the effects of insulin in reducing blood sugar and promoting wound healing. These effects, however, should be considered preliminary, and high-dose zinc supplements are not recommended for diabetics except on the advice of their personal physicians.

Exercise performance has been associated with adequate zinc status, especially in athletes who avoid red meat, concentrate their diets too much on carbohydrates, or follow an overly restricted dietary regime. Low zinc intake (below 3 mg/day) has been linked to reduced activity of a zinc-containing enzyme in red blood cells, carbonic anhydrase, which helps red blood cells transport carbon dioxide from tissues to the lungs to be exhaled. Mild-to-moderate zinc deficiency can lead to significant reductions in the body's ability to take up and use oxygen, remove carbon dioxide, and generate energy during high-intensity exercise.

SAFETY/DOSAGE

The short-term use of zinc at therapeutic doses for cold relief (see next paragraph) is assumed to be safe, and chronic supplementation with zinc at levels 2–3 times the current RDA should not be expected to pose any significant adverse effects. High doses of zinc are not recommended for periods of more than two weeks, however, owing to concerns of immune system suppression, interference with copper absorption, increased risk for heart disease, and other long-term health effects. High doses of zinc (gram levels) can cause nausea, diarrhea, and vomiting (Salzman et al., 2002).

The DV for zinc is 15 mg/day, which should be adequate for support of bone metabolism and optimal physical performance. As therapy for colds, however, higher levels are required, with levels in the range of 13–23 mg (in lozenge form) taken every 2–4 hours for no more than 2 weeks. These levels appear to be quite effective for reducing the duration and severity of cold symptoms compared with not taking zinc lozenges. It is also important to note that high levels of other supplements, particularly calcium and iron, can decrease zinc absorption, while complexation (chelation) with various amino acids (such as glycine, histidine, and aspartate) or other organic compounds (such as gluconate or picolinate) may increase zinc bioavailability. Zinc supplementation can reduce absorption of copper (Bonham et al., 2003) and iron (Donangelo et al., 2002) but may also potentiate the effect of supplemental vitamin A on night vision and immune parameters (Christian et al., 2001).

REFERENCES

Bogden JD, Oleske JM, Lavenhar MA, Munves EM, Kemp FW, Bruening KS, Holding KJ, Denny TN, Guarino MA, Holland BK. Effects of one year of supplementation with zinc and other micronutrients on cellular immunity in the elderly. J Am Coll Nutr 1990;9(3):214–225.

Bonham M, O'Connor JM, Alexander HD, Coulter J, Walsh PM, McAnena LB, Downes CS, Hannigan BM, Strain JJ. Zinc supplementation has no effect on circulating levels of peripheral blood leucocytes and lymphocyte subsets in healthy adult men. Br J Nutr 2003;89(5):695–703.

Bunker VW, Stansfield MF, Deacon-Smith R, Marzil RA, Hounslow A, Clayton BE. Dietary supplementation and immunocompetence in housebound elderly subjects. Br J Biomed Sci 1994;51(2):128–135.

Christian P, Khatry SK, Yamini S, Stallings R, LeClerq SC, Shrestha SR, Pradhan EK, West KP Jr. Zinc supplementation might potentiate the effect of vitamin A in restoring night vision in pregnant Nepalese women. Am J Clin Nutr 2001;73(6):1045–1051.

Donangelo CM, Woodhouse LR, King SM, Viteri FE, King JC. Supplemental zinc lowers measures of iron status in young women with low iron reserves. J Nutr 2002;132(7):1860–1864.

Eby GA. Zinc ion availability--the determinant of efficacy in zinc lozenge treatment of common colds. J Antimicrob Chemother 1997;40(4):483–493.

Eby GA, Davis DR, Halcomb WW. Reduction in duration of common colds by zinc gluconate lozenges in a double-blind study. Antimicrob Agents Chemother 1984;25(1):20–24.

Garland ML, Hagmeyer KO. The role of zinc lozenges in treatment of the common cold. Ann Pharmacother 1998;32(1):63–69.

Johnson MA, Porter KH. Micronutrient supplementation and infection in institutionalized elders. Nutr Rev 1997;55(11 pt 1):400–404.

Mahalanabis D, Chowdhury A, Jana S, Bhattacharya MK, Chakrabarti MK, Wahed MA, Khaled MA. Zinc supplementation as adjunct therapy in children with measles accompanied by pneumonia: a double-blind, randomized controlled trial. Am J Clin Nutr 2002;76(3):604–607.

McElroy BH, Miller SP. Effectiveness of zinc gluconate glycine lozenges (Cold-Eeze) against the common cold in school-aged subjects: a retrospective chart review. Am J Ther 2002;9(6):472–475.

Penny ME, Peerson JM, Marin RM, Duran A, Lanata CF, Lonnerdal B, Black RE, Brown KH. Randomized, community-based trial of the effect of zinc supplementation, with and without other micronutrients, on the duration of persistent childhood diarrhea in Lima, Peru. J Pediatr 1999;135(2 pt 1):208–217.

Salzman MB, Smith EM, Koo C. Excessive oral zinc supplementation. J Pediatr Hematol Oncol 2002;24(7):582–584.

Sazawal S, Black RE, Jalla S, Mazumdar S, Sinha A, Bhan MK. Zinc supplementation reduces the incidence of acute lower respiratory infections in infants and preschool children: a double-blind, controlled trial. Pediatrics 1998;102(1 pt 1):1–5.

Singh A, Failla ML, Deuster PA. Exercise-induced changes in immune function: effects of zinc supplementation. J Appl Physiol 1994;76(6):2298–2303.

ADDITIONAL RESOURCES

Abbasi AA, Prasad AS, Rabbani P, DuMouchelle E. Experimental zinc deficiency in man. Effect on testicular function. J Lab Clin Med 1980;96(3):544–550.

Bogden JD, Oleske JM, Lavenhar MA, Munves EM, Kemp FW, Bruening KS, Holding KJ, Denny TN, Guarino MA, Krieger LM, et al. Zinc and immunocompetence in elderly people: effects of zinc supplementation for 3 months. Am J Clin Nutr 1988;48(3):655–663.

Couzy F, Lafargue P, Guezennec CY. Zinc metabolism in the athlete: influence of training, nutrition and other factors. Int J Sports Med 1990;11(4):263–266.

Hunt CD, Johnson PE, Herbel J, Mullen LK. Effects of dietary zinc depletion on seminal volume and zinc loss, serum testosterone concentrations, and sperm morphology in young men. Am J Clin Nutr 1992;56(1):148–157.

Lukaski HC. Magnesium, zinc, and chromium nutriture and physical activity. Am J Clin Nutr 2000;72(2 suppl):585S–593S.

Nishi Y. Anemia and zinc deficiency in the athlete. J Am Coll Nutr 1996;15(4):323–324.

Sazawal S, Jalla S, Mazumder S, Sinha A, Black RE, Bhan MK. Effect of zinc supplementation on cell-mediated immunity and lymphocyte subsets in preschool children. Indian Pediatr 1997;34(7):589–597.

Smith JC, Makdani D, Hegar A, Rao D, Douglass LW. Vitamin A and zinc supplementation of preschool children. J Am Coll Nutr 1999;18(3):213–222.

CHAPTER

Antioxidant and Eye Health Supplements

Antioxidants
β Carotene
Bilberry (*Vaccinium myrtillus* L.)
Grape Seed (*Vitis vinifera*)
Green Tea (*Camellia sinensis*)
Lutein and Zeaxanthin
Lycopene
N-Acetylcysteine (NAC)

Pine Bark (*Pinus* spp.)
Quercetin
Schisandra (*Schisandra chinensis*)
Selenium
Spirulina (*Spirulina maxima, S. platensis*)
Vitamin C
Vitamin E

ANTIOXIDANTS

Overall Rank

★★★★★   for cellular protection
★★★★   for antiaging benefits

OVERVIEW

The term *antioxidant* refers to the activity of numerous vitamins, minerals, and other phytochemicals to protect against the damaging effects of highly reactive molecules known as free radicals. Free radicals can chemically react with, and damage, many structures in the body. Particularly susceptible to oxidative damage are the cellular membranes, mitochondrial membranes, and DNA of virtually all cells. Free-radical reactions and oxidative damage have been linked to many of the "diseases of aging," such as heart disease and cancer. Antioxidant dietary supplements are routinely marketed with direct and implied claims for cellular protection, antiaging effects, prevention of cancer and heart disease, reduction of wrinkles, enhancement of immune function, and promotion of vision.

272

The free-radical theory of aging (and disease promotion) holds that through a gradual accumulation of microscopic damage to our cell membranes, DNA, tissue structures, and enzyme systems, we begin to lose function and are predisposed to disease. In response to free-radical exposure, the body increases its production of endogenous antioxidant enzymes (glutathione peroxidase, catalase, superoxide dismutase), but it has been theorized that supplemental levels of dietary antioxidants may be warranted in some situations to help prevent excessive oxidative damage to muscles, mitochondria, and other tissues (such as during and following intense exercise and exposure to pollutants such as secondhand smoke and oxidizing radiation such as sunlight).

COMMENTS

The four key nutritional antioxidants—vitamins C and E, β carotene, and selenium—are well studied, relatively inexpensive, and widely available as dietary supplements. In addition, a multitude of fruit and vegetable phytonutrient extracts also possess significant antioxidant activity. In most cases, phytonutrient extracts are quite expensive, although their potent antioxidant activity may allow dosages to be fairly small. Popular antioxidant nutrients found in commercial dietary supplements include zinc, copper, *Ginkgo biloba* extract, grape seed extract, pine bark extract, lycopene, lutein, quercetin, and α-lipoic acid, among dozens of others.

When it comes to antioxidant supplementation, it is the overall collection of several antioxidants that is important (rather than any single "super" antioxidant). This concept of balancing supplemental antioxidants is referred to as the "antioxidant network" and is generally composed of five major classes of antioxidants: carotenoids, tocopherols and tocotrienols (vitamin E), vitamin C, thiols (e.g., sulfur-containing compounds such as α-lipoic acid and cysteine), and bioflavonoids. In theory, smaller doses of these antioxidant agents, when given in combination, help regenerate one another following free-radical quenching, thus delivering a more effective and safer antioxidant regimen than with higher doses of isolated antioxidant nutrients. This combined approach to antioxidant supplementation is logical because certain antioxidants work primarily against certain free radicals and in specific parts of the body (e.g., vitamin E against hydroxyl radicals within cell membranes, or vitamin C against superoxide within aqueous spaces).

SCIENTIFIC SUPPORT

Thousands of studies have clearly documented the beneficial effects of dozens of antioxidant nutrients, and thousands of nutrients and phytochemicals possess significant antioxidant activity in the test tube. Increased dietary intake of antioxidant nutrients like vitamins C and E, minerals like selenium, and various phytonutrients like extracts from grape seed, pine bark, and green tea have been linked to reduced rates of oxidative damage and may help reduce the incidence of chronic diseases such as heart disease and cancer. Readers are referred to the relevant section of this chapter for a full discussion of these.

SAFETY/DOSAGE

At the typically recommended levels, most antioxidants appear to be quite safe. For example, vitamin E, one of the most powerful membrane-bound antioxidants, also has one of the best safety profiles. Doses of 100–400 IU of vitamin E have been linked to significant cardiovascular benefits with no side effects. Vitamin C, another powerful antioxidant, can help protect and restore the antioxidant activity of vitamin E and is considered safe in doses of 500–1,000 mg. Higher doses of vitamin C are not recommended because of concerns that such levels may cause an "unbalancing" of the oxidative systems and actually promote oxidative damage instead of preventing it. Another popular antioxidant, β carotene, is somewhat controversial as a dietary supplement. Although diets high in fruits and vegetables deliver approximately 5–6 mg of carotenes daily, these carotenes comprise a mixture of β carotene and other naturally occurring carotenoids. Concern was raised several years ago by studies in which high-dose β carotene supplements appeared to promote lung cancer in heavy smokers. Those studies provided β carotene supplements of 20–60 mg/day—about 5–10 times the levels that could reasonably be expected in the diet (Comstock et al., 1997; Goodman et al., 1996; Albanes et al., 1996).

Based on the available scientific evidence, daily supplementation with vitamin E (100 to 400 IU), vitamin C (250 to 1,000 mg), β carotene (5 to 6 mg), and selenium (70 to 200 μg) appears to be prudent (Age-Related Eye Disease, 2001; Evans and Henshaw, 2000; Ji, 1995; Wolters, 2004).

REFERENCES

Age-Related Eye Disease Study (AREDS) Research Group. A randomized, placebo-controlled, clinical trial of high-dose supplementation with vitamins C and E and beta carotene for age-related cataract and vision loss: AREDS Report No. 9. Arch Ophthalmol 2001;119(10):1439–1452.

Albanes D, Heinonen OP, Taylor PR, Virtamo J, Edwards BK, Rautalahti M, Hartman AM, Palmgren J, Freedman LS, Haapakoski J, Barrett MJ, Pietinen P, Malila N, Tala E, Liippo K, Salomaa ER, Tangrea JA, Teppo L, Askin FB, Taskinen E, Erozan Y, Greenwald P, Huttunen JK. Alpha-Tocopherol and beta-carotene supplements and lung cancer incidence in the alpha-tocopherol, beta-carotene cancer prevention study: effects of base-line characteristics and study compliance. J Natl Cancer Inst 1996;88(21):1560–1570.

Comstock GW, Alberg AJ, Huang HY, Wu K, Burke AE, Hoffman SC, Norkus EP, Gross M, Cutler RG, Morris JS, Spate VL, Helzlsouer KJ. The risk of developing lung cancer associated with antioxidants in the blood: ascorbic acid, carotenoids, alpha-tocopherol, selenium, and total peroxyl radical absorbing capacity. Cancer Epidemiol Biomarkers Prev 1997;6(11):907–916.

Evans JR, Henshaw K. Antioxidant vitamin and mineral supplementation for preventing age-related macular degeneration. Cochrane Database Syst Rev 2000;(2):CD000253.

Goodman GE, Thornquist M, Kestin M, Metch B, Anderson G, Omenn GS. The association between participant characteristics and serum concentrations of beta-carotene, retinol, retinyl palmitate, and alpha-tocopherol among participants in the Carotene and Retinol Efficacy Trial (CARET) for prevention of lung cancer. Cancer Epidemiol Biomarkers Prev 1996;5(10):815–821.

Ji LL. Oxidative stress during exercise: implication of antioxidant nutrients. Free Radic Biol Med 1995;18(6):1079–1086.

Wolters M, Hermann S, Hahn A. Effects of 6-month multivitamin supplementation on serum concentrations of alpha-tocopherol, beta-carotene, and vitamin C in healthy elderly women. Int J Vitam Nutr Res 2004;74(2):161–168.

ADDITIONAL RESOURCES

Age-Related Eye Disease Study (AREDS) Research Group. The effect of five-year zinc supplementation on serum zinc, serum cholesterol and hematocrit in persons randomly assigned to treatment group in the age-related eye disease study: AREDS Report No. 7. J Nutr 2002;132(4):697–702.

Balakrishnan SD, Anuradha CV. Exercise, depletion of antioxidants and antioxidant manipulation. Cell Biochem Funct 1998;16(4):269–275.

Dragan I, Dinu V, Mohora M, Cristea E, Ploesteanu E, Stroescu V. Studies regarding the antioxidant effects of selenium on top swimmers. Rev Roum Physiol 1990;27(1):15–20.

Girodon F, Blache D, Monget AL, Lombart M, Brunet-Lecompte P, Arnaud J, Richard MJ, Galan P. Effect of a two-year supplementation with low doses of antioxidant vitamins and/or minerals in elderly subjects on levels of nutrients and antioxidant defense parameters. J Am Coll Nutr 1997;16(4):357–365.

Grievink L, Zijlstra AG, Ke X, Brunekreef B. Double-blind intervention trial on modulation of ozone effects on pulmonary function by antioxidant supplements. Am J Epidemiol 1999;149(4):306–314.

Hammond BR Jr, Johnson MA. The Age-Related Eye Disease Study (AREDS). Nutr Rev 2002;60(9):283–238.

Jacques PF, Halpner AD, Blumberg JB. Influence of combined antioxidant nutrient intakes on their plasma concentrations in an elderly population. Am J Clin Nutr 1995;62(6):1228–1233.

Kanter M. Free radicals, exercise and antioxidant supplementation. Proc Nutr Soc 1998;57(1):9–13.

Marangon K, Herbeth B, Lecomte E, Paul-Dauphin A, Grolier P, Chancerelle Y, Artur Y, Siest G. Diet, antioxidant status, and smoking habits in French men. Am J Clin Nutr 1998;67(2):231–239.

McBee WL, Lindblad AS, Ferris FL III. Who should receive oral supplement treatment for age-related macular degeneration? Curr Opin Ophthalmol 2003;14(3):159–162.

McQuillan BM, Hung J, Beilby JP, Nidorf M, Thompson PL. Antioxidant vitamins and the risk of carotid atherosclerosis. The Perth Carotid Ultrasound Disease Assessment Study (CUDAS). J Am Coll Cardiol 2001;38(7):1788–1794.

Mitchell P, Smith W, Cumming RG, Flood V, Rochtchina E, Wang JJ. Nutritional factors in the development of age-related eye disease. Asia Pac J Clin Nutr 2003;12(suppl):S5.

Rousseau AS, Hininger I, Palazzetti S, Faure H, Roussel AM, Margaritis I. Antioxidant vitamin status in high exposure to oxidative stress in competitive athletes. Br J Nutr 2004;92(3):461–468.

Sackett CS, Schenning S. The age-related eye disease study: the results of the clinical trial. Insight 2002;27(1):5–7.

Schunemann HJ, Grant BJ, Freudenheim JL, Muti P, Browne RW, Drake JA, Klocke RA, Trevisan M. The relation of serum levels of antioxidant vitamins C and E, retinol and carotenoids with pulmonary function in the general population. Am J Respir Crit Care Med 2001;163(5):1246–1255.

Singh RB, Ghosh S, Niaz MA, Singh R, Beegum R, Chibo H, Shoumin Z, Postiglione A. Dietary intake, plasma levels of antioxidant vitamins, and oxidative stress in relation to coronary artery disease in elderly subjects. Am J Cardiol 1995;76(17):1233–1238.

Singh RB, Niaz MA, Bishnoi I, Sharma JP, Gupta S, Rastogi SS, Singh R, Begum R, Chibo H, Shoumin Z. Diet, antioxidant vitamins, oxidative stress and risk of coronary artery disease: the Peerzada Prospective Study. Acta Cardiol 1994;49(5):453–467.

Ward JA. Should antioxidant vitamins be routinely recommended for older people? Drugs Aging 1998;12(3):169–175.

Wolters M, Hermann S, Hahn A. Effects of 6-month multivitamin supplementation on serum concentrations of alpha-tocopherol, beta-carotene, and vitamin C in healthy elderly women. Int J Vitam Nutr Res 2004;74(2):161–168.

Wood LG, Fitzgerald DA, Lee AK, Garg ML. Improved antioxidant and fatty acid status of patients with cystic fibrosis after antioxidant supplementation is linked to improved lung function. Am J Clin Nutr 2003;77(1):150–159.

Yu BP, Kang CM, Han JS, Kim DS. Can antioxidant supplementation slow the aging process? Biofactors 1998;7(1–2):93–101.

β CAROTENE

Overall Rank

★★★★★ for correcting vitamin A deficiency
★★★★ for cellular protection (antioxidant effect)
★★★ for anticancer effects

OVERVIEW

β Carotene is one of the carotenoids, a large family of compounds with more than 600 members, including lycopene and lutein. Carotenoids are widely distributed in fruits and vegetables and are responsible, along with flavonoids, for contributing the color to many plants (a rule of thumb is the brighter the fruit or vegetable, the higher the content of flavonoids and carotenoids). In terms of nutrition, β carotene's primary role is as a precursor to vitamin A (the body can convert β carotene into vitamin A as it is needed). It is important to note that although β carotene and vitamin A are described together in many nutrition texts, they are not the same compound and they have vastly different effects in the body and important differences in terms of safety. β Carotene, like most carotenoids, is also a powerful antioxidant; therefore, it has been recommended to protect against various diseases, including cancer, cataracts, and heart disease. The best food sources are brightly colored fruits and vegetables, such as cantaloupe, apricots, carrots, red peppers, sweet potatoes, and dark leafy greens.

Evidence from population studies suggests that obtaining carotenoids from various food sources (i.e., eating lots of fruits and vegetables) can help protect against many forms of cancer and heart disease as well as slow the progression of eye diseases such as cataracts and macular degeneration (Daviglus, 1996; van Poppel, 1996). It is logical (perhaps) to assume that β carotene (which is the primary carotenoid in the diet), an antioxidant, may be responsible for a significant portion of the observed beneficial health effects of carotenoid-rich diets. It is not logical, however, to then assume that high doses of isolated β-carotene supplements will deliver the same anticancer and cardioprotective effects observed with diets high in fruits and vegetables.

COMMENTS

β-Carotene supplements are relatively inexpensive and widely available. The source of a β carotene supplement can be either natural or synthetic. The natural forms typically come from algae (*Dunaliella salina*), fungi (*Blakeslea trispora*), or palm oil. In terms of conversion to vitamin A, the "trans" form of β carotene has the maximum conversion rate. Synthetic β carotene is nearly all in the trans form (98%), while natural forms vary in the form of β carotene that they provide (the different forms are known as isomers). Among natural forms of β carotene, the fungal form provides the highest concentration of trans β carotene (94%), followed by algae sources (64%) and palm oil sources (34%). Therefore, from the perspective of vitamin A conversion, either the synthetic form or the fungal form of β carotene will provide the highest conversion into active vitamin A. From a "mixed" carotenoid perspective, however, β carotene derived from algae also provides the "cis" isomer of β carotene (about 31%) as well as α carotene (3–4%) and other carotenoids (1–2%). β Carotene derived from palm oil provides the most "balanced" mixture of carotenoid isomers (34% trans-β, 27% cis-β, 30% α, and 9% other carotenoids), but it also has the lowest vitamin A conversion (because it provides only 34% as the trans form).

Based on current evidence (Nelson, 2003; Paolini, 2003; Pryor, 2000), β carotene supplements should be used primarily as a way to supply adequate levels of vitamin A for proper nutrition, not for prevention of cancer, heart disease, or eye problems (although a "dietary" level of mixed carotenoids of up to 10 mg/day probably poses no significant health risk). There may also be some benefit in consuming β carotene supplements for skin protection (reduced risk of sunburn), but this effect may be more pronounced when taken in conjunction with other antioxidants such as lycopene, lutein, selenium, and vitamins C and E.

SCIENTIFIC SUPPORT

It is important to note that most of the scientific evidence for the health benefits of β carotene comes from studies that looked at food sources of β carotene (and other carotenoids, often referred to as "mixed" carotenoids), not supplements. From population (epidemiological) studies, we know that a high consumption of fruits and vegetables is associated with a significant reduction in many diseases, especially several forms of cancer (lung, stomach, colon, breast, prostate, and bladder). Because the data suggest that the "active" components in a plant-based diet may be carotenoids, and because β carotene is the chief carotenoid in our diets, it was widely believed (until about the mid-1990s) that most of the health benefits attributable to fruits and vegetables may be owing to β carotene.

One of the largest epidemiological studies, the Physicians' Health Study (PHS, comprising more than 22,000 male physicians) found that although high levels of carotenoids obtained from the diet were associated with reduced cancer risk, β carotene from supplements (about 25 mg/day) had no effect on cancer risk (Comstock et al., 1997). A possible explanation for this finding may be that although purified β carotene may contribute some antioxidant benefits, a blend of carotenoids (and/ or other compounds in fruits and vegetables) is probably even more important for preventing cancer. It may even be possible that isolated β carotene supplements interfere with absorption or metabolism of other beneficial carotenoids from the diet.

Unfortunately, intervention studies that have looked at purified β carotene supplements (not mixed carotenoids) have not cleared up any of the confusion. In 1994, the results from a large (almost 30,000 subjects) supplementation study (Alpha-Tocopherol and Beta-Carotene [ATBC] Study) showed that β carotene supplements (20 mg/day for 5–8 years) not only failed to prevent lung cancer in high-risk subjects (long-time male smokers) but actually caused an increase in lung cancer risk by almost 20% (Pietinen et al., 1997). The ATBC Study also found a 10% increase in heart disease and a 20% increase in strokes among the β carotene users. In 1996, another large study (Carotene and Retinol Efficacy Trial [CARET]) found virtually the same thing, with subjects receiving β carotene showing almost 50% more cases of lung cancer (Goodman et al., 1996). These results were so alarming that the National Cancer Institute decided to halt the $40 million study nearly 2 years early. The ATBC Study examined long-time heavy smokers, while the CARET looked at present and former smokers as well as workers exposed to asbestos—all of whom can be considered at high risk for developing lung cancer (which may or may not have contributed to the surprising study results).

On the positive side, β carotene has been successfully used for nearly 20 years to treat photosensitivity diseases, such as erythropoietic protoporphyria and other skin conditions (Malvy et al., 2001). Therefore, β carotene has found its way into a variety of topical and internally consumed products meant for skin protection. In Europe, one of the most popular uses for carotenoid supplements (primarily β carotene and lycopene) is for skin protection during the summer sunbathing months (for "inside-out" sun protection).

Overall, it is interesting to note that all three large-scale clinical trials on β carotene supplementation and cancer risk (PHS, ATBC, and CARET) concluded that β carotene provided no protection against lung cancer and two found a higher risk for lung cancer. The association between eating a diet high in fruits and vegetables and a reduced risk for cancer and heart disease remains strong, however, and there is no current evidence that small amounts of supplemental β carotene (such as a multivitamin) is unsafe. A prudent approach to carotenoid supplementation for disease prevention may be to strive to obtain a balanced blend of mixed carotenoids from foods, while reserving purified β carotene supplements for skin protection and as a source of vitamin A (see dosage suggestions in the next section).

SAFETY/DOSAGE

At recommended dosages, β carotene is thought to be quite safe, although at least two large studies have shown that high-dose β carotene (20–50 mg/day) can increase the risk of heart disease and cancer in smokers (Goodmanm, 1996; Pietinen, 1997). Other reported side effects from high-dose β carotene supplements (100,000 IU or 60 mg daily) include nausea, diarrhea, and a yellow-orange tinge to the skin (especially hands and feet), which fades at lower doses. The safest way to obtain β carotene and other carotenoids is from eating a wide variety of fruits and vegetables.

The trans form of β carotene can be converted to vitamin A (3 mg of β carotene supplies 5,000 IU of vitamin A). Although β carotene supplements are commonly available in doses of 25,000 IU (15 mg) per day, and many people consume as much as 100,000 IU (60 mg) per day, the scientific literature does not support doses of β carotene much higher than the levels recommended for supplying vitamin A precursors (about 5,000–10,000 IU/day of β carotene, or 3–6 mg/day).

REFERENCES

Comstock GW, Alberg AJ, Huang HY, Wu K, Burke AE, Hoffman SC, Norkus EP, Gross M, Cutler RG, Morris JS, Spate VL, Helzlsouer KJ. The risk of developing lung cancer associated with antioxidants in the blood: ascorbic acid, carotenoids, alpha-tocopherol, selenium, and total peroxyl radical absorbing capacity. Cancer Epidemiol Biomarkers Prev 1997;6(11):907–916.

Daviglus ML, Dyer AR, Persky V, Chavez N, Drum M, Goldberg J, Liu K, Morris DK, Shekelle RB, Stamler J. Dietary beta-carotene, vitamin C, and risk of prostate cancer: results from the Western Electric Study. Epidemiology 1996;7(5):472–477.

Goodman GE, Thornquist M, Kestin M, Metch B, Anderson G, Omenn GS. The association between participant characteristics and serum concentrations of beta-carotene, retinol, retinyl palmitate, and alpha-tocopherol among participants in the Carotene and Retinol Efficacy Trial (CARET) for prevention of lung cancer. Cancer Epidemiol Biomarkers Prev 1996;5(10):815–821.

Malvy DJ, Favier A, Faure H, Preziosi P, Galan P, Arnaud J, Roussel AM, Briancon S, Hercberg S. Effect of two years' supplementation with natural antioxidants on vitamin and trace element status biomarkers: preliminary data of the SU.VI.MAX study. Cancer Detect Prev 2001;25(5):479–485.

Nelson JL, Bernstein PS, Schmidt MC, Von Tress MS, Askew EW. Dietary modification and moderate antioxidant supplementation differentially affect serum carotenoids, antioxidant levels and markers of oxidative stress in older humans. J Nutr 2003;133(10):3117–3123.

Paolini M, Abdel-Rahman SZ, Sapone A, Pedulli GF, Perocco P, Cantelli-Forti G, Legator MS. Beta-carotene: a cancer chemopreventive agent or a co-carcinogen? Mutat Res 2003;543(3):195–200.

Pietinen P, Ascherio A, Korhonen P, Hartman AM, Willett WC, Albanes D, Virtamo J. Intake of fatty acids and risk of coronary heart disease in a cohort of Finnish men. The Alpha-Tocopherol, Beta-Carotene Cancer Prevention Study. Am J Epidemiol 1997;145(10):876–887.

Pryor WA, Stahl W, Rock CL. Beta carotene: from biochemistry to clinical trials. Nutr Rev 2000;58(2 pt 1):39–53.

ADDITIONAL RESOURCES

Collins AR, Olmedilla B, Southon S, Granado F, Duthie SJ. Serum carotenoids and oxidative DNA damage in human lymphocytes. Carcinogenesis 1998;19(12):2159–2162.

Hininger IA, Meyer-Wenger A, Moser U, Wright A, Southon S, Thurnham D, Chopra M, Van Den Berg H, Olmedilla B, Favier AE, Roussel AM. No significant effects of lutein, lycopene or beta-carotene supplementation on biological markers of oxidative stress and LDL oxidizability in healthy adult subjects. J Am Coll Nutr 2001;20(3):232–238.

Kiokias S, Gordon MH. Dietary supplementation with a natural carotenoid mixture decreases oxidative stress. Eur J Clin Nutr 2003;57(9):1135–1140.

Malila N, Virtamo J, Virtanen M, Pietinen P, Albanes D, Teppo L. Dietary and serum alpha-tocopherol, beta-carotene and retinol, and risk for colorectal cancer in male smokers. Eur J Clin Nutr 2002;56(7):615–621.

Vainio H. Chemoprevention of cancer: lessons to be learned from beta-carotene trials. Toxicol Lett 2000;112–113:513–517.

van Poppel G. Epidemiological evidence for beta-carotene in prevention of cancer and cardiovascular disease. Eur J Clin Nutr 1996;50(suppl 3):S57–S61.

Woodall AA, Britton G, Jackson MJ. Dietary supplementation with carotenoids: effects on alpha-tocopherol levels and susceptibility of tissues to oxidative stress. Br J Nutr 1996;76(2):307–317.

Woutersen RA, Wolterbeek AP, Appel MJ, van den Berg H, Goldbohm RA, Feron VJ. Safety evaluation of synthetic beta-carotene. Crit Rev Toxicol 1999;29(6):515–542.

BILBERRY (*VACCINIUM MYRTILLUS* L.)

Overall Rank

★★★★ as an antioxidant
★★★★ for peripheral vascular disorders
★★★★ for eye health
★★★ for diabetic retinopathy
★★ for diarrhea

OVERVIEW

Bilberry is a good example of an herbal medicine that is representative of a trend in the interest in fruits with high anthocyanin content. Not only are these supplements and foods safe, but they are potent antioxidants of a class that are just beginning to be understood and appreciated. Many anthocyanin antioxidant compounds also help maintain vascular, cardiovascular, and eye health. Bilberry's main active components are the flavonoids called anthocyanidins, of which there are many in bilberry, and the carotenoids (zeaxanthin and lutein; McKenna et al., 2001).

Bilberry has been used in several therapeutic applications because of its wide range of activities. Bilberry has been reported to be vasoprotective, antiedemic, antioxidant, anti-inflammatory, antiulcer, and astringent. The anthocyanosides in bilberry are known to exhibit many functions, including stabilizing and reinforcing collagen, decreasing capillary permeability, relaxing smooth musculature, increasing urinary output, and increasing the contractile strength of the myocardium. A few of the key preclinical studies are listed here (McKenna et al., 2001):

- An extract of bilberry was tested for its effects on microvascular permeability in a hamster cheek pouch model of ischemia reperfusion injury. Bilberry caused a significant reduction in microvascular impairment, preservation of arteriolar tone, reduced number of leukocytes adhering to venular walls, preservation of capillary perfusion, and an increase in microvascular permeability (Bertuglia et al., 1995).
- Detre et al. (1986) tested the effect of bilberry on vascular permeability in rats with induced hypertension. Bilberry was found to bring the vascular permeability, which is increased in hypertensive states, back to normal levels in the hypertensive rat model.
- Bilberry has been shown to have antiaggregation activity similar to acetylsalicylic acid. In a study with 30 volunteers, bilberry was shown to inhibit aggregation at days 30 and 60 but return to normal after day 120. This study supported the theory that bilberry's action depends on an increase in cyclic adenosine monophosphate and/or platelet thromboxane A_2 (Pulliero et al., 1989).
- Bilberry has been found to exhibit a protective effect on the capillary walls by stabilizing membrane phospholipids and by increasing connective tissue biosynthesis (Mian et al., 1977).
- Bilberry has exhibited antioxidant activity in a number of antioxidant models. An extract in mice with induced liver peroxidation showed significant antioxidant activity at doses of 250 and 500 mg/kg administered orally (Martín-Aragón et al., 1999).

COMMENTS

Bilberry seems to be a safe and efficacious preventative to degenerating vascular illnesses, and an excellent dietetic aid for diabetics for the prevention of macular degeneration. As people in the United States age, they are sure to need safe, effective supplements to help prevent age-related degeneration, and bilberry appears to be such a supplement.

SCIENTIFIC SUPPORT

When administered to pregnant patients exhibiting venous insufficiency of the lower limbs or acute hemorrhoids, bilberry extract (Tegens, 160 mg, 240 mg, or 340 mg daily) caused a progressive amelioration of symptoms during the 3 month of treatment. The symptoms were reduced by 94.6% for pruritus, 87.5% for paresthesias, 80.1% for cramps, 78.5% for pain, 60% for exhaustion and the sensation of heaviness, and 75–83% for hemorrhoids. No side effects or adverse reactions were found for either mothers or babies included in the study (Teglio et al., 1987).

Boniface et al. (1985) confirmed pharmacological evidence in experimental studies that bilberry's anthocyanosides reduce the biosynthesis of polymeric collagen and glycoproteins (which are responsible for the vascular complications in diabetics) and compared this with a couple of clinical studies involving diabetics. The clinical studies administered bilberry anthocyanosides to diabetics and found increases in vascular health, thus confirming the pharmacological findings.

Bilberry anthocyanosides (Tegens, 480 mg/day for 30 days) administered to patients with venous diseases characterized by phlebopathic stasis significantly improved measures of venous health compared with conventional treatments. Symptoms monitored were limb heaviness, pain levels, dyschromic and dystrophic skin phenomena, and limb edema (Ghiringhelli et al., 1978).

Patients with retinopathies were administered bilberry anthocyanosides (Tegens, 160 mg/day) in a preliminary study. In the treatment phase of the study, 50% showed improvements versus only 20% in the control group. In patients with hard exudates in the back pole, 35% in the control phase worsened over the course of the study compared with 20% of the treatment group. In patients with circinate disposition of the hard exudates, 15% worsened in the control group versus 10% in the treatment group (Repossi et al., 1987).

Bravetti et al. (1987) examined the effects of anthocyanosides from bilberry extract administered with vitamin E (180 mg of a 25% standardized extract and 100 mg of vitamin E) in patients with mild senile cortical cataracts. The treatment was found to reduce lens opacity in 97% of the cases examined.

A double-blind, placebo-controlled, crossover study examined the effect of bilberry extract (Tegens, 160 mg 2 times daily) in 14 patients with diabetes or hypertension. An improvement of 77–90% in clinical symptoms was found for the patients after 1 month, and bilberry was concluded to be a safe and effective therapy (Perossini et al., 1987).

Anthocyanosides from bilberry (Tegens, 480 mg 3 times daily) were administered to 10 patients with diabetic retinopathy in a pilot study. In the course of the study (6 months) improvements were seen in the retinal picture of all patients. The authors concluded that bilberry has strong promise in the therapy of diabetic retinopathy (Orsucci et al., 1983).

Patients with various retinopathies were administered bilberry (Difarel 100 at 200 mg 3 times daily) and showed improvements in their conditions. The authors noted that improvements in the hemorrhagic tendency and vascular permeability were seen in all participants but were most evident in those with diabetic retinopathy (Scharrer and Ober, 1981).

Bilberry extract was administered to normal subjects at 300 mg/day in a placebo-controlled study. Significant improvements were found in measures of visual health: adaptive ability to light and dark, macular recuperation time, and chromatic discrimination (Sala et al., 1979).

An anthocyanoside-rich extract of bilberry was administered to 40 normal subjects in a placebo-controlled trial to test its effect on various aspects of visual health. In the treatment group, improvements were found in all tested visual functions, including darkness adaptation, macular sensitivity, and adaptocinematographic thresholds compared with placebo (Jayle and Aubert, 1964).

Under conditions of food rationing and little or no fruits available during World War II, British Royal Air Force pilots were reported to use bilberry to improve their night vision. Subsequently, numerous clinical studies were performed to try to confirm this effect (McKenna et al., 2001). In one study, the long-term administration of a bilberry extract (Difrarel 100, 100 mg of anthocyanosides and 0.005 β carotene, 4 tablets daily for 8 days) showed improvements in the visual functions of 14 air traffic controllers. The results found decreased dazzling effect, decreased visual fatigue, and a quicker adaptation of scotopic vision (Belleoud et al., 1966).

SAFETY/DOSAGE

Bilberry dosages are usually recommended in the range of 240–640 mg/day for most uses (usually 500 mg) and less than 300 mg/day for eye health. Bilberry extracts are typically based on anthocyanoside content, and a 25% standardized extract is the standard preparation (McKenna et al., 2001):

Bilberry is quite safe because it is a traditional food. The only reported side effects of bilberry have been digestive disturbances; these effects, however, have not yet been clearly investigated, and it is possible that most of these reports were idiosyncratic. Furthermore, bilberry is often formulated with minerals, which are known to cause some digestive disturbance when taken without food (McKenna et al., 2001).

Very high doses of bilberry have a blood-thinning action and should be avoided by patients using warfarin or antiplatelet drugs (McKenna et al., 2001).

REFERENCES

Belleoud L, Leluan D, Boyer Y. Study on the effects of anthocyanin glucosides on the nocturnal vision of air traffic controllers. Revue de Medecine Aeronautique et Spatiale 1966;3:45.

Bertuglia S, Malandrino S, Colantuoni A. Effect of Vaccinium myrtillus anthocyanosides on ischaemia reperfusion injury in hamster cheek pouch microcirculation. Pharmacol Res 1995;31(3–4):183–187.

Boniface R, Miskulin M, Robert L. Pharmacological properties of myrtillus anthocyanosides: correlation with results of treatment of diabetic microangiopathy. In: Farkas, L, Gabor M, and Kallay F, eds. Flavonoids and Bioflavonoids. Ireland: Elsevier, 1985:293–301.

Bravetti GO, Fraboni E, Maccolini E. Preventive medical treatment of senile cataract with vitamin E and Vaccinium myrtillus anthocyanosides: clinical evaluation. Annali di Ottalmologia e Clinica Oculistica 1987;115:109–116.

Detre Z, Jellinek H, Miskulin M, Robert AM. Studies on vascular permeability in hypertension: action of anthocyanosides. Clin Physiol Biochem 1986;4(2):143–149.

Ghiringhelli C, Gregoratti L, Marastoni F. Capillarotropic action of anthocyanosides in high dosage in phlebopathic statis. Minerva Cardioangiol 1978;26(4):255–276.

Jayle GE, Aubert L. Action of anthocyanin glycosides on the scotopic and mesopic vision of the normal subject. Therapie 1964;19:171–185.

Martín-Aragón S, Basabe B, Benedi JM et al. In vitro and in vivo antioxidant properties of Vaccinium myrtillus. Pharmaceutical Biology1999; 37:109–113.

McKenna DJ, Jones K, Hughes K, eds. Botanical Medicines: A Desktop Reference for the Major Herbal Supplements. New York: Haworth Press, 2001.

Mian E, Curri SB, Lietti A, et al. Anthocyanosides and microvessels wall: new findings on the mechanism of action of their protective effect in syndromes caused by abnormal capillary fragility. Minerva Medica 1977;68:3565–3581.

Orsucci, PL, et al. Treatment of diabetic retinopathy with anthocyanosides: a preliminary report. Clin Oc 1983;5:377.

Perossini M, Guidi G, Chiellini S. et al. Diabetic and hypertensive retinopathy therapy with Vaccinium myrtillus anthocyanosides (Tegens): double-blind, placebo-controlled clinical trial. Annali di Ottalmologia e Clinica Oculistica 1987;113:1173–1190.

Pulliero G, Montin S, Bettini V, et al. Ex vivo study of the inhibitory effects of Vaccinium myrtillus anthocyanosides on human platelet aggregation. Fitoterapia 1989;55:69–74.

Repossi P, Malagola R, De Cadilhac C. The role of anthocyanosides on vascular permeability in diabetic retinopathy. Annali di Ottalmologia e Clinica Oculistica 1987;113:357.

Sala D, Rolando M, Rossi PL, et al. Effect of anthocyanosides on visual performance at low illumination. Minerva Oftalmol 1979;21:283–285.

Scharrer A, Ober M. Anthocyanosides in the treatment of retinopathies. Klinische Monatsblatter für Augenheilkunde 1981;178:386–389.

Teglio L, Mazzanti C, Tronconi T, et al. Vaccinium myrtillus anthocyanosides (Tegens) in the treatment of venous insufficiency of the lower limbs and acute hemorrhoids in pregnancy. Quaderni di Clinica Ostertrica e Ginecologica 1987;42:221–231.

GRAPE SEED (*VITIS VINIFERA*)

Overall Rank

★★★★ as an antioxidant

★★★★ for cardioprotective and circulatory benefits (capillary reinforcement, collagen protection, vasorelaxation)

★★★★ for treating and preventing varicose veins

OVERVIEW

Grape seed extract is mostly used for its antioxidant qualities and for its numerous cardioprotective and circulatory benefits. In 2003, grape seed extract attained generally recognized as safe (GRAS) status with the Food and Drug Administration and is therefore expected to become more popular in functional foods. The active constituents of grape seed extract are proanthocyanidins, the procyanidin oligomers (PCOs). Grape seed or PCO extracts normally contain a mixture of PCOs of varying lengths (dimers, trimers, tetramers, and oligomers of up to seven units).

Grape seed extract has been confirmed in both preclinical and clinical studies to be a potent antioxidant, and it has good clinical evidence of its usefulness in preventing and ameliorating cardiovascular and circulatory disorders. Grape seed extract and the PCOs from grape seed have been studied in animals and in vitro to confirm the cardioprotective, circulatory, and antioxidant benefits found from traditional use. Some of the key preclinical studies are listed here:

- Rabbits fed grape seed extracts in cholesterol-enriched diets showed significant decrease in cholesteryl ester hydroperoxides compared with the controls fed cholesterol-enriched diets alone. The rabbits in the grape seed extract group also showed significantly fewer atherosclerotic plaques in their aortic arch, a significant decrease in the total cholesterol and malondialdehyde contents in the aortic arch and thoracic aorta, and a decrease in the number of foam cells in oxidized low-density lipoprotein (LDL)–positive cells of the atherosclerotic lesions (Yamakoshi et al., 1999).
- The cardioprotective effects of PCOs were found to be mediated by scavenging of oxygen-centered radicals (hydroxyl and peroxyl) and sequestering of the cations Fe+2 and Cu+2, which enhance the formation of harmful hydroxyl radicals when triggered by superoxide/hydrogen peroxide (Maffei Facinó et al., 1996).
- The cardioprotective benefits of grape seed extract were shown in rats. Compared with controls, the rats fed the grape seed extract showed a significantly faster recovery time from myocardial infarction, significantly smaller infarct mass and size, and higher aortic flow (Sato et al., 1999).
- Jonadet et al. (1983) found that grape seed showed the highest in vitro elastase-inhibiting activities compared with bilberry and pine park. Elastase is involved with the destruction of elastic fibers and conjunctive tissue.
- Procyanidins from grape seed are known to inhibit lipid peroxidation because they are effective scavengers of superoxide anion, hydroxyl radical anion, and lipid peroxyl radicals (Maffei Facinó et al., 1996; Meunier et al., 1989).
- Procyanidins also indirectly have antioxidant functions by inhibiting oxidation of LDL catalyzed by Cu+2 (Frankel et al., 1993).

COMMENTS

Grape seed is a good example of a nontoxic (GRAS) botanical that has several benefits in supplementing the diet. It has confirmed use as an antioxidant, as a cardioprotectant, and for circulatory health and would make an excellent daily addition to the standard American diet.

SCIENTIFIC SUPPORT

Peripheral Vascular Benefits

Retinopathies were studied by (1) a controlled study of 75 patients with ocular stress caused by a visual display unit and (2) a study of 91 myopic patients. Procyanidins (300 mg/day for 60 days) caused significant improvement of subjective symptoms and contrast sensitivity relative to the control group in study 1. In study 2, retinal function was reported to have improved from administration of 300 mg/day of procyanidins for 28 days (Bombardelli and Morazzoni, 1995).

A double-blind, placebo-controlled study of 92 patients with peripheral venous insufficiency found procyanidins (300 mg/day for 28 days) effective in 75% of the patients. Procyanidin treatment was found to improve the functional measures of venous insufficiency (pain, paresthesias, nocturnal cramps, edema, etc.) by more than 50% (Bombardelli and Morazzoni, 1995).

Visual adaptation to low-intensity light (night morphoscopic vision) and visual performance following glare was improved in patients given a grape seed extract (Endotelon, 200 mg/day for 5 weeks). The placebo-controlled study enrolled 100 subjects without ophthalmological pathology (Corbe et al., 1988).

Lesbre and Tigaude (1983) conducted a randomized, placebo-controlled study in 20 patients diagnosed with capillary hyperpermeability and hepatic cirrhosis. The capillary fragility index in the patients given the grape seed extract (150 mg of proanthocyanidins 2 times a day for 8 weeks) was significantly higher than in those given a placebo.

Sarrat (1981) conducted a study on 30 patients without varicose veins for the effect of grape seed extract (150 mg/day for 30 days), Diosamine (a semisynthetic flavonoid product), or placebo on the possible indications that could develop into varicose veins later in life. The grape seed extract significantly lowered the occurrence of indications such as heaviness of the legs, cramps, itching, and abnormal sensations like burning and prickling and the sensation of swelling. The author concluded that grape seed extract might be effective in preventing varicose veins from developing.

In a double-blind study, grape seed extract (Endotelon, 150 mg/day for 30 days) was compared with Diosamine (450 mg/day for 30 days) for its effect on 50 female patients with chronic venous insufficiency (mostly pregnancy related). Although both treatments were effective in reducing the symptoms of chronic venous insufficiency, grape seed extract showed a faster and longer-lasting action. Also, only 45% of the Diosamine group became symptom free compared with 65% of the grape seed extract group (Delacroix, 1981). Royer and Schmidt (1981) showed in a preliminary study that a single oral dose of procyanidins increased objectively the venous tone in patients with widespread varicose veins.

The effect of procyanidins (150 mg/day) in 25 diabetic and hypertensive patients in a double-blind, placebo-controlled study was investigated. Capillary resistance increased 23% in the treatment group. In another study of 28 diabetic and hypertensive patients, capillary resistance was found to increase 18% using a similar dose of procyanidins (Lagrue et al., 1981).

Dartenuc et al. (1980) conducted a double-blind study with standardized grape seed extract in 37 hospitalized patients with capillary fragility. Endotelon was administered at the rate of 50 mg of proanthocyanidins 2 times daily over 15 days. In 10 of 21 patients given the extract and in 3 of 12 on placebo, capillary resistance was improved.

A double-blind, placebo-controlled study of a standardized grape seed extract on 71 patients with peripheral venous insufficiency found grape seed extract to have a significant beneficial effect. Grape seed extract treatment (Endotelon, 100 mg 3 times daily for 28 days) caused significant improvement in symptoms of nocturnal cramps, leg heaviness, edema, and tingling. Improvements were found for 75% of the active treatment group compared with 41% on placebo (Thébaut et al., 1985).

Visual acuity was improved or remained stable in 29 of 30 patients diagnosed with atherosclerotic retinopathy. In this double-blind, placebo-controlled study, the patients were given 100 mg/day of proanthocyanidins or placebo for 1 year (Vérin et al., 1978).

Antioxidant Activity

The antioxidant activity of grape seed extract (300 mg/day for 5 days of a standardized extract with 150 mg of grape procyanidins per capsule) was studied in 20 healthy, nonsmoking adults who all followed a standardized dietary pattern in a single-blinded, randomized, placebo-controlled, crossover study. The mean total antioxidant capacity of the serum of the treatment group was significantly improved compared with baseline and showed no significant change in the placebo group (Nuttall et al., 1998).

SAFETY/DOSAGE

The dosage recommendation of grape seed extract (containing 80–85% procyanidin oligomers) depends on whether the treatment is for preventative or therapeutic purposes. For prevention, 50 mg is recommended (or 125 mg of a bound form such as PCO-phosphatidylcholine). For therapeutic purposes, the dosage should range between 30 mg and 150 mg. Procyanidins have been found to have a synergistic effect with vitamin C (McKenna et al., 2001).

Mild and transient side effects have been found in clinical trials, including mild gastrointestinal discomfort, vertigo, nausea, allergic reactions, and headaches. Some PCOs can produce a platelet antiaggregation activity and therefore would be contraindicated for patients on anticoagulant medications or those about to enter surgery (McKenna et al., 2001).

Procyanidins are thought to be safe during pregnancy because no teratogenic effects were found in pregnant chicks, mice, or rabbits at doses 10 times the normal, and no contraindications were found from clinical studies in humans. No safety data are available on grape seed extract use during lactation (McKenna et al., 2001).

REFERENCES

Bombardelli E, Morazzoni P. Vitis vinifera L. Fitoterapia 1995;66:291–317.

Corbe C, Boissin JP, Siou A. Light vision and chorioretinal circulation. Study of the effect of procyanidolic oligomers (Endotelon). J Fr Ophtalmol 1988;11(5):453–460.

Dartenuc JY, Marache P, Choussat H. Capillary resistance in geriatrics. A study of a microangioprotector = Endotelon. Bordeaux Médical 1980;13:903–907.

Delacroix, P. Double-blind trial of Endotelon in chronic venous insufficiency. La Revue de Médecine 1981;27–28:1793–1802.

Frankel EN, Kanner J, German JB, Parks E, Kinsella JE. Inhibition of oxidation of human low-density lipoprotein by phenolic substances in red wine. Lancet 1993;341(8843):454–457.

Jonadet M, Meunier MT, Bastide J, Bastide P. Anthocyanosides extracted from Vitis vinifera, Vaccinium myrtillus and Pinus maritimus. I. Elastase-inhibiting activities in vitro, II: compared angioprotective activities in vivo. J Pharm Belg 1983;38(1):41–46.

Lagrue G, Olivier-Martin F, Grillot A. A study of the effects of procyanidol oligomers on capillary resistance in hypertension and in certain nephropathies. Sem Hop 1981;57(33–36):1399–1401.

Lesbre FX, Tigaud JD. The effect of Endotelon on the capillary fragility index of a specified controlled group: cirrhosis patients. Gazette Medicale 1983;90:24–28.

Maffei Facinó R, Carini M, Aldini G, Berti F, Rossoni G, Bombardelli E, Morazzoni P. Procyanidines from Vitis vinifera seeds protect rabbit heart from ischemia/reperfusion injury: antioxidant intervention and/or iron and copper sequestering ability. Planta Med 1996;62(6):495–502.

McKenna DJ, Jones K, Hughes K, eds. Botanical Medicines: A Desktop Reference for the Major Herbal Supplements. New York: Haworth Press, 2001.

Meunier MT, Duroux E, Bastide, P. Free-radical scavenging activity of procyanidolic oligomers and anthocyanosides with respect to superoxide anion and lipid peroxidation. Plantes Medicinales et Phytotherapie 1989;23:267–274.

Nuttall SL, Kendall MJ, Bombardelli E, Morazzoni P. An evaluation of the antioxidant activity of a standardized grape seed extract, Leucoselect. J Clin Pharm Ther 1998;23(5):385–389.

Royer RJ, Schmidt CL. Evaluation of venotropic drugs by venous gas plethysmography. A study of procyanidolic oligomers. Sem Hop 1981;57(47–48):2009–2013.

Sato M, Maulik G, Ray PS, Bagchi D, Das DK Cardioprotective effects of grape seed proanthocyanidin against ischemic reperfusion injury. J Mol Cell Cardiol 1999;31(6):1289–1297.

Sarrat L. Therapeutic approach to functional disorders of lower extremities. Bordeaux Medical 1981;14:685.

Thébaut JF, Thébaut P, Vin F. Study of Endotelon in functional manifesations of peripheral venous insufficiency. Results of one double-blind carried out on 92 patients. Gazette Médicale 1985;92:96–100.

Vérin MMP, Vildy A, Maurin JF. Retinopathies and O.P.C. Bordeaux Médical 1978;11:1467–1474.

Yamakoshi J, Kataoka S, Koga T, Ariga T. Proanthocyanidin-rich extract from grape seeds attenuates the development of aortic atherosclerosis in cholesterol-fed rabbits. Atherosclerosis 1999;142(1):139–149.

GREEN TEA (*CAMELLIA SINENSIS*)

Overall Rank

★★★★★ as an antioxidant
★★★★ for anticancer effects
★★★★ for thermogenic benefits (weight loss)
★★★ for energy (as a source of caffeine)

OVERVIEW

Green tea (*Camellia sinensis*) is the second most consumed beverage in the world (water is the first) and has been used medicinally for centuries in India and China. A number of beneficial health effects are attributed to regular consumption of green tea, and dried or powdered extracts of green tea are available as dietary supplements. Green tea is prepared by picking the leaves, lightly steaming them, and allowing them to dry. Black tea, the most popular type of tea in the United States, is made by allowing the leaves to ferment before drying. The fermentation process destroys a portion of the active compounds in black tea, but the compounds in green tea remain active. The active constituents in green tea are a family of polyphenols (catechins) with potent antioxidant activity. Tannins, large polyphenol molecules, form the bulk of the active compounds in green tea, with catechins comprising nearly 90%. Several catechins are present in significant quantities: epicatechin (EC), epigallocatechin (EGC), epicatechin gallate (ECG), and epigallocatechin gallate (EGCG). EGCG makes up about 10–50% of the total catechin content of green tea and appears to be the most powerful of the catechins, with antioxidant activity about 25–100 times more potent than that of vitamins C and E. A cup of green tea may provide 10–40 mg of polyphenols and has antioxidant activity greater than a serving of broccoli, spinach, carrots, or strawberries. A number of commercial green tea extracts are standardized to total polyphenol content and/or EGCG content, and many are marketed with claims for preventing cancer, enhancing immune function, boosting antioxidant protection, reducing cholesterol, and stimulating weight loss.

COMMENTS

Green tea consumed either as a beverage or as a daily dietary supplement is especially beneficial for persons at high risk for cancer (e.g., family history) or those undergoing or recovering from chemotherapy or radiation treatment. Green tea is also beneficial as a general protective measure and dietary "insurance" of adequate polyphenol intake (which would otherwise be obtained from a diet high in fruits and vegetables). Recent data provide strong evidence that green tea may be effective in stimulating thermogenesis, increasing caloric expenditure, promoting fat oxidation, and controlling body weight (Chantre, 2002; Dulloo, 1999; Dulloo, 2000; Komatsu, 2003; Kovacs, 2004).

SCIENTIFIC SUPPORT

Because the active compounds, the catechins, found in green tea are known to possess potent antioxidant activity, they may provide beneficial health effects by protecting the body from oxidative damage from free radicals. A number of chronic disease states have been associated with free radical–induced oxidative damage, including cancer, heart disease, suppressed immune function, and accelerated aging.

Although numerous laboratory investigations have shown the powerful antioxidant activity of green tea and green tea extracts (August et al., 1999; Benzie et al., 1999), prospective clinical studies in humans are few (Hakim et al., 2003, 2004). From the laboratory findings, it is clear that green tea is an effective antioxidant, that it provides clear protection from experimentally induced DNA damage, and that it can slow or halt the initiation and progression of cancerous tumor growth (Ahn et al., 2003). There is also evidence from some studies that green tea provides significant immunoprotective qualities, particularly in the case of cancer patients undergoing radiation or chemotherapy (Elmets et al., 2001; Pisters et al., 2001). White blood cell counts appear to be maintained more effectively in cancer patients consuming green tea compared with nonsupplemented patients.

Several epidemiological studies show an association between consumption of total flavonoids in the diet and the risk for cancer and heart disease. Men with the highest consumption of flavonoids (from fruits and vegetables) have approximately half the risk of heart disease and cancer compared with those with the lowest intake. The primary catechin in green tea, EGCG, appears to inhibit the growth of cancer cells as well as play a role in stimulating apoptosis (programmed cell death), both of which are crucial aspects for cancer prevention (Pisters et al., 2001; Weisburger et al., 1998).

In terms of heart disease protection, the potent antioxidant properties of polyphenols would be expected to reduce free-radical damage to cells and prevent the oxidation of LDL cholesterol, both of which would be expected to inhibit the formation of atherosclerotic plaques (Hodgson et al., 2000).

Aside from the clear benefits of green tea as an antioxidant, studies have suggested a role of catechins in promoting weight loss. Animal studies have shown green tea (and oolong tea) to suppress food intake, body weight gain, and fat tissue accumulation, while human studies have shown increases in metabolic rate and better weight maintenance following weight loss (Komatsu et al., 2003; Kovacs et al., 2004).

In some studies, green tea is associated with a mild increase in thermogenesis (increased caloric expenditure), which is generally attributed to its caffeine content. A handful of studies, however, have shown that green tea extract stimulates thermogenesis to an extent much greater than can be attributed directly to its caffeine content alone, meaning that the thermogenic properties of green tea may be the result of an interaction between caffeine and its high content of catechin polyphenols (Chantre and Lairon et al., 2002; Dulloo et al., 1999). A probable reason for the thermogenic effect of green tea is an increase in levels of norepinephrine, because catechin polyphenols are known to inhibit catechol-O-methyl-transferase (the enzyme that degrades norepinephrine). One study examined this possibility and the effect of green tea extract on 24-hour energy expenditures in 10 healthy men, each of whom consumed three treatments of green tea extract (50 mg of caffeine and 90 mg of epigallocatechin gallate), caffeine (50 mg), or a placebo at breakfast, lunch, and dinner (Dulloo et al., 1999). The results of the study showed that, compared with the placebo, the green tea extract resulted in a significant (4%) increase in 24-hour energy expenditure (approximately 80 calories per day) and a significant increase in the body's use of fat as an energy source (24-hour respiratory quotient). In addition, the 24-hour urinary norepinephrine excretion was 40% higher during treatment with the green tea extract than with the placebo. It is interesting to note that treatment with caffeine in amounts equivalent to those found in the green tea extract (50 mg) had no effect on energy expenditure or fat oxidation, suggesting that the thermogenic properties of green tea stem from compounds other than its caffeine content alone (Komatsu et al., 2003; Kovacs et al., 2004).

SAFETY/DOSAGE

Green tea consumption of as much as 20 cups per day has not been associated with any significant side effects. In high doses, however, teas that contain caffeine may lead to restlessness, insomnia, heart palpitations, and tachycardia (rapid heartbeat). Decaffeinated versions of green tea and green tea extracts are available, but owing to differences in caffeine extraction methods, the amounts of phenolic and catechin compounds can vary among extracts. In addition, people taking aspirin or other anticoagulant agents (including vitamin E and *Ginkgo biloba*) on a daily basis should be aware of the possible inhibition of platelet aggregation (blood clotting) associated with green tea (in some cases, green tea may prolong bleeding times). Typical dosage recommendations are for 100–500 mg/day, preferably of an extract standardized to at least 40% polyphenols and/or EGCG as a marker compound (roughly equivalent to 4–10 cups of brewed green tea).

REFERENCES

Ahn WS, Yoo J, Huh SW, Kim CK, Lee JM, Namkoong SE, Bae SM, Lee IP. Protective effects of green tea extracts (polyphenon E and EGCG) on human cervical lesions. Eur J Cancer Prev 2003;12(5):383–390.

August DA, Landau J, Caputo D, Hong J, Lee MJ, Yang CS. Ingestion of green tea rapidly decreases prostaglandin E2 levels in rectal mucosa in humans. Cancer Epidemiol Biomarkers Prev 1999;8(8):709–713.

Benzie IF, Szeto YT, Strain JJ, Tomlinson B. Consumption of green tea causes rapid increase in plasma antioxidant power in humans. Nutr Cancer 1999;34(1):83–87.

Chantre P, Lairon D. Recent findings of green tea extract AR25 (Exolise) and its activity for the treatment of obesity. Phytomedicine 2002;9(1):3–8.

Dulloo AG, Duret C, Rohrer D, Girardier L, Mensi N, Fathi M, Chantre P, Vandermander J. Efficacy of a green tea extract rich in catechin polyphenols and caffeine in increasing 24-h energy expenditure and fat oxidation in humans. Am J Clin Nutr 1999;70(6):1040–1045.

Dulloo AG, Seydoux J, Girardier L, Chantre P, Vandermander J. Green tea and thermogenesis: interactions between catechin-polyphenols, caffeine and sympathetic activity. Int J Obes Relat Metab Disord 2000;24(2):252–258.

Elmets CA, Singh D, Tubesing K, Matsui M, Katiyar S, Mukhtar H. Cutaneous photoprotection from ultraviolet injury by green tea polyphenols. J Am Acad Dermatol 2001;44(3):425–432.

Hakim IA, Harris RB, Brown S, Chow HH, Wiseman S, Agarwal S, Talbot W. Effect of increased tea consumption on oxidative DNA damage among smokers: a randomized controlled study. J Nutr 2003;133(10):3303S–3309S.

Hakim IA, Harris RB, Chow HH, Dean M, Brown S, Ali IU. Effect of a 4-month tea intervention on oxidative DNA damage among heavy smokers: role of glutathione S-transferase genotypes. Cancer Epidemiol Biomarkers Prev 2004;13(2):242–249.

Hodgson JM, Puddey IB, Croft KD, Burke V, Mori TA, Caccetta RA, Beilin LJ. Acute effects of ingestion of black and green tea on lipoprotein oxidation. Am J Clin Nutr 2000;71(5):1103–1107.

Komatsu T, Nakamori M, Komatsu K, Hosoda K, Okamura M, Toyama K, Ishikura Y, Sakai T, Kunii D, Yamamoto S. Oolong tea increases energy metabolism in Japanese females. J Med Invest 2003;50(3–4):170–175.

Kovacs EM, Lejeune MP, Nijs I, Westerterp-Plantenga MS. Effects of green tea on weight maintenance after body-weight loss. Br J Nutr 2004;91(3):431–437.

Pisters KM, Newman RA, Coldman B, Shin DM, Khuri FR, Hong WK, Glisson BS, Lee JS. Phase I trial of oral green tea extract in adult patients with solid tumors. J Clin Oncol 2001;19(6):1830–1838.

Weisburger JH, Rivenson A, Aliaga C, Reinhardt J, Kelloff GJ, Boone CW, Steele VE, Balentine DA, Pittman B, Zang E. Effect of tea extracts, polyphenols, and epigallocatechin gallate on azoxymethane-induced colon cancer. Proc Soc Exp Biol Med 1998;217(1):104–108.

ADDITIONAL RESOURCES

Chow HH, Cai Y, Alberts DS, Hakim I, Dorr R, Shahi F, Crowell JA, Yang CS, Hara Y. Phase I pharmacokinetic study of tea polyphenols following single-dose administration of epigallocatechin gallate and polyphenon E. Cancer Epidemiol Biomarkers Prev 2001;10(1):53–58.

Gupta S, Ahmad N, Mohan RR, Husain MM, Mukhtar H. Prostate cancer chemoprevention by green tea: in vitro and in vivo inhibition of testosterone-mediated induction of ornithine decarboxylase. Cancer Res 1999;59(9):2115–2120.

Lin JK, Liang YC, Lin-Shiau SY. Cancer chemoprevention by tea polyphenols through mitotic signal transduction blockade. Biochem Pharmacol 1999;58(6):911–915.

Maron DJ, Lu GP, Cai NS, Wu ZG, Li YH, Chen H, Zhu JQ, Jin XJ, Wouters BC, Zhao J. Cholesterol-lowering effect of a theaflavin-enriched green tea extract: a randomized controlled trial. Arch Intern Med 2003;163(12):1448–1453.

LUTEIN AND ZEAXANTHIN

Overall Rank

★★★★ for general eye health
★★★★ for prevention of age-related macular degeneration (ARMD)

OVERVIEW

Lutein and zeaxanthin are carotenoids found in highest concentrations in the macular region of the eyes (the back of the eye where the retina is located), where they are believed to help filter out damaging blue light and prevent free-radical damage to the delicate structures in the back of the eye. Dietary supplements containing lutein and zeaxanthin are commonly recommended to help prevent age-related macular degeneration (ARMD) and the development of glaucoma and cataracts.

Because antioxidants can provide increased protection against the oxidizing ultraviolet (UV) radiation of the sun, anybody that spends time outdoors exposed to the sun should be concerned about the potential for UV radiation to damage eye health and impact vision. Lutein and zeaxanthin are the only carotenoids that become concentrated in the retinal region of the eye known as the macula. High dietary intake of lutein-rich fruits and vegetables (yellow and dark green) has been associated with a significant reduction in macular degeneration, the leading cause of blindness in Americans over the age of 65.

COMMENTS

Dietary supplements containing lutein and zeaxanthin are available from a number of manufacturers as an alternative for people not able or willing to increase their consumption of brightly colored fruits and vegetables. The supplement should deliver an effective level of lutein (about 4–6 mg/day). Lutein is now being added to national brands of multivitamins, but most provide only 250 µg or less of lutein—more than 20 times less than the levels shown to be effective in preventing ARMD and even several times below levels that could reasonably be achieved in the diet from a high intake of fruits and vegetables.

SCIENTIFIC SUPPORT

Lutein and zeaxanthin are yellow pigments found in high concentrations in egg yolks and yellow fruits and vegetables, as well as in dark green, leafy vegetables. In particular, spinach, kale, and collard greens contain high levels of these two carotenoids, and numerous dietary survey studies (Castenmiller et al., 1999; Sommerburg et al., 1998) have shown that persons with the highest consumption of spinach (a rich source of lutein) have the lowest risk of developing ARMD (reductions of as much as 90%, in some cases).

Both lutein and zeaxanthin seem to reduce the risk of ARMD and protect overall eye health by at least two different routes. First, both carotenoids are absorbed from the diet into the circulation and eventually concentrate specifically in the eye (in the macular region of the retina). It is interesting to note that lutein and zeaxanthin are the only carotenoids known to concentrate specifically in the eye tissues. The high levels of these carotenoids in the eye serve to protect tissues by minimizing free-radical damage and by absorbing damaging blue light rays (Landrum et al., 1997).

It is thought that a low macular pigment density may increase the risk of ARMD and cataracts by allowing more damage from blue light (Sommerburg et al., 1999). Several observational studies have shown that high dietary intakes of lutein and zeaxanthin (from spinach, broccoli, and eggs) are associated with a significant (20%) reduction in the risk for cataracts (Moeller et al., 2000) and an approximate 40% reduction in the risk for ARMD (Bartlett and Esperjesi, 2003; Mozaffarieh et al., 2003). Studies have shown that dietary supplementation with lutein

(30 mg/day for 140 days) elevates serum lutein levels by 10 times, increases macular pigment density by 20–40%, and reduces transmission of blue light to the eye's photoreceptors by 30–40% (Hammond et al., 1997; Johnson et al., 2000). Other studies have shown that daily egg yolk consumption can increase plasma levels of lutein by 28–50% and zeaxanthin by 114–142%. Multicenter clinical studies of patients with advanced ARMD (ranging in age from 55 to 80 years) have found the risk for ARMD to be reduced by more than 40% by a high dietary intake of carotenoids (Pratt, 1999). In particular, both lutein and zeaxanthin were strongly associated with a reduced risk for macular degeneration (Seddon et al., 1994).

SAFETY/DOSAGE

There are no known adverse side effects associated with dietary supplements containing lutein or zeaxanthin when used at recommended levels. Most supplements should be taken with a meal to lessen the chance of stomach upset and increase digestion and absorption (bioavailability). From studies of ARMD rates and dietary intake, it appears that diets providing about 6 mg of lutein per day can reduce ARMD prevalence by nearly half (Bartlett, 2003; Beatty, 2004; Bone, 2000; Koh, 2004; Landrum, 1997). Eating more of the carotenoid-rich foods previously mentioned should be the first step to increase lutein intake. Unfortunately, diet surveys have indicated that consumption of these foods has dropped more than 20% in the two groups at highest risk for ARMD (women and older persons) (Granado, 2003; Gruber, 2004). Because many carotenoids are rapidly cleared from the body, it is logical to consider splitting daily intake into two doses (3 mg with breakfast and 3 mg with dinner).

REFERENCES

Bartlett H, Eperjesi F. Age-related macular degeneration and nutritional supplementation: a review of randomised controlled trials. Ophthalmic Physiol Opt 2003;23(5):383–399.

Beatty S, Nolan J, Kavanagh H, O'Donovan O. Macular pigment optical density and its relationship with serum and dietary levels of lutein and zeaxanthin. Arch Biochem Biophys 2004;430(1):70–76.

Bone RA, Landrum JT, Dixon Z, Chen Y, Llerena CM. Lutein and zeaxanthin in the eyes, serum and diet of human subjects. Exp Eye Res 2000;71(3):239–245.

Castenmiller JJ, West CE, Linssen JP, van het Hof KH, Voragen AG. The food matrix of spinach is a limiting factor in determining the bioavailability of beta-carotene and to a lesser extent of lutein in humans. J Nutr 1999;129(2):349–355.

Granado F, Olmedilla B, Blanco I. Nutritional and clinical relevance of lutein in human health. Br J Nutr 2003;90(3):487–502.

Gruber M, Chappell R, Millen A, LaRowe T, Moeller SM, Iannaccone A, Kritchevsky SB, Mares J. Correlates of serum lutein + zeaxanthin: findings from the Third National Health and Nutrition Examination Survey. J Nutr 2004;134(9):2387–2394.

Hammond BR Jr, Johnson EJ, Russell RM, Krinsky NI, Yeum KJ, Edwards RB, Snodderly DM. Dietary modification of human macular pigment density. Invest Ophthalmol Vis Sci 1997;38(9):1795–1801.

Johnson EJ, Hammond BR, Yeum KJ, Qin J, Wang XD, Castaneda C, Snodderly DM, Russell RM. Relation among serum and tissue concentrations of lutein and zeaxanthin and macular pigment density. Am J Clin Nutr 2000;71(6):1555–1562.

Koh HH, Murray IJ, Nolan D, Carden D, Feather J, Beatty S. Plasma and macular responses to lutein supplement in subjects with and without age-related maculopathy: a pilot study. Exp Eye Res 2004;79(1):21–27.

Landrum JT, Bone RA, Joa H, Kilburn MD, Moore LL, Sprague KE. A one year study of the macular pigment: the effect of 140 days of a lutein supplement. Exp Eye Res 1997;65(1):57–62.

Moeller SM, Jacques PF, Blumberg JB. The potential role of dietary xanthophylls in cataract and age-related macular degeneration. J Am Coll Nutr 2000;19(5 suppl):522S–527S.

Mozaffarieh M, Sacu S, Wedrich A. The role of the carotenoids, lutein and zeaxanthin, in protecting against age-related macular degeneration: A review based on controversial evidence. Nutr J 2003;2(1):20.

Pratt S. Dietary prevention of age-related macular degeneration. J Am Optom Assoc 1999;70(1):39–47.

Seddon JM, Ajani UA, Sperduto RD, Hiller R, Blair N, Burton TC, Farber MD, Gragoudas ES, Haller J, Miller DT, et al. Dietary carotenoids, vitamins A, C, and E, and advanced age-related macular degeneration. Eye Disease Case-Control Study Group. JAMA 1994;272(18):1413–20.

Sommerburg O, Keunen JE, Bird AC, van Kuijk FJ. Fruits and vegetables that are sources for lutein and zeaxanthin: the macular pigment in human eyes. Br J Ophthalmol 1998;82(8):907–910.

Sommerburg OG, Siems WG, Hurst JS, Lewis JW, Kliger DS, van Kuijk FJ. Lutein and zeaxanthin are associated with photoreceptors in the human retina. Curr Eye Res 1999;19(6):491–495.

ADDITIONAL RESOURCES

Alves-Rodrigues A, Shao A. The science behind lutein. Toxicol Lett 2004;150(1):57–83.

Blodi BA. Nutritional supplements in the prevention of age-related macular degeneration. Insight 2004;29(1):15–16, quiz 17–18.

Bone RA, Landrum JT, Friedes LM, Gomez CM, Kilburn MD, Menendez E, Vidal I, Wang W. Distribution of lutein and zeaxanthin stereoisomers in the human retina. Exp Eye Res 1997;64(2):211–218.

Davies NP, Morland AB. Macular pigments: their characteristics and putative role. Prog Retin Eye Res 2004;23(5):533–559.

Handelman GJ, Nightingale ZD, Lichtenstein AH, Schaefer EJ, Blumberg JB. Lutein and zeaxanthin concentrations in plasma after dietary supplementation with egg yolk. Am J Clin Nutr 1999;70(2):247–251.

Molldrem KL, Li J, Simon PW, Tanumihardjo SA. Lutein and beta-carotene from lutein-containing yellow carrots are bioavailable in humans. Am J Clin Nutr 2004;80(1):131–136.

Riso P, Brusamolino A, Ciappellano S, Porrini M. Comparison of lutein bioavailability from vegetables and supplement. Int J Vitam Nutr Res 2003;73(3):201–205.

Roodenburg AJ, Leenen R, van het Hof KH, Weststrate JA, Tijburg LB. Amount of fat in the diet affects bioavailability of lutein esters but not of alpha-carotene, beta-carotene, and vitamin E in humans. Am J Clin Nutr 2000;71(5):1187–1193.

LYCOPENE

Overall Rank

★★★★★ as an antioxidant
★★★★ for reducing the risk of prostate and cervical cancers
★★ for skin health

OVERVIEW

Lycopene is the carotenoid responsible for giving tomatoes their red color. Among the roughly 600 known carotenoids, lycopene is the most abundant form found in the U.S. diet (β carotene is number two). More than 80% of the lycopene consumed in the United States comes from tomato sauce, pizza, and ketchup. The lycopene content of tomatoes can be influenced dramatically during the ripening process, and large differences are noted among various types of tomatoes (e.g., red varieties have more lycopene than yellow). The bioavailability of lycopene is increased following cooking, so processed tomato products such as ketchup, tomato juice, and pizza sauce have more bioavailable lycopene than do fresh tomatoes. Because of the epidemiological evidence that diets high in lycopene-rich foods are associated with a reduced risk of many cancers, lycopene supplements are often promoted for cancer protection, for heart health, and as a general antioxidant (Agarwal, 2000; Gann, 1999; Giovannucci, 1999).

COMMENTS

In the past, virtually all lycopene supplements were extremely expensive—and many still are. In 2001, however, supplement manufacturers introduced a synthetic lycopene that should cut the cost of lycopene-containing supplements about 5 times and still deliver the same effectiveness. As an antioxidant, lycopene is twice as potent as β carotene in protecting white blood cells from membrane damage caused by free radicals. For patients undergoing pharmaceutical treatment of high cholesterol or triglycerides, it is important to be aware that common treatments such as cholestyramine and Probucol have been shown to reduce plasma lycopene levels by 30–40%. The most cost-effective method for obtaining lycopene daily is unquestionably a diet high in tomato-based foods.

SCIENTIFIC SUPPORT

You may have seen some bottles of ketchup labeled "Lycopene may help reduce the risk of prostate and cervical cancer"—not a bad claim for a bottle of ketchup. Lycopene is a potent antioxidant and seems to inhibit growth of cancer cells, so it is logical that a higher intake of this carotenoid may indeed be associated with a reduced incidence of cancer (Norrish et al., 2000). In addition, lycopene may also help prevent heart disease through this same antioxidant mechanism by inhibiting LDL cholesterol oxidation (Arab and Steck, 2000). Finally, lycopene is known to play a role, along with β carotene, in protecting the skin from the damaging effects of UV radiation (Dorgan et al., 2004).

The theory behind lycopene's cancer preventive benefits is logical. Indeed, plasma lycopene levels are clearly reduced by about 40–50% in smokers whose lungs are exposed to a high degree of oxidative damage (Dietrich et al., 2003), and several epidemiologic studies have shown that consumption of foods high in lycopene (tomatoes, pizza sauce, and tomato juice) is associated with lower rates of prostate cancer (Gann et al., 1999). Dietary supplements containing 10–40 mg of lycopene have been shown to reduce DNA damage in white blood cells (Porrini et al., 2000), probably by reducing oxidative damage to DNA and lipoproteins. It is important to remember the recent history concerning lycopene's carotenoid cousin, β carotene, which was associated with reduced disease incidence when consumed in foods but appeared less effective, and in some cases detrimental, when consumed as isolated high-dose dietary supplements.

In a study of patients suffering from prostate cancer, lycopene supplements have been shown to slow tumor growth (Kucuk et al., 2002). In subjects consuming the lycopene supplement, prostate tumors shrunk and produced lower levels of prostate-specific antigen, a marker compound produced by active prostate cancer cells (Kelloff et al., 1999). An interesting note with this study was that the supplement used was not a purified lycopene supplement but a high-lycopene tomato concentrate, suggesting that other tomato compounds in addition to lycopene may contribute to the protective effect. Another study concluded that regular consumption of various processed tomato products—like ketchup, tomato juice and tomato sauce—significantly raises blood levels of lycopene (Paetau et al., 1999).

SAFETY/DOSAGE

No significant adverse side effects are associated with regular consumption of supplemental levels of lycopene, but owing to the controversy surrounding high doses of supplemental β carotene (which appears to increase lung cancer risk when supplemented at high and unbalanced doses in lifelong heavy smokers), doses of lycopene should remain in the range of levels attainable from a diet high in tomato-based products (10–40 mg/day). The most compelling cancer prevention data suggest that 10 servings of tomato products per week (approximately 20–100 mg of lycopene, depending on food choices and preparation methods) can reduce the risk of prostate cancer by approximately 35% (Giovannucci, 1999).

REFERENCES

Agarwal S, Rao AV. Tomato lycopene and its role in human health and chronic diseases. CMAJ 2000;163(6):739–744.

Arab L, Steck S. Lycopene and cardiovascular disease. Am J Clin Nutr 2000;71(6 suppl):1691S–1695S, discussion 1696S–1697S.

Dietrich M, Block G, Norkus EP, Hudes M, Traber MG, Cross CE, Packer L. Smoking and exposure to environmental tobacco smoke decrease some plasma antioxidants and increase gamma-tocopherol in vivo after adjustment for dietary antioxidant intakes. Am J Clin Nutr 2003;77(1):160–166.

Dorgan JF, Boakye NA, Fears TR, Schleicher RL, Helsel W, Anderson C, Robinson J, Guin JD, Lessin S, Ratnasinghe LD, Tangrea JA. Serum carotenoids and alpha-tocopherol and risk of nonmelanoma skin cancer. Cancer Epidemiol Biomarkers Prev 2004;13(8):1276–1282.

Gann PH, Ma J, Giovannucci E, Willett W, Sacks FM, Hennekens CH, Stampfer MJ. Lower prostate cancer risk in men with elevated plasma lycopene levels: results of a prospective analysis. Cancer Res 1999;59(6):1225–1230.

Giovannucci E. Tomatoes, tomato-based products, lycopene, and cancer: review of the epidemiologic literature. J Natl Cancer Inst 1999;91(4):317–331.

Kelloff GJ, Lieberman R, Steele VE, Boone CW, Lubet RA, Kopelovitch L, Malone WA, Crowell JA, Sigman CC. Chemoprevention of prostate cancer: concepts and strategies. Eur Urol 1999;35(5–6):342–350.

Kucuk O, Sarkar FH, Djuric Z, Sakr W, Pollak MN, Khachik F, Banerjee M, Bertram JS, Wood DP Jr. Effects of lycopene supplementation in patients with localized prostate cancer. Exp Biol Med (Maywood) 2002;227(10):881–885.

Norrish AE, Jackson RT, Sharpe SJ, Skeaff CM. Prostate cancer and dietary carotenoids. Am J Epidemiol 2000;151(2):119–123.

Paetau I, Rao D, Wiley ER, Brown ED, Clevidence BA. Carotenoids in human buccal mucosa cells after 4 wk of supplementation with tomato juice or lycopene supplements. Am J Clin Nutr 1999;70(4):490–494.

Porrini M, Riso P. Lymphocyte lycopene concentration and DNA protection from oxidative damage is increased in women after a short period of tomato consumption. J Nutr 2000;130(2):189–192.

ADDITIONAL RESOURCES

Bramley PM. Is lycopene beneficial to human health? Phytochemistry 2000;54(3):233–236.

Briviba K, Schnabele K, Rechkemmer G, Bub A. Supplementation of a diet low in carotenoids with tomato or carrot juice does not affect lipid peroxidation in plasma and feces of healthy men. J Nutr 2004;134(5):1081–1083.

Casso D, White E, Patterson RE, Agurs-Collins T, Kooperberg C, Haines PS. Correlates of serum lycopene in older women. Nutr Cancer 2000;36(2):163–169.

De Stefani E, Oreggia F, Boffetta P, Deneo-Pellegrini H, Ronco A, Mendilaharsu M. Tomatoes, tomato-rich foods, lycopene and cancer of the upper aerodigestive tract: a case-control in Uruguay. Oral Oncol 2000;36(1):47–53.

Grant WB. Calcium, lycopene, vitamin D and prostate cancer. Prostate 2000;42(3):243.

Heber D. Colorful cancer prevention: alpha-carotene, lycopene, and lung cancer. Am J Clin Nutr 2000;72(4):901–902.

Hughes DA, Wright AJ, Finglas PM, Polley AC, Bailey AL, Astley SB, Southon S. Effects of lycopene and lutein supplementation on the expression of functionally associated surface molecules on blood monocytes from healthy male nonsmokers. J Infect Dis 2000;182(suppl 1):S11–S15.

John JH, Ziebland S, Yudkin P, Roe LS, Neil HA; Oxford Fruit and Vegetable Study Group. Effects of fruit and vegetable consumption on plasma antioxidant concentrations and blood pressure: a randomised controlled trial. Lancet 2002;359(9322):1969–1974.

Kucuk O, Sarkar FH, Sakr W, Djuric Z, Pollak MN, Khachik F, Li YW, Banerjee M, Grignon D, Bertram JS, Crissman JD, Pontes EJ, Wood DP Jr. Phase II randomized clinical trial of lycopene supplementation before radical prostatectomy. Cancer Epidemiol Biomarkers Prev 2001;10(8):861–868.

Michaud DS, Feskanich D, Rimm EB, Colditz GA, Speizer FE, Willett WC, Giovannucci E. Intake of specific carotenoids and risk of lung cancer in 2 prospective US cohorts. Am J Clin Nutr 2000;72(4):990–997.

Pellegrini N, Riso P, Porrini M. Tomato consumption does not affect the total antioxidant capacity of plasma. Nutrition 2000;16(4):268–271.

Rao AV, Agarwal S. Role of antioxidant lycopene in cancer and heart disease. J Am Coll Nutr 2000;19(5):563–569.

Rao AV, Fleshner N, Agarwal S. Serum and tissue lycopene and biomarkers of oxidation in prostate cancer patients: a case-control study. Nutr Cancer 1999;33(2):159–164.

Riso P, Pinder A, Santangelo A, Porrini M. Does tomato consumption effectively increase the resistance of lymphocyte DNA to oxidative damage? Am J Clin Nutr 1999;69(4):712–718.

Sengupta A, Das S. The anti-carcinogenic role of lycopene, abundantly present in tomato. Eur J Cancer Prev 1999;8(4):325–330.

Singh M, Krishanappa R, Bagewadi A, Keluskar V. Efficacy of oral lycopene in the treatment of oral leukoplakia. Oral Oncol 2004;40(6):591–596.

Slattery ML, Benson J, Curtin K, Ma KN, Schaeffer D, Potter JD. Carotenoids and colon cancer. Am J Clin Nutr 2000;71(2):575–582.

N-ACETYLCYSTEINE (NAC)

Overall Rank

★★★★ for antioxidant benefits (glutathione related)
★★★ for general immune support

OVERVIEW

N-acetylcysteine (NAC) is a derivative of the sulfur-containing amino acid cysteine. It is produced naturally in the body and is found in many protein-containing foods. NAC is an intermediary, along with glutamic acid and glycine, in the conversion of cysteine into glutathione (GTH), the body's primary cellular antioxidant. Dietary supplements containing NAC are recommended as general antioxidants and specifically to increase cellular glutathione levels, enhance immune system function, and treat bronchitis and other respiratory conditions.

NAC's proposed benefits in human health are thought to originate from either of its two primary actions in the body. First, NAC is rapidly metabolized to intracellular glutathione. GTH and the enzyme complexes that it forms act as reducing agents and antioxidants in the body. GTH also helps "detoxify" (in the liver) many chemicals into less harmful compounds and accelerates the body's removal of heavy metals such as mercury and lead. Additionally, GTH is known to protect cell membranes, especially those of lymphocytes and phagocytes, two of the major classes of immune cells. Although purified glutathione is sold as a dietary supplement, absorption is notoriously low, and NAC is thought to be a better source method of boosting cellular GTH levels. NAC's second beneficial action in the body is to cleave protein disulfide bonds by converting them to two sulfhydryl groups. In the case of smoker's cough and bronchitis, this action results in the breakup of mucoproteins in lung mucus, reducing their chain lengths, thinning the mucus, and easing breathing.

COMMENTS

Research on NAC has clearly shown value in the treatment of chronic bronchitis and lung ailments as well as for persons desiring an increase in generalized antioxidant protection and immune system support.

SCIENTIFIC SUPPORT

Several studies have been performed to confirm that NAC is converted to glutathione in the body (Faintuch et al., 1999). A review of these studies showed that oral NAC supplementation was successful in enhancing the levels of glutathione in the liver, in plasma, and in the bronchioles of the lungs (Walsh and Lee, 1999). Lack of glutathione has been shown to contribute to various health conditions, including adult respiratory distress syndrome and idiopathic pulmonary fibrosis (Malorni et al., 1998).

In a double-blind, placebo-controlled study of 116 subjects with chronic bronchitis, the therapeutic effects of NAC were investigated over a 6-month period (Pela et al., 1999). The group receiving NAC experienced a significant reduction (by almost one third) in the number of sick days from December to March (173 for the NAC group versus 456 for placebo) as well as a greater reduction (by almost half) in days of coughing (204 for the NAC group versus 399 for placebo). NAC has also been shown to help reduce levels of fatigue and improve the ability to contract muscles during exhaustive exercise, possibly owing to reduced levels of oxidative stress (Droge, 1999).

A clinical trial of NAC and immune function evaluated the response of the CD4-CD8 lymphocyte system in HIV-positive patients (for whom falling CD4 counts are an indicator of disease progression). The 15 patients were divided into two groups, one receiving two 400-mg doses of NAC parenterally twice daily and the other receiving 600 mg orally twice daily (Molnar et al., 1998; Puerto et al., 2002). During the experiment, eight patients receiving NAC were considered "successful," including two patients who became serum negative for the illness and 6 patients who experienced no opportunistic infections. The researchers involved concluded that NAC is a useful adjunct to antiviral and immunotherapy (Malorni et al., 1998).

SAFETY/DOSAGE

Toxicological data show that NAC is safe for consumption in its therapeutic dosage ranges. High intakes of approximately 60–80 g/day are not associated with significant adverse effects, although extended supplementation with high levels of NAC could lead to minor zinc depletion. Typical dosage recommendations for NAC are in the range of 250–1,500 mg/day daily for the majority of therapeutic benefits.

REFERENCES

Droge W. Cysteine and glutathione in catabolic conditions and immunological dysfunction. Curr Opin Clin Nutr Metab Care 1999;2(3):227–233.

Faintuch J, Aguilar PB, Nadalin W. Relevance of N-acetylcysteine in clinical practice: fact, myth or consequence? Nutrition 1999;15(2):177–179.

Malorni W, Rivabene R, Lucia BM, Ferrara R, Mazzone AM, Cauda R, Paganelli R. The role of oxidative imbalance in progression to AIDS: effect of the thiol supplier N-acetylcysteine. AIDS Res Hum Retroviruses 1998;14(17):1589–1596.

Molnar Z, MacKinnon KL, Shearer E, Lowe D, Watson ID. The effect of N-acetylcysteine on total serum anti-oxidant potential and urinary albumin excretion in critically ill patients. Intensive Care Med 1998;24(3):230–235.

Pela R, Calcagni AM, Subiaco S, Isidori P, Tubaldi A, Sanguinetti CM. N-acetylcysteine reduces the exacerbation rate in patients with moderate to severe COPD. Respiration 1999;66(6):495–500.

Puerto M, Guayerbas N, Victor V, De la Fuente M. Effects of N-acetylcysteine on macrophage and lymphocyte functions in a mouse model of premature ageing. Pharmacol Biochem Behav 2002;73(4):797–804.

Walsh TS, Lee A. N-acetylcysteine administration in the critically ill. Intensive Care Med 1999;25(5):432–434.

ADDITIONAL RESOURCES

Malins DC, Hellstrom KE, Anderson KM, Johnson PM, Vinson MA. Antioxidant-induced changes in oxidized DNA. Proc Natl Acad Sci USA 2002;99(9):5937–5941.

Marchetti G, Lodola E, Licciardello L, Colombo A. Use of N-acetylcysteine in the management of coronary artery diseases. Cardiologia 1999;44(7):633–637.

Martinez M, Martinez N, Hernandez AI, Ferrandiz ML. Hypothesis: can N-acetylcysteine be beneficial in Parkinson's disease? Life Sci 1999;64(15):1253–1257.

Miquel J. Can antioxidant diet supplementation protect against age-related mitochondrial damage? Ann N Y Acad Sci 2002;959:508–516.

PINE BARK (*PINUS* SPP.)

Overall Rank

★★★★ as an antioxidant
★★★★ for cardiovascular health
★★★★ for venous health (venous insufficiency and capillary health)
★★★   for complications of diabetes (diabetic retinopathy)
★★   for asthma
★★   for skin health
★★   for improving cognitive function

OVERVIEW

The active components in pine bark are similar to those of grape seed extract (PCOs) as well as phenolic acids (derivatives of benzoic and cinnamic acids). Virtually all the clinical work done on pine bark has been performed on Pycnogenol, the proprietary extract of the French maritime pine. Pycnogenol has been found to be a potent antioxidant, and much of its pharmacologic function comes from this activity. Not only can Pycnogenol enhance the synthesis of antioxidative enzymes and the regeneration of vitamins C and E, but also it acts as a free-radical scavenger. In addition, Pycnogenol exhibits anti-inflammatory and immunomodulatory activity: it antagonizes vasoconstriction caused by epinephrine and norepinephrine by increasing the activity of nitric oxide synthase, thus improving cognitive function and cardioprotective effects, such as dilation of small blood vessels, a mild hypertensive effect (through the inhibition of angiotensin-converting enzyme), and the prevention of smoking-induced platelet aggregation (Rohdewald, 2002). Besides pine bark's previously known clinical efficacy for improving diabetic retinopathy, animal studies confirm that Pycnogenol reduces oxidative stress in diabetic states (Maritim et al., 2003).

COMMENTS

Pine bark extract is a good example of an herbal medicine that exerts so many pharmacologic activities that it starts to sound like an unfounded panacea. The clinical work that is mounting on pine bark extract— primarily in the form of Pycnogenol—is proving that it is an effective herbal supplement (Arcangeli, 2000; Devaraj, 2002; Petrassi, 2000; Rohdewald, 2002).

SCIENTIFIC SUPPORT

In a review of the many clinical studies on Pycnogenol (a standardized extract of French maritime pine bark), it has been found to be beneficial for many conditions and to have numerous pharmacologic properties. The review included clinical data published in peer-reviewed articles as well as results that had been presented at meetings and foreign-language studies not widely available. Pycnogenol has shown clinical efficacy in venous insufficiency and retinal microhemorrhages, protection against erythema induced by UV radiation, asthma, lupus erythematosus (through immunomodulatory activity), cardiovascular disease, smoking-induced damage, and premenstrual symptoms (Rohdewald, 2002).

Attention-Deficit/Hyperactivity Disorder (ADHD)
Tenenbaum et al. (2002) performed a double-blind, placebo-controlled, crossover study of Pycnogenol and methylphenidate for the treatment of ADHD. Neither Pycnogenol nor methylphenidate outperformed placebo for the treatment of 24 adults with ADHD.

Asthma
Hosseini et al. (2001) conducted a randomized, double-blind, placebo-controlled, crossover study to ascertain if Pycnogenol was helpful in treating asthma. The 26 participants were administered either 1 mg/lb per day (maximum 200 mg/day) of Pycnogenol or a placebo for 4 weeks and then crossed over to get the alternative treatment. Almost all the participants responded to Pycnogenol treatment compared with the placebo, and no adverse effects were observed.

Erectile Dysfunction and Fertility
A clinical study was performed to investigate the effect of Pycnogenol and L-arginine in erectile dysfunction. The 40 participants were supplemented with an L-arginine supplement (Sargenor, a solution of dipeptide arginyl aspartate providing 1.7 g/day of L-arginine) for 3 months. Starting the second month, Pycnogenol (40 mg 2 times daily) was added to the

treatment. After 1 month of treatment with L-arginine, only 5% of patients experienced normal erections, but in the second month, after Pycnogenol was added to the therapy, the portion rose to 80%. By the end of the third month of treatment, 92.5% of the participants experienced normal erections (Stanislavov and Nikolova, 2003).

Roseff (2002) conducted a nonrandomized, prospective, clinical study to determine the effects of Pycnogenol on sperm function parameters in subfertile men. The 19 participants were given 200 mg of Pycnogenol for 90 days, and their semen was analyzed before and after treatment for sperm count, motility scores, and morphology. After Pycnogenol treatment, sperm morphology increased by 38%, and the mannose receptor binding assay scores improved by 19%.

Diabetic Retinopathy

Pycnogenol was studied in several clinical studies for the treatment of diabetic retinopathy because of its known ability to increase capillary resistance. In a systematic review of the literature on the treatment of diabetic retinopathy by Pycnogenol, Schonlau and Rohdewald (2001) found five clinical studies published since the late 1960s with a total of 1,289 patients. The authors noted that the impetus for the review was that three of the five studies were published in foreign languages. They found that all the studies clearly exhibited Pycnogenol's ability to stop the progression of retinopathy and to partly recover visual acuity. Additionally, they found tolerance to be very good and side effects rare (mostly gastrointestinal discomfort).

Blood Lipid and Antioxidant Capacity

To test the effect of Pycnogenol on oxidative stress and blood lipid levels, Devaraj et al. (2002) administered 150 mg/day of Pycnogenol for 6 weeks to 25 healthy volunteers. A significant increase of the blood oxygen radical absorbance capacity (ORAC) was found, indicating beneficial antioxidant effects on oxidative stress. Pycnogenol treatment also significantly decreased LDL cholesterol levels in the blood and increased HDL levels.

Silliman et al. (2003) conducted a nonrandomized clinical study to determine the effect of Pycnogenol on the antioxidant capacity of serum and urine. The 27 participants were administered either Pycnogenol or a placebo in a beverage. Blood samples were collected and analyzed for vitamin C and ORAC, and urine samples were collected and analyzed for total phenolics, ferric-reducing antioxidant potential, and ORAC. No significant differences were found in the vitamin C or antioxidant status of young healthy adults taking Pycnogenol.

Skin Health

Ni et al. (2002) performed a clinical examination to see if Pycnogenol had an effect on melasma (a common cutaneous hyperpigmentation disorder that primarily affects the sun-exposed areas on women). The study of Pycnogenol in this indication was performed because in earlier studies, Pycnogenol had been reported to be an antioxidant several times more effective than vitamin C or E and to protect against UV radiation. The 30 women with melasma were administered 25 mg of Pycnogenol with meals 3 times daily for 30 days. Pycnogenol was found to be 80% effective in reducing melasma with no adverse side effects observed. The authors noted that many of the participants reported that the positive side effects of Pycnogenol treatment improved other symptoms or conditions, such as fatigue, constipation, anxiety, and pains in the body.

Gingival and Dental Health

Kimbrough et al. (2002) tested the effect of a chewing gum with and without Pycnogenol on gingival bleeding and plaque formation in a randomized, double-blind, placebo-controlled study. The 40 participants were instructed to chew gum with or without 5 mg of Pycnogenol for 14 days. The Pycnogenol chewing gum significantly reduced gingival bleeding and plaque accumulation.

Smoking-Induced Platelet Aggregation

Putter et al. (1999) tested the effect of Pycnogenol on platelet aggregation induced by cigarette smoking. Measures of increased heart rate and blood pressure caused by cigarette smoking were not affected by either Pycnogenol or aspirin in a group of German smokers. After 500 mg of aspirin or 125 mg of Pycnogenol, however, the increased platelet aggregation induced by smoking in German subjects was prevented. The same study performed on American smokers found that it took 200 mg of aspirin to reduce platelet aggregation significantly compared with 100–140 mg of Pycnogenol. One advantage of Pycnogenol over aspirin (besides the lower dosage needed to produce effect) was that Pycnogenol did not increase bleeding time, whereas aspirin significantly increased it from 167 to 236 seconds.

Venous Insufficiency

Koch (2002) performed an open, controlled, comparative study on Venostasin (horse chestnut seed extract) versus Pycnogenol for the treatment of chronic venous insufficiency (CVI). The 40 participants with CVI were treated with either 600 mg of Venostasin or 360 mg of Pycnogenol daily for 4 weeks. In addition to assessments of CVI, blood lipid levels were monitored in the study. Pycnogenol was found to be more efficacious than Venostasin for CVI; additionally, Pycnogenol improved blood lipid levels but Venostasin did not.

Petrassi et al. (2000) conducted a clinical study with two phases (a randomized double-blind, placebo-controlled phase and an open phase) to assess the efficacy of Pycnogenol for the treatment of CVI. Treatment of Pycnogenol in each phase was 100 mg 2–3 times daily for 2 months. Of the 40 participants, 30 were treated with Pycnogenol and 10 were treated with the placebo. Pycnogenol was found to significantly reduce the clinical symptoms of CVI, with a lack of side effects or change in blood chemistry and hematologic parameters. The authors concluded Pycnogenol to be a safe and effective therapy for both CVI and related venocapillary disturbances.

In a double-blind, placebo-controlled study, Pycnogenol was investigated for its efficacy for treating CVI. The 40 patients in the study were given either Pycnogenol (100 mg 3 times daily) or a placebo for 2 months. The author concluded that Pycnogenol safely and significantly reduced the symptoms of CVI compared with the placebo (Arcangeli, 2000).

Systemic Lupus Erythematosus
In a pilot study on Pycnogenol for the treatment of systemic lupus erythematosus (SLE), 11 patients were administered Pycnogenol or a placebo in addition to the regular treatment protocol. The study found that with Pycnogenol treatment, production of reactive oxygen species, apoptosis, p56(*lck*) activity, and erythrocyte sedimentation rate were reduced. The authors concluded that Pycnogenol could be useful in treating the inflammatory aspects of SLE (Stefanescu et al., 2001).

SAFETY/DOSAGE

The dosages of pine bark extract, in the form of Pycnogenol, that have been used in clinical studies range from approximately 75 mg/day to 360 mg/day, with 200 mg/day being the most common dosage for oxidative stress and asthma and 300 mg/day being most common for venous insufficiency. Dosages as low as 75 mg/day have shown good results on improving melasma in women.

Pycnogenol has been found to exhibit low acute and chronic toxicity and mild side effects. Side effects were experienced in clinical studies in only a small percentage of participants (Rohdewald, 2002).

REFERENCES
Arcangeli P. Pycnogenol in chronic venous insufficiency. Fitoterapia 2000;71(3):236–244.
Devaraj S, Vega-Lopez S, Kaul N, Schonlau F, Rohdewald P, Jialal I. Supplementation with a pine bark extract rich in polyphenols increases plasma antioxidant capacity and alters the plasma lipoprotein profile. Lipids 2002;37(10):931–934.
Hosseini S, Pishnamazi S, Sadrzadeh SM, Farid F, Farid R, Watson RR. Pycnogenol in the management of asthma. J Med Food 2001;4(4):201–209.
Kimbrough C, Chun M, dela Roca G, Lau BH. Pycnogenol chewing gum minimizes gingival bleeding and plaque formation. Phytomedicine 2002;9(5):410–413.
Koch R. Comparative study of Venostasin and Pycnogenol in chronic venous insufficiency. Phytother Res 2002;16(suppl 1):S1–S5.
Maritim A, Dene BA, Sanders RA, Watkins JB III. Effects of pycnogenol treatment on oxidative stress in streptozotocin-induced diabetic rats. J Biochem Mol Toxicol 2003;17(3):193–199.
Ni Z, Mu Y, Gulati O. Treatment of melasma with Pycnogenol. Phytother Res 2002;16(6):567–571.
Petrassi C, Mastromarino A, Spartera C. Pycnogenol in chronic venous insufficiency. Phytomedicine 2000;7(5):383–388.

Putter M, Grotemeyer KH, Wurthwein G, Araghi-Niknam M, Watson RR, Hosseini S, Rohdewald P. Inhibition of smoking-induced platelet aggregation by aspirin and Pycnogenol. Thromb Res 1999;95(4):155–161.

Rohdewald P. A review of the French maritime pine bark extract (Pycnogenol), a herbal medication with a diverse clinical pharmacology. Int J Clin Pharmacol Ther 2002;40(4):158–168.

Roseff SJ. Improvement in sperm quality and function with French maritime pine tree bark extract. J Reprod Med 2002;47(10):821–824.

Schonlau F, Rohdewald P. Pycnogenol for diabetic retinopathy. A review. Int Ophthalmol 2001;24(3):161–171.

Silliman K, Parry J, Kirk LL, Prior RL. Pycnogenol does not impact the antioxidant or vitamin C status of healthy young adults. J Am Diet Assoc 2003;103(1):67–72.

Stanislavov R, Nikolova V. Treatment of erectile dysfunction with pycnogenol and L-arginine. J Sex Marital Ther 2003;29(3):207–213.

Stefanescu M, Matache C, Onu A, Tanaseanu S, Dragomir C, Constantinescu I, Schonlau F, Rohdewald P, Szegli G. Pycnogenol efficacy in the treatment of systemic lupus erythematosus patients. Phytother Res 2001;15(8):698–704.

Tenenbaum S, Paull JC, Sparrow EP, Dodd DK, Green L. An experimental comparison of Pycnogenol and methylphenidate in adults with attention-deficit/hyperactivity disorder (ADHD). J Atten Disord 2002;6(2):49–60.

QUERCETIN

Overall Rank

★★★★ as an antioxidant
★★★★ for cardiovascular disease
★★★★ for venous and capillary health
★★ to support eye health (antioxidant)
★ to enhance thermogenesis

OVERVIEW

Quercetin is a phytochemical found naturally in many foods, such as red wine, green tea, onions, apples, and leafy vegetables. Most of what we know about quercetin has been derived from preclinical studies, because few studies on quercetin as a monotherapy have been conducted. Quercetin exhibits strong antioxidant, anti-inflammatory, and possibly some antihistamine and antitumor activities. Quercetin also inhibits the activity of an enzyme that breaks down norepinephine. These activities are theorized to be at least partially responsible for some of the healthy benefits of foods like red wine and green tea. Quercetin is often included in dietary supplement formulations for its antioxidant, cellular protective, and cardiovascular effects. Because quercetin exhibits antioxidant benefits, it is also considered beneficial for prevention of oxidative stress and macular degeneration.

COMMENTS

Quercetin is rarely used as a monotherapy, but as a component of our foods, and possibly a component of dietary supplement formulations, is thought to promote a strong antioxidant effect. We still know little about quercetin's clinical effectiveness or even its pharmacokinetics, but there are promising preclinical and early clinical studies indicating that it is one of the synergistic components of our foods that bring multiple health benefits (Pignatelli et al., 2000).

SCIENTIFIC SUPPORT

The effect of quercetin was studied in two clinical studies in combination with other substances (sodium nucleinate in one study, and tocopherol acetate in the other) for treatment of Flexner dysentery. In combination with sodium nucleinate, it was found to reduce symptoms of dyspepsia, promote the arrest of bacterial isolation, and normalize immune status. In combination with tocopherol acetate, it promoted healthy clinical indices and immune status (Frolov et al., 1993; Iushchuk et al., 1991).

Cardiovascular Disease
Another clinical study investigated the effects of two of the flavonoids from red wine, quercetin (10–20 μmol/L) and catechin (50–100 μmol/L), on platelet aggregation. The study was designed to test whether flavonoids had a synergistic effect through their antioxidant function in producing collagen-induced platelet aggregation, which in turn stimulates the phospholipase C pathway. Neither substance on its own has been found to affect platelet function. The study found that the combination of flavonoids caused a blunting of hydrogen peroxide production, which in turn inhibited platelet function and activated phospholipase C. The authors suggested that the results of this study indicate a possible explanation of the decreased risk of cardiovascular disease that comes with moderate consumption of red wine (Pignatelli et al., 2000).

Inflammatory Diseases of the Parotid Glands
Timofeev et al. (1990) found high effectiveness in the quercetin treatment of inflammatory diseases of the parotid glands. The study involved 26 patients who received a 0.1% quercetin solution, and the effectiveness of treatment was assessed through clinical examination and cytologic study of the saliva.

Pharmacokinetics
Graefe et al. (1999) performed two clinical studies to determine the pharmacokinetics of quercetin. The elimination half-life of quercetin was found to be 2.4 hours and 0.7 hour, the volume of distribution at steady state was 92.6 L and 6.2 L, and total body clearance was 34.6 L/hour and 28.1 L/hour. The absorption of quercetin was found to be 0–

50% of the dose. The authors admitted the data so far were inconsistent and inconclusive and could be attributed to highly sensitive assay methodology.

Ferry et al. (1996) performed a phase I dosing clinical trial with quercetin. The recommendation for phase 2 clinical trial was a 1,400 mg/m^2 bolus dose in 3-week or 1-week intervals. The authors concluded that quercetin is safe at those levels and observed lymphocyte tyrosine kinase activity and evidence of antitumor activity.

SAFETY/DOSAGE

No widely accepted dosage has been determined for quercetin. As an antioxidant, vasodilator and blood thinner, quercetin has been used with intakes ranging from 100–1,000 mg (in divided doses) with no apparent side effects, but it is thought to be active at the lower levels of usage. Because it has been shown to have vasodilatory and blood-thinning properties, quercetin is contraindicated for those with risk of bleeding.

REFERENCES

Ferry DR, Smith A, Malkhandi J, Fyfe DW, deTakats PG, Anderson D, Baker J, Kerr DJ. Phase I clinical trial of the flavonoid quercetin: pharmacokinetics and evidence for in vivo tyrosine kinase inhibition. Clin Cancer Res 1996;2(4):659–668.

Frolov VM, Peresadin NA, Khomutianskaia NI, Pshenichnyi IIa. The efficacy of quercetin and tocopherol acetate in treating patients with Flexner's dysentery. Lik Sprava 1993;(4):84–86.

Graefe EU, Derendorf H, Veit M. Pharmacokinetics and bioavailability of the flavonol quercetin in humans. Int J Clin Pharmacol Ther 1999;37(5):219–233.

Iushchuk ND, Frolov VM, Peresadin NA. The treatment of protracted forms of Flexner dysentery. Ter Arkh 1991;63(11):19–22.

Pignatelli P, Pulcinelli FM, Celestini A, Lenti L, Ghiselli A, Gazzaniga PP, Violi F. The flavonoids quercetin and catechin synergistically inhibit platelet function by antagonizing the intracellular production of hydrogen peroxide. Am J Clin Nutr 2000;72(5):1150–1155.

Timofeev AA, Maksiutina NP, Topchii DV, Voitenko GN, Balanda PP. The use of a solution of quercetin for the treatment of inflammatory diseases of the parotid glands. Klin Khir 1990;(12):20–22.

SCHISANDRA (*SCHISANDRA CHINENSIS*)

Overall Rank

★★★★ as an antioxidant
★★★ for cardiovascular disease
★★★ as an adaptogen
★★★ for liver support
★★ for central nervous system (CNS) dysfunctions related to old age
★★ for treating and preventing diabetes
★★ for treating and preventing cancer

OVERVIEW

Schisandra (or schizandra) has long been used in Traditional Chinese Medicine (TCM) for promoting well-being and vitality. Today, schisandra is used in many medicinal and nutraceutical preparations as an antioxidant and adaptogen; for cardiovascular disease, liver disease, and CNS dysfunctions related to old age; and to treat and help prevent cancer and diabetes. The activity of schisandra is thought to be the result of a complementary and potentiating action between its principal active components, including lignans (Opletal et al., 2001). This theory makes sense if schisandra is viewed as an adaptogen—an herb thought to balance the body functions and response to stress.

COMMENTS

Schisandra is an ancient herb that is just becoming known by the larger world market. Numerous case reports have been documented in TCM, but so far schisandra is lacking clinical support, and little is known of its potential for adverse reactions.

SCIENTIFIC SUPPORT

Schisandra has been the subject of numerous uncontrolled clinical trials in China for the treatment of hepatic disorders (hepatitis), athletic performance, Parkinson disease, neuroses, and pregnancy and labor disorders (to strengthen uterine contraction; McKenna et al., 2001). Additionally, schisandra in herbal formulations has been included in a couple of clinical trials, but it is not known how much schisandra contributed to the result of the trials.

One trial included only one other active treatment. Panossian et al. (1999) conducted a double-blind, placebo-controlled clinical study on the effects of the adaptogens *Shisandra chinensis* and *Bryonia alba* in athletes. It was shown that the treatment with adaptogens raised the concentration of nitric oxide and cortisol in the blood plasma and saliva in a similar manner in athletes undergoing heavy physical exercise. Furthermore, it was noted that after the treatment with the adaptogens, when the athletes underwent heavy physical exercise, nitric oxide and cortisol were not elevated, in contrast to the placebo group, which showed increased nitric oxide. The authors concluded that nitric oxide could be used for the evaluation of physical loading as well as an adaptogen exhibiting stress protection.

SAFETY/DOSAGE

The usual dosage of schisandra for liver health and adaptogenic support is between 200–800 mg/day. Schisandra is generally regarded as safe, even though toxicity and adverse reaction testing has not been well documented. The only reported side effects have been dizziness and diarrhea, which can be mitigated by reducing the dosage. Schisandra may induce uterine contraction and therefore should be avoided by pregnant women (McKenna et al., 2001).

REFERENCES
McKenna DJ, Jones K, Hughes K, eds. Botanical Medicines: A Desktop Reference for the Major Herbal Supplements. New York: Haworth Press, 2001.

Opletal L, Krenkova M, Havlickova P. Phytotherapeutic aspects of diseases of the circulatory system. 7. Schisandra chinensis (Turcz. Baill.): its composition and biological activity. Ceska Slov Farm 2001;50(4):173–180.

Panossian AG, Oganessian AS, Ambartsumian M, Gabrielian ES, Wagner H, Wikman G. Effects of heavy physical exercise and adaptogens on nitric oxide content in human saliva. Phytomedicine 1999;6(1):17–26.

SELENIUM

Overall Rank

★★★★★ for correcting selenium deficiency
★★★★ as an antioxidant
★★★★ for anticancer effects

OVERVIEW

Selenium is a trace mineral found in supplements in several forms, such as sodium selenite, selenomethionine, and high-selenium yeast (which contains selenomethionine). In general, the organic form of selenium (selenomethionine) is absorbed somewhat better than the inorganic (selenite) form, but not all evidence supports this generality. In the body, selenium functions as part of an antioxidant enzyme called glutathione peroxidase and is necessary for normal growth and proper utilization of iodine in thyroid function. Selenium also supports the antioxidant effect of vitamin E. The best dietary sources of selenium include nuts, unrefined grains, brown rice, wheat germ, and seafood. Dietary supplements containing selenium are generally promoted as antioxidants and for their proposed effects in cancer prevention.

Population studies in China have shown that people living in areas in which the soil is depleted of selenium have higher rates of certain cancers, leading to the obvious suggestion that optimal selenium consumption may help protect against cancer (Taylor, 1994; Zhou, 1999). As part of the system of the antioxidant glutathione peroxidase, selenium plays a direct role in the body's ability to protect cells from damage by free radicals and thus would be a logical adjunct to protection of cells throughout the body.

COMMENTS

Although most people do not consume enough selenium, gross deficiencies are rare (except where fruits and vegetables are grown in selenium-depleted soil). The recommended dietary allowance (RDA) for selenium is in the range of 55–70 μg/day for adults. As part of an overall antioxidant support regimen, selenium should be included at 50–200 μg/day. Virtually all multivitamin/mineral supplements include selenium, and even a "basic" product should provide 20 μg or so.

SCIENTIFIC SUPPORT

A number of animal studies have shown that selenium supplementation can reduce tumor growth in mice and rats (Hamilton, 2001). The strongest scientific evidence for a beneficial effect of selenium supplementation comes from studies of cancer risk. In one of the largest well-controlled studies (Taylor et al., 1994), 200 μg of selenium (from high-selenium yeast) was found to reduce the risk of several cancers, including cancer of the prostate (66%), colon (50%), and lung (40%), compared with a placebo. There was no significant difference in the risk of skin cancer between groups (which is what the study was originally designed to look at). Selenium supplementation was also found to reduce total mortality, mortality from all cancers combined, and the combined incidence of three cancers—lung cancer, colorectal cancer, and prostate cancer (Combs et al., 1997).

A randomized, double-blind, placebo-controlled study was conducted to determine if selenium played a clinical role in intrinsic asthma. The 24 participants were given either 100 μg of sodium selenite or placebo for 14 weeks. The selenium-treated group showed significant clinical improvement, as well as increases in serum selenium and in the activity of the platelet selenium–dependent enzyme glutathione peroxidase. A reduction of platelet aggregation in the treatment group was also found (Hasselmark et al., 1993).

The Qidong province of China shows a high incidence of hepatitis B virus (HBV) and primary liver cancer (PLC). An 8-year intervention trial on the effect of selenium supplementation on HBV and PLC incidence was conducted. Selenium was administered to segments of the population in the form of selenized table salt, which caused a reduction in PLC by 35.1%. In a more focused group of citizens who were found positive for the HBV surface antigen, 200 µg of selenium (as a selenized yeast tablet) or a placebo were administered. In the placebo group, 7 of the 113 participants presented with PLC, whereas no one in the selenium treatment group developed PLC (Yu et al., 1997).

In a double-blind, placebo-controlled intervention that measured the effects of supplementation of vitamins and trace minerals on immunity and infections resistance, 725 older patients were given either trace elements (zinc and selenium sulfide); vitamins (β carotene, ascorbic acid, and vitamin E); or a placebo. The institutionalized older patients participating in the study were found to have a significant improvement in humoral response after vaccinations and reduced incidence of respiratory tract infections from supplementation of trace minerals (Girodon et al., 1999).

SAFETY/DOSAGE

Although selenium can be considered quite toxic at high doses, its important role in supporting the body's own internal antioxidant defense systems cannot be disputed. At the recommended dosage, 50–200 µg/day, selenium is considered safe, whereas doses of 900–1,000 µg/day may cause selenium toxicity (nausea, vomiting, depression, irritability, nervousness, skin rashes, and loss of hair and fingernails). The dietary reference intake for selenium is 55–70 µg for adults and 65–75 µg for pregnant and nursing women. In most clinical trials of selenium, doses are in the range of 100–200 µg/day. Daily selenium intake should be limited to 200 µg.

REFERENCES

Combs GF Jr, Clark LC, Turnbull BW. Reduction of cancer risk with an oral supplement of selenium. Biomed Environ Sci 1997;10(2–3):227–234.

Girodon F, Galan P, Monget AL, Boutron-Ruault MC, Brunet-Lecomte P, Preziosi P, Arnaud J, Manuguerra JC, Herchberg S. Impact of trace elements and vitamin supplementation on immunity and infections in institutionalized elderly patients: a randomized controlled trial. MIN. VIT. AOX. geriatric network. Arch Intern Med 1999;159(7):748–754.

Hamilton KK. Antioxidant supplements during cancer treatments: where do we stand? Clin J Oncol Nurs 2001;5(4):181–182.

Hasselmark L, Malmgren R, Zetterstrom O, Unge G. Selenium supplementation in intrinsic asthma. Allergy 1993;48(1):30–36.

Taylor PR, Li B, Dawsey SM, Li JY, Yang CS, Guo W, Blot WJ. Prevention of esophageal cancer: the nutrition intervention trials in Linxian, China. Linxian Nutrition Intervention Trials Study Group. Cancer Res 1994;54(7 suppl):2029S–2031S.

Yu SY, Zhu YJ, Li WG. Protective role of selenium against hepatitis B virus and primary liver cancer in Qidong. Biol Trace Elem Res 1997;56(1):117–124.

Zhou B, Wang T, Sun G, Guan P, Wu JM. A case-control study of the relationship between dietary factors and risk of lung cancer in women of Shenyang, China. Oncol Rep 1999;6(1):139–143.

ADDITIONAL RESOURCES

Clark LC, Dalkin B, Krongrad A, Combs GF Jr, Turnbull BW, Slate EH, Witherington R, Herlong JH, Janosko E, Carpenter D, Borosso C, Falk S, Rounder J. Decreased incidence of prostate cancer with selenium supplementation: results of a double-blind cancer prevention trial. Br J Urol 1998;81(5):730–734.

Comstock GW, Alberg AJ, Huang HY, Wu K, Burke AE, Hoffman SC, Norkus EP, Gross M, Cutler RG, Morris JS, Spate VL, Helzlsouer KJ. The risk of developing lung cancer associated with antioxidants in the blood: ascorbic acid, carotenoids, alpha-tocopherol, selenium, and total peroxyl radical absorbing capacity. Cancer Epidemiol Biomarkers Prev 1997;6(11):907–916.

Holben DH, Smith AM, Ilich JZ, Landoll JD, Holcomb JP, Matkovic V. Selenium intakes, absorption, retention, and status in adolescent girls. J Am Diet Assoc 2002;102(8):1082–1087.

Knekt P, Jarvinen R, Seppanen R, Rissanen A, Aromaa A, Heinonen OP, Albanes D, Heinonen M, Pukkala E, Teppo L. Dietary antioxidants and the risk of lung cancer. Am J Epidemiol 1991;134(5):471–479.

Lamberg L. Diet may affect skin cancer prevention. JAMA 1998;279(18):1427–1428.

van den Brandt PA, Goldbohm RA, van't Veer P, Bode P, Dorant E, Hermus RJ, Sturmans F. A prospective cohort study on selenium status and the risk of lung cancer. Cancer Res 1993;53(20):4860–4865.

SPIRULINA (*SPIRULINA MAXIMA, S. PLATENSIS*)

Overall Rank

★★★ as an antioxidant
★★★ to stimulate the immune system
★★ as a "holistic" vitamin or nutritional supplement
★★ for heart disease prevention (cholesterol lowering)
★ for promoting healthy energy levels and mood
★ for promoting weight loss

OVERVIEW

Spirulina is a blue-green algae that grows naturally in lakes and has been part of the diet supplementation of people in South America, Central America, and Africa for centuries. Spirulina has gained popularity as a dietary and food supplement and for its numerous health benefits, including as a "holistic" multivitamin; for promoting health, wellness, and energy; to stimulate the immune system; for improving blood lipid levels, as a chemoprotective; and for promoting weight loss. Spirulina is indeed showing good results in preliminary trials for many of these indications, and it has been proven to be a highly nutritive source of vitamins and minerals (Blinkova et al., 2001; Chamorro et al., 2002).

For example, spirulina is a source of a highly bioavailable form of iron and has been found to provide an adequate supply of iron (Puyfoulhoux et al., 2001). Additionally, spirulina contains unusually high levels of γ-linolenic acid (GLA), one of the essential fatty acids (Otles and Pire, 2001).

COMMENTS

Although it is much more expensive than most multivitamins, spirulina also is proving to have more bioavailable forms of nutrients than the average multivitamin. Caution should be exercised, however, that it is not completely substituting a multivitamin regime, because it does not contain all the nutrients that a multivitamin does. Overall, the research behind spirulina is showing promising results in various health conditions, making it a very attractive addition to the diet—if you can get over the green color it adds to food.

SCIENTIFIC SUPPORT

Liver Disease
Gorban et al. (2000) performed a clinical trial involving the use of spirulina in 60 patients with chronic diffuse disorders of the liver. The authors found clinical effectiveness in the treatment and suggested that the hepatoprotective effects were the result of its anti-inflammatory, antioxidant, membrane-stabilizing, and immunocorrecting actions.

Malnutrition
In an attempt to fight infant malnutrition using spirulina as a nutritious food, a study was conducted on infants in Burkina Faso, West Africa. The study included 182 malnourished infants with a Z-score of less than 2 for their age. The participants were divided into three groups: (1) those receiving the usual nutritional rehabilitation program, (2) those receiving the usual nutritional rehabilitation program plus 5 g/day of spirulina, and (3) those receiving the usual nutritional rehabilitation program plus spirulina and fish. The study lasted 3 months, and the outcome assessment criteria were group evolution in length for age and weight for length, and the corresponding Z-score at 60 and 90 days. No noticeable differences were found in the assessment criteria among the three groups (Branger et al., 2003).

Cholesterol and Heart Disease
Based on previous study findings that GLA prevents the accumulation of cholesterol in the body, and because a good amount of GLA is found in spirulina, a study was conducted to determine if spirulina had a beneficial effect on secondary hyperlipidemia caused by nephrotic syndrome. Twenty-three patients were included in the study and were given

either their usual medication or their medication plus 1 g/day of spirulina. The addition of spirulina to the treatment of nephrotic syndrome resulted in significantly improved blood lipid levels (Samuels et al., 2002).

Oral Cancer

Mathew et al. (1995) conducted a study on the effect of spirulina (*Spirulina fusiformis*) as a chemopreventative among tobacco chewers in Kerala, India. The participants, already diagnosed with oral leukoplakia, were given 1 g/day of spirulina or a placebo for 12 months. In 20 of the 44 participants, complete regression of the lesions was found, as opposed to 3 of 43 in the placebo group. No toxicity reactions were reported, and no increase in serum concentration of retinol or β carotene was found.

Immune Stimulation

To determine the molecular mechanism for which spirulina is able to potentiate the immune system, the blood cells of volunteers before and after oral administration of spirulina (hot water) extracts were analyzed. The results of the study indicate that spirulina acts directly on myeloid lineages and has an effect (either direct or indirect) on natural killer cells (Hirahashi et al., 2002).

SAFETY/DOSAGE

The typical dosage of spirulina is 2–3 g/day. It is usually taken in multiple capsules or tablets daily or as a powder added to juice or foods. Spirulina is generally considered safe, but not many toxicity studies have documented its safety. Chamorro et al. (1996) reviewed the safety of spirulina and found that it did not cause body or organ toxicity in animal experiments with dosages much higher than expected in human consumption. Detailed analysis has led to toxic metal, biogenic toxin, and organic chemical analysis, showing spirulina to be either absent in these substances or to have them in tolerable levels.

REFERENCES

Blinkova LP, Gorobets OB, Baturo AP. Biological activity of Spirulina. Zh Mikrobiol Epidemiol Immunobiol 2001;(2):114–118.

Branger B, Cadudal JL, Delobel M, Ouoba H, Yameogo P, Ouedraogo D, Guerin D, Valea A, Zombre C, Ancel P; personnels des CREN. Spiruline as a food supplement in case of infant malnutrition in Burkina-Faso. Arch Pediatr 2003;10(5):424–431.

Chamorro G, Salazar M, Araujo KG, dos Santos CP, Ceballos G, Castillo LF. Update on the pharmacology of Spirulina (Arthrospira), an unconventional food. Arch Latinoam Nutr 2002;52(3):232–240.

Chamorro G, Salazar M, Favila L, Bourges H. Pharmacology and toxicology of Spirulina alga. Rev Invest Clin 1996;48(5):389–399.

Gorban' EM, Orynchak MA, Virstiuk NG, Kuprash LP, Panteleimonova TM, Sharabura LB. Clinical and experimental study of spirulina efficacy in chronic diffuse liver diseases. Lik Sprava 2000;(6):89–93.

Hirahashi T, Matsumoto M, Hazeki K, Saeki Y, Ui M, Seya T. Activation of the human innate immune system by Spirulina: augmentation of interferon production and

NK cytotoxicity by oral administration of hot water extract of Spirulina platensis. Int Immunopharmacol 2002;2(4):423–434.

Mathew B, Sankaranarayanan R, Nair PP, Varghese C, Somanathan T, Amma BP, Amma NS, Nair MK. Evaluation of chemoprevention of oral cancer with Spirulina fusiformis. Nutr Cancer 1995;24(2):197–202.

Otles S, Pire R. Fatty acid composition of Chlorella and Spirulina microalgae species. J AOAC Int 2001;84(6):1708–1714.

Puyfoulhoux G, Rouanet JM, Besancon P, Baroux B, Baccou JC, Caporiccio B. Iron availability from iron-fortified spirulina by an in vitro digestion/Caco-2 cell culture model. J Agric Food Chem 2001;49(3):1625–1629.

Samuels R, Mani UV, Iyer UM, Nayak US. Hypocholesterolemic effect of spirulina in patients with hyperlipidemic nephrotic syndrome. J Med Food 2002;5(2):91–96.

VITAMIN C

Overall Rank

★★★★★ for correcting vitamin C deficiency
★★★★ for preventing and treating colds and flu
★★★★ for antioxidant support

OVERVIEW

Vitamin C, also known as ascorbic acid, is a water-soluble vitamin needed by the body for hundreds of vital metabolic reactions. Scurvy, the disease caused by vitamin C deficiency, is prevented by adequate intake of ascorbic acid (*ascorbic* literally means "without scurvy"). As a dietary supplement, vitamin C is consumed by more people than any other vitamin, mineral, or herbal product. Good food sources of vitamin C include all citrus fruits (oranges, grapefruit, lemons) as well as many other fruits and vegetables such as strawberries, tomatoes, broccoli, brussels sprouts, peppers, and cantaloupe. Vitamin C is a fairly "fragile" vitamin and can be easily destroyed by cooking or exposure of food to oxygen. Dietary supplements containing vitamin C are generally promoted as antioxidants and specifically for preventing colds, boosting immunity, and reducing the risk of certain cancers.

As a water-soluble vitamin, ascorbic acid performs its antioxidant functions within the aqueous compartments of the blood and inside cells and can help restore the antioxidant potential of vitamin E (a fat-soluble antioxidant). Vitamin C also functions as an essential cofactor for the enzymes involved in the synthesis of collagen—the chief structural protein in connective tissues such as bones, cartilage, and skin. Thus, vitamin C is often recommended for wound healing and as an ingredient in supplements designed for healthy skin.

As a preventive against infections such as influenza and other viruses, vitamin C is thought to strengthen cell membranes, thereby preventing entrance of the virus to the interior of the cell. Support of immune cell function is also a key role performed by vitamin C and an effect that may help fight infections in their early stages. The combined effects of cellular strengthening, collagen synthesis, and antioxidant protection are thought to account for the multifaceted approach by which vitamin C helps to maintain health.

COMMENTS

As a dietary supplement, vitamin C is the most popular single nutrient supplement. It is typically included in all multivitamin blends but at widely varying levels. As a single nutrient supplement, typical doses range from 100–500 mg/tablet. Because the body can absorb and retain only about 250 mg of vitamin C at one time, any amount over that is quickly washed out in the urine. Therefore, the most effective approach to supplementing with vitamin C is to take it in divided doses throughout the day.

Vitamin C is one of the least expensive dietary supplements available, with a monthly supply costing no more than a few dollars. In fact, no reliable evidence has shown that expensive "natural" forms of ascorbic acid are cost-effective, because the body absorbs or uses these forms (derived from rose hips or acerola and containing varying levels of bioflavonoids in addition to ascorbic acid) no more efficiently than it does synthetic vitamin C (by contrast, the natural form of vitamin E is clearly superior to the synthetic form).

SCIENTIFIC SUPPORT

As a way to prevent or reduce the symptoms associated with the common cold, more than 100 studies of vitamin C have been conducted. In several of the largest studies, no effect on the incidence of the common cold was observed, indicating to many scientists that vitamin C has no preventive effects in normally nourished subjects (Douglas et al., 2004). Several smaller targeted studies, however, conducted in subjects under heavy acute physical stress, show that vitamin C decreases the incidence of the common cold by half (Douglas et al., 2004). In other studies, healthy subjects consuming low levels of vitamin C (less than 60 mg/day) have a cold incidence that is about one-third lower following vitamin C supplementation (Wolters et al., 2004).

In general, regular vitamin C supplementation at levels at or slightly greater than 1,000 mg/day has consistently reduced the incidence and duration of colds (although the degree of benefit has varied significantly). For example, in some of the larger studies, duration of infection was reduced by only about 5%, but absentee reports were reduced by nearly 20% (Fletcher et al., 2003). At least three controlled studies have shown an 80% reduction in the incidence of pneumonia among vitamin C users (Sasazuki et al., 2005). In one large study with more than 700 students participating, vitamin C (1,000 mg/hour for the first 6 hours followed by 3,000 mg/day) reduced cold and flu symptoms by 85% (Audera et al., 2001).

Although it appears that persons with low vitamin C intakes experience the most important and dramatic preventive effects of vitamin C supplementation, those with average daily consumption from foods may also benefit from supplemental levels. In support of an elevated vitamin C intake, an expert scientific panel recently recommended increasing the current RDA for vitamin C from 60 mg to at least 100–200 mg/day. The panel also cautioned that taking more than 1,000 mg of vitamin C daily could have adverse effects (read more in the next section) and recommended that "whenever possible, vitamin C intake should come from fruits and vegetables" (at least five servings of fruits and vegetables daily). The current RDA of 60 mg/day was established in 1980, but since the last RDA review (in 1989), scientists have learned much more about the functions of vitamin C in the body and the need for elevated vitamin C consumption (Institute of Medicine, 2000).

SAFETY/DOSAGE

As a water-soluble vitamin, ascorbic acid is extremely safe even at relatively high doses (because most of the excess is excreted in the urine). At high doses (more than 1,000 mg/day), some people can experience gastrointestinal side effects such as stomach cramps, nausea, and diarrhea. In addition, vitamin C intakes exceeding 1,000 mg/day may increase the risk of developing kidney stones in some people. Although the RDA for vitamin C was raised in 2000 from 60 mg to 75–90 mg (higher for men), it is well established that almost everybody can benefit from higher levels (Ames, 2003; Halliwell, 1999; Malvy, 2001). For example, the vitamin C recommendation for cigarette smokers is 100–200 mg/day because smoking destroys vitamin C in the body (Schectman et al., 1991). The vitamin C deficiency disease, scurvy, can be prevented by consumption of as little as 10 mg/day of vitamin C, but somewhat higher levels are prudent during exposure to stress (physical or psychological) or infection (e.g., a sick friend or family member).

Although vitamin C is well absorbed, the percentage absorbed from supplements decreases with increasing dosages, and optimal absorption is achieved by taking several small doses throughout the day (100–200 mg/dose for a total daily intake of 200–1,000 mg). Full blood and tissue saturation is typically achieved with daily intakes of 200–500 mg/day (in two or three divided doses).

REFERENCES

Audera C, Patulny RV, Sander BH, Douglas RM. Mega-dose vitamin C in treatment of the common cold: a randomised controlled trial. Med J Aust 2001;175(7):359–362.
Douglas RM, Hemila H, D'Souza R, Chalker EB, Treacy B. Vitamin C for preventing and treating the common cold. Cochrane Database Syst Rev 2004;(4):CD000980.
Fletcher AE, Breeze E, Shetty PS. Antioxidant vitamins and mortality in older persons: findings from the nutrition add-on study to the Medical Research Council Trial of

Assessment and Management of Older People in the Community. Am J Clin Nutr 2003;78(5):999–1010.

Sasazuki S, Sasaki S, Tsubono Y, Okubo S, Hayashi M, Tsugane S. Effect of vitamin C on common cold: randomized controlled trial. Eur J Clin Nutr 2006;60(1):9–17.

Schectman G, Byrd JC, Hoffmann R. Ascorbic acid requirements for smokers: analysis of a population survey. Am J Clin Nutr 1991;53(6):1466–1470.

Wolters M, Hermann S, Hahn A. Effects of 6-month multivitamin supplementation on serum concentrations of alpha-tocopherol, beta-carotene, and vitamin C in healthy elderly women. Int J Vitam Nutr Res 2004;74(2):161–168.

ADDITIONAL RESOURCES

Ames BN, Shigenaga MK, Hagen TM. Oxidants, antioxidants, and the degenerative diseases of aging. Proc Natl Acad Sci U S A 1993;90(17):7915–7922.

Fuller CJ, Grundy SM, Norkus EP, Jialal I. Effect of ascorbate supplementation on low density lipoprotein oxidation in smokers. Atherosclerosis 1996;119(2):139–150.

Giugliano D. Dietary antioxidants for cardiovascular prevention. Nutr Metab Cardiovasc Dis 2000;10(1):38–44.

Halliwell B. Antioxidant defence mechanisms: from the beginning to the end (of the beginning). Free Radic Res 1999;31(4):261–272.

Halliwell B. Oxidative stress, nutrition and health. Experimental strategies for optimization of nutritional antioxidant intake in humans. Free Radic Res 1996;25(1):57–74.

Institute of Medicine, Food and Nutrition Board. DRI – Dietary Reference Intakes for Vitamin C, Vitamin E, Selenium, and Carotenoids. A Report of the Panel on Dietary Antioxidants and Related Compounds. Washington, DC: National Academy Press, 2000.

Jacob RA, Aiello GM, Stephensen CB, Blumberg JB, Milbury PE, Wallock LM, Ames BN. Moderate antioxidant supplementation has no effect on biomarkers of oxidant damage in healthy men with low fruit and vegetable intakes. J Nutr 2003;133(3):740–743.

Jialal I, Grundy SM. Effect of combined supplementation with alpha-tocopherol, ascorbate, and beta carotene on low-density lipoprotein oxidation. Circulation 1993;88(6):2780–2786.

Johnston CS, Meyer CG, Srilakshmi JC. Vitamin C elevates red blood cell glutathione in healthy adults. Am J Clin Nutr 1993;58(1):103–105.

Kim MK, Sasazuki S, Sasaki S, Okubo S, Hayashi M, Tsugane S. Effect of five-year supplementation of vitamin C on serum vitamin C concentration and consumption of vegetables and fruits in middle-aged Japanese: a randomized controlled trial. J Am Coll Nutr 2003;22(3):208–216.

Klipstein-Grobusch K, Geleijnse JM, den Breeijen JH, Boeing H, Hofman A, Grobbee DE, Witteman JC. Dietary antioxidants and risk of myocardial infarction in the elderly: the Rotterdam Study. Am J Clin Nutr 1999;69(2):261–266.

Lykkesfeldt J, Christen S, Wallock LM, Chang HH, Jacob RA, Ames BN. Ascorbate is depleted by smoking and repleted by moderate supplementation: a study in male smokers and nonsmokers with matched dietary antioxidant intakes. Am J Clin Nutr 2000;71(2):530–536.

Malvy DJ, Favier A, Faure H, Preziosi P, Galan P, Arnaud J, Roussel AM, Briancon S, Hercberg S. Effect of two years' supplementation with natural antioxidants on vitamin and trace element status biomarkers: preliminary data of the SU.VI.MAX study. Cancer Detect Prev 2001;25(5):479–485.

Meydani SN, Leka LS, Fine BC, Dallal GE, Keusch GT, Singh MF, Hamer DH. Vitamin E and respiratory tract infections in elderly nursing home residents: a randomized controlled trial. JAMA 2004;292(7):828–836.

Nyyssonen K, Parviainen MT, Salonen R, Tuomilehto J, Salonen JT. Vitamin C deficiency and risk of myocardial infarction: prospective population study of men from eastern Finland. BMJ 1997;314(7081):634–638.

Record IR, Dreosti IE, McInerney JK. Changes in plasma antioxidant status following consumption of diets high or low in fruit and vegetables or following dietary supplementation with an antioxidant mixture. Br J Nutr 2001;85(4):459–464.

Valero MP, Fletcher AE, De Stavola BL, Vioque J, Alepuz VC. Vitamin C is associated with reduced risk of cataract in a Mediterranean population. J Nutr 2002;132(6):1299–1306.

VITAMIN E

Overall Rank
★★★★★ for correcting vitamin E deficiency
★★★★ for heart health
★★★★ for antioxidant support

OVERVIEW

Vitamin E is actually a family of related compounds known as tocopherols and tocotrienols. Although α tocopherol is the most common form found in dietary supplements, vitamin E also exists in foods with slightly different chemical structures, such as β, γ- and δ-tocopherol as well as α, β, γ, and δ tocotrienols. Vitamin E was discovered in the early 1930s when rats fed a diet free of vegetable oils (the primary dietary source of vitamin E) developed reproductive problems. Although vitamin E does not have exactly the same reproductive effects in humans, it is commonly thought of as a "virility" vitamin for men.

Vitamin E can be obtained as a supplement in natural or synthetic form. In most cases, the natural and synthetic forms of vitamins and minerals are identical, but in the case of vitamin E, the natural form is clearly superior in terms of absorption and retention in the body. The natural form of α tocopherol is known as d-α tocopherol, whereas the synthetic form is called dl-α tocopherol. The synthetic "dl" form is the most common form found in dietary supplements, although many manufacturers are switching over to the more potent (and expensive) natural "d" form because consumers are learning to look for it.

Dietary sources of vitamin E include vegetable oils, margarine, nuts, seeds, avocados, and wheat germ. Safflower oil contains a good amount of vitamin E, but corn oil and soybean oil contain very little. For people watching their dietary fat consumption, vitamin E intake is likely to be low, owing to a reduced intake of high-fat foods. As a point of reference, 60 almonds are needed to supply the recommended amount of vitamin E, and about 400–800 almonds would be needed to provide the amount of vitamin E (200–400 IU) associated with heart health benefits in most studies.

Dietary supplements containing vitamin E are generally promoted as antioxidants and specifically to reduce the risk of cardiovascular disease and cancer. Vitamin E has also been shown to play a role in immune function, DNA repair, and other metabolic processes.

COMMENTS

Natural d-α tocopherol is clearly more bioavailable and preferentially retained by the body compared with the more common synthetic ("dl") form of vitamin E. Unfortunately, although the natural form is 2–3 times more potent than the synthetic form, it is also about twice the price. It may be preferable to choose products that offer a balanced source of "mixed tocopherols," including the natural forms of all eight of the vitamin E isomers (d-α, d-β, d-γ, and d-δ forms of both the tocopherols and tocotrienols).

A meta-analysis that generated a great deal of media attention combined the results of 19 clinical trials of vitamin E supplementation for various diseases, including heart disease, end-stage renal failure, and Alzheimer disease, and reported that adults who took supplements of 400 IU/day or more were 6% more likely to die from any cause than those who did not take vitamin E supplements (Miller et al., 2005). Further breakdown of the risk by vitamin E dose and adjustment for other vitamin and mineral supplements, however, revealed that the increased risk of death was statistically significant only at a dose of 2,000 IU/day, which is higher than the tolerable upper limit for adults (1,500 IU/day). This study is at odds with at least three other meta-analytical studies that combined the results of randomized, controlled trials designed to evaluate the efficacy of vitamin E supplementation for the prevention or treatment of cardiovascular disease and found no evidence that vitamin E supplementation of up to 800 IU/day significantly increased or decreased cardiovascular disease mortality or all-cause mortality (Morris and Carson, 2003; Shekelle, 2004; Stone, 2000; Swain, 1999). At present, there is no convincing evidence that vitamin E supplementation of up to 800 IU/day increases the risk of death from cardiovascular disease or other causes.

Some of the reasons that Miller et al. (2005) reached their conclusions are that the research reviewed was conducted with older subjects who had chronic illnesses and that various types and compounds of vitamin E are available, including synthetic and natural forms, which research shows to have varying effects (and are not addressed in the meta-analysis or in most of the studies included in the analysis). Overall, it is important to understand that the Miller et al. (2005) study, like all studies of nutrition and dietary supplements, needs to be placed in context—that vitamin E has been studied for many years and in hundreds of clinical trials with solid evidence showing the benefits of 400–800 IU of natural vitamin E in the reduction of heart attacks.

SCIENTIFIC SUPPORT

Of the various isomers of vitamin E, the α-tocopherol form is typically considered the "gold standard" in terms of antioxidant activity, although the most recent but dated in vitro research suggests that the other chemical forms may possess equivalent or superior antioxidant protection (Moyad et al., 1999). Vitamin E deficiencies are related to a wide variety of health problems, including cataracts, heart disease, lung problems, and liver damage.

Several studies published over the last several years have clearly shown that natural vitamin E, the "d" form, is about 2–3 times more bioavailable than synthetic "dl" vitamin E (Morris and Carson, 2003). The natural form of the vitamin is extracted from vegetable oils, mostly from soybeans, which are cheap and plentiful in the United States. Synthetic vitamin E, in contrast, is manufactured from petroleum byproducts, resulting in a chemical mixture in which only one-eighth of the mixture is the powerful "d" isomer (the other seven-eighths are weaker vitamin E isomers).

A wide variety of epidemiological and prospective studies have shown health benefits associated with higher-than-average vitamin E consumption (Miller et al., 1997, 2005; Morris and Carson, 2003). In most cases, the level of vitamin E intake required for heart, lung, eye, and cancer protection are 10–30 times higher than the current RDA levels. Although high-dose α-tocopherol supplements are clearly a powerful antioxidant measure, concern has been raised because such supplements may displace body stores of the other naturally occurring forms of vitamin E.

There is a strong inverse relationship between plasma vitamin E levels (which almost exclusively measure only α tocopherol) and the incidence of coronary heart disease (Muntwyler et al., 2002; Shekelle et al., 2004; Stone, 2000). Several supplementation studies, however, have failed to demonstrate a protective effect when α tocopherol alone has been supplemented. In two large studies (Kushi et al., 1996; Yusuf et al., 2000), vitamin E appeared to offer greater protection when obtained from the diet (which is primarily γ tocopherol) and not as dramatically when taken in supplements (which are primarily α tocopherol). The strongest correlation was shown with the consumption of margarine, nuts, and seeds—all of which are excellent sources of γ tocopherol. In addition, serum levels of γ tocopherol (but not α tocopherol) are reduced in heart disease patients and rise rapidly when chronic smokers quit. Because α-tocopherol supplementation reduces tissue levels of the γ-tocopherol form, a mixed tocopherol that better reflects the ratios found in our diet may be more useful as a supplement than the formulations of vitamin E currently available.

In other studies, heart disease patients have been shown to have normal serum α-tocopherol levels but much lower γ-tocopherol levels compared with a group of healthy control subjects. In one of the largest epidemiological studies (21,809 women), vitamin E consumption was inversely associated with the risk of death from coronary heart disease, but this link was strongest in the women who did not consume vitamin E supplements but got their vitamin E from foods (Eidelman et al., 2004).

Overall, it appears that at least some studies indicate that a balanced intake of each of the naturally occurring forms of vitamin E may be the most prudent approach in terms of overall health benefits. For example, high-dose α-tocopherol supplements can reduce body stores of γ tocopherol, whereas a 50/50 intake of each maintains elevated tissues stores of both (Moyad et al., 1999). Such findings are potentially important, given that γ tocopherol is the major form of vitamin E in the U.S. diet and has been found to inhibit lipid peroxidation (cell membrane damage) more effectively than α tocopherol (Moyad et al., 1999). This may mean that the various forms of vitamin E may complement each other in the body.

SAFETY/DOSAGE

Side effects associated with vitamin E supplements are exceedingly rare. Unlike other fat-soluble vitamins, such as A, D, and K, vitamin E is relatively nontoxic, even at doses many times the current daily value of 30 IU. A caution is advised, however, in persons at risk for prolonged bleeding, such as those taking anticoagulant medications, because vitamin E supplements can decrease blood-clotting ability (reduced platelet aggregation) and prolong bleeding time. Despite vitamin E's 30-IU daily value, most research studies show that optimal intakes associated with health benefits are in the range of 100–800 IU—an amount that cannot be obtained from foods. The Institute of Medicine has set an upper tolerable intake level for vitamin E at 1,000 mg/day (1,500 IU/day) for any form of supplementary α tocopherol because the nutrient can act as an anticoagulant and may increase the risk of bleeding problems. Upper tolerable intake levels "represent the maximum intake of a nutrient that is likely to pose no risk of adverse health effects in almost all healthy people in the general population."

REFERENCES

Eidelman RS, Hollar D, Hebert PR, Lamas GA, Hennekens CH. Randomized trials of vitamin E in the treatment and prevention of cardiovascular disease. Arch Intern Med 2004;164(14):1552–1556.

Kushi LH, Folsom AR, Prineas RJ, Mink PJ, Wu Y, Bostick RM. Dietary antioxidant vitamins and death from coronary heart disease in postmenopausal women. N Engl J Med 1996;334(18):1156–1162.

Miller ER III, Appel LJ, Levander OA, Levine DM. The effect of antioxidant vitamin supplementation on traditional cardiovascular risk factors. J Cardiovasc Risk 1997;4(1):19–24.

Miller ER III, Pastor-Barriuso R, Dalal D, Riemersma RA, Appel LJ, Guallar E. Meta-analysis: high-dosage vitamin E supplementation may increase all-cause mortality. Ann Intern Med 2005;142(1):37–46.

Morris CD, Carson S. Routine vitamin supplementation to prevent cardiovascular disease: a summary of the evidence for the U.S. Preventive Services Task Force. Ann Intern Med 2003;139(1):56–70.

Moyad MA, Brumfield SK, Pienta KJ. Vitamin E, alpha- and gamma-tocopherol, and prostate cancer. Semin Urol Oncol 1999;17(2):85–90.

Muntwyler J, Hennekens CH, Manson JE, Buring JE, Gaziano JM. Vitamin supplement use in a low-risk population of US male physicians and subsequent cardiovascular mortality. Arch Intern Med 2002;162(13):1472–1476.

Shekelle PG, Morton SC, Jungvig LK, Udani J, Spar M, Tu W, J Suttorp M, Coulter I, Newberry SJ, Hardy M. Effect of supplemental vitamin E for the prevention and treatment of cardiovascular disease. J Gen Intern Med 2004;19(4):380–389.

Stone NJ. The Gruppo Italiano per lo Studio della Sopravvivenza nell'Infarto Miocardio (GISSI)-Prevenzione Trial on fish oil and vitamin E supplementation in myocardial infarction survivors. Curr Cardiol Rep 2000;2(5):445–451.

Swain RA, Kaplan-Machlis B. Therapeutic uses of vitamin E in prevention of atherosclerosis. Altern Med Rev 1999;4(6):414–423.

Yusuf S, Dagenais G, Pogue J, Bosch J, Sleight P. Vitamin E supplementation and cardiovascular events in high-risk patients. The Heart Outcomes Prevention Evaluation Study Investigators. N Engl J Med 2000;342(3):154–160.

ADDITIONAL RESOURCES

Miller JW. Vitamin E and memory: is it vascular protection? Nutr Rev 2000;58(4):109–111.

Morris MC, Beckett LA, Scherr PA, Hebert LE, Bennett DA, Field TS, Evans DA. Vitamin E and vitamin C supplement use and risk of incident Alzheimer disease. Alzheimer Dis Assoc Disord 1998;12(3):121–126.

Pietinen P, Ascherio A, Korhonen P, Hartman AM, Willett WC, Albanes D, Virtamo J. Intake of fatty acids and risk of coronary heart disease in a cohort of Finnish men. The Alpha-Tocopherol, Beta-Carotene Cancer Prevention Study. Am J Epidemiol 1997;145(10):876–887.

Virtamo J, Rapola JM, Ripatti S, Heinonen OP, Taylor PR, Albanes D, Huttunen JK. Effect of vitamin E and beta carotene on the incidence of primary nonfatal myocardial infarction and fatal coronary heart disease. Arch Intern Med 1998;158(6):668–675.

Willett WC, Stampfer MJ, Underwood BA, Taylor JO, Hennekens CH. Vitamins A, E, and carotene: effects of supplementation on their plasma levels. Am J Clin Nutr 1983;38(4):559–566.

Woodall AA, Britton G, Jackson MJ. Dietary supplementation with carotenoids: effects on alpha-tocopherol levels and susceptibility of tissues to oxidative stress. Br J Nutr 1996;76(2):307–317.

CHAPTER 10

Gastrointestinal Support Supplements

Aloe (Aloe Vera)
Cayenne or Chili (*Capsicum annuum, C. frutescens*)
Fiber
Ginger (*Zingiber officinale*)
Mastic (from *Pistacia lentiscus*)

Milk Thistle (*Silybum marianum*)
Prebiotics or Fructo-Oligosaccharides (FOS)
Probiotics (Acidophilus, Bifidus)
Slippery Elm (*Ulmus rubra, U. fulva*)
Yellow Dock (*Rumex crispus*)

ALOE (ALOE VERA)

Overall Rank
★★★★ for healing wounds, burns, and minor skin irritations (topically)
★★★ as a laxative
★★ for blood sugar reduction
★★ for immune system support
★ for blood lipid reduction

OVERVIEW

Almost everybody is familiar with the use of aloe for soothing sunburns, but the internal use of aloe is not well known. The active substances in aloe are thought to be the immunomodulatory gel polysaccharides (especially the acetylated mannans) and glycoproteins. The mucilaginous gel derived from aloe's parenchymatous cells is used for numerous curative purposes, and the bitter yellow exudate from the bundle sheath cells is mainly used for its purgative properties (Grindlay and Reynolds, 1986). Topically, aloe is used for skin irritations, to prevent irritation or skin injury from radiation, for mouth ulcers, for herpes, to minimize frostbite, and for periodontal uses (McCauley et al., 1990; Rieger and Carson, 2002). Used internally, aloe may regulate blood sugar levels and control diabetes, treat mouth and stomach ulcers, lower cholesterol,

325

provide immune system support, treat inflammatory bowel disease, and act as a laxative (Borrelli and Izzo, 2000; Reynolds and Dweck, 1999).

COMMENTS

Despite relatively little scientific support, the use of aloe is very popular. Creams and lotions containing extracts of the plant are particularly favored. Regarding internal applications for aloe, more time and clinical research are needed to determine the plant's effectiveness and to teach people how to use aloe correctly.

SCIENTIFIC SUPPORT

Blood Sugar Regulation, Diabetes Control, and Wound Healing

A systematic review of the clinical data in published research on aloe vera was conducted to assess its clinical effectiveness. Only controlled trials were included in the review, and all indications were included. Ten studies were found, and they indicated that oral administration of aloe could be beneficial for reducing blood lipid levels in patients with hyperlipidemia. Topical administration was found not to be an effective preventative for radiation-induced injuries. Although topical administration might be effective for genital herpes and psoriasis, it was unclear if aloe vera promoted wound healing. The authors cautioned that the results of the trials were very preliminary and still needed clinical work to define the parameters and effectiveness of treatments (Vogler and Ernst, 1999).

Skin Irritations and Burns

A systematic review of literature on complementary and alternative medicine in dermatology provides a brief overview of two conditions, atopic dermatitis and chronic venous insufficiency, treated with aloe vera gel and tea tree oil. The authors concluded that no compelling evidence supports the effectiveness of either the aloe vera gel or the tea tree oil for those two conditions (Ernst et al., 2002).

A prospective, randomized, blinded, clinical trial was conducted to ascertain whether aloe vera might help decrease skin reactions to radiation therapy. Patients were divided into two groups and randomized and used either aloe vera plus a mild detergent or the mild detergent alone. A protective effect for adding aloe to the treatment regimen was found only at high levels of radiation (more than 2,700 centi-Gray units) and only over time (Olsen et al., 2001).

In an open, uncontrolled, clinical study to investigate the efficacy of a bioadhesive patch (Aloex, containing aloe vera hydrogel) for aphthous stomatitis (mouth ulcers), 31 patients were administered at least three patches daily for 4 days. The study found that treatment with the patches resulted in large improvements in symptoms and pain, and the compliance was also markedly high (Andriani et al., 2000).

Two phase 3 studies were conducted to ascertain if aloe vera gel could be helpful for preventing radiation therapy–induced dermatitis. The first was a randomized, double-blind, placebo-controlled (with a placebo gel) study involving 194 women receiving breast or chest wall irradiation. The second was a placebo-controlled, randomized study involving 108 patients receiving radiation treatment along with either aloe vera gel or nothing. Neither study found that aloe vera gel protected against radiation-induced dermatitis (Williams et al., 1996).

Syed et al. (1996) studied the efficacy of aloe vera extract 0.5% in a hydrophilic cream for its effectiveness in treating psoriasis vulgaris. The 60 patients with slight to moderate chronic plaque-type psoriasis and Psoriasis Area and Severity Index (PASI) scores between 4.8 and 16.7 were randomized into two parallel groups receiving either a 100-g tube of aloe or a placebo. The patients were told to self-administer the cream topically at home 3 times daily for 5 consecutive days each week (for a maximum of 4 weeks). Treatment was well tolerated, and no adverse effects were reported. The aloe vera extract 0.5% in the hydrophilic cream was statistically more effective than the placebo in curing psoriasis lesions and lowering PASI scores.

Visuthikosol et al. (1995) compared the effectiveness in healing burn wounds with aloe vera gel compared with Vaseline gauze. Aloe vera gel healed the burn wounds statistically faster than did the Vaseline gauze, with a healing time of 11.89 days for the aloe treatment versus 18.19 days for the gauze. Histological examinations of the healing wounds revealed earlier epithelialization in the aloe group.

Immunity and Cancer

Lissoni et al. (1998) studied the immunomodulating effect of aloe vera when used along with pineal indole melatonin (MLT) in patients with advanced solid tumors for which no effective standard anticancer techniques are available. The 50 participants were given either MLT alone (20 mg/day orally in the dark period) or MLT plus aloe vera tincture (1 mL 2 times daily). Compared with the group treated with MLT alone, the aloe treatment group had a higher 1-year survival rate and a higher portion of people achieving stable disease. The authors concluded that MLT plus aloe vera extract may produce therapeutic benefits, including stabilization of disease and survival, in patients with advanced solid tumors.

SAFETY/DOSAGE

The dosage of aloe depends on the preparation and the usage, of which there are many. Generally, as a laxative, aloe is used in the range of 50–200 mg/day or about 1–3 oz orally. For topical applications, the gel is generally applied throughout the day as needed.

No significant side effects of aloe vera gel have been noted, except the occasional allergy. One study found anthranoid laxative abuse (such as aloe vera gel) to be linked to colorectal cancer (Siegers et al., 1993).

REFERENCES

Andriani E, Bugli T, Aalders M, Castelli S, De Luigi G, Lazzari N, Rolli GP. The effectiveness and acceptance of a medical device for the treatment of aphthous stomatitis. Clinical observation in pediatric age. Minerva Pediatr 2000;52(1–2):15–20.

Borrelli F, Izzo AA. The plant kingdom as a source of anti-ulcer remedies. Phytother Res 2000;14(8):581–591.

Ernst E, Pittler MH, Stevinson C. Complementary/alternative medicine in dermatology: evidence-assessed efficacy of two diseases and two treatments. Am J Clin Dermatol 2002;3(5):341–348.

Grindlay D, Reynolds T. The Aloe vera phenomenon: a review of the properties and modern uses of the leaf parenchyma gel. J Ethnopharmacol 1986;16(2–3):117–151.

Lissoni P, Giani L, Zerbini S, Trabattoni P, Rovelli F. Biotherapy with the pineal immunomodulating hormone melatonin versus melatonin plus aloe vera in untreatable advanced solid neoplasms. Nat Immun 1998;16(1):27–33.

McCauley RL, Heggers JP, Robson MC. Frostbite. Methods to minimize tissue loss. Postgrad Med 1990;88(8):67–68, 73–77.

Olsen DL, Raub W Jr, Bradley C, Johnson M, Macias JL, Love V, Markoe A. The effect of aloe vera gel/mild soap versus mild soap alone in preventing skin reactions in patients undergoing radiation therapy. Oncol Nurs Forum 2001;28(3):543–547.

Reynolds T, Dweck AC. Aloe vera leaf gel: a review update. J Ethnopharmacol 1999;68(1–3):3–37.

Rieger L, Carson RE. The clinical effects of saline and aloe vera rinses on periodontal surgical sites. J Okla Dent Assoc 2002;92(3):40–43.

Siegers CP, von Hertzberg-Lottin E, Otte M, Schneider B. Anthranoid laxative abuse—a risk for colorectal cancer? Gut 1993;34(8):1099–1101.

Syed TA, Ahmad SA, Holt AH, Ahmad SA, Ahmad SH, Afzal M. Management of psoriasis with Aloe vera extract in a hydrophilic cream: a placebo-controlled, double-blind study. Trop Med Int Health 1996;1(4):505–509.

Visuthikosol V, Chowchuen B, Sukwanarat Y, Sriurairatana S, Boonpucknavig V. Effect of aloe vera gel to healing of burn wound a clinical and histologic study. J Med Assoc Thai 1995;78(8):403–409.

Vogler BK, Ernst E. Aloe vera: a systematic review of its clinical effectiveness. Br J Gen Pract 1999;49(447):823–828.

Williams MS, Burk M, Loprinzi CL, Hill M, Schomberg PJ, Nearhood K, O'Fallon JR, Laurie JA, Shanahan TG, Moore RL, Urias RE, Kuske RR, Engel RE, Eggleston WD. Phase III double-blind evaluation of an aloe vera gel as a prophylactic agent for radiation-induced skin toxicity. Int J Radiat Oncol Biol Phys 1996;36(2):345–349.

ADDITIONAL RESOURCES

Robinson M. Medical therapy of inflammatory bowel disease for the 21st century. Eur J Surg Suppl 1998;(582):90–98.

CAYENNE OR CHILI (*CAPSICUM ANNUUM* AND *C. FRUTESCENS*)

Overall Rank

★★★ for digestive health
★★★ for pain (internally and topically)
★★ for headache
★★ for skin health (topically)
★★ for incontinence

OVERVIEW

Chili peppers are well known and in foods are usually strongly liked or disliked by people. The hotness of chili peppers comes from a group of compounds called the capsaicinoids, of which capsaicin is the most well studied because of its higher prevalence and potency. Chili peppers have a long traditional use in many cultures for several dysfunctions and for aiding in and protecting normal processes, such as digestion. Capsaicin or chili peppers of many varieties have both internal and topical uses, including gastrointestinal health, headache, pain (both rheumatoid arthritis and osteoarthritis), and psoriasis and dermatitis. Capsaicin is theorized to wok on pain because it depletes substance P, which has been implicated in the development of pain and inflammation.

COMMENTS

Cayenne or chili peppers are a good example of a botanical medicine and food that is so prevalent in so many cultures—and often for similar uses—that the good clinical results seem inevitable. It is not surprising then, that most of the clinical work on capsaicin and chili peppers have revealed beneficial results in numerous disorders.

SCIENTIFIC SUPPORT

Gastrointestinal Health

To demonstrate in humans the early results of animal studies that showed capsaicin aids in protecting against gastric mucosal injury, 18 healthy volunteers were recruited for two studies, 2 weeks apart. The subjects were administered 20 g of chili orally with 200 mL of water or just water. Each group followed the initial treatment with 600 mg of aspirin taken with 200 mL of water. The gastric injury in the treatment group as determined by endoscopy was 1.5 compared with 4.0 in the control group, indicating a significant gastroprotective effect of the chili in humans (Yeoh et al., 1995).

Gonzalez et al. (1998) performed a controlled trial to investigate whether a capsaicin-containing red pepper sauce (Tabasco) could activate the afferent nerves in the regulation of gastrointestinal motility. After baseline recordings, red pepper or saline solution was administered intraesophageally in seven healthy volunteers. Red pepper was found to have significant effects on gastrointestinal motility: prolonging gastric emptying, decreasing the perception and discomfort threshold of intra-esophageal balloon distension, and reducing the percentage of normal electrical activity on the electrogastrogram. The authors theorized that these profound changes in gastrointestinal motility could be the result of retaining the pepper irritant in the stomach and then faster intestinal transit (as found in the study) to improve clearance and protection of the esophagus.

Skin Health

To determine the role of substance P (an undecapeptide neuro-transmitter) in the development of psoriasis and pruritus, a double-blind, placebo-controlled study was conducted on the effect of capsaicin (a substance P depleter) in patients with pruritic psoriasis. The patients were instructed to apply capsaicin (0.025%) cream or a placebo cream 4 times daily for 6 weeks. The capsaicin cream resulted in significant improvements of global evaluation and pruritus relief and in psoriasis severity scores. The most frequent but transient side effect reported was a burning sensation when the cream was applied. The authors concluded that these results also supported a role for substance P in psoriasis and pruritus (Ellis et al., 1993).

Bernstein et al. (1986) performed a double-blind study on the effect of capsaicin on psoriasis. The 44 participants with psoriasis applied capsaicin topically on lesions on one side of their bodies and a placebo cream on the other side for 6 weeks. The capsaicin application produced significant improvements in the psoriasis throughout the study. In almost half of the patients, reported side effects of burning, stinging, itching, or redness occurred on initial application but diminished or were absent for the rest of the study on further applications.

Exercise and Metabolism

Yoshioka et al. (1999) conducted two studies to investigate the effect of capsaicin on feeding behavior and energy intake. In the first study, the capsaicin was added to high-fat and high-carbohydrate diets, and the subsequent effect on energy and macronutrient intake was studied. The capsaicin was found to significantly reduce the desire to eat after breakfast when added to a high-carbohydrate diet, and this effect was found for the high-carbohydrate breakfast alone. Both capsaicin-added diets were found to significantly decrease protein and fat intakes during lunch. In the second study, an appetizer with capsaicin was studied in 10 males. The red pepper significantly reduced the energy and carbohydrate intakes in the meals consumed a few hours later. A power spectral analysis was performed and indicated that these results were related to an increase in the ratio of sympathetic to parasympathetic nervous system activity.

To determine the effect of red pepper on energy metabolism, a clinical study was performed involving long-distance runners (18–23 years old). A breakfast with or without 10 g of hot red pepper was consumed, and the expired gases and venous blood were collected both during rest (2.5 hours after the meal) and during exercise. The hot red pepper was found to significantly elevate the respiratory quotient and blood lactate both at rest and during exercise. Oxygen consumption at rest (30 minutes after the meal) showed a nonsignificant increase, and a significant increase in plasma epinephrine and norepinephrine levels occurred 30 minutes after the meal. The authors concluded that the hot red pepper stimulates carbohydrate oxidation both at rest and during exercise (Lim et al., 1997).

Headache
The acute effects of capsaicin (300 μg per 100 μL) on human nasal mucosa of cluster headache sufferers were studied by Sicuteri et al. (1989). The capsaicin was applied on both healthy participants and cluster headache sufferers and found to produce desensitization to the initial painful sensations to treatment (pain, sneezing, and nasal secretion) in both groups after 5 days of treatment. After capsaicin treatment, the number of cluster headache attacks was significantly decreased for 60 days following treatment. Sicuteri et al. (1990) performed a subsequent study to determine the features of pain transmission in cluster headache sufferers.

Pain (Osteoarthritis, Rheumatoid Arthritis, Postherpetic Neuralgia, Headache)
Capsaicin is theorized to be effective on pain relief due to its substance P depleting ability. As mentioned in the previous section, capsaicin has been found effective for relief of pain from cluster headaches (Sicuteri et al., 1989, 1990).

Keitel et al. (2001) performed a randomized, double-blind, parallel group study on the effect of a capsicum plaster (CAS 404–86–4) on patients with nonspecific back pain. The 154 patients were administered the cream or a placebo for 3 weeks. Three pain scales were used as primary outcome assessments, and secondary assessments included tests of motility, a disability index, and global assessments by patients and physicians. The capsicum group produced significant decreases in the sums of all pain scores compared with placebo. Efficacy ratings by both physicians and patients were significantly higher for the capsicum treatment. The tolerance ratings for the capsicum plaster were higher than placebo, and the adverse effects reported in this study were mostly mild and transient.

McCarthy and McCarty (1992) performed a randomized, double-blind, clinical trial on the effect of topical 0.075% capsaicin cream on the painful joints of rheumatoid arthritis and osteoarthritis sufferers.

The 21 patients were instructed to apply the capsaicin cream or a placebo 4 times daily for 4 weeks. Capsaicin was found to reduce tenderness and pain significantly in patients with osteoarthritis, but not for those with rheumatoid arthritis. A local burning sensation was the only minor side effect noted.

Deal et al. (1991) performed a randomized, double-blind, placebo-controlled study on the effect of capsaicin cream on 70 patients with either osteoarthritis or rheumatoid arthritis. The patients were instructed to apply the 0.025% capsaicin cream or a placebo to painful knees 4 times daily for 2 weeks. Both pain scales and global evaluations were used as primary outcome assessments. Significantly more pain relief was experienced by the capsaicin-treated patients than by the placebo group throughout and at the end of the study. Both rheumatoid arthritis (57%) and osteoarthritis (33%) patients reported significant improvements from the treatment. Transient burning sensations were reported as a side effect of application of the cream.

Bernstein et al. (1989) performed a double-blind, placebo-controlled study on postherpetic neuralgia after uncontrolled studies had reported success with capsaicin treatment of this disorder. The 32 older patients with chronic postherpetic neuralgia were treated with either capsaicin cream or a placebo for 6 weeks. Pain scales and global evaluation were used for outcome assessments. In all efficacy variables, capsaicin cream proved to be significantly better than placebo. Additionally, after the 6 weeks of treatment, approximately 80% of the participants using capsaicin experienced some pain relief. The authors recommended capsaicin treatment for postherpetic neuralgia as an initial management therapy because of the low possibility of drug interaction or systemic toxicity.

Incontinence

Cruz (1998) reviewed the findings of a category of unmyelinated type C bladder afferent fibers in the pelvic nerves that were extremely sensitive to capsaicin. Capsaicin was able to desensitize these fibers by intravesical administration, reduce involuntary micturition, increase urinary capacity, and reduce intensity of pain in patients with bladder pain.

SAFETY/DOSAGE

The usual dosage for internal use of capsicum is in the range of 30–120 mg, with 60 mg most common. Patients should be advised not to bite or chew on the capsules. For topical applications for pain or skin irritation, the content of creams in clinical studies has been 0.025–0.075% capsaicin, with application 4–5 times daily.

For the topical use of capsaicin cream, the frequent and transient but not serious side effect of a burning sensation is reported. Capsaicin and the capsaicinoids are strong irritants to the mucous membranes and can produce dermatitis.

REFERENCES

Bernstein JE, Korman NJ, Bickers DR, Dahl MV, Millikan LE. Topical capsaicin treatment of chronic postherpetic neuralgia. J Am Acad Dermatol 1989;21(2 pt 1):265–270.

Bernstein JE, Parish LC, Rapaport M, Rosenbaum MM, Roenigk HH Jr. Effects of topically applied capsaicin on moderate and severe psoriasis vulgaris. J Am Acad Dermatol 1986;15(3):504–507.

Cruz F. Desensitization of bladder sensory fibers by intravesical capsaicin or capsaicin analogs. A new strategy for treatment of urge incontinence in patients with spinal detrusor hyperreflexia or bladder hypersensitivity disorders. Int Urogynecol J Pelvic Floor Dysfunct 1998;9(4):214–220.

Deal CL, Schnitzer TJ, Lipstein E, Seibold JR, Stevens RM, Levy MD, Albert D, Renold F. Treatment of arthritis with topical capsaicin: a double-blind trial. Clin Ther 1991;13(3):383–395.

Ellis CN, Berberian B, Sulica VI, Dodd WA, Jarratt MT, Katz HI, Prawer S, Krueger G, Rex IH Jr, Wolf JE. A double-blind evaluation of topical capsaicin in pruritic psoriasis. J Am Acad Dermatol 1993;29(3):438–442.

Gonzalez R, Dunkel R, Koletzko B, Schusdziarra V, Allescher HD. Effect of capsaicin-containing red pepper sauce suspension on upper gastrointestinal motility in healthy volunteers. Dig Dis Sci 1998;43(6):1165–1171.

Keitel W, Frerick H, Kuhn U, Schmidt U, Kuhlmann M, Bredehorst A. Capsicum pain plaster in chronic non-specific low back pain. Arzneimittelforschung 2001;51(11):896–903.

Lim K, Yoshioka M, Kikuzato S, Kiyonaga A, Tanaka H, Shindo M, Suzuki M. Dietary red pepper ingestion increases carbohydrate oxidation at rest and during exercise in runners. Med Sci Sports Exerc 1997;29(3):355–361.

McCarthy GM, McCarty DJ. Effect of topical capsaicin in the therapy of painful osteoarthritis of the hands. J Rheumatol 1992;19(4):604–607.

Sicuteri F, Fanciullacci M, Nicolodi M, Geppetti P, Fusco BM, Marabini S, Alessandri M, Campagnolo V. Substance P theory: a unique focus on the painful and painless phenomena of cluster headache. Headache 1990;30(2):69–79.

Sicuteri F, Fusco BM, Marabini S, Campagnolo V, Maggi CA, Geppetti P, Fanciullacci M. Beneficial effect of capsaicin application to the nasal mucosa in cluster headache. Clin J Pain 1989;5(1):49–53.

Yeoh KG, Kang JY, Yap I, Guan R, Tan CC, Wee A, Teng CH. Chili protects against aspirin-induced gastroduodenal mucosal injury in humans. Dig Dis Sci 1995;40(3):580–583.

Yoshioka M, St-Pierre S, Drapeau V, Dionne I, Doucet E, Suzuki M, Tremblay A. Effects of red pepper on appetite and energy intake. Br J Nutr 1999;82(2):115–123.

FIBER

Overall Rank

★★★★★ for gut health
★★★★★ for cholesterol control
★★★★ for gut regularity and constipation

OVERVIEW

Fiber is found in the stems, seeds, and leaves of plants. Fiber is made up of long chains of sugar, but as humans, we lack the digestive enzymes to break down these complex polysaccharides (although a small amount of ingested fiber can be partially broken down by enzymes produced by bacteria in the intestines). Most of the fiber, however, is not broken down and exits the body in the feces. *Fiber* is a very broad term. More precise terms are *soluble fiber* and *insoluble fiber*. Soluble fiber dissolves in water and can be broken down by bacterial enzymes; insoluble fiber does not dissolve or break down. The distinction is important because the solubility of the fiber determines its health benefit. Fiber found in food is usually a mixture of both types; purified fiber supplements, however, may contain just one type of fiber.

Dietary sources of fiber are plentiful. Fruits, vegetables, seeds, and legumes (i.e., dried peas and beans such as lentils, split peas, red beans, and pinto beans) contain both types of fiber. Barley, oats, oat bran, and rye contain predominantly soluble fiber. Wheat bran, brown rice, and whole grains (grains that have not been refined) are excellent sources of insoluble fiber.

Supplemental sources of fiber include psyllium, methylcellulose, and polycarbophil, as well as fiber extracted from fruits, vegetables, and grains. Psyllium is a concentrated source of fiber from the husks of the psyllium plant. Methylcellulose and polycarbophil are chemically altered forms of cellulose (the cell wall of many plants). The chemical alterations make them resistant to bacterial breakdown. The Food and Drug Administration (FDA) has approved health claims for two dietary fibers: β glucan (0.75 g/serving) and psyllium (1.78 g/serving), based on evidence that 4 servings/day can reduce cardiovascular disease risk by reducing total cholesterol by an average of 2% and overall cardiovascular disease risk by about 4% (Jenkins et al., 2002).

General health recommendations call for a daily consumption of 20–40 g of fiber, but the average American consumes less than 15 g. Although the amount of soluble and insoluble fiber is not specified, it is assumed that people will receive both types of fiber. In general, claims made for supplemental forms of dietary fiber are based on scientific evidence showing that soluble fiber reduces the risk of heart disease by lowering total and low-density lipoprotein (LDL) cholesterol levels, and insoluble fiber reduces the risk of colon cancer by reducing the concentrations of fecal bile acids (American Medical Association, 1989; Anderson, 1994; Stampfer, 2000; Wolk, 1999).

COMMENTS

Clearly, adequate fiber is necessary for good health. Consumption of 20–40 g/day of fiber is possible from food sources alone but requires a high consumption of legumes and whole grains. At the same time, it is recognized that in the United States, the average fiber intake is less than 15 g/day. In light of average intake, fiber supplements are often recommended and warranted.

SCIENTIFIC SUPPORT

Soluble Fiber and Heart Disease Risk
Hundreds of studies have been conducted to examine the role of soluble fiber in reducing the risk of heart disease by lowering cholesterol levels.

Although it is difficult to compare the studies because of differences in the type and amount of soluble fiber, the number of people studied, and the initial cholesterol levels of the subjects, some general conclusions can be drawn. It is generally accepted by nutrition scientists that approximately 2–10 g/day of soluble fiber appears to reduce blood cholesterol and LDL cholesterol (Jenkins et al., 1993, 2001, 2002). The reduction is small but makes a substantial contribution to reducing heart disease risk. The source of the fiber (oats, pectin found in fruits, or psyllium) seems to make little difference because all types have been shown to be effective (Jenkins et al., 2002; Lampe et al., 1992). The inclusion of soluble fiber in the diet is both practical and safe as long as the individual is not allergic to the source of the fiber.

Soluble fiber reduces the risk of heart disease by lowering cholesterol and LDL (Jenkins et al., 1993, 2001). Although the mechanism is not entirely known, soluble fiber is thought to decrease the absorption of bile. Bile, which contains cholesterol, is necessary for the digestion of fat. It is secreted into the intestine in response to food intake, and most is reabsorbed after digestion is complete. When soluble fiber is present in the digestive tract, not as much bile is reabsorbed and more must be made by the liver. Some of the cholesterol that would have circulated in the blood is used to make the bile. In addition, soluble fiber can be partially broken down by intestinal bacteria, producing fatty acids that keep the liver from making cholesterol. It is generally accepted by nutrition scientists that soluble fiber intake can help reduce cholesterol levels. In one study, a high-fiber fruit and vegetable diet was shown to reduce LDL cholesterol levels by 33% within 1 week (Jenkins et al., 2001), and several studies have shown that the drop in total and LDL cholesterol from a diet high in fiber is nearly 50% greater than would be predicted by differences in dietary fat and cholesterol (Haack et al., 1998; Jenkins et al., 1993, 1997).

Insoluble Fiber and Colon Cancer Risk

For nearly 30 years, researchers have been studying the effect of fiber on colon cancer. People who consume diets high in fiber tend to also consume diets that are low in total fat, low in animal fat, and high in fruits and vegetables—all of which are factors that might reduce colon cancer risk. Fiber is also a vehicle for other compounds, such as phytic acid, an antioxidant thought to prevent colon cancer. Researchers are trying to determine whether fiber should be considered an independent factor in reducing colon cancer risk or whether the effect of fiber stems from a combination of other factors. Results of human studies have been mixed, but some large studies suggest that fiber is not protective against colon cancer (Hung et al., 2004; McCullough et al., 2003; Michels et al., 2000; Sellers et al., 1998). In particular, McCullough and Michels looked at very large populations (62,609 men and 70,554 women in the Cancer Prevention Study II Nutrition Cohort, 88,764 women in the

Nurses Health Study, and 47,325 men in the Health Professionals Follow-up Study), finding that higher intakes of plant foods or fiber were not related to lower risk of colon cancer (but that low intakes were related to a higher cancer risk).

On the other hand, numerous studies have suggested that diets high in insoluble fiber reduce the risk of colon cancer (Alberts et al., 1996; Kesaniemi et al., 1990; Lampe et al., 1992). If and how fiber reduces the risk of cancer is not completely known and is undoubtedly complicated. The theory that supports the role of a high-fiber diet in the prevention of colon cancer is controversial. It is suggested that insoluble fiber may work by helping to excrete bile from the body. Bile, which is necessary for the digestion of fat, is also thought to promote tumor growth. Insoluble fiber may bind with the bile, thus preventing it from being a promoter. Insoluble fiber also reduces the amount of time that fecal material is in the colon. Exposure to potential cancer-causing compounds is reduced because the fiber binds and removes these compounds quickly.

Researchers who question whether insoluble fiber actually reduces colon cancer risk do so because they are not convinced that the fiber itself is responsible. They suggest that foods that contain insoluble dietary fiber also contain substances such as antioxidants, folate, or dozens of other phytonutrients that protect the body from colon cancer (McCullough et al., 2003; Slattery et al., 1997; Voorrips et al., 2000). They argue that it is these compounds, rather than the dietary fiber, that help to protect against colon cancer.

Constipation

Constipation is a condition where bowel movements (feces) are hard and dry. The strain of trying to pass the hard, dry feces may result in hemorrhoids (swollen veins in the rectum). Adequate fiber, fluid, and exercise help prevent constipation. Both soluble and insoluble fibers help the feces stay moist because fiber attracts water. A well-accepted theory is that the laxative effect of insoluble fiber is also a result of its ability to speed up the time it takes for feces to move out of the body. Scientific studies support the role of dietary fiber to relieve constipation, especially when combined with adequate fluid intake and exercise. Both dietary fiber and fiber supplements are beneficial (Kritchevsky, 1986; Sandler, 1993).

SAFETY/DOSAGE

The intake of dietary fiber or fiber supplements within the recommended doses is considered safe. To prevent dehydration, adequate fluid must be consumed. Side effects such as excessive gas or bloating may occur. Some sources of the fiber are common allergens—for example, wheat and psyllium.

Total daily fiber consumption should be within the range of 20–40 g, with supplemental sources of fiber advised when dietary sources (fruits, vegetables, whole grains, legumes, and seeds) are below recommended levels. Popular fiber supplements (taken with 8 oz of water) are psyllium (7 g up to 3 times daily), methylcellulose (10 g up to 3 times daily), and polycarbophil (1 g up to 4 times daily).

REFERENCES

Alberts DS, Ritenbaugh C, Story JA, Aickin M, Rees-McGee S, Buller MK, Atwood J, Phelps J, Ramanujam PS, Bellapravalu S, Patel J, Bextinger L, Clark L. Randomized, double-blinded, placebo-controlled study of effect of wheat bran fiber and calcium on fecal bile acids in patients with resected adenomatous colon polyps. J Natl Cancer Inst 1996;88(2):81–92.

American Medical Association Council on Scientific Affairs. Dietary fiber and health. Conn Med 1989;53(9):529–534.

Anderson JW, Smith BM, Gustafson NJ. Health benefits and practical aspects of high-fiber diets. Am J Clin Nutr 1994;59(5 suppl):1242S–1247S.

Haack VS, Chesters JG, Vollendorf NW, Story JA, Marlett JA. Increasing amounts of dietary fiber provided by foods normalizes physiologic response of the large bowel without altering calcium balance or fecal steroid excretion. Am J Clin Nutr 1998;68(3):615–622.

Hung HC, Joshipura KJ, Jiang R, Hu FB, Hunter D, Smith-Warner SA, Colditz GA, Rosner B, Spiegelman D, Willett WC. Fruit and vegetable intake and risk of major chronic disease. J Natl Cancer Inst 2004;96(21):1577–1584.

Jenkins DJ, Kendall CW, Popovich DG, Vidgen E, Mehling CC, Vuksan V, Ransom TP, Rao AV, Rosenberg-Zand R, Tariq N, Corey P, Jones PJ, Raeini M, Story JA, Furumoto EJ, Illingworth DR, Pappu AS, Connelly PW. Effect of a very-high-fiber vegetable, fruit, and nut diet on serum lipids and colonic function. Metabolism 2001;50(4):494–503.

Jenkins DJ, Kendall CW, Vuksan V, Vidgen E, Parker T, Faulkner D, Mehling CC, Garsetti M, Testolin G, Cunnane SC, Ryan MA, Corey PN. Soluble fiber intake at a dose approved by the US Food and Drug Administration for a claim of health benefits: serum lipid risk factors for cardiovascular disease assessed in a randomized controlled crossover trial. Am J Clin Nutr 2002;75(5):834–839.

Jenkins DJ, Popovich DG, Kendall CW, Vidgen E, Tariq N, Ransom TP, Wolever TM, Vuksan V, Mehling CC, Boctor DL, Bolognesi C, Huang J, Patten R. Effect of a diet high in vegetables, fruit, and nuts on serum lipids. Metabolism 1997;46(5):530–537.

Jenkins DJ, Wolever TM, Rao AV, Hegele RA, Mitchell SJ, Ransom TP, Boctor DL, Spadafora PJ, Jenkins AL, Mehling C, et al. Effect on blood lipids of very high intakes of fiber in diets low in saturated fat and cholesterol. N Engl J Med 1993;329(1):21–26.

Kesaniemi YA, Tarpila S, Miettinen TA. Low vs high dietary fiber and serum, biliary, and fecal lipids in middle-aged men. Am J Clin Nutr 1990;51(6):1007–1012.

Kritchevsky D. The role of dietary fiber in health and disease. J Environ Pathol Toxicol Oncol 1986;6(3–4):273–284.

Lampe JW, Slavin JL, Melcher EA, Potter JD. Effects of cereal and vegetable fiber feeding on potential risk factors for colon cancer. Cancer Epidemiol Biomarkers Prev 1992;1(3):207–211.

McCullough ML, Robertson AS, Chao A, Jacobs EJ, Stampfer MJ, Jacobs DR, Diver WR, Calle EE, Thun MJ. A prospective study of whole grains, fruits, vegetables and colon cancer risk. Cancer Causes Control 2003;14(10):959–970.

Michels KB, Edward Giovannucci, Joshipura KJ, Rosner BA, Stampfer MJ, Fuchs CS, Colditz GA, Speizer FE, Willett WC. Prospective study of fruit and vegetable consumption and incidence of colon and rectal cancers. J Natl Cancer Inst 2000;92(21):1740–1752.

Sellers TA, Bazyk AE, Bostick RM, Kushi LH, Olson JE, Anderson KE, Lazovich D, Folsom AR. Diet and risk of colon cancer in a large prospective study of older women: an analysis stratified on family history (Iowa, United States). Cancer Causes Control 1998;9(4):357–367.

Sandler RS, Lyles CM, Peipins LA, McAuliffe CA, Woosley JT, Kupper LL. Diet and risk of colorectal adenomas: macronutrients, cholesterol, and fiber. J Natl Cancer Inst 1993;85(11):884–891.

Slattery ML, Potter JD, Coates A, Ma KN, Berry TD, Duncan DM, Caan BJ. Plant foods and colon cancer: an assessment of specific foods and their related nutrients (United States). Cancer Causes Control 1997;8(4):575–590.

Stampfer MJ, Hu FB, Manson JE, Rimm EB, Willett WC. Primary prevention of coronary heart disease in women through diet and lifestyle. N Engl J Med 2000;343(1):16–22.

Voorrips LE, Goldbohm RA, van Poppel G, Sturmans F, Hermus RJ, van den Brandt PA. Vegetable and fruit consumption and risks of colon and rectal cancer in a prospective cohort study: The Netherlands Cohort Study on Diet and Cancer. Am J Epidemiol 2000;152(11):1081–1092.

Wolk A, Manson JE, Stampfer MJ, Colditz GA, Hu FB, Speizer FE, Hennekens CH, Willett WC. Long-term intake of dietary fiber and decreased risk of coronary heart disease among women. JAMA 1999;281(21):1998–2004.

ADDITIONAL RESOURCES

Correa P. Epidemiological correlations between diet and cancer frequency. Cancer Res 1981;41(9 pt 2):3685–3690.

Jacobs DR Jr, Meyer KA, Kushi LH, Folsom AR. Whole-grain intake may reduce the risk of ischemic heart disease death in postmenopausal women: the Iowa Women's Health Study. Am J Clin Nutr 1998;68(2):248–257.

GINGER (ZINGIBER OFFICINALE)

Overall Rank

★★★★ for nausea prevention
★★★★ for control of inflammation
★★★   for pain relief
      as an antioxidant

OVERVIEW

Ginger has a long history of traditional use in many cultures and has been cultivated in India since before written history. In many countries, ginger is considered a spice, a flavor, and a medicine. Traditional medicine indications for ginger include indigestion, flatulence, diarrhea, malaria, fever, and low libido. In Traditional Chinese Medicine, it is used for diarrhea, abdominal pain, vomiting, abnormal uterine bleeding, cough, and dyspnea, and topically for inflamed joints. In traditional Indian medicine, it is used for strengthening the memory and as an aphrodisiac, a digestive, and a carminative (McKenna et al., 2002).

The pungent components in ginger, the gingerols, give it its aroma. Among the other compounds present are terpenoids and phenolic compounds, such as the shogaols. Western science has confirmed many of the traditional indications for ginger and has found that it possesses antiemetic, anti-inflammatory, and spasmolytic activities; promotes gastric secretion and saliva stimulant; stimulates peripheral circulation; and increases gastric motility (McKenna et al., 2002). The mechanisms of action of ginger for nausea are not fully understood but may be the result of ginger's ability to prevent gastric dysrhythmias by inhibiting the production but not the function of prostaglandins (Gonlachanvit et al., 2003). In 1992, Qian and Liu performed preclinical studies that indicated ginger's antimotion sickness action may be caused by central and peripheral anticholinergic and antihistaminic effects. Regardless, ginger is quickly gaining more clinical confirmation as a safe and effective treatment for nausea and gastric distress.

COMMENTS

Ginger is a good example of a food that is also an effective medicine. Ginger has been proven, both through a long traditional use and in clinical studies, to be effective in relieving nausea from various origins and may be found effective in the future for other indications, such as pain relief and inflammation.

SCIENTIFIC SUPPORT

Gastric Disorders

To understand the mechanism by which ginger is able to prevent motion sickness, a double-blind, randomized, placebo-controlled, crossover, clinical study was conducted subjecting 13 people (with a history of motion sickness) to circular vection. The authors had previously theorized that the mechanism results from ginger's preventing the development of gastric dysrhythmias and the elevation of plasma vasopressin. The outcome measures were nausea (score 0–3), electrogastrographic recordings, and plasma vasopressin levels. Ginger (1,000 and 2,000 mg) was able to reduce nausea, tachygastria and plasma vasopressin. It also prolonged the time before the onset of nausea and shortened recovery time (Lien et al., 2003).

In an exploration of the mechanism by which ginger is able to prevent nausea, it was hypothesized that ginger prevents disruption of slow-wave rhythm by acute hyperglycemia via inhibition of prostaglandin production. Twenty-two volunteers were administered ginger (1 g) or placebo and then subjected to fasting electrogastrography during hyperglycemic clamping to 250–290 mg/dL. It was confirmed that ginger was able to prevent slow-wave dysrhythmias evoked by acute hyperglycemia but had no effect on dysrhythmias elicited by the prostaglandin E1 analog. This confirmed that ginger was able to inhibit the production but not action of the prostaglandins (Gonlachanvit et al., 2003).

In a study on the gastric emptying rate of ginger, ginger root (1 g) or a placebo was given to 16 volunteers. The authors found that ginger did not affect gastric emptying (Phillips et al., 1993).

A placebo-controlled study was conducted to characterize the effects of ginger on gastric function and to evaluate the antimotion sickness activity of ginger. Ginger was given as either a dry powder (500 mg or

1,000 mg) or fresh ginger root (1,000 mg). Subjects were tested by making timed head movements in a rotating chair until they reached an endpoint of motion sickness that was short of vomiting. Ginger was found not to possess antimotion sickness activity or the ability to alter gastric function during motion sickness (Stewart et al., 1991).

Several clinical studies have investigated ginger for its use in alleviating pregnancy-related nausea (Portnoi et al., 2003; Smith et al., 2004; Sripramote and Lekhyananda, 2003; Willetts et al., 2003). In a randomized, placebo-controlled, double-blind, parallel design, Vutyavanich et al. (2001) studied the efficacy of ginger powder against nausea and vomiting in 67 pregnant women characterized as having pregnancy-related nausea and vomiting. After 4 days of treatment, the ginger group had 37.5% incidence in vomiting versus 65.7% in the placebo group. The subjective outcomes had the highest difference between groups, with 87.5% of the ginger group reporting improved symptoms versus 28.6% of the placebo group.

Inflammatory Response

In a clinical study on the effect of ginger consumption on thromboxane B_2 (TXB_2) production, seven volunteers ingested 5 g of fresh ginger for 7 days. A significant decrease in TXB_2 production was found in six of the volunteers (Srivastava and Mustafa, 1989). Lumb (1994) performed a randomized, double-blind, placebo-controlled study on ginger powder (2 g in capsules) in eight volunteers and measured whole blood platelet aggregation, platelet count, and bleeding time before and at 3 hours and 24 hours after administration. No significant differences were found in measurements. Janssen et al. (1996) studied the effects on ginger (both cooked and raw) on TBX_2 production in a randomized, placebo-controlled, multiple crossover study and found no significant difference in TBX_2 production.

Pain Relief

Srivastava and Mustafa (1992) conducted a questionnaire-based open study on ginger in a group of 46 patients with osteoarthritis or rheumatoid arthritis who had taken ginger for 3 months to 2.5 years. Significant pain relief was reported by 55% of the osteoarthritis patients and 74% of the rheumatoid arthritis patients.

Bliddal et al. (2000) performed a randomized, double-blind, placebo-controlled study on the effect of a ginger extract (Eurovita Extract 33, standardized to contain hydroxy-methoxy-phenyl compounds) on pain relief. No significant differences in pain relief were found for ginger. The authors, however, questioned whether carryover effects from the washout period produced confounding results and whether the amount of time for treatment was sufficient.

SAFETY/DOSAGE

The dosage of ginger is typically 1–2 g of fresh or powdered root daily. Ginger extracts are on the market, but fresh ginger root is thought to be superior (McKenna et al., 2002).

Side effects from ginger are unknown. In some of the studies, side effects such as headache were reported but could have resulted from motion sickness rather than ginger (Lien, 2003; Stewart, 1991). Ginger should only be used in the case of gallstones after consulting a physician. Small-scale studies on the use of ginger during pregnancy or lactation have found no adverse effects (McKenna et al., 2002).

REFERENCES

Bliddal H, Rosetzsky A, Schlichting P, Weidner MS, Andersen LA, Ibfelt HH, Christensen K, Jensen ON, Barslev J. A randomized, placebo-controlled, cross-over study of ginger extracts and ibuprofen in osteoarthritis. Osteoarthritis Cartilage 2000;8(1):9–12.

Gonlachanvit S, Chen YH, Hasler WL, Sun WM, Owyang C. Ginger reduces hyperglycemia-evoked gastric dysrhythmias in healthy humans: possible role of endogenous prostaglandins. J Pharmacol Exp Ther 2003;307(3):1098–1103.

Janssen PL, Meyboom S, van Staveren WA, de Vegt F, Katan MB. Consumption of ginger (Zingiber officinale roscoe) does not affect ex vivo platelet thromboxane production in humans. Eur J Clin Nutr 1996;50(11):772–774.

Lien HC, Sun WM, Chen YH, Kim H, Hasler W, Owyang C. Effects of ginger on motion sickness and gastric slow-wave dysrhythmias induced by circular vection. Am J Physiol Gastrointest Liver Physiol 2003;284(3):G481–G489.

Lumb AB. Effect of dried ginger on human platelet function. Thromb Haemost 1994;71(1):110–111.

McKenna D, Jones K, Hughes K, eds. Botanical Medicines: The Desk Reference for Major Herbal Supplements. 2nd Ed. New York: Haworth Press, 2002.

Phillips S, Hutchinson S, Ruggier R. Zingiber officinale does not affect gastric emptying rate. A randomised, placebo-controlled, crossover trial. Anaesthesia 1993;48(5):393–395.

Portnoi G, Chng LA, Karimi-Tabesh L, Koren G, Tan MP, Einarson A. Prospective comparative study of the safety and effectiveness of ginger for the treatment of nausea and vomiting in pregnancy. Am J Obstet Gynecol 2003;189(5):1374–1377.

Qian DS, Liu ZS. Pharmacologic studies of antimotion sickness actions of ginger. Zhongguo Zhong Xi Yi Jie He Za Zhi 1992;12(2):95–98, 70.

Smith C, Crowther C, Willson K, Hotham N, McMillian V. A randomized controlled trial of ginger to treat nausea and vomiting in pregnancy. Obstet Gynecol 2004;103(4):639–645.

Sripramote M, Lekhyananda N. A randomized comparison of ginger and vitamin B6 in the treatment of nausea and vomiting of pregnancy. J Med Assoc Thai 2003;86(9):846–853.

Srivastava KC, Mustafa T. Ginger (Zingiber officinale) and rheumatic disorders. Med Hypotheses 1989;29(1):25–28.

Srivastava KC, Mustafa T. Ginger (Zingiber officinale) in rheumatism and musculoskeletal disorders. Med Hypotheses 1992;39(4):342–348.

Stewart JJ, Wood MJ, Wood CD, Mims ME. Effects of ginger on motion sickness susceptibility and gastric function. Pharmacology 1991;42(2):111–120.

Vutyavanich T, Kraisarin T, Ruangsri R. Ginger for nausea and vomiting in pregnancy: randomized, double-masked, placebo-controlled trial. Obstet Gynecol 2001;97(4):577–582.

Willetts KE, Ekangaki A, Eden JA. Effect of a ginger extract on pregnancy-induced nausea: a randomised controlled trial. Aust N Z J Obstet Gynaecol 2003;43(2):139–144.

ADDITIONAL RESOURCES

Fischer-Rasmussen W, Kjaer SK, Dahl C, Asping U. Ginger treatment of hyperemesis gravidarum. Eur J Obstet Gynecol Reprod Biol 1991;38(1):19–24.

MASTIC (FROM *PISTACIA LENTISCUS*)

Overall Rank

★★ for treating and preventing ulcers
★★ for alleviating gastrointestinal discomfort (heartburn)
★★ for treating and preventing bad breath

OVERVIEW

Mastic is a resin, or gum, extracted from a tree grown in Mediterranean or Middle Eastern regions. Long used as a chewing gum and a traditional medicine, mastic resin also has been developed for use in numerous industrial applications (Milov et al., 1998). Preliminary clinical evidence has confirmed that mastic resins are useful in the treatment of ulcers. Further, mastic has been shown to exhibit antibacterial activity against *Helicobacter pylori*, explaining its efficacy in ulcers. Mastic has also shown antibacterial, antiplaque, and antigingival activity in the saliva and on the teeth (Takahashi et al., 2003).

COMMENTS

Although mastic has not yet been well studied as an herbal medicine, preliminary clinical evidence is promising to confirm the efficacy of its historical use in treating ulcers (Al-Habbal, 1984; Huwez, 1986).

SCIENTIFIC SUPPORT

Duodenal Ulcer

Al-Habbal et al. (1984) performed a double-blind, clinical study on mastic for treatment of duodenal ulcer. Twenty patients were given mastic (1 g/day) and 18 received a placebo (lactose, 1 g/day) to for 2 weeks. Mastic treatment resulted in highly statistically significant improvements in both the symptomatic relief (80% of the treatment group versus 50% of the placebo group) and the clinical manifestation of disease as proven by endoscopic examination (70% of the treatment group versus 22% of the placebo patients). Additionally, mastic was found to be well tolerated with no side effects.

Antiplaque, Antigingival, and Antibacterial Activity of Mastic Chewing Gum

A chewing gum of mastic resin was tested in two double-blind, randomized, placebo-controlled studies for the control of dental plaque. In the first study, saliva was collected from the mouths of participants after mechanical brushing and chewing gum and examined for its antibacterial activity by mastic or placebo gum. The mastic chewing gum group showed statistically significant reductions in bacterial growth compared with the placebo group during the 4 hours of chewing gum. In the second study, mastic and placebo gum chewing (and no brushing) were tested over 7 days for their ability to control new plaque formation on tooth surfaces and on gingival inflammation. The mastic group showed significantly reduced plaque index measures and gingival index compared with the placebo group (Takahashi et al., 2003).

SAFETY/DOSAGE

For treating ulcers and gastrointestinal discomfort, 1 g of mastic is used. Mastic is not known to produce any side effects and is thought to be safe (Al-Habbal et al., 1984).

REFERENCES

Al-Habbal MJ, Al-Habbal Z, Huwez FU. A double-blind controlled clinical trial of mastic and placebo in the treatment of duodenal ulcer. Clin Exp Pharmacol Physiol 1984;11(5):541–544.

Huwez FU, Al-Habbal MJ. Mastic in treatment of benign gastric ulcers. Gastroenterol Jpn 1986;21(3):273–274.

Milov DE, Andres JM, Erhart NA, Bailey DJ. Chewing gum bezoars of the gastrointestinal tract. Pediatrics 1998;102(2):e22.

Takahashi K, Fukazawa M, Motohira H, Ochiai K, Nishikawa H, Miyata T. A pilot study on antiplaque effects of mastic chewing gum in the oral cavity. J Periodontol 2003;74(4):501–505.

MILK THISTLE (SILYBUM MARIANUM)

Overall Rank

★★★★★ for detoxification and liver health
★★★★★ for liver protection (against toxins)
★★★★ as a restorative from liver disorders

OVERVIEW

Milk thistle is a common weed that has a long history as a traditional medicine and food. Its potent activity in restoring and protecting the liver has been confirmed in numerous studies, and it is often included in herbal medicines intended to act as "detoxification" formulas. The main active constituents of milk thistle are the flavonolignans; the bioactive flavonolignans are generally called silymarin. Silymarin has three isomers: silybin (also called silibinin), silydianin, and silychristin (McKenna et al., 2001).

Silymarin has exhibited cholesterol-lowering and normalizing activity, blood pressure–lowering activity in hypertensive patients, antiproliferative activity in cancer cells, and chemoprotective activity. The preclinical data that most relate to both the traditional and current herbal uses of milk thistle, however, are focused on hepatic functions and antioxidant activity (McKenna et al., 2001). Some highlights of this preclinical data follows:

- Silymarin has shown hepatoprotective activity against a number of toxins, including carbon tetrachloride, galactosamine, ethanol, paracetamol, Amanita toxins, thioacetamide, microcystin-LR, heavy metals, poisons of lanthamden (from lanthanum), sulfur acetamide, and the FU3 virus (a hepatotoxic virus of cold blooded animals; Bone, 1996; Morazzoni and Bombardelli, 1995).
- Silymarin has shown activity against peroxidation in liver microsomes of rats (Bosisio et al., 1992).
- Silymarin has hepatorestorative properties, primarily through the stimulation of protein synthesis. Silymarin stimulates the activity of RNA polymerase, which synthesizes ribosomal RNA (Sonnenbichler and Zetl, 1988).
- In the process of liver cirrhosis and damage caused by ethyl alcohol and paracetamol, the depletion of glutathione levels causes most of the damage to the liver. Silymarin has been found to increase glutathione levels, thus protecting the liver (Valenzuela et al., 1985).
- Also involved in the hepatoprotective activity of silymarin, certain cytosol enzymes (including alanine aminotransferase [ALT] and lactic dehydrogenase) are inhibited by silymarin, preventing the destruction of the cell membranes. In addition, certain intoxicants have been found to block phospholipid synthesis on rat livers, and silymarin is capable of counteracting this effect (Castigli et al., 1977).
- Silybin was found to partially or completely block the toxic effects of cisplatin on the kidney functions of rats (Gaedeke et al., 1996).
- Silymarin (especially silybin) acts as scavengers of free radicals and reactive oxygen species. Free-radical formation is known to be one of the key processes in hepatotoxicity, contributing to lipid peroxidation on the cellular membranes (Valenzuela et al., 1989).

COMMENTS

Milk thistle is safe and efficacious in a therapeutic area that lacks many good pharmaceutical alternatives: liver restoration and protection. Although it is not in the forefront of public awareness, liver health may be one of the most pertinent issues surrounding our evolving unhealthy lifestyles and our growing concern about the effect of toxins from the environment on our health.

SCIENTIFIC SUPPORT

A study by Lang et al. (1990a) investigated the effect of milk thistle extract (Legalon, 140 mg orally 3 times daily) in cirrhotic patients (from alcohol consumption). The randomized, double-blind, placebo-controlled study was conducted in 4 weeks and used a second active treatment for comparison (Acia-P, 200 mg orally 3 times daily). Both active treatments showed significant improvements in hepatic functions, and no change was found for the placebo group. In the milk thistle group, bilirubin, aspartate aminotransferase (AST), and ALT had normalized during treatment (they were moderately elevated before the study). Another study by Lang et al. (1990b) found similar results.

A 2-year, double-blind, placebo-controlled study examined the effect of an oral dose of 200 mg of 70% silymarin extract 3 times daily in 170 cirrhotic patients (alcohol was the cause of the disease in 91 patients and was not the cause in 79 patients). At the end of the study, the treatment group had a 23% mortality rate and a cumulative survival rate of 58% compared with the 33% mortality rate and 38% cumulative survival rate of the placebo group (Ferenci et al., 1989).

Further studies have found that silymarin exhibits a hepatoprotective action in people prior to alcohol consumption and improves hepatic function in alcoholic patients. Silymarin has been found to be most effective for milder cases of alcohol cirrhosis (McKenna et al., 2001; Salmi and Sarna, 1982).

In a double-blind, crossover, clinical study on the effect of silymarin (420 mg/day) versus ursodeoxycholic acid (UDCA, 600 mg/day) in chronic hepatitis patients, significant improvements were found in both treatment groups. Significant declines in the serum levels of several elevated liver enzymes were noted for both groups, and the group receiving UDCA also had a significant reduction in levels of γ–glutamyl-transpeptidase (γ–GT). The crossover phase of the study used a combination therapy of UDCA and silymarin versus placebo, but the combined treatment showed no advantage over either single treatment (Lirussi and Okolicsanyi, 1992).

A review of clinical studies performed by Hikino and Kiso (1988) found silymarin to work therapeutically through three main activities in protecting the liver from toxic agents: stabilizing the cell membrane, stimulating protein synthesis, and accelerating the regeneration of damaged liver tissue. An open-label study involving 975 patients with liver damage from various causes examined the effect of 140 mg of a 70% standardized milk thistle extract administered orally 2–3 times daily for 12 weeks. Five hundred seventy of the patients were diagnosed with a fatty liver, with 143 confirmed to have fatty liver hepatitis and 214 confirmed to have hepatic cirrhosis. A mean reduction in the levels of serum liver enzymes (AST dropped from 46.0 µg/L to 28.8 µg/L; ALT from 48.0 µg/L to 31.0 µg/L; and γ–GT from 112.0 µg/L to 60.6 µg/L), and a normalization of total bilirubin concentration was found at the end of the study (Grungreiff et al., 1995).

A double-blind study using silymarin (800 mg/day orally for 90 days) found therapeutic effects in female patients with hepatopathies who had been taking psychopharmaceutical drugs such as phenothiazines or butrophenones for 5 years. A decline in the level of malodialdehyde was found in the treatment group (Palasciano et al., 1994). A study involving 2,169 patients with hepatotoxicities found improved or normalized clinical readings after taking silymarin orally for 8 weeks (at an average of 264 mg/day) (Frerick et al., 1990).

A study involving 49 workers who had been exposed to toluene and/or xylene vapors on the job for 5–20 years tested the therapeutic effect of silymarin on liver function. All the patients had low blood platelet counts and abnormal liver function before the study, and after taking silymarin for 30 days (at 140 mg orally 3 times daily) showed significant improvement in liver and hematological tests. Symptoms reported as headaches were ameliorated after treatment, as well as parameters of leukocytosis, relative lymphocytosis, serum, γ–GT, ALT, and AST. In addition, platelet counts were increased after treatment (Szilard et al., 1988).

A 12-month, open-controlled study involving diabetic patients with alcoholic liver cirrhosis examined the therapeutic effect of silymarin (600 mg/day) with standard therapy for 4 months. Significant improvements in those receiving silymarin were found: a significant decrease in fasting and daily blood glucose levels, daily glycated hemoglobin levels, and glucosuria levels. Levels of malodialdehyde were also decreased. In addition, blood insulin levels were improved significantly, as well as the amount of insulin needed by injection (Velussi et al., 1997).

SAFETY/DOSAGE

Dosage of milk thistle is 175 mg/day and is usually based on an extract standardized to 80% silymarin flavonoids (silybin, silydianin, and silychristin). Other daily dosage recommendations vary depending on the preparation: 200–400 mg (70% silymarin standardized extract, calculated as silybin); 600 mg (of a 70:1 extract for advanced cirrhosis); and 3–5 mL (1:1 liquid extract; McKenna et al., 2001).

Milk thistle is known to be safe and well tolerated because of its long history as a food. Most of the side effects reported in clinical trials are considered not significantly different from placebo or of a mild and transient nature. A few cases have been reported of a mild laxative effect and pruritic skin rash produced by milk thistle (McKenna et al., 2001).

REFERENCES

Bone K. Silybum marianum. MediHerb 1996; 2: 22–23:1322–1375.

Bosisio E, Benelli C, and Pirola O. Effect of the flavonolignans of Silybum marianum L. on lipid peroxidation in rat liver microsomes and freshly isolated hepatocytes. Pharmacol Res 1992;25:147–154.

Castigli E, Montanini I, Roberti R, Porcellati G. The activity of silybin on phospholipid metabolism of normal and fatty liver in vivo. Pharmacol Res Comm 1977;9:59–69.

Ferenci P, Dragosics B, Dittroch H, Frank H, Benda L, Lochs H, Meryn S, Base W, Schneider B. Randomized controlled trial of silymarin treatment in patients with cirrhosis of the liver. J Hepatol 1989;9:105–113.

Frerick H, Kuhn U, Strenge-Hesse A. Silymarin—ein phytopharmakon zur behandlung von toxischen leberschäden. Der Kassenarzt 1990;33–34:36–41.

Gaedeke J, Fels LM, Bokemeyer C, Mengs U, Stolte H, Lentzen H. Cisplatin nephrotoxicity and protection by silibinin. Nephrol Dial Transplant 1996;11(1):55–62.

Grungreiff K, Albrecht M, Strenge-Hesse A. The value of drug therapy for liver disease in general practice. Medizinische Welt 1995;46:222–227.

Hikino H, Kiso Y. Natural products for liver disease. In: Wagner H, Hikino H, Farnsworth NR, eds. Economic and Medicinal Plant Research. 2nd Ed. London: Academic Press, 1988.

Lang I, Nekam K, Deak G, Muzes G, Gonzales-Cabello R, Gergely P, Csomos G, Feher J. Immunomodulatory and hepatoprotective effects of in vivo treatment with free radical scavengers. Ital J Gastroenterol 1990a;22(5):283–287.

Lang I, Nekam K, Gonzalez-Cabello R, Muzes G, Gergely P, Feher J. Hepatoprotective and immunological effects of antioxidant drugs. Tokai J Exp Clin Med 1990b;15(2–3):123–127.

Lirussi F, Okolicsanyi L. Cytoprotection in the nineties. Experience with ursodeoxycholic acid and silymarin in chronic liver disease. Acta Physiologica Hungarica 1992;80:363–367.

McKenna DJ, Jones K, Hughes K, eds. Botanical Medicines: A Desktop Reference for the Major Herbal Supplements. New York: Haworth Press, 2001.

Morazzoni P, Bombardelli E. Silybum marianum (Carduus marianus) Fitoterapia 1995;66:3–42.

Palasciano G, Portincasa P, Palmieri V, Ciani D, Vendemiale G, Altomare E. The effect of silymarin on plasma levels of malondialdehyde in patients receiving long-term treatment with psychotropic drugs. Curr Ther Res 1994;55:537–545.

Salmi H, Sarna S. Effect of silymarin on chemical, functional and morphological alterations of the liver: a double-blind controlled study. Scand J Gastroenterol 1982;17(4):517–521.

Sonnenbichler J, Zetl, I. Specific binding of a flavonolignane derivative to an estradiol receptor. In: Cody V, Middleton E Jr, Harborne JB, eds. Plant Flavonoids in Biology and Medicine: Biochemical, Pharmacological and Structure-Activity Relationships. New York: Alan R. Liss, 1988.

Szilard S, Szentgyorgyi D, Demeter D. Protective effect of Legalon in workers exposed to organic solvents. Acta Medica Hungarica 1988;45:249–246.

Valenzuela A, Aspillaga M, Vial S, Guerra R. Selectivity of silymarin on the increase of the glutathione content in different tissues of the rat. Planta Medica 1989;55(5):420–442.

Valenzuela A, Lagos C, Schmidt K, Videla LA. Silymarin protection against hepatic lipid peroxidation induced by acute ethanol intoxication in the rat. Biochem Pharmacol 1985;34(12):2209–2212.

Velussi M, Cernigoi AM, De Monte A, Dapas F, Caffau C, Zilli M. Long-term (12 months) treatment with an anti-oxidant drug (silymarin) is effective on hyperinsulinemia, exogenous insulin need and malondialdehyde levels in cirrhotic diabetic patients. J Hepatol 1997;26(4):871–879.

PREBIOTICS OR FRUCTO-OLIGOSACCHARIDES (FOS)

Overall Rank

★★★ for gut health
★★ for immune system support

OVERVIEW

Fructo-oligosaccharides (FOS), also called prebiotics, are a group of undigestible compounds that stimulate the growth of beneficial microflora. (Note that *probiotics*, discussed in the next section, are the actual beneficial bacteria, such as acidophilus and bifidum). Chemically, an FOS is a glucose molecule bonded to multiple fructose molecules. Because these bonds cannot be broken down by enzymes in the human small intestine, the FOS molecule is intact when it reaches the large intestine, where it becomes a substrate for colonic bacteria. The effects of short-chain FOS have been studied for nearly two decades. Groups of oligosaccharides can be found in foods like beans, blueberries, and onions; a liquid supplement is available in Japan; and FOS is available in capsule form in the United States.

COMMENTS

FOS has been shown to selectively stimulate the growth and activity of beneficial bacteria in the colon. Found naturally in many foods—like wheat, onions, bananas, honey, garlic, and leeks—FOS can also be isolated from chicory root or synthesized enzymatically from sucrose (both more commonly found in FOS dietary supplements). Fermentation of FOS in the colon results in numerous physiologic effects, including increasing the numbers of the beneficial bifidobacteria in the colon, increasing calcium absorption, increasing fecal weight, shortening gastrointestinal transit time, and possibly lowering blood lipid levels.

Based on the available scientific evidence, FOS supplements are generally claimed to boost levels and activity of beneficial gut bacteria and thus promote general gut health, reduce serum lipids, increase intestinal calcium absorption, alleviate antibiotic-induced diarrhea, and reduce both the severity of irritable bowel syndromes and the risk of colon cancer.

SCIENTIFIC SUPPORT

Short-chain FOS is metabolized in the colon (by colonic bacteria) into short-chain fatty acids (Giacco et al., 2004). These short-chain fatty acids cause a drop in pH, which may inhibit the growth of pathogenic bacteria, facilitate intestinal calcium absorption, and act as an energy substrate for colonic epithelial cells (Bouhnik et al., 1999; Tahiri et al., 2001). By manipulating colonic pH and microflora content, FOS may play a protective role against colon cancer (Giacco et al., 2004; Swanson et al., 2002; Ten Bruggencate et al., 2003, 2004). Research also points to a reduction in liver fatty acid synthesis as a possible mechanism for serum lipid reduction (Giacco et al., 2004; Swanson et al., 2002).

Human studies have shown significant increases in bifidobacteria from ingestion of as little as 6–8 g of short-chain FOS per day (Chow, 2002). Research has also shown decreases in pathogenic colonic bacteria from FOS ingestion (Chow, 2002). There is evidence that short-chain FOS can lower cholesterol and triglycerides, but most of this research has involved animal models. Colon tumors and indicators of cancer have also been reduced in animal models. Although animal studies have given promising results, relatively few human studies have shown that mineral absorption can be enhanced from FOS ingestion (Tahiri et al., 2001).

SAFETY/DOSAGE

Because the bonds of FOS are not digestible, bacterial metabolism in the large intestine produces gas and bloating. Flatulence is a common symptom associated with FOS ingestion and can be worse in people who are lactose intolerant (depending on how the FOS is processed). Studies have shown that the severity of symptoms is dose-dependent (less FOS, fewer symptoms). Ingestion of 20–30 g/day has been associated with the onset of severe discomfort, but symptoms may be alleviated by starting with a small dose and increasing gradually to the desired amount (Bouhnik et al., 1999). The "optimal" dose of FOS—the amount that produces a significant increase in bifidobacteria and is fairly well tolerated—appears to be 10 g/day.

REFERENCES

Bouhnik Y, Flourie B, Riottot M, Bisetti N, Gailing MF, Guibert A, Bornet F, Rambaud JC. Effects of fructo-oligosaccharides ingestion on fecal bifidobacteria and selected metabolic indexes of colon carcinogenesis in healthy humans. Nutr Cancer 1996;26(1):21–29.

Bouhnik Y, Vahedi K, Achour L, Attar A, Salfati J, Pochart P, Marteau P, Flourie B, Bornet F, Rambaud JC. Short-chain fructo-oligosaccharide administration dose-dependently increases fecal bifidobacteria in healthy humans. J Nutr 1999;129(1):113–116.

Chow J. Probiotics and prebiotics: A brief overview. J Ren Nutr 2002;12(2):76–86.

Giacco R, Clemente G, Luongo D, Lasorella G, Fiume I, Brouns F, Bornet F, Patti L, Cipriano P, Rivellese AA, Riccardi G. Effects of short-chain fructo-oligosaccharides on glucose and lipid metabolism in mild hypercholesterolaemic individuals. Clin Nutr 2004;23(3):331–340.

Swanson KS, Grieshop CM, Flickinger EA, Bauer LL, Wolf BW, Chow J, Garleb KA, Williams JA, Fahey GC Jr. Fructooligosaccharides and Lactobacillus acidophilus modify bowel function and protein catabolites excreted by healthy humans. J Nutr 2002;132(10):3042–3050.

Tahiri M, Tressol JC, Arnaud J, Bornet F, Bouteloup-Demange C, Feillet-Coudray C, Ducros V, Pepin D, Brouns F, Rayssiguier AM, Coudray C. Five-week intake of short-chain fructo-oligosaccharides increases intestinal absorption and status of magnesium in postmenopausal women. J Bone Miner Res 2001;16(11):2152–2160.

Ten Bruggencate SJ, Bovee-Oudenhoven IM, Lettink-Wissink ML, Katan MB, Van Der Meer R. Dietary fructo-oligosaccharides and inulin decrease resistance of rats to salmonella: protective role of calcium. Gut 2004;53(4):530–535.

Ten Bruggencate SJ, Bovee-Oudenhoven IM, Lettink-Wissink ML, Van der Meer R. Dietary fructo-oligosaccharides dose-dependently increase translocation of salmonella in rats. J Nutr 2003;133(7):2313–2318.

ADDITIONAL RESOURCES

Alles MS, Hautvast JG, Nagengast FM, Hartemink R, Van Laere KM, Jansen JB. Fate of fructo-oligosaccharides in the human intestine. Br J Nutr 1996;76(2):211–221.

Djouzi Z, Andrieux C. Compared effects of three oligosaccharides on metabolism of intestinal microflora in rats inoculated with a human faecal flora. Br J Nutr 1997;78(2):313–324.

Flickinger EA, Hatch TF, Wofford RC, Grieshop CM, Murray SM, Fahey GC Jr. In vitro fermentation properties of selected fructooligosaccharide-containing vegetables and in vivo colonic microbial populations are affected by the diets of healthy human infants. J Nutr 2002;132(8):2188–2194.

Gibson GR. Dietary modulation of the human gut microflora using prebiotics. Br J Nutr 1998;80(4):S209–S212.

Luo J, Van Yperselle M, Rizkalla SW, Rossi F, Bornet FR, Slama G. Chronic consumption of short-chain fructooligosaccharides does not affect basal hepatic glucose production or insulin resistance in type 2 diabetics. J Nutr 2000;130(6):1572–1577.

Moore N, Chao C, Yang LP, Storm H, Oliva-Hemker M, Saavedra JM. Effects of fructo-oligosaccharide-supplemented infant cereal: a double-blind, randomized trial. Br J Nutr 2003;90(3):581–587.

Piche T, des Varannes SB, Sacher-Huvelin S, Holst JJ, Cuber JC, Galmiche JP. Colonic fermentation influences lower esophageal sphincter function in gastroesophageal reflux disease. Gastroenterology 2003;124(4):894–902.

Rao AV. Dose-response effects of inulin and oligofructose on intestinal bifidogenesis effects. J Nutr 1999;129(7 suppl):1442S–1445S.

Roberfroid MB. Dietary fiber, inulin, and oligofructose: a review comparing their physiological effects. Crit Rev Food Sci Nutr 1993;33(2):103–148.

Roberfroid MB. Prebiotics and synbiotics: concepts and nutritional properties. Br J Nutr 1998;80(4):S197–S202.

Roberfroid MB, Van Loo JA, Gibson GR. The bifidogenic nature of chicory inulin and its hydrolysis products. J Nutr 1998;128(1):11–19.

Schaafsma G, Meuling WJ, van Dokkum W, Bouley C. Effects of a milk product, fermented by Lactobacillus acidophilus and with fructo-oligosaccharides added, on blood lipids in male volunteers. Eur J Clin Nutr 1998;52(6):436–440.

van Dokkum W, Wezendonk B, Srikumar TS, van den Heuvel EG. Effect of nondigestible oligosaccharides on large-bowel functions, blood lipid concentrations and glucose absorption in young healthy male subjects. Eur J Clin Nutr 1999;53(1):1–7.

PROBIOTICS (ACIDOPHILUS, BIFIDUS)

Overall Rank

★★★★ for gut health
★★★★ for gut immunity
★★★ for systemic immunity
★★★ for reducing the risk of colon cancer

OVERVIEW

Probiotics is a term used to refer to a group of beneficial bacteria that help maintain the health and function of the gastrointestinal tract. Probiotics have been defined as viable microorganisms that, when ingested, help prevent and treat specific pathologic conditions. These microorganisms are believed to exert biological effects through a phenomenon known as colonization resistance, whereby the indigenous anaerobic flora limits the concentration of potentially pathogenic (mostly aerobic) flora in the digestive tract. Other modes of action, such as supplying enzymes or influencing enzyme activity in the gastrointestinal tract, may also account for some of the other physiologic effects that have been attributed to probiotics.

Acidophilus (*Lactobacillus acidophilus*) and bifidus (*Bifidobacterium lactis*) of varying strains are popular forms of beneficial bacteria found in dietary supplements. By displacing other bacteria and yeast, acidophilus and other lactic acid bacteria may also play an important role in immune system function and prevention of gastrointestinal problems, including cancer. A wide variety of beneficial bacterial strains can be found in cultured yogurts and in freeze-dried form as dietary supplements. Claims for these products are generally for reducing cholesterol levels (marginal evidence), supporting immune system function (solid evidence), maintaining a healthy digestive system (solid evidence), and preventing colon cancer (preliminary evidence) (Bengmark, 2000, 1998; Collins and Gibson, 1999; de Roos, 2000).

COMMENTS

Dietary supplements providing acidophilus in combination with other beneficial probiotics are fairly inexpensive. Given the strong evidence for their beneficial effects on immune system function and the possibility that regular consumption may reduce colon cancer risk, these supplements would be a good choice for anybody looking for a general immune system booster (Dupont, 2000; Erickson, 2000; LaMont, 2000; Sanders, 2000).

SCIENTIFIC SUPPORT

The digestive system is home to millions of bacteria that help digest, modify, and convert the food we eat. Any alteration in the gastrointestinal environment is likely to influence the activity of these beneficial bacteria, sometimes posing health problems. Maintaining the "normal" populations of these good bacteria in the intestines by consuming them as supplements or in cultured yogurt can help displace disease-promoting bacteria and yeast that may gain a foothold when the levels of good bacteria drop.

Acidophilus and other beneficial bacteria are both acid and bile resistant and thus capable of surviving transit through the gastrointestinal tract after they are ingested. These bacteria are sometimes called probiotics because regular consumption is linked to health benefits such as reducing cholesterol, preventing microbial growth, modulating the immune system, and possibly preventing colon cancer.

Both human and animal studies have shown direct benefits of regular consumption of acidophilus and other beneficial bacteria on immune system function (Arunachalam et al., 2000; Gill et al., 2000, 2001a, 2001b; Sheih et al., 2001). Overall, probiotics tend to result in an enhanced ability of the immune system to recognize and destroy invading organisms. Several key components of the immune system, including macrophages, immunoglobulins, and cytokines, are altered by regular intake of beneficial bacteria. Populations of white blood cells are known to increase in number and activity following 1–2 weeks of consuming beneficial bacteria (Gill et al., 2001a, 2001b; Sheih et al., 2001). Importantly, resistance to viral and bacterial infections is significantly improved following regular intake of probiotics.

Epidemiological studies support the possibility that consumption of beneficial bacteria (from fermented milk and yogurt) may play a role in the prevention of colon cancer and inflammatory conditions (Gill et al., 2000, 2001a, 2001b; Isolauri et al., 2000; Sheih et al., 2001). Test-tube studies have shown that acidophilus can decrease the cancer-causing potential (mutagenic activity) of various carcinogens, possibly because of a direct interaction between the carcinogens and the bacteria (Brady, 2000; Dugas, 1999; Gibson, 1998). Consumption of acidophilus (and other lactic acid bacteria) has also been shown to reduce levels of cancer-causing enzymes in the digestive tract, supporting the possibility that probiotics do indeed play a role in the prevention of colon cancer.

SAFETY/DOSAGE

No safety issues are associated with regular consumption of acidophilus or other probiotics at recommended levels, although people with severe gastrointestinal ailments (e.g., Crohn disease, ulcerative colitis) should consult with their personal physician before consuming probiotic supplements. Most probiotic products will typically list the type of bacteria and the number of "live cells" on the label or side panel. There are no strict guidelines for dosage intake, but 1–10 billion colony forming units (CFUs) is a general rule of thumb and corresponds to effective levels used in human studies.

REFERENCES

Arunachalam K, Gill HS, Chandra RK. Enhancement of natural immune function by dietary consumption of Bifidobacterium lactis (HN019). Eur J Clin Nutr 2000;54(3):263–267.

Bengmark S. Bacteria for optimal health. Nutrition 2000;16(7–8):611–615.

Bengmark S. Ecological control of the gastrointestinal tract. The role of probiotic flora. Gut 1998;42(1):2–7.

Brady LJ, Gallaher DD, Busta FF. The role of probiotic cultures in the prevention of colon cancer. J Nutr 2000;130(2 suppl):410S–414S.

Collins MD, Gibson GR. Probiotics, prebiotics, and synbiotics: approaches for modulating the microbial ecology of the gut. Am J Clin Nutr 1999;69(5):1052S–1057S.

de Roos NM, Katan MB. Effects of probiotic bacteria on diarrhea, lipid metabolism, and carcinogenesis: a review of papers published between 1988 and 1998. Am J Clin Nutr 2000;71(2):405–411.

Dugas B, Mercenier A, Lenoir-Wijnkoop I, Arnaud C, Dugas N, Postaire E. Immunity and probiotics. Immunol Today 1999;20(9):387–390.

Dupont C. Bacterial flora in the infant and intestinal immunity: Implication and prospects for infant food with probiotics. Arch Pediatr 2000;7(suppl 2):252S–255S.

Erickson KL, Hubbard NE. Probiotic immunomodulation in health and disease. J Nutr 2000;130(2 suppl):403S–409S.

Gibson GR, McCartney AL. Modification of the gut flora by dietary means. Biochem Soc Trans 1998;26(2):222–228.

Gill HS, Rutherfurd KJ, Cross ML. Dietary probiotic supplementation enhances natural killer cell activity in the elderly: an investigation of age-related immunological changes. J Clin Immunol 2001a;21(4):264–271.

Gill HS, Rutherfurd KJ, Cross ML, Gopal PK. Enhancement of immunity in the elderly by dietary supplementation with the probiotic Bifidobacterium lactis HN019. Am J Clin Nutr 2001b;74(6):833–839.

Gill HS, Rutherfurd KJ, Prasad J, Gopal PK. Enhancement of natural and acquired immunity by Lactobacillus rhamnosus (HN001), Lactobacillus acidophilus (HN017) and Bifidobacterium lactis (HN019). Br J Nutr 2000;83(2):167–176.

Isolauri E, Arvola T, Sutas Y, Moilanen E, Salminen S. Probiotics in the management of atopic eczema. Clin Exp Allergy 2000;30(11):1604–1610.

LaMont JT. The renaissance of probiotics and prebiotics. Gastroenterology 2000;119(2):291.

Sanders ME. Considerations for use of probiotic bacteria to modulate human health. J Nutr 2000;130(2 suppl):384S–390S.

Sheih YH, Chiang BL, Wang LH, Liao CK, Gill HS. Systemic immunity-enhancing effects in healthy subjects following dietary consumption of the lactic acid bacterium Lactobacillus rhamnosus HN001. J Am Coll Nutr 2001;20(2 suppl):149–156.

ADDITIONAL RESOURCES

Agerholm-Larsen L, Raben A, Haulrik N, Hansen AS, Manders M, Astrup A. Effect of 8 week intake of probiotic milk products on risk factors for cardiovascular diseases. Eur J Clin Nutr 2000;54(4):288–297.

Bengmark S. Colonic food: pre- and probiotics. Am J Gastroenterol 2000;95(1 suppl):S5–S7.

Chin J, Turner B, Barchia I, Mullbacher A. Immune response to orally consumed antigens and probiotic bacteria. Immunol Cell Biol 2000;78(1):55–66.

Cunningham-Rundles S, Ahrne S, Bengmark S, Johann-Liang R, Marshall F, Metakis L, Califano C, Dunn AM, Grassey C, Hinds G, Cervia J. Probiotics and immune response. Am J Gastroenterol 2000;95(1 suppl):S22–S25.

D'Argenio G, Mazzacca G. Short-chain fatty acid in the human colon. Relation to inflammatory bowel diseases and colon cancer. Adv Exp Med Biol 1999;472:149–158.

Davidson GP, Butler RN. Probiotics in pediatric gastrointestinal disorders. Curr Opin Pediatr 2000;12(5):477–481.

Del Piano M, Ballare M, Montino F, Orsello M, Garello E, Ferrari P, Masini C, Strozzi GP, Sforza F. Clinical experience with probiotics in the elderly on total enteral nutrition. J Clin Gastroenterol 2004;38(6 suppl):S111–S114.

Folwaczny C. Probiotics for prevention of ulcerative colitis recurrence: alternative medicine added to standard treatment? Z Gastroenterol 2000;38(6):547–550.

Friedrich MJ. A bit of culture for children: probiotics may improve health and fight disease. JAMA 2000;284(11):1365–1366.

Gibson GR, Fuller R. Aspects of in vitro and in vivo research approaches directed toward identifying probiotics and prebiotics for human use. J Nutr 2000;130(2 suppl):391S–395S.

Gismondo MR, Drago L, Lombardi A. Review of probiotics available to modify gastrointestinal flora. Int J Antimicrob Agents 1999;12(4):287–292.

Goldin BR. Health benefits of probiotics. Br J Nutr 1998;80(4):S203–S207.

Gorbach SL. Probiotics and gastrointestinal health. Am J Gastroenterol 2000;95(1 suppl):S2–S4.

Guslandi M. The relationship between gut microflora and intestinal inflammation. Can J Clin Gastroenterol 2000;14(1):32.

Hirayama K, Rafter J. The role of probiotic bacteria in cancer prevention. Microbes Infect 2000;2(6):681–686.

Hoerr RA, Bostwick EF. Bioactive proteins and probiotic bacteria: modulators of nutritional health. Nutrition 2000;16(7–8):711–713.

Holzapfel WH, Haberer P, Snel J, Schillinger U, Huis in't Veld JH. Overview of gut flora and probiotics. Int J Food Microbiol 1998;41(2):85–101.

Hove H, Norgaard H, Mortensen PB. Lactic acid bacteria and the human gastrointestinal tract. Eur J Clin Nutr 1999;53(5):339–350.

Kirjavainen PV, Apostolou E, Salminen SJ, Isolauri E. New aspects of probiotics—a novel approach in the management of food allergy. Allergy 1999;54(9):909–915.

Klaenhammer TR. Probiotic bacteria: today and tomorrow. J Nutr 2000;130(2 suppl):415S–416S.

Kochhar KP. Probiotics and gastrointestinal function in health and disease. Trop Gastroenterol 2000;21(1):8–11.

Macfarlane GT, Cummings JH. Probiotics and prebiotics: can regulating the activities of intestinal bacteria benefit health? BMJ 1999;318(7189):999–1003.

Makelainen H, Tahvonen R, Salminen S, Ouwehand AC. In vivo safety assessment of two Bifidobacterium longum strains. Microbiol Immunol 2003;47(12):911–914.

Matsuzaki T, Chin J. Modulating immune responses with probiotic bacteria. Immunol Cell Biol 2000;78(1):67–73.

Orrhage K, Nord CE. Bifidobacteria and lactobacilli in human health. Drugs Exp Clin Res 2000;26(3):95–111.

Roberfroid MB. Prebiotics and probiotics: are they functional foods? Am J Clin Nutr 2000;71(6 suppl):1682S–1687S; discussion 1688S–1690S.

Rolfe RD. The role of probiotic cultures in the control of gastrointestinal health. J Nutr 2000;130(2 suppl):396S–402S.

Santos MS, Leka LS, Ribaya-Mercado JD, Russell RM, Meydani M, Hennekens CH, Gaziano JM, Meydani SN. Short- and long-term beta-carotene supplementation do not influence T cell-mediated immunity in healthy elderly persons. Am J Clin Nutr 1997;66(4):917–924.

Sheu BS, Wu JJ, Lo CY, Wu HW, Chen JH, Lin YS, Lin MD. Impact of supplement with Lactobacillus- and Bifidobacterium-containing yogurt on triple therapy for Helicobacter pylori eradication. Aliment Pharmacol Ther 2002;16(9):1669–1675.

Wang KY, Li SN, Liu CS, Perng DS, Su YC, Wu DC, Jan CM, Lai CH, Wang TN, Wang WM. Effects of ingesting Lactobacillus- and Bifidobacterium-containing yogurt in subjects with colonized Helicobacter pylori. Am J Clin Nutr 2004;80(3):737–741.

SLIPPERY ELM (*ULMUS RUBRA, U. FULVA*)

Overall Rank

★★★ for soothing effect on mucous membranes (sore throat)
★★ for digestive health
★ for dry coughs
★ as a skin moisturizer in minor skin irritations

OVERVIEW

Slippery elm contains mucilaginous compounds that are the reason why *slippery* is in its name and why it has herbal therapeutic uses. The mucilaginous effect of slippery elm has been used traditionally and safely for soothing irritated mucous membranes in the throat and sinuses during colds and sore throat, in the digestive system during digestive complaints (e.g., diarrhea, constipation, Crohn disease), and on the skin during minor irritations (e.g., poison oak and wound healing).

COMMENTS

Although slippery elm lacks clinical support, the soothing effect of the mucilaginous components is well known. Additionally, related elm species have shown evidence of antimicrobial activity and promise for inflammation and diseases of the mucous membranes (Jun et al., 1998; Song et al., 2003; Ye et al., 1990; Youn et al., 2003).

SCIENTIFIC SUPPORT

No direct clinical support could be found on slippery elm as a single phytotherapeutic agent.

SAFETY/DOSAGE

Slippery elm lacks clinical and toxicity testing, but it has been used as a traditional remedy without any adverse reports. It is generally thought to be completely safe and nontoxic, with no drug interactions. Slippery elm is available in different preparations, such as lozenges, capsules, tablets, and teas. Generally, 800 mg is taken 3–4 times daily for the soothing of mucous membranes.

REFERENCES

Jun CD, Pae HO, Kim YC, Jeong SJ, Yoo JC, Lee EJ, Choi BM, Chae SW, Park RK, Chung HT. Inhibition of nitric oxide synthesis by butanol fraction of the methanol extract of Ulmus davidiana in murine macrophages. J Ethnopharmacol 1998;62(2):129–135.

Song SE, Choi BK, Kim SN, Yoo YJ, Kim MM, Park SK, Roh SS, Kim CK. Inhibitory effect of procyanidin oligomer from elm cortex on the matrix metalloproteinases and proteases of periodontopathogens. J Periodontal Res 2003;38(3):282–289.

Ye G, Cao Q, Chen X, Li S, Jia B. Ulmus macrocarpa hance for the treatment of ulcerative colitis—a report of 36 cases. J Tradit Chin Med 1990;10(2):97–98.

Youn HJ, Lakritz J, Kim DY, Rottinghaus GE, Marsh AE. Anti-protozoal efficacy of medicinal herb extracts against Toxoplasma gondii and Neospora caninum. Vet Parasitol 2003;116(1):7–14.

ADDITIONAL RESOURCES

Oiseth D. Study on carbohydrate constituents of mucilage of Ulmus glabra Huds. Pharm Acta Helv 1954;29(8):251–256.

YELLOW DOCK (*RUMEX CRISPUS*)

Overall Rank

★★ as a laxative
★ for digestive health
★ for liver support (to stimulate bile flow)
★ for skin conditions

OVERVIEW

Yellow dock, also called curly dock and sour dock, is a member of the buckwheat family that can be found naturalized in many parts of the world. Originally from northern Europe and Asia, it has a long history of use in traditional medicines as a digestive aid, for skin conditions, and for liver health. Yellow dock is known as an astringent because of its content of tannins, which may be the reason for its use in skin conditions. Yellow dock extracts have been confirmed to have antioxidant and antimicrobial activity. Additionally, yellow dock contains the anthraquinone glycosides, a group of compounds that are known for their laxative activity. The anthraquinone glycosides are also the primary active components in other popular herbal laxatives, such as senna, cascara, and aloe. The bitterness of yellow dock leaves makes them useful as digestive aids. Yellow dock is also rich in iron (Bruneton, 1995).

COMMENTS

Yellow dock lacks clinical backing as a single phytotherapeutic agent, but the anthraquinone glycosides in yellow dock are well known and have clinically confirmed activity.

SCIENTIFIC SUPPORT

No clinical studies could be found that used yellow dock alone as a therapeutic agent. Several clinical studies, however, confirm the activity of the anthraquinone glycosides in other herbal laxatives (Gunaydin, 2002; de Witte, 1993).

SAFETY/DOSAGE

The laxative effect of yellow dock appears to be mild and safe. The fresh leaves are high in oxalates, and there have been a few reports of yellow dock toxicity in grazing sheep and at least one report of a human toxicity. If the oxalates are taken in high amounts, they may inhibit nutrient absorption. Root preparations are typical, and the dosage is generally 1 g/day of the dried root or 3–4 mL of the root extract 3 times daily. As with any laxative product, caution should be used by anyone who is pregnant or nursing.

REFERENCES

Bruneton, J. Pharmacognosy, Phytochemistry, Medicinal Plants. New York: Lavoisier Publishing, 1995.

de Witte P. Metabolism and pharmacokinetics of anthranoids. Pharmacology 1993;47 Suppl 1:86–97.

Gunaydin K, Topcu G, Ion RM. 1,5-dihydroxyanthraquinones and an anthrone from roots of Rumex crispus. Nat Prod Lett 2002;16(1):65–70.

ADDITIONAL RESOURCES

Panciera RJ, Martin T, Burrows GE, Taylor DS, Rice LE. Acute oxalate poisoning attributable to ingestion of curly dock (Rumex crispus) in sheep. J Am Vet Med Assoc 1990;196(12):1981–1984.

Reig R, Sanz P, Blanche C, Fontarnau R, Dominguez A, Corbella J. Fatal poisoning by Rumex crispus (curled dock): pathological findings and application of scanning electron microscopy. Vet Hum Toxicol 1990;32(5):468–470.

Yildirim A, Mavi A, Kara AA. Determination of antioxidant and antimicrobial activities of Rumex crispus L. extracts. J Agric Food Chem 2001;49(8):4083–4089.

CHAPTER 11

Supplements for "Male" and "Female" Health

Supplements for "Male" Health	Damiana (*Turnera diffusa*)
Maca (*Lepidium meyenii*)	Dong Quai (*Angelica sinensis*)
Pygeum	Evening Primrose Oil
Saw Palmetto	Flaxseed Oil and Linseed Oil
Yohimbine from Yohimbe and	Gotu Kola
Quebracho (*Pausinystalia yohimbe*,	Horse Chestnut (*Aesculus*
Aspidosperma quebracho-blanco)	*hippocastanum* L.)
Supplements for "Female" Health	Red Clover (*Trifolium pratense*)
Black Cohosh (*Actaea racemosa* L.,	Uva Ursi or Bearberry (*Arctostaphylos*
Cimicifuga racemosa [L.] Nutt)	*uva-ursi*)
Blue Cohosh (*Caulophyllum*	Vitex or Chasteberry (*Vitex agnus-*
thalictroides)	*castus* L.)
Cranberry (*Vaccinium macrocarpon*)	

SUPPLEMENTS FOR "MALE" HEALTH

Maca (*LEPIDIUM MEYENII*)

Overall Rank
★★ for sexual performance and libido
★★ for increasing energy and endurance
★★ for increasing memory and mood

OVERVIEW

Maca is a South American tuber that has been used since ancient times as a staple food crop in the Andes. Although maca has been long known
358

as a folkloric medicine and food for increasing energy, physical and mental endurance, and stamina, it has more recently been in the spotlight for its use in altering sexual function (Balick and Lee, 2002). Maca is thought to be able to increase libido in both men and women, although this effect has been clinically tested only in men. Preliminary clinical studies have shown that maca increases libido and fertility independent of sexual hormone functioning and parameters of mood (depression and anxiety). Several positive studies performed in animals (mice, rats) found increased sexual performance, libido, and fertility parameters (Cicero et al., 2001, 2002; Gonzales et al., 2001b; Zheng et al., 2000).

It is interesting to note that the tall physical height and strength of the Andes people, who live at very high elevations and include maca among their food staples, has been theorized as linked to their consumption of maca (Canales et al., 2000). Maca is rich in nutrients, such as amino acids and glucosinolates, that have been linked to its activity (Piacente et al., 2002).

COMMENTS

The jury is still out as to the best dosage form of maca and the health conditions that may benefit from it, although the clinical evidence of its effect in altering libido and fertility is promising. In either case, maca enjoys a long history of use as a food that makes people feel good and strong, and it continues to do so in Peru and in the Andes of South America.

SCIENTIFIC SUPPORT

Hormonal Regulation, Mood, and Libido

In a randomized, double-blind, placebo-controlled, parallel study, maca was tested for its effect on hormone levels when administered for libido and fertility enhancement. Maca was given in either 1,500-mg or 3,000-mg daily doses for 12 weeks, and hormone levels were tested: serum luteinizing (LH), follicle stimulating hormone (FSH), prolactin (PRL), testosterone (T), estradiol (E2), and 17-alpha hydroxyprogesterone. Maca was found not to have any effect on reproductive hormone levels (Gonzales et al., 2003).

The reported effect of maca on libido was examined to see if it was related to serum testosterone or mood levels in a randomized, double-blind, placebo-controlled study. Either 1,500 mg or 3,000 mg of maca was given for 12 weeks, and the self-perception of sexual desire and the Hamilton tests for anxiety were measured at 4, 8, and 12 weeks of treatment. At week 8, maca produced an improvement in sexual desire, but serum testosterone and oestradiol levels were found to be unchanged.

Additionally, no correlations were found in Hamilton scores for depression or anxiety. The effect of maca on libido was found to be separate from testosterone or mood regulation (Gonzales et al., 2002).

Semen Production

The effect of maca supplementation on semen function and health parameters was studied in a preliminary clinical study. Nine men were administered maca (*L. meyenii*; 1,500 or 3,000 mg/day) for four months and seminal analysis was performed along with hormonal analysis on LH, FSH, PRL, T, and E2. Seminal analysis followed guidelines of the World Health Organization. Maca was found to improve sperm production in a non–dose dependent manner by mechanisms not related to hormonal production (Gonzales et al., 2001a).

SAFETY/DOSAGE

Because it has a long historical use as a staple food, maca is thought to be very safe and free of side effects and drug interactions. Maca is generally recommended in dosages of 1.5–5 g/day of dried tuber or approximately 900 mg/day of extract. Different manufacturers have different preparations, so it is best to read the label recommendations.

REFERENCES

Balick MJ, Lee R. Maca: from traditional food crop to energy and libido stimulant. Altern Ther Health Med 2002;8(2):96–98.

Canales M, Aguilar J, Prada A, Marcelo A, Huaman C, Carbajal L. Nutritional evaluation of Lepidium meyenii (MACA) in albino mice and their descendants. Arch Latinoam Nutr 2000;50(2):126–133.

Cicero AF, Bandieri E, Arletti R. Lepidium meyenii Walp. improves sexual behaviour in male rats independently from its action on spontaneous locomotor activity. J Ethnopharmacol 2001;75(2–3):225–229.

Cicero AF, Piacente S, Plaza A, Sala E, Arletti R, Pizza C. Hexanic maca extract improves rat sexual performance more effectively than methanolic and chloroformic Maca extracts. Andrologia 2002;34(3):177–179.

Gonzales GF, Cordova A, Gonzales C, Chung A, Vega K, Villena A. Lepidium meyenii (Maca) improved semen parameters in adult men. Asian J Androl 2001a;3(4):301–303.

Gonzales GF, Cordova A, Vega K, Chung A, Villena A, Gonez C. Effect of Lepidium meyenii (Maca), a root with aphrodisiac and fertility-enhancing properties, on serum reproductive hormone levels in adult healthy men. J Endocrinol 2003;176(1):163–168.

Gonzales GF, Cordova A, Vega K, Chung A, Villena A, Gonez C, Castillo S. Effect of Lepidium meyenii (MACA) on sexual desire and its absent relationship with serum testosterone levels in adult healthy men. Andrologia 2002;34(6):367–372.

Gonzales GF, Ruiz A, Gonzales C, Villegas L, Cordova A. Effect of Lepidium meyenii (maca) roots on spermatogenesis of male rats. Asian J Androl 2001b;3(3):231–233.

Piacente S, Carbone V, Plaza A, Zampelli A, Pizza C. Investigation of the tuber constituents of maca (Lepidium meyenii Walp.). J Agric Food Chem 2002;50(20):5621–5625.

Zheng BL, He K, Kim CH, Rogers L, Shao Y, Huang ZY, Lu Y, Yan SJ, Qien LC, Zheng QY. Effect of a lipidic extract from Lepidium meyenii on sexual behavior in mice and rats. Urology 2000;55(4):598–602.

PYGEUM

Overall Rank

★★★★ for alleviating symptoms of benign prostatic hyperplasia (BPH)

OVERVIEW

Pygeum (*Pygeum africanum*), also known as African plum (a related plant, African cherry or *Prunus africana*, is also used as pygeum), is a large evergreen tree that grows in the high plateaus of southern Africa. The pygeum bark is traditionally powdered and drunk as a tea for genitourinary complaints, including bladder pain and urinary difficulty. As with saw palmetto, pygeum has been used and tested predominantly in Europe for the treatment of benign prostatic hyperplasia and its most common symptoms, including frequent nocturnal urination, low urine volume, incomplete bladder emptying, and prostate enlargement. In France and Italy, pygeum is the main course of natural treatment for BPH and is usually used in combination products that contain other herbal BPH treatments such as saw palmetto (the most popular in Germany) and nettle root. Increased demand for pygeum has led to overharvesting and is threatening the survival of the species, with international trade currently being monitored.

COMMENTS

Although the mechanism of action of pygeum is largely unknown, it is theorized to inhibit fibroblast hyperproliferation and prevent bladder contractile dysfunction through effects on 5-α-reductase, an important enzyme shown to play a role in prostate growth (Cristoni et al., 2000; Levin and Das, 2000). As a result, pygeum may decrease excessive prostate growth (hyperplasia) and could allow for better contraction of the bladder for more productive urination. Both of these actions could improve the quality of life of men with BPH. The chemical composition of pygeum bark extracts are known to be rich in phytosterols, such as β sitosterol, β sitosterone, and campesterol; ferulic acid esters, including n-docosanol; and triterpenes, including oleanolic acid, crataegolic acid, and ursolic acid.

SCIENTIFIC SUPPORT

Animal studies indicate that partial bladder obstruction can lead to bladder contractile problems but that BPH-like symptoms can be prevented by pretreatment with pygeum extract. In humans, several clinical trials have demonstrated the benefits of pygeum extract in alleviating symptoms of BPH (Breza et al., 1998; Chatelain et al., 1999; Ishani et al., 2000; Krzeski et al., 1993; Wilt et al., 2000, 2002). In general, daily doses of pygeum bark extract at 25–100 mg have demonstrated significant reductions in measures of the International Prostate Symptom Score (IPSS) of about 40% and increased quality of life of about 30% (Breza et al., 1998). In one study, 209 patients with symptomatic BPH consumed 50 mg or 100 mg of pygeum extract for 2 months; results showed similar effects in both dosage groups, including 35% improvement in IPSS and 28% improvement in quality of life (Chatelain et al., 1999). Other studies (18 controlled trials involving 1,562 men) have shown pygeum supplementation to reduce nocturnal urination frequency by 19–32%, reduce residual urine volume by 24%, increase peak urine flow by 23%, and reduce nocturnal frequency by 32% (Breza et al., 1998; Ishani et al., 2000; Krzeski et al., 1993; Wilt et al., 2000).

The ferulic acid component of pygeum bark extracts has been noted to possess some modest antiandrogenic activity, leading bodybuilding enthusiasts to supplement with pygeum as a way to reduce conversion of testosterone to dihydrotestosterone (DHT) and thus enhance muscle cell exposure to free testosterone. Such an effect has not been demonstrated in human trials. Likewise, the phytosterol component of pygeum bark extracts appear to compete with androgen precursors and in turn may be able to inhibit prostaglandin synthesis and provide a modest anti-inflammatory action (along with the triterpene components).

SAFETY/DOSAGE

The side effects of pygeum are relatively rare and mild and are generally gastrointestinal in nature. No drug interactions have been reported. It is important for any man with an enlarged prostate to consult with his personal physician to determine the cause of prostate enlargement and to rule out prostate cancer.

Pygeum africanum bark extract is generally taken twice a day in 50-mg capsules, although taking 100 mg in a single dose has been shown to be just as effective and safe. The extract consists of three groups of active constituents: phytosterols, pentacyclic triterpenoids, and ferulic esters of long-chained fatty alcohols. Thus, this oily extract is typically sold as softgel capsules standardized to 14% triterpenes and 0.5% n-docosanol.

REFERENCES

Breza J, Dzurny O, Borowka A, Hanus T, Petrik R, Blane G, Chadha-Boreham H.
    Efficacy and acceptability of tadenan (Pygeum africanum extract) in the treatment of benign prostatic hyperplasia (BPH): a multicentre trial in central Europe. Curr Med Res Opin 1998;14(3):127–139.
Chatelain C, Autet W, Brackman F. Comparison of once and twice daily dosage forms of Pygeum africanum extract in patients with benign prostatic hyperplasia: a randomized, double-blind study, with long-term open label extension. Urology 1999;54(3):473–478.
Cristoni A, Di Pierro F, Bombardelli E. Botanical derivatives for the prostate. Fitoterapia 2000;71(suppl 1):S21–S28.

Ishani A, MacDonald R, Nelson D, Rutks I, Wilt TJ. Pygeum africanum for the treatment of patients with benign prostatic hyperplasia: a systematic review and quantitative meta-analysis. Am J Med 2000;109(8):654–664.

Krzeski T, Kazon M, Borkowski A, Witeska A, Kuczera J. Combined extracts of Urtica dioica and Pygeum africanum in the treatment of benign prostatic hyperplasia: double-blind comparison of two doses. Clin Ther 1993;15(6):1011–1020.

Levin RM, Das AK. A scientific basis for the therapeutic effects of Pygeum africanum and Serenoa repens. Urol Res 2000;28(3):201–209.

Wilt T, Ishani A, Mac Donald R, Rutks I, Stark G. Pygeum africanum for benign prostatic hyperplasia. Cochrane Database Syst Rev 2002;(1):CD001044.

Wilt TJ, Ishani A, Rutks I, MacDonald R. Phytotherapy for benign prostatic hyperplasia. Public Health Nutr 2000;3(4A):459–472.

ADDITIONAL RESOURCES

Barry M. Review: Pygeum africanum extracts improve symptoms and urodynamics in symptomatic benign prostatic hyperplasia. ACP J Club 2002;137(2):61.

Buck AC. Is there a scientific basis for the therapeutic effects of serenoa repens in benign prostatic hyperplasia? Mechanisms of action. J Urol 2004;172(5 pt 1):1792–1799.

Mathe G, Hallard M, Bourut CH, Chenu E. A Pygeum africanum extract with so-called phyto-estrogenic action markedly reduces the volume of true and large prostatic hypertrophy. Biomed Pharmacother 1995;49(7–8):341–343.

McQueen CE, Bryant PJ. Pygeum. Am J Health Syst Pharm 2001 Jan 15;58(2):120–123.

Strong KM. African plum and benign prostatic hypertrophy. J Herb Pharmcother 2004;4(1):41–46.

SAW PALMETTO

Overall Rank

★★★★★ for alleviating symptoms of BPH
★★ for treating male-pattern baldness
★★ for enhancing sexual performance

OVERVIEW

Saw palmetto (*Serenoa repens*) is a dwarf (2–4 feet in height) palm tree found in the United States from the Carolinas to Texas. For centuries, the crude extracts of saw palmetto have been used to improve sperm production and to increase breast size and sexual vigor, but its most effective use—and the only use with a scientific basis—is to improve the symptoms of benign prostatic hyperplasia.

The premise for using saw palmetto is that it maintains normal prostate health by decreasing the metabolism and action of male steroids. Saw palmetto has been demonstrated to decrease the activity of 5-α-reductase, which stimulates the conversion of testosterone to dihydrotestosterone, its more active form. Because DHT is necessary for excessive growth (hyperplasia) of the prostate and is elevated in men with BPH, inhibition of 5-alpha reductase, and therefore DHT production, may alleviate BPH and the associated compression of the urethra (the tube that runs through the prostate gland to carry urine from the bladder). Additionally, studies have shown that saw palmetto helps inhibit the production of various inflammatory factors, probably because of an effect of the fatty acids, thus serving to decrease overall prostate inflammation. The prescription medication for treating BPH, finasteride, is available under the brand name Proscar; a lower-potency version called Propecia is used for treating hair loss in men (because the same conversion of testosterone to DHT is thought to result in thinning and loss of hair in men).

COMMENTS

Considering that the possible health benefits are similar to the prescription drugs Proscar for BPH and Propecia for hair loss, and because saw palmetto appears to be safe, effective, and without side effects, saw palmetto should be considered an outstanding choice for natural therapy in diagnosed cases of BPH.

SCIENTIFIC SUPPORT

Although studies of saw palmetto as a treatment for prostatitis have been disappointing (Kaplan et al., 2004), its effectiveness in treating BPH is supported by numerous well-controlled clinical trials. In one study of 155 men with BPH, International Prostate Symptom Scores and quality of life were improved, as were measures of sexual function and prostate size following 6 months of supplementation with 320 mg/day of saw palmetto extract (Pytel et al., 2002). In another study of 100 male outpatients, both 320 mg/day and 480 mg/day of saw palmetto extract for 3 months had similar significant effects in improving quality-of-life scores, maximum and mean urinary flow rates, and residual urinary volume (Gerber et al., 2001; Giannakopoulos et al., 2002). Several smaller studies of saw palmetto extracts (160 mg twice daily) have shown significant improvements in symptoms of BPH (Gerber et al., 1998). Saw palmetto has shown effects comparable to those seen in drug treatment with the synthetic 5-α-reductase inhibitor finasteride, such as improvements in maximum urinary flow rates, reduced trips to the bathroom, a greater ability to fully empty the bladder, and an increased quality of life (Sokeland, 2000).

SAFETY/DOSAGE

Because saw palmetto has primarily been tested in adult males, it is not recommended for children or for women who are pregnant or lactating. No drug interactions have been reported for saw palmetto (Markowitz et al., 2003). It is important to note that because saw palmetto extract may alleviate only BPH symptoms, patients with enlarged prostates should consult with their physicians on a regular basis to rule out prostate cancer or other causes of hypertrophy. Doses in clinical studies have typically used 160 mg of the oil-based (lipophilic) berry extract taken twice a day (morning and evening) for at least 30 days (total daily dose of 320 mg). Effective products are standardized for fatty acid and sterol content; approximately 80–90% total fatty acids and sterols is recommended.

REFERENCES

Gerber GS, Kuznetsov D, Johnson BC, Burstein JD. Randomized, double-blind, placebo-controlled trial of saw palmetto in men with lower urinary tract symptoms. Urology 2001;58(6):960–964, discussion 964–965.

Gerber GS, Zagaja GP, Bales GT, Chodak GW, Contreras BA. Saw palmetto (Serenoa repens) in men with lower urinary tract symptoms: effects on urodynamic parameters and voiding symptoms. Urology 1998;51(6):1003–1007.

Giannakopoulos X, Baltogiannis D, Giannakis D, Tasos A, Sofikitis N, Charalabopoulos K, Evangelou A. The lipidosterolic extract of Serenoa repens in the treatment of benign prostatic hyperplasia: a comparison of two dosage regimens. Adv Ther 2002;19(6):285–296.

Kaplan SA, Volpe MA, Te AE. A prospective, 1-year trial using saw palmetto versus finasteride in the treatment of category III prostatitis/chronic pelvic pain syndrome. J Urol 2004;171(1):284–288.

Markowitz JS, Donovan JL, Devane CL, Taylor RM, Ruan Y, Wang JS, Chavin KD. Multiple doses of saw palmetto (Serenoa repens) did not alter cytochrome P450 2D6 and 3A4 activity in normal volunteers. Clin Pharmacol Ther 2003;74(6):536–542.

Pytel YA, Vinarov A, Lopatkin N, Sivkov A, Gorilovsky L, Raynaud JP. Long-term clinical and biologic effects of the lipidosterolic extract of Serenoa repens in patients with symptomatic benign prostatic hyperplasia. Adv Ther 2002;19(6):297–306.

Sokeland J. Combined sabal and urtica extract compared with finasteride in men with benign prostatic hyperplasia: analysis of prostate volume and therapeutic outcome. BJU Int 2000;86(4):439–442.

ADDITIONAL RESOURCES

Bauer HW, Casarosa C, Cosci M, Fratta M, Blessmann G. Saw palmetto fruit extract for treatment of benign prostatic hyperplasia. Results of a placebo-controlled double-blind study. MMW Fortschr Med 1999;141(25):62.

Brown GA, Vukovich MD, Martini ER, Kohut ML, Franke WD, Jackson DA, King DS. Effects of androstenedione-herbal supplementation on serum sex hormone concentrations in 30- to 59-year-old men. Int J Vitam Nutr Res 2001;71(5):293–301.

Brown GA, Vukovich MD, Martini ER, Kohut ML, Franke WD, Jackson DA, King DS. Endocrine and lipid responses to chronic androstenediol-herbal supplementation in 30- to 58-year-old men. J Am Coll Nutr 2001;20(5):520–528.

Brown GA, Vukovich MD, Reifenrath TA, Uhl NL, Parsons KA, Sharp RL, King DS. Effects of anabolic precursors on serum testosterone concentrations and adaptations to resistance training in young men. Int J Sport Nutr Exerc Metab 2000;10(3):340–359.

Gerber GS. Saw palmetto for the treatment of men with lower urinary tract symptoms. J Urol 2000;163(5):1408–1412.

Marks LS, Partin AW, Epstein JI, Tyler VE, Simon I, Macairan ML, Chan TL, Dorey FJ, Garris JB, Veltri RW, Santos PB, Stonebrook KA, deKernion JB. Effects of a saw palmetto herbal blend in men with symptomatic benign prostatic hyperplasia. J Urol 2000;163(5):1451–1456.

McPartland JM, Pruitt PL. Benign prostatic hyperplasia treated with saw palmetto: a literature search and an experimental case study. J Am Osteopath Assoc 2000;100(2):89–96.

Preuss HG, Marcusen C, Regan J, Klimberg IW, Welebir TA, Jones WA. Randomized trial of a combination of natural products (cernitin, saw palmetto, B-sitosterol, vitamin E) on symptoms of benign prostatic hyperplasia (BPH). Int Urol Nephrol 2001;33(2):217–225.

Segars LW. Saw palmetto extracts for benign prostatic hyperplasia. J Fam Pract 1999;48(2):88–89.

Veltri RW, Marks LS, Miller MC, Bales WD, Fan J, Macairan ML, Epstein JI, Partin AW. Saw palmetto alters nuclear measurements reflecting DNA content in men with symptomatic BPH: evidence for a possible molecular mechanism. Urology 2002;60(4):617–622.

Wilt TJ, Ishani A, Stark G, MacDonald R, Lau J, Mulrow C. Saw palmetto extracts for treatment of benign prostatic hyperplasia: a systematic review. JAMA 1998;280(18):1604–1609.

YOHIMBINE FROM YOHIMBE AND QUEBRACHO (*PAUSINYSTALIA YOHIMBE, ASPIDOSPERMA QUEBRACHO-BLANCO*)

Overall Rank

★★★★ for enhancing sexual performance
★★★★ for improving erectile dysfunction (ED)
★★★ as a stimulant
★★ as an aphrodisiac
★★ for increasing muscle mass (by increasing testosterone)
★★ for promoting weight loss
★ for alleviating depression

OVERVIEW

Yohimbe is an African traditional medicinal herb that is almost legendary in the United States for its reputation as aphrodisiac and sexual performance enhancer. Although it has been on the market in the United States for much longer than prescription medications like Viagra, most people think little is known clinically about this herbal drug. Quebracho, a South American herb also known for its effects as an aphrodisiac and sexual performance enhancer, contains small amounts of the same active component of yohimbe, yohimbine (Tam et al., 2001). Both herbs are commonly marketed in the United States as components of "herbal Viagra" supplements, and for bodybuilding and athletic performance.

Yohimbe is an alkaloid stimulant that has central nervous system activity and blocks the α-2-adrenergic receptors. These actions are the basis of the claims that yohimbe can increase energy levels and promote weight loss. Yohimbine is also a monoamine oxidase inhibitor and thus increases norepinephrine, actions that suggest the herb may help in treating depression. It is also a vasodilator and has been shown to increase blood flow to the genitals in both men and women (Riley, 1994).

COMMENTS

There is much concern about the safety and purity of yohimbine products on the market, concern that is bolstered by one study that found that the amount of yohimbine in commercial products was wide ranging (Ernst, 1998). Additionally, there is little clinical proof of yohimbine's effectiveness in sexual performance or any of its several other claims. Because yohimbine's possible side effects are consistent with its pharmacological action, it may be a safe herb if used under the right conditions, and with the right quality, but it currently has much potential for abuse and adulteration (Abebe, 2003; Tam, 2001).

SCIENTIFIC SUPPORT

Yohimbine has been tested for erectile dysfunction in many uncontrolled clinical trials, but this section includes only a review of the key controlled studies, including one review. Ernst and Pittler (1998) conducted a systematic review of the literature on yohimbine's use in ED. They found seven trials that fit the inclusion criteria of randomized, placebo-controlled trials for yohimbine monotherapy. They found the trials to be of satisfactory quality, and that these trials demonstrated yohimbine to be better than placebo for treatment of ED. They found serious side effects to be infrequent and reversible in nature. Yohimbine was concluded to be a reasonable therapeutic option for early consideration of treatment for ED.

Mann et al. (1996) conducted a randomized, double-blind, placebo-controlled study on the use of yohimbine for ED. The 31 patients included in the trial were given either 15 mg/day of yohimbine or a placebo for 7 weeks. The Clinical Global Impression Scale was used to assess erectile function as a primary outcome. Additional parameters included nocturnal penile tumescence and rigidity (NPTR). The yohimbine group showed a significantly greater improvement in nonorganic ED; however, no difference was found between the placebo and the yohimbine group in organic ED. The NPTR was unchanged in both groups.

In a double-blind, placebo-controlled, crossover trial, yohimbine was examined for its efficacy in ED. The 48 subjects received daily administrations of either 18 mg of yohimbine or a placebo for 10 weeks. Overall, 46% of those on the yohimbine treatment reported beneficial results. The authors concluded that yohimbine is a safe and effective treatment for ED of either organic or nonorganic cause (Reid et al., 1987).

Rowland et al. (1997) investigated the effect of yohimbine on ED in a double-blind, placebo-controlled, crossover study. The trial included a group of men with ED and a group of sexually functional men for comparison. Yohimbine was administered at a dosage of up to 30 mg/day, and assessments were recorded on several objective and subjective measures of ED through daily logs and psychophysiological laboratory procedures involving response to visual sexual stimulation (VSS). In the sexually functional men, the study found that yohimbine had no effect on sexual response. In the men with ED, the results on sexual function were mixed. Frequency of sexual activities increased, along with genital response to VSS and masturbation. However, sexual arousal did not change during intercourse.

In a double-blind, placebo-controlled, crossover study on the use of yohimbine for ED, mixed results were found. Of the 215 participants in the study with ED that took yohimbine, 38% reported subjective improvement, with only 5% being completely satisfied. The authors noted that the effect appeared to occur in the central nervous system and that the usual dose of yohimbine had little effect, whereas higher doses were needed to achieve better results (Sonda et al., 1990).

Susset et al. (1989) conducted a double-blind, partial crossover study on the effect of yohimbine hydrochloride in ED patients. Assessment was multifactorial and included cavernosography, penile brachial blood pressure index, sacral evoked response, testosterone and prolactin determination, and the DeRogatis Sexual Functioning Inventory and daytime arousal test. Treatment of the 82 patients consisted of 42 mg/day of yohimbine hydrochloride orally for 1 month. Fourteen percent of the patients underwent full restoration of erectile function, 20% reported partial improvement, and 65% reported no improvement. A positive effect was reported in only three of the placebo patients. The action of yohimbine seemed to take 2–3 weeks to reach full potential. The authors noted that the results of the study were encouraging, especially because the participants, from the Veterans Administration population, had a high incidence of diabetes and vascular pathological conditions not found in the regular population. The few side effects reported were of a benign nature.

Vogt et al. (1997) conducted a double-blind, placebo-controlled, clinical trial of yohimbine hydrochloride in patients with ED of both organic and nonorganic cause. The 85 patients were given either 30 mg/day of yohimbine or a placebo for 8 weeks. Subjective and objective criteria to assess ED were included in the outcome parameters. Yohimbine was found to be significantly more effective than the placebo (71% versus 45%) and overall was well tolerated. No serious side effects were reported, and only 7% of the patients rated tolerability of yohimbine to be fair or poor.

Yohimbine was tested in a placebo-controlled study for its effectiveness in treating organic ED. The 22 patients were given a high dose of yohimbine hydrochloride (100 mg/day) orally for 30 days or a placebo. No significant difference was found between the yohimbine treatment and the placebo, even though 3% reported complete restoration of erectile function and 12% reported partial response (Teloken et al., 1998).

SAFETY/DOSAGE

Typical dosage recommendations are 10–30 mg of alkaloids in a yohimbe extract. No widely accepted standardization level for yohimbe has been established, and dosage recommendations are generally based on yohimbine or total alkaloid content. However, a wide variety of products are on the market, and caution should be exercised in finding one that is reputable.

Adverse effects are a concern and have been reported with yohimbe use, including dizziness, headaches, loss of coordination, anxiety, high blood pressure, and hallucinations. Yohimbe is not recommended for patients with diabetes, high blood pressure, or kidney disease or for women who are pregnant or likely to become pregnant. Caution is also advised for people taking nasal decongestants, diet aids, ephedrine, phenylpropanolamine, or other antidepressants (because yohimbe can potentiate their effect). Further, yohimbe should not be taken in combination with foods containing tyramine (Abebe, 2003; Sandler and Aronson, 1993; Tam, 2001).

REFERENCES

Abebe W. An overview of herbal supplement utilization with particular emphasis on possible interactions with dental drugs and oral manifestations. J Dent Hyg 2003;77(1):37–46.

Ernst E, Pittler MH. Yohimbine for erectile dysfunction: a systematic review and meta-analysis of randomized clinical trials. The Journal of Urology 1998;159:433–436.

Mann K, Klingler T, Noe S, Roschke J, Muller S, Benkert O. Effects of yohimbine on sexual experiences and nocturnal penile tumescence and rigidity in erectile dysfunction. Arch Sex Behav 1996;25(1):1–16.

Reid K, Surridge DH, Morales A et al. Double-blind trial of yohimbine in treatment of psychogenic impotence. Lancet 1987;2(8556):421–423.

Riley AJ. Yohimbine in the treatment of erectile disorder. Br J Clin Pract 1994;48(3):133–136.

Rowland DL, Kallan K, Slob AK. Yohimbine, erectile capacity, and sexual response in men. Arch Sex Behav 1997;26(1):49–62.

Sandler B, Aronson P. Yohimbine-induced cutaneous drug eruption, progressive renal failure, and lupus-like syndrome. Urology 1993;41(4):343–345.

Sonda LP, Mazo R, Chancellor MB. The role of yohimbine for the treatment of erectile impotence. J Sex Marital Ther 1990;16(1):15–21.

Susset JG, Tessier CD, Wincze J, Bansal S, Malhotra C, Schwacha MG. Effect of yohimbine hydrochloride on erectile impotence: a double-blind study. J Urol 1989; 141(6):1360–1363.

Tam SW, Worcel M, Wyllie M. Yohimbine: a clinical review. Pharmacol Ther 2001;91(3):215–243.

Teloken C, Rhoden EL, Sogari P, Dambros M, Souto CA. Therapeutic effects of high dose yohimbine hydrochloride on organic erectile dysfunction. J Urol 1998;159(1):122–124.

Vogt HJ, Brandl P, Kockott G et al. Double-blind, placebo-controlled safety and efficacy trial with yohimbine hydrochloride in the treatment of nonorganic erectile dysfunction. Int J Impot Res 1997;9(3):155–161.

SUPPLEMENTS FOR "FEMALE" HEALTH

BLACK COHOSH (*ACTAEA RACEMOSA* L., *CIMICIFUGA RACEMOSA* [L.] NUTT)

Overall Rank

★★★★★   for relief of menopausal symptoms
★★★★   for hormone balancing
★★★   for premenstrual syndrome (PMS)

OVERVIEW

Black cohosh is a traditional herbal medicine with a long history of use by Native Americans; today it is used primarily for the treatment of menopausal symptoms. However, black cohosh is also used in herbal hormone-balancing formulas, including those for premenstrual syndrome. Other uses include replenishing postoperative deficits following ovariectomy or hysterectomy, treating juvenile menstrual disorders, promoting menstrual flow (emmenagogue), and relieving dysmenorrhea or painful menstruation.

The main active constituents of black cohosh are considered to be the triterpene glycosides, and the standardized preparation of Remifemin—the brand that has the most clinical research—is calculated using the triterpene glycoside 27-deoxyactein. Other chemical constituents found in black cohosh include quinolizidine alkaloids; formononetin; isoferulic and salicylic acids (low concentrations); tannins; resins; volatile oils; palmitic, gallic, butyric, and oleic acids; starches; and sucrose (McKenna et al., 2001).

Black cohosh has been studied for cardiovascular and circulatory functions in animals, for osteoporosis in rats and tissue culture, and for certain immune and inflammatory functions (McKenna et al., 2001); however, this summary will be limited to reproductive and hormonal functions. Although a review of the preclinical studies to assess estrogenic activity of black cohosh have produced a range of conflicting results, the activity of black cohosh is not thought to result from estrogenic activity. Some of the key preclinical studies are listed here:

- Uterine weight and serum ceruloplasmin levels were increased in ovariectomized rats fed an alcoholic extract of black cohosh (Eagon et al., 1997).
- A 25% decrease in LH was produced by a black cohosh extract (Eagon et al., 1998).
- Black cohosh was shown not to produce a proliferation of estrogen receptor–positive MCF-7 breast cancer cells (Foster, 1999).

- No estrogenic effects of black cohosh were found in mice or rats (Einer-Jensen et al., 1996).
- No significant decrease in LH or other hormonal changes have been found for the new lower recommended doses of Remifemin cases (Remifemin, 1997).

COMMENTS

Black cohosh has become the "superstar" of the women's health herbs and will no doubt increase in popularity as a result of its strong clinical support and the recent controversy surrounding the risks in using standard hormone replacement therapy (HRT).

SCIENTIFIC SUPPORT

An open multicenter, multiclinic, retrospective study was published in Germany in 1982 that assessed Remifemin therapy in 629 females with menopausal complaints. Clear improvements were found in neurovegetative and psychological complaints. In 40–50% of patients, all symptoms abated, and an additional 30–40% of patients showed notable improvement (Foster, 1999). A product surveillance survey of 911 postmenopausal, premenopausal, and perimenopausal women found putative synergistic effects for the combination of black cohosh and St. John's wort (*Hypericum perforatum*; Liske et al., 1997).

A multicenter, controlled, randomized, double-blind, clinical study compared the results of treatments with two doses of Remifemin in 152 women with neurovegetative climacteric complaints of premenopause or postmenopause. The decrease in the Kupperman Menopause Index and Self-Assessment Depression Scale was statistically significant, and the efficacy was rated as good or very good by both doctors and patients in 80% of cases (Remifemin, 1997). The effect of Remifemin on LH and FSH secretion was examined in 110 menopausal women. After 8 weeks of therapy, the levels of LH (but not FSH) were found to be significantly reduced; pulsatile LH release is related to hot flash symptoms (Düker et al., 1991).

In an open study of 60 female patients who had postoperative ovarian functional deficits following hysterectomy (but at least one functional ovary remaining), Remifemin was compared with estriol, conjugated estrogens, and an estrogen-gestagen combination. There was improvement in the profile of postoperative ovarian functional complaints, significant declines in the Kupperman Menopause Index, and a moderate but insignificant decline in serum gonadotropin concentration; there were no significant differences in the positive responses among the four groups (Lehmann-Willenbrock and Riedal, 1988).

A 6-month study investigated switching treatments for patients with severe menopausal complaints from estrogen injection to a regime of oral Remifemin. Clear improvements were noted in the Menopausal

Index, and over half (56%) of the patients required no further injections (Pethö, 1987). In a randomized, double-blind study of menopausal complaints in 80 women, Remifemin was compared with conjugated estrogens or placebo for 12 weeks of therapy. Compared with the estrogens and placebo, the Remifemin group showed significant increases in the proliferation of vaginal epithelium and improvements of somatic and psychological parameters (Stoll, 1987).

In an open study of 60 women with menopausal symptoms, Remifemin was compared with conjugated estrogens or diazepam. All three therapies showed comparable positive responses in neurovegetative and psychological symptoms; however, only Remifemin and conjugated estrogens produced a proliferation and maturation of the vaginal epithelial cells (Warnecke, 1985). Two open studies measured the response of black cohosh in women who had refused hormone therapy or for whom hormone therapy was contraindicated. In both studies, neurovegetative and psychological symptoms were improved (Daiber, 1983; Vorberg, 1984).

SAFETY/DOSAGE

Most studies of black cohosh have used Remifemin (a standardized extract containing triterpene glycosides calculated as 27-deoxyactein, 1 mg/tablet). The dosage used in most studies—and the one that the makers of Remifemin suggest is needed for relief of climacteric symptoms—is two 1-mg tablets 2 times daily (Remifemin, 1997), although some studies have used double that dosage. Other recommended dosage forms have been cited: 40–200 mg of dried rhizome; 0.4–2.0 mL of a 1:10 60% ethanol tincture; 2–4 mL of a 1:10 60% ethanol tincture; 0.3–2.0 mL of a liquid extract of 1:1 in 90% alcohol; or 0.3 to 2.0 g of the decoction of the rhizome 3 times daily (McKenna et al., 2001).

Occasional gastric discomfort is the only side effect noted in the clinical studies. Overdoses may produce nausea, vomiting, dizziness, reduced pulse rate, increased perspiration, and premature birth during pregnancy (McKenna et al., 2001).

Although certain estrogens have been associated with the increased risk of female cancers, the actions of black cohosh have been described as "estradiol-like," and no contraindication has been described between black cohosh and people with estrogen-dependent tumors. There has been some evidence that black cohosh may be helpful (in combination with tamoxifen) in the treatment of breast cancer (Foster, 1999; McKenna, 2001). Opinions about the mechanism of action of black cohosh do not attribute the activity to hormonal (estrogenic) effects (McKenna et al., 2001).

Black cohosh does not have an established safe dosage during pregnancy or labor. The *American Herbal Products Association's Botanical Safety Handbook* lists black cohosh as an herb that should not be taken during pregnancy or nursing (McGuffin et al., 1997); however, there have been reports of herbalists using black cohosh along with blue cohosh (Caulophyllum thalictroides) to induce and aid labor (McKenna et al., 2001).

REFERENCES

Daiber W. Klimakterische heschwerden: ohne hormone. Ärztliche Praxis 1983;35:1946–1947.

Duker EM, Kopanski L, Jarry H, Wuttke W. Effects of extracts from Cimicifuga racemosa on gonadotropin release in menopausal women and ovariectomized rats. Planta Med 1991;57(5):420–424.

Eagon CL, Teepe MS, Eagon PK. Medicinal botanicals: estrogenicity in rat uterus and liver. Proceedings of the American Association for Cancer Research 1997;38:293.

Eagon PK, Swafford DS, Elm MS. Estrongenicity of medicinal botanicals [Abstract]. Proceedings of the American Association for Cancer Research 1998;39:2624.

Einer-Jensen N, Zhao J, Andersen KP, Kristoffersen K. Cimicifuga and Melbrosia lack oestrogenic effects in mice and rats. Maturitas 1996;25(2):149–153.

Foster S. Black cohosh: Cimicifuga racemosa, a literature review. HerbalGram 1999;(45):35–50.

Lehmann-Willenbrock E, Riedal HH. Clinical and endocrinologic examinations of climacteric symptoms following hysterectomy with remaining ovaries. Zentralblatt für Gynäkologie 1988;110:611–618.

Liske E, Gerhard I, Wüstenberg P. Menopause: herbal combination product for psychovegatative complaints. Therapiewosche Gynäkologie 1997;10:172–175.

McGuffin M, Hobbs C, Upton R, Goldberg A. American Herbal Products Association's Botanical Safety Handbook. Boca Raton, FL: CRC Press, 1997.

McKenna DJ, Jones K, Hughes K, eds. Botanical Medicines: A Desktop Reference for the Major Herbal Supplements. New York: Haworth Press, 2001.

Pethö A. Klimakterische beschwerden. Ärztliche Praxis 1987;47:1551–1553.

Remifemin: A Plant-based Gynecological Agent [Scientific brochure]. Salzgitter, Germany: Schaper and Brümmer GmbH, 1997.

Stoll W. Phytopharmacon influences atrophic vaginal epithelium. Double-blind study—Cimicifuga vs. estrogenic substances. Therapeuticon 1987;1:23–31.

Vorberg, G. Therapie kilmaktarischer beschwerden. Erfolgreiche hormonfreie therapie mit Remifemin. Zeitschrift für Allegemeinmedizin 1984;60:626–629.

Warnecke G. Influencing menopausal symptoms with a phytotherapeutic agent. Medizinische Welt 1985;36:871–874.

BLUE COHOSH (*CAULOPHYLLUM THALICTROIDES*)

Overall Rank

WARNING: Blue cohosh may be dangerous if used by the general public. Only qualified herbalists or midwives with the appropriate traditional training should administer blue cohosh, because no clinical evidence warrants or guides its use.

★★ for inducing labor
★ for menstrual pain

OVERVIEW

Blue cohosh is a plant native to North America that was used by Native American women to help ease pain in menstruation and childbirth. Blue cohosh is mostly used today in combination with black cohosh or other herbs. With black cohosh, it is thought to make a balanced antispasmodic, calming nervous and muscular spasms. With other herbs, it may be used to treat anxiety, bronchitis, sore throat, and urinary disorders. Blue cohosh is used for its uterine stimulatory action in inducing labor, but it must be used cautiously because it may constrict blood vessels and be toxic to the myocardium. It is thought to have uterine tonic activity and to be useful when the uterus has lost tone. Additionally, it may have an antispasmodic action that helps ease false labor pains or menstrual pains.

COMMENTS

As previously noted, blue cohosh should be used only by qualified herbalists or trained midwives. No clinical evidence warrants or guides its use.

SCIENTIFIC SUPPORT

A large-scale survey was conducted on the use of herbal preparations for cervical ripening, induction, and augmentation of labor by 500 certified nurse-midwives (CNMs) and nurse-midwifery education programs. The herbal preparations used by the responding CNMs for inducing labor were as follows: 64% used blue cohosh, 45% used black cohosh, 63% used red raspberry leaf, 93% used castor oil, and 60% used evening primrose oil. None of the CNMs found out about these herbs through their formal education programs, 69% learned about them from other CNMs, and 4% learned through formal research publications (McFarlin et al., 1999).

SAFETY/DOSAGE

Blue cohosh is normally taken as a nonstandardized herbal preparation. As a decoction, 1 teaspoon of the dried root in 1 cup of water can be boiled and simmered for 10 minutes and drunk 3 times daily. As a tincture, the recommended dosage is 0.5–2.0 mL 3 times daily. As an antispasmodic, it is often combined with other herbs, such as skullcap and/or black cohosh. Blue cohosh should not be taken by people with high blood pressure. Women should not take blue cohosh during pregnancy or lactation unless under the care of a qualified health professional.

Blue cohosh has serious safety concerns and should not be used by anyone who does not know its proper use. Blue cohosh contains compounds, such as callophyllosaponin, methylcytisin, and caulosaponin, that may constrict coronary vessels (Jones and Lawson, 1998). One case was reported of a woman who took blue cohosh to induce uterine contraction and gave birth to an infant with acute myocardial infarction associated with profound congestive heart failure and shock. Other causes of myocardial infarction were ruled out, and because the herb contains vasoactive glycosides and one alkaloid known to have toxic effects on the myocardium, blue cohosh was indicated as the possible culprit. This is the first known reported case on the toxic effects of blue cohosh on a newborn (Jones and Lawson, 1998).

In a case study of women with developed tachycardia, diaphoresis, abdominal pain, vomiting, and muscle weakness after trying to induce abortion by taking blue cohosh, it was suspected that nicotinic toxicity from methylcytisin produced the symptoms (Rao and Hoffman, 2002).

REFERENCES

Jones TK, Lawson BM. Profound neonatal congestive heart failure caused by maternal consumption of blue cohosh herbal medication. J Pediatr 1998;132(3 pt 1):550–552.

McFarlin BL, Gibson MH, O'Rear J, Harman P. A national survey of herbal preparation use by nurse-midwives for labor stimulation. Review of the literature and recommendations for practice. J Nurse Midwifery 1999;44(3):205–216.

Rao RB, Hoffman RS. Nicotinic toxicity from tincture of blue cohosh (Caulophyllum thalictroides) used as an abortifacient. Vet Hum Toxicol 2002;44(4):221–222.

CRANBERRY (*VACCINIUM MACROCARPON*)

Overall Rank

★★★★★ for urinary tract infections (UTIs)
★★★★   for antioxidant activity
★★★★   as an antibacterial

OVERVIEW

Cranberries come from shrubs that grow in swamps in North America or Europe. Cranberries are famous in American cuisine as part of the traditional Thanksgiving fare. Native Americans ate the berries for various reasons, such as to cure "bad fever," to cleanse the stomach, relieve nausea, and treat bladder complaints. In the 1840s, German chemists found that cranberry consumption could produce urine containing hippuric acid. In about 1900 in the United States, it was discovered that the continual consumption of cranberries could prevent urinary tract infections. Since that time, women have used cranberries for this purpose. Everybody seems to know about using cranberry juice for UTIs, yet clinical evidence has been slow in catching up to this reputation (McKenna et al., 2002).

Originally, it was thought that cranberry juice only worked by producing acidic urine. However, after there were doubts of this mechanism, it was found that cranberries prevent *Escherichia coli* from adhering to the lining of the urinary tract. Cranberries are available in many forms, including juice (sweetened and unsweetened), fresh berries, dehydrated fruit juice concentrate in capsules, berry tea, and extracts. It is important for efficacy that the form of cranberry not be too diluted (as is the case of many commercial cranberry juice drinks) (McKenna et al., 2002).

COMMENTS

The reviews by Jepson et al. (2000, 2001, and 2004) are telling in that early on, little clinical evidence could be found to confirm cranberry's efficacy. However, since 2000, clinical trials have been of higher quality.

SCIENTIFIC SUPPORT

Urinary Tract Infection

In a review of the clinical studies on the effectiveness of cranberry products for UTIs, Raz et al. (2004) found that approximately a dozen trials had been performed, but the trials suffered a number of limitations. One of the limitations was stated as the use of many cranberry products, such as cranberry juice concentrate, cranberry juice cocktail, and cranberry capsules with different dosing regimens.

In a systematic review of cranberries (especially cranberry juice) on urinary tract infections (UTIs), data were collected consisting of randomized or semirandomized, controlled trials of cranberry juice and other cranberry products. Seven trials met the criteria; in six trials, the effectiveness of cranberry juice versus water or placebo was tested, and in two trials, the effectiveness of cranberry tablets versus placebo was tested. Two of the well-designed randomized clinical trials provided evidence of the efficacy of cranberry juice (with significant results) over 12 months of use in women. However, whether cranberry juice was efficacious in the other groups was unclear, as was the optimum dosage or method of administration (Jepson et al., 2004). In an earlier review with the same inclusion criteria, only five trials were found to meet the criteria. The reviewers concluded that size of the trials available at that time was too small and their quality too poor to interpret reliable results (Jepson et al., 2001). Just 1 year earlier, in a similar systematic review, no trials were found to fit the inclusion criteria (Jepson, 2000).

A randomized, double-blind, placebo-controlled trial was conducted to determine whether the antibacterial effects of cranberry juice are effective in reducing or eliminating bacteriuria and pyuria in people with spinal cord injury. Each participant was administered 2 g of concentrated cranberry juice in capsule form or a placebo for 6 months. Cranberry extract was found not to produce significant differences in urinary bacterial colonies compared with the placebo (Waites et al., 2004).

In a randomized, placebo-controlled trial, cranberry tablets (concentrated juice) were compared with cranberry juice and a placebo for efficacy and cost-effectiveness. The participants (women) were divided into three groups: placebo juice plus placebo tablets, placebo juice plus cranberry tablets, and cranberry juice plus placebo tablets. Tablets were administered 2 times daily, and 250 mL of the juice 3 times daily. Cost-effectiveness was calculated as dollar cost per urinary tract infection. Both cranberry juice and tablets were found to significantly reduce the number of patients experiencing at least one symptomatic UTI per year. The cost of prophylaxis was $624 for cranberry tablets and $1,400 for cranberry juice. Cost-effectiveness ratios showed cranberry tablets to be 2 times more cost-effective than juice for UTIs (Stothers, 2002).

Habash et al. (1999) conducted a study comparing water consumption and ascorbic acid or cranberry supplements on urine acidity and other measures. Ascorbic acid was the only treatment to consistently produce acidic urine. Urine collected after cranberry or ascorbic acid had lower initial deposition rates and numbers of E. coli and Enterococcus faecalis but not other antimicrobials, whereas water increased deposition rates and numbers of E. coli and E. faecalis. In a randomized, double-blind, placebo-controlled trial of cranberry juice on bacteriuria and pyuria in elderly women, 153 elderly women were administered either cranberry juice (300 mL/day) or placebo. The cranberry juice reduced the frequency of bacteriuria with pyuria in older women (Avorn et al., 1994).

Antioxidant Activity

Pedersen et al. (2000) conducted a placebo-controlled comparison of blueberry juice to cranberry juice for increasing plasma phenolic content and antioxidant activity. The participants were given 500 mL of blueberry juice, cranberry juice, or a sucrose solution. Blood and urine samples were collected and analyzed after juice consumption. Cranberry juice, but not blueberry juice, produced an increase in the plasma antioxidant capacity that may be explained by an increase in vitamin C that was absent in blueberry juice.

SAFETY/DOSAGE

A typical daily dosage that has been recommended for cranberry is 1/2 cup of fresh fruit, 15 mL of dried fruit, or 90 mL of juice cocktail (1/3 of which is pure juice). For an active UTI, the dosage is increased to 12–32 fl oz, or 390–960 mL. Some products available on the market are standardized to total organic acids or polyphenolic content (McKenna et al., 2002).

Cranberry juice, when taken at the recommended levels, has no known side effects. People with the tendency to develop kidney stones should limit their intake of cranberry juice to no more than 1 L/day (McKenna et al., 2002).

REFERENCES

Avorn J, Monane M, Gurwitz JH, Glynn RJ, Choodnovskiy I, Lipsitz LA. Reduction of bacteriuria and pyuria after ingestion of cranberry juice. JAMA 1994;271(10):751–754.

Habash MB, Van der Mei HC, Busscher HJ, Reid G. The effect of water, ascorbic acid, and cranberry derived supplementation on human urine and uropathogen adhesion to silicone rubber. Can J Microbiol 1999;45(8):691–694.

Jepson RG, Mihaljevic L, Craig J. Cranberries for preventing urinary tract infections. Cochrane Database Syst Rev 2004;(2):CD001321.

Jepson RG, Mihaljevic L, Craig J. Cranberries for preventing urinary tract infections. Cochrane Database Syst Rev 2001;(3):CD001321.

Jepson RG, Mihaljevic L, Craig J. Cranberries for treating urinary tract infections. Cochrane Database Syst Rev 2000;(2):CD001322.

McKenna D, Jones K, Hughes K, eds. Botanical Medicines: The Desk Reference for Major Herbal Supplements. 2nd Ed. Binghamton, NY: Haworth Press, 2002.

Pedersen CB, Kyle J, Jenkinson AM, Gardner PT, McPhail DB, Duthie GG. Effects of blueberry and cranberry juice consumption on the plasma antioxidant capacity of healthy female volunteers. Eur J Clin Nutr 2000;54(5):405–408.

Raz R, Chazan B, Dan M. Cranberry juice and urinary tract infection. Clin Infect Dis 2004;38(10):1413–1419.

Stothers L. A randomized trial to evaluate effectiveness and cost effectiveness of naturopathic cranberry products as prophylaxis against urinary tract infection in women. Can J Urol 2002;9(3):1558–1562.

Waites KB, Canupp KC, Armstrong S, DeVivo MJ. Effect of cranberry extract on bacteriuria and pyuria in persons with neurogenic bladder secondary to spinal cord injury. J Spinal Cord Med 2004;27(1):35–40.

DAMIANA (*TURNERA DIFFUSA*)

Overall Rank

★★ for enhancing sexual performance and desire
★★ for inducing relaxation and decreasing anxiety
★ for alleviating depression
★ for promoting blood sugar regulation and weight loss

OVERVIEW

Damiana is a traditional medicine of Mexico and southern United States that has gained some popularity as an herbal aphrodisiac. Damiana has been claimed to produce a mild euphoria and thus to alleviate depression, induce relaxation, and decrease anxiety. Perhaps it is this activity that also gives damiana its use in enhancing sexual performance. In animal studies, damiana has exhibited antidiabetic activity and antihyperglycemic activity (Alarcon-Aguilara et al., 1998; Arletti et al., 1999). Other speculations of damiana's usefulness relate to its content of terpenes, and one study demonstrates its ability to bind to the progesterone receptor in human breast cancer cells, although no other clinical work has elucidated damiana's mechanism of action (Zava et al., 1998).

COMMENTS

Damiana is a component in a branded herbal preparation called Argin-Max, which its manufacturer claims can improve sexual function for women. One clinical study showed beneficial results of this formulation, but whether damiana contributed to its efficacy is unknown (Ito et al., 2001). Another mixed herbal formulation containing damiana was clinically tested and found to promote weight loss and delay gastric emptying (Andersen and Fogh, 2001).

SCIENTIFIC SUPPORT

No clinical support on the single phytotherapeutic preparation is available.

SAFETY/DOSAGE

Generally, damiana is recommended in the dosages of 400–800 mg 3 times daily if used singly. Not much is known about the long-term safety of damiana, but it has been noted to cause a euphoric and mild laxative effect at high dosages.

REFERENCES

Alarcon-Aguilara FJ, Roman-Ramos R, Perez-Gutierrez S, Aguilar-Contreras A, Contreras-Weber CC, Flores-Saenz JL. Study of the anti-hyperglycemic effect of plants used as antidiabetics. J Ethnopharmacol 1998;61(2):101–110.
Andersen T, Fogh J. Weight loss and delayed gastric emptying following a South American herbal preparation in overweight patients. J Hum Nutr Diet 2001;14(3):243–250.
Arletti R, Benelli A, Cavazzuti E, Scarpetta G, Bertolini A. Stimulating property of Turnera diffusa and Pfaffia paniculata extracts on the sexual-behavior of male rats. Psychopharmacology (Berl) 1999;143(1):15–19.
Ito TY, Trant AS, Polan ML. A double-blind placebo-controlled study of ArginMax, a nutritional supplement for enhancement of female sexual function. J Sex Marital Ther 2001;27(5):541–549.
Zava DT, Dollbaum CM, Blen M. Estrogen and progestin bioactivity of foods, herbs, and spices. Proc Soc Exp Biol Med 1998;217(3):369–378.

DONG QUAI (ANGELICA SINENSIS)

Overall Rank

★★★ for hormonal balance and easing symptoms of menopause and PMS
★ for increasing libido

OVERVIEW

Dong quai has a long history of use in both Traditional Chinese Medicine and Native American medicine, and it continues to be used for female conditions to balance the effects of menopause (hot flashes and night sweats) and PMS (cramping). The active components in dong quai are thought to be the coumarins, ferulic acid, and ligustilide. The coumarins are known to increase blood flow, and ferulic acid and ligustilide are known to have muscle-relaxing effects. Although there have been no known estrogenic compounds found in dong quai, it has been confirmed to have both estrogenic and antiestrogenic activity in vitro (Amato et al., 2002). Dong quai is sometimes used in "bust-enhancing" herbal products, but no clinical studies have been conducted on it for this purpose (Fugh-Berman, 2003). Dong quai has been shown to possess nonspecific immunomodulatory activity in vitro (Wilasrusmee et al., 2002a, 2002b).

COMMENTS

Dong quai was included in a phytoestrogen combination that a clinical study found to be beneficial in treating migraines associated with the menstrual cycle, but how much dong quai contributed to its efficacy is unknown (Burke et al., 2002). After only one negative clinical study, dong quai was abandoned from clinical practice by many in the United States; however, considering its long history of use and reported success in alternative medicine settings, it seems dong quai deserves more clinical research and more credit.

SCIENTIFIC SUPPORT

Hirata et al. (1997) examined the use of dong quai in postmenopausal women in a double-blind, randomized, placebo-controlled clinical trial. Outcome parameters measured its effects on endometrial thickness (by ultrasonography), cellular maturation of vaginal cells, the Kupperman index (for determining menopausal symptoms), and frequency of hot flashes. Seventy-one women were included in the study and given either dong quai or a placebo for 24 weeks. No statistically significant differences were found between the treatment and placebo groups for any of the parameters measured. The authors concluded that dong quai does not produce estrogen-like responses in postmenopausal women for the parameters measured.

SAFETY/DOSAGE

Generally, dong quai is administered in the dosage range of 250–1,000 mg/day (taken in divided doses) for the relief of menopausal or menstrual symptoms. There is no consensus on the standardization of dong quai because activity has been found in different fractions of the plant extracts. Dong quai is considered quite safe, but there is some concern of its potential to increase photosensitivity because of the coumarins it contains. Another concern is a potential drug interaction with aspirin because of dong quai's antiplatelet activity (Abebe, 2002, 2003).

REFERENCES

Abebe W. Herbal medication: potential for adverse interactions with analgesic drugs. J Clin Pharm Ther 2002;27(6):391–401.

Abebe W. An overview of herbal supplement utilization with particular emphasis on possible interactions with dental drugs and oral manifestations. J Dent Hyg 2003 Winter;77(1):37–46.

Amato P, Christophe S, Mellon PL. Estrogenic activity of herbs commonly used as remedies for menopausal symptoms. Menopause 2002;9(2):145–150.

Burke BE, Olson RD, Cusack BJ. Randomized, controlled trial of phytoestrogen in the prophylactic treatment of menstrual migraine. Biomed Pharmacother 2002;56(6):283–288.

Fugh-Berman A. "Bust enhancing" herbal products. Obstet Gynecol 2003;101(6):1345–1349.

Hirata JD, Swiersz LM, Zell B, Small R, Ettinger B. Does dong quai have estrogenic effects in postmenopausal women? A double-blind, placebo-controlled trial. Fertil Steril 1997;68(6):981–986.

Wilasrusmee C, Kittur S, Siddiqui J, Bruch D, Wilasrusmee S, Kittur DS. In vitro immunomodulatory effects of ten commonly used herbs on murine lymphocytes. J Altern Complement Med 2002;8(4):467–475.

Wilasrusmee C, Siddiqui J, Bruch D, Wilasrusmee S, Kittur S, Kittur DS. In vitro immunomodulatory effects of herbal products. Am Surg 2002;68(10):860–864.

ADDITIONAL RESOURCES

Rosenberg Zand RS, Jenkins DJ, Diamandis EP. Effects of natural products and nutraceuticals on steroid hormone-regulated gene expression. Clin Chim Acta 2001;312(1–2):213–219.

EVENING PRIMROSE OIL

See also the discussion in the "Essential Fatty Acids" section of Chapter 7.

Overall Rank

★★★★ for alleviating symptoms of PMS

OVERVIEW

Evening primrose oil is made from the seeds of the herb *Oenothera biennis*, which grows wild in arid environments like sand dunes. True to its name, the bright yellow evening primrose flowers open in the evening and fade in bright sunlight. First documented medicinally in England, evening primrose oil is most commonly used for relieving premenstrual syndrome, fibrocystic breasts, and menopausal symptoms such as hot flashes.

COMMENTS

It appears that evening primrose oil may be a useful alternative to prescription medications for symptoms of PMS, especially breast pain associated with the menstrual cycle. Perhaps the most promising use for evening primrose oil is its cardioprotective effect delivered by its profile of anti-inflammatory fatty acids.

SCIENTIFIC SUPPORT

The essential (not produced by the body) fatty acid linoleic acid makes up 60–80% of evening primrose oil. γ-Linoleic acid (GLA) is synthesized by the body from linoleic acid and comprises 8–14% of the oil. GLA is a precursor of prostaglandin E1 (PGE1), the deficiency of which has been documented in some women with premenstrual syndrome and cyclical breast pain (Bendich, 2000; Bordoni et al., 1987). Because decreased levels of PGE1 can increase the pain-inducing effects of the hormone prolactin on breast tissue, it is thought that low PGE1 levels may be a primary cause of many of the symptoms associated with premenstrual syndrome (Cheung, 1999).

In addition to its applications for specific detrimental effects of the menstrual cycle, theories for non-gender-related uses for evening primrose oil are prevalent. PGE1 has beneficial anti-inflammatory, blood-thinning, and vasodilating properties (Dirks et al., 1998). Also, GLA's action in increasing PGE1 levels suggests that supplementation with evening primrose oil theoretically could provide benefits in rheumatoid arthritis and coronary artery disease (Laivuori et al., 1993). Because essential fatty acids are claimed to have positive effects on certain skin diseases, supplementation with evening primrose oil, composed mostly of essential fatty acids, could also alleviate eczema and dermatitis. Finally, people with GLA deficiencies are thought to produce more fat in their bodies—so theories abound for evening primrose oil supplements to promote fat loss.

Most scientific literature related to evening primrose oil supplementation involves its use for promoting well-being during the menstrual cycle. In two controlled studies, subjects received 4–6 grams of evening primrose oil or a placebo for 3–4 months—but neither trial was able to demonstrate a significant benefit of the supplements (Horrobin 1983, 1993). It is worth noting that other placebo-controlled studies have shown significant benefits of supplementation with evening primrose oil, but only after 6 months of treatment (Chenoy et al., 1994; Collins et al., 1993). In the treatment of cyclic breast pain, evening primrose oil has been found to be more effective than a placebo (44% versus 19%, respectively); and when compared with prescription drugs (bromocriptine and danazol), evening primrose oil was as effective as bromocriptine but less effective than danazol in alleviating breast pain (Huntley and Ernst, 2003). In one well-controlled study to evaluate the use of evening primrose oil for the relief of hot flashes associated with meno-pause, 56 women were treated for 6 months with either 4 g of evening primrose oil or a placebo, but no significant benefits were attributed to taking evening primrose oil for treatment of menopausal symptoms (Huntley and Ernst, 2003).

Perhaps the most convincing evidence for supplementing with evening primrose oil involves its use in patients with coronary artery disease. A study in 10 patients with high cholesterol levels showed that 3.6 g of evening primrose oil taken daily for 8 weeks significantly decreased low-density lipoprotein (LDL, the "bad" cholesterol) by 9% (Cerin et al., 1993). However, for patients with high triglyceride and cholesterol levels, no such reductions occurred. In a double-blind, crossover study in men taking either fish oil alone or fish oil plus evening primrose oil, the combination led to a significant (12%) decrease in atherogenic markers, whereas fish oil alone led to a nonsignificant (6%) decrease in the same markers (Brzeski et al., 1991).

Many other claims have been made for the use of evening primrose oil, but the scientific findings are rather disappointing. In a 6-week, double-blind, placebo-controlled study of 58 children who required treatment with topical skin steroids for atopic dermatitis (22 of whom also had asthma), no significant difference was found between the pla-cebo group and the group treated with evening primrose oil (Schafer and Kragballe, 1991). Likewise, no effect was seen in terms of asthma symptoms. In a 24-week, double-blind, placebo-controlled study of 39 patients with chronic hand dermatitis (Whitaker et al., 1996), no thera-peutic value was shown following administration of 600 mg/day GLA supplements (compared with the placebo). No scientific evidence is available to support any benefit of evening primrose oil in alleviating rheumatoid arthritis or in aiding weight loss.

SAFETY/DOSAGE

Evening primrose oil appears to be quite safe. Potential adverse effects include gastrointestinal upset and headache. Because evening primrose oil hinders platelet aggregation, the supplement may increase the antico-agulant effect of drugs like warfarin. Therefore, people taking anticoagu-lants should consult with their personal physicians before taking evening primrose oil. The most common dose of evening primrose oil is 1–4 g/day of a supplement with approximately 10% GLA.

REFERENCES

Bendich A. The potential for dietary supplements to reduce premenstrual syndrome (PMS) symptoms. J Am Coll Nutr 2000;19(1):3–12.

Bordoni A, Biagi PL, Turchetto E, Serroni P, De Jaco AP, Orlandi C. Treatment of premenstrual syndrome with essential fatty acids. G Clin Med 1987;68(1):23–28.

Brzeski M, Madhok R, Capell HA. Evening primrose oil in patients with rheumatoid arthritis and side-effects of non-steroidal anti-inflammatory drugs. Br J Rheumatol 1991;30(5):370–372.

Cerin A, Collins A, Landgren BM, Eneroth P. Hormonal and biochemical profiles of premenstrual syndrome. Treatment with essential fatty acids. Acta Obstet Gynecol Scand 1993;72(5):337–343.

Chenoy R, Hussain S, Tayob Y, O'Brien PM, Moss MY, Morse PF. Effect of oral gamolenic acid from evening primrose oil on menopausal flushing. BMJ 1994;308(6927):501–503.

Cheung KL. Management of cyclical mastalgia in oriental women: pioneer experience of using gamolenic acid (Efamast) in Asia. Aust N Z J Surg 1999;69(7):492–494.

Collins A, Cerin A, Coleman G, Landgren BM. Essential fatty acids in the treatment of premenstrual syndrome. Obstet Gynecol 1993;81(1):93–98.

Dirks J, van Aswegen CH, du Plessis DJ. Cytokine levels affected by gamma-linolenic acid. Prostaglandins Leukot Essent Fatty Acids 1998;59(4):273–277.

Horrobin DF. The effects of gamma-linolenic acid on breast pain and diabetic neuropathy: possible non-eicosanoid mechanisms. Prostaglandins Leukot Essent Fatty Acids 1993;48(1):101–104.

Horrobin DF. The role of essential fatty acids and prostaglandins in the premenstrual syndrome. J Reprod Med 1983;28(7):465–468.

Huntley AL, Ernst E. A systematic review of herbal medicinal products for the treatment of menopausal symptoms. Menopause 2003;10(5):465–476.

Laivuori H, Hovatta O, Viinikka L, Ylikorkala O. Dietary supplementation with primrose oil or fish oil does not change urinary excretion of prostacyclin and thromboxane metabolites in pre-eclamptic women. Prostaglandins Leukot Essent Fatty Acids 1993;49(3):691–694.

Schafer L, Kragballe K. Supplementation with evening primrose oil in atopic dermatitis: effect on fatty acids in neutrophils and epidermis. Lipids 1991;26(7):557–560.

Whitaker DK, Cilliers J, de Beer C. Evening primrose oil (Epogam) in the treatment of chronic hand dermatitis: disappointing therapeutic results. Dermatology 1996;193(2):115–120.

ADDITIONAL RESOURCES

Blommers J, de Lange-De Klerk ES, Kuik DJ, Bezemer PD, Meijer S. Evening primrose oil and fish oil for severe chronic mastalgia: a randomized, double-blind, controlled trial. Am J Obstet Gynecol 2002;187(5):1389–1394.

Budeiri D, Li Wan Po A, Dornan JC. Is evening primrose oil of value in the treatment of premenstrual syndrome? Control Clin Trials 1996;17(1):60–68.

Douglas S. Premenstrual syndrome. Evidence-based treatment in family practice. Can Fam Physician 2002;48:1789–1797.

Girman A, Lee R, Kligler B. An integrative medicine approach to premenstrual syndrome. Am J Obstet Gynecol 2003;188(5 suppl):S56–S65.

Goldfien A. Premenstrual syndrome. Curr Ther Endocrinol Metab 1994;5:219–222.

Hardy ML. Herbs of special interest to women. J Am Pharm Assoc (Wash) 2000;40(2):234–242.

Hederos CA, Berg A. Epogam evening primrose oil treatment in atopic dermatitis and asthma. Arch Dis Child 1996;75(6):494–497.

Horrobin DF. Evening primrose oil and premenstrual syndrome. Med J Aust 1990;153(10):630–631.

Horrobin DF, Morse PF. Evening primrose oil and atopic eczema. Lancet 1995;345(8944):260–261.

Johnson SR. Premenstrual syndrome therapy. Clin Obstet Gynecol 1998;41(2):405–421.

Khoo SK, Munro C, Battistutta D. Evening primrose oil and treatment of premenstrual syndrome. Med J Aust 1990;153(4):189–192.

Kleijnen J. Evening primrose oil. BMJ 1994;309(6958):824–825.

Martens-Lobenhoffer J, Meyer FP. Pharmacokinetic data of gamma-linolenic acid in healthy volunteers after the administration of evening primrose oil (Epogam). Int J Clin Pharmacol Ther 1998;36(7):363–366.

Veale DJ, Torley HI, Richards IM, O'Dowd A, Fitzsimons C, Belch JJ, Sturrock RD. A double-blind placebo controlled trial of Efamol Marine on skin and joint symptoms of psoriatic arthritis. Br J Rheumatol 1994;33(10):954–958.

FLAXSEED OIL AND LINSEED OIL

See also the discussion in the "Essential Fatty Acids" section of Chapter 7.

Overall Rank

★★★★ for treating inflammatory conditions
★★★★ for promoting heart health

OVERVIEW

Flaxseed (also known as linseed) is just what it sounds like, the seed of the flax plant. The typical use of flaxseed is as a source (from the oil of the seeds) of the essential fatty acids linolenic acid (LN) and linoleic acid (LA). Flaxseed oil is about 57% LN (an ω-3) and about 17% LA (an ω-6). LN can be converted into eicosapentaenoic acid (EPA) and docosahexanoic acid (DHA), fatty acids that are precursors to anti-inflammatory and antiatherogenic prostaglandins. Another beneficial ingredient found in abundance in flaxseed is lignan, a phytochemical with potential for cancer prevention.

COMMENTS

Flaxseed oil is typically used as a dietary supplement for reducing symptoms of PMS and menopause (for which the evidence is thin) and for reducing inflammation and treating various inflammatory conditions such as pain, heart disease, eczema, and psoriasis (for which the evidence is modest but the theory strong, based on findings with other fatty acids such as those from fish oil).

SCIENTIFIC SUPPORT

Some of the health benefits associated with flaxseed consumption may be due to the presence of compounds called lignans, which are known to possess various proestrogenic and antiestrogenic properties. Studies have shown that large doses (several grams per day) of flaxseed oil can reduce blood clotting by reducing platelet aggregation (Allman et al., 1995). Regular flaxseed consumption has also been associated with improvements in the ratio of ω-3 to ω-6 fatty acids in the blood, which may offer protection from atherogenesis and relief from inflammatory conditions (Layne et al., 1996). Numerous animal studies have shown a beneficial role of flaxseed oil in delaying breast cancer progression and protecting against colon cancer, sometimes providing as much as a 50% reduction compared with control groups not fed flaxseed. A clear and consistent reduction in proinflammatory markers (tumor necrosis factor and interleukin) has been noted in human subjects supplemented with flaxseed oil (Mest et al., 1983), but long-term studies showing reductions in disease risk are lacking (McManus et al., 1996).

SAFETY/DOSAGE

Effective doses of flaxseed or flaxseed oil of 30–60 g/day (2–4 tablespoons or 1–2 oz) are unlikely to pose any adverse side effects. A note of caution is warranted, however, in cases of compromised blood clotting owing to the tendency of flaxseed oil to reduce platelet aggregation and prolong bleeding times. A similar cautionary note is advisable for patients undergoing surgical procedures that predispose the patient to excessive bleeding.

REFERENCES

Allman MA, Pena MM, Pang D. Supplementation with flaxseed oil versus sunflower seed oil in healthy young men consuming a low fat diet: effects on platelet composition and function. Eur J Clin Nutr 1995;49(3):169–178.

Layne KS, Goh YK, Jumpsen JA, Ryan EA, Chow P, Clandinin MT. Normal subjects consuming physiological levels of 18:3(n-3) and 20:5(n-3) from flaxseed or fish oils have characteristic differences in plasma lipid and lipoprotein fatty acid levels. J Nutr 1996;126(9):2130–2140.

McManus RM, Jumpson J, Finegood DT, Clandinin MT, Ryan EA. A comparison of the effects of n-3 fatty acids from linseed oil and fish oil in well-controlled type II diabetes. Diabetes Care 1996;19(5):463–467.

Mest HJ, Beitz J, Heinroth I, Block HU, Forster W. The influence of linseed oil diet on fatty acid pattern in phospholipids and thromboxane formation in platelets in man. Klin Wochenschr 1983;61(4):187–191.

ADDITIONAL RESOURCES

Beitz J, Mest HJ, Forster W. Influence of linseed oil diet on the pattern of serum phospholipids in man. Acta Biol Med Ger 1981;40(7–8):K31–K35.

Francois CA, Connor SL, Bolewicz LC, Connor WE. Supplementing lactating women with flaxseed oil does not increase docosahexaenoic acid in their milk. Am J Clin Nutr 2003;77(1):226–233.

Mantzioris E, James MJ, Gibson RA, Cleland LG. Dietary substitution with an alpha-linolenic acid-rich vegetable oil increases eicosapentaenoic acid concentrations in tissues. Am J Clin Nutr 1994;59(6):1304–1309.

Mantzioris E, James MJ, Gibson RA, Cleland LG. Differences exist in the relationships between dietary linoleic and alpha-linolenic acids and their respective long-chain metabolites. Am J Clin Nutr 1995;61(2):320–324.

Morton MS, Wilcox G, Wahlqvist ML, Griffiths K. Determination of lignans and isoflavonoids in human female plasma following dietary supplementation. J Endocrinol 1994;142(2):251–259.

Pang D, Allman-Farinelli MA, Wong T, Barnes R, Kingham KM. Replacement of linoleic acid with alpha-linolenic acid does not alter blood lipids in normolipidaemic men. Br J Nutr 1998;80(2):163–167.

St-Onge MP, Lamarche B, Mauger JF, Jones PJ. Consumption of a functional oil rich in phytosterols and medium-chain triglyceride oil improves plasma lipid profiles in men. J Nutr 2003;133(6):1815–1820.

Tarpila S, Aro A, Salminen I, Tarpila A, Kleemola P, Akkila J, Adlercreutz H. The effect of flaxseed supplementation in processed foods on serum fatty acids and enterolactone. Eur J Clin Nutr 2002;56(2):157–165.

Wallace FA, Miles EA, Calder PC. Comparison of the effects of linseed oil and different doses of fish oil on mononuclear cell function in healthy human subjects. Br J Nutr 2003;89(5):679–689.

GOTU KOLA

Overall Rank

★★★   for enhancing wound healing
★★★   for treating and preventing varicose veins and hemorrhoids
★★   for antianxiety effects
★★   for enhancing memory and cognitive function

OVERVIEW

Gotu kola (*Centella asiatica*) is a creeping vine-like plant native to India and Southeast Asia. In India and Indonesia, gotu kola has long been used to promote wound healing and treat skin diseases. In Europe, extracts of *Centella asiatica* are used as drugs for the treatment of wound healing defects. Gotu kola should not be confused with the kola nut, which is completely unrelated and is often used in dietary supplements as a "natural" source of caffeine. Modern dietary supplements of gotu kola are generally marketed to help prevent varicose veins and hemorrhoids; heal scars, burns, and wounds; reduce skin inflammation; and smooth skin wrinkles. In addition to the benefits of gotu kola on connective tissue, there also appear to be some benefits for the central nervous system, with potential improvements in energy levels, memory, anxiety, and sleep patterns.

COMMENTS

The primary benefits of gotu kola appear to be an enhancement of wound healing and an improvement in overall vein function (especially for varicose veins and hemorrhoids). Antianxiety effects are also interesting and warrant additional study. Based on traditional usage patterns and clinical findings, gotu kola represents a good value for people who suffer from varicose veins or swollen ankles as well as for anybody recovering from a connective tissue injury such as a muscle or tendon strain, ligament sprain, or skin abrasion.

SCIENTIFIC SUPPORT

Gotu kola contains a blend of compounds, including at least three triterpenes (asiatic acid, madecassic acid, and asiaticoside) that appear to have antioxidant benefits and an ability to stimulate collagen synthesis for tissue regeneration (Tenni et al., 1988). Perhaps the best data for gotu kola are shown by its ability to improve symptoms of varicose veins, particularly overall discomfort, tiredness, and swelling (Cataldi et al., 2001). In human studies, gotu kola extract (30–180 mg/day for 4 weeks) leads to improvements in various measurements of vein function (foot swelling, ankle edema, and fluid leakage from the veins) compared with a placebo (Cesarone et al., 1994). Gotu kola appears to have a generally beneficial effect on connective tissues, possibly improving the structure and function of the connective tissue in the body, keeping veins stronger, and reducing the symptoms of other connective tissue diseases. In one animal study, asiatic acid and asiaticoside were the most active of the three triterpenes, but all three were effective in stimulating collagen synthesis and glycosaminoglycan synthesis (Maquart et al., 1999). Radiation injury to the skin of laboratory rats was reduced by treatment with madecassol (one of the triterpene compounds in gotu kola), suggesting a skin regeneration and anti-inflammatory activity (Suguna et al., 1996).

The activity of asiaticoside has been studied in normal as well as delayed-type wound healing. In one study, administration of asiaticoside produced significant increases in hydroxyproline content tensile strength and collagen content of wounds. In addition, other studies have indicated an antioxidant effect of asiaticoside and triterpenes contained in gotu kola (Shukla et al., 1999a, 1999b), with significant increases in both enzymatic and nonenzymatic antioxidants, such as superoxide dismutase, catalase, glutathione peroxidase, vitamin E, and ascorbic acid in newly formed tissues, as well as a several-fold decrease in free-radical damage and lipid peroxide levels. This enhancement of antioxidant levels at the initial stage of healing may be an important contributory factor in the healing properties of gotu kola.

SAFETY/DOSAGE

Orally, gotu kola appears to be nontoxic, and it seldom causes any side effects other than the occasional allergic skin rash. There are some concerns that gotu kola may be carcinogenic if applied topically to the skin, but this has been reported in only one laboratory study and has not appeared as a major concern in human studies or in animal models of wound healing. Typical dosage recommendations are in the range of 60–180 mg/day, usually consumed in divided doses of 20–60 mg 3 times daily for at least 4 weeks. It is important to look for an extract standardized to contain triterpene compounds, typically 30–40%, and including asiaticoside, asiatic acid, madecassic acid, and madecassoside (which typically occur at only 1–4% in the whole herb).

REFERENCES

Cataldi A, Gasbarro V, Viaggi R, Soverini R, Gresta E, Mascoli F. Effectiveness of the combination of alpha tocopherol, rutin, melilotus, and centella asiatica in the treatment of patients with chronic venous insufficiency. Minerva Cardioangiol 2001;49(2):159–163.

Cesarone MR, Laurora G, De Sanctis MT, Incandela L, Grimaldi R, Marelli C, Belcaro G. The microcirculatory activity of Centella asiatica in venous insufficiency. A double-blind study. Minerva Cardioangiol 1994;42(6):299–304.

Maquart FX, Chastang F, Simeon A, Birembaut P, Gillery P, Wegrowski Y. Triterpenes from Centella asiatica stimulate extracellular matrix accumulation in rat experimental wounds. Eur J Dermatol 1999;9(4):289–296.

Shukla A, Rasik AM, Dhawan BN. Asiaticoside-induced elevation of antioxidant levels in healing wounds. Phytother Res 1999a;13(1):50–54.

Shukla A, Rasik AM, Jain GK, Shankar R, Kulshrestha DK, Dhawan BN. In vitro and in vivo wound healing activity of asiaticoside isolated from Centella asiatica. J Ethnopharmacol 1999b;65(1):1–11.

Suguna L, Sivakumar P, Chandrakasan G. Effects of Centella asiatica extract on dermal wound healing in rats. Indian J Exp Biol 1996;34(12):1208–1211.

Tenni R, Zanaboni G, De Agostini MP, Rossi A, Bendotti C, Cetta G. Effect of the triterpenoid fraction of Centella asiatica on macromolecules of the connective matrix in human skin fibroblast cultures. Ital J Biochem 1988;37(2):69–77.

ADDITIONAL RESOURCES

Bradwejn J, Zhou Y, Koszycki D, Shlik J. A double-blind, placebo-controlled study on the effects of Gotu Kola (Centella asiatica) on acoustic startle response in healthy subjects. J Clin Psychopharmacol 2000;20(6):680–684.

Sastravaha G, Yotnuengnit P, Booncong P, Sangtherapitikul P. Adjunctive periodontal treatment with Centella asiatica and Punica granatum extracts. A preliminary study. J Int Acad Periodontol 2003;5(4):106–115.

HORSE CHESTNUT (*AESCULUS HIPPOCASTANUM* L.)

Overall Rank

★★★★★ for vein health (venotonic)
★★★ for treating and preventing hemorrhoids
★★ for treating and preventing inflammatory conditions
★★ for reducing and preventing postoperative edema

OVERVIEW

Horse chestnut is used in the form of an extract of the seed of the plant. Horse chestnut itself is a beautiful ornamental tree, with lush palmate leaves and spikes of creamy-white and red spotted flowers. With other members of the *Aesculus* genus, horse chestnut is considered toxic and only to be used in the standardized extract form. Native Americans, however, leached the nuts for several days to make a meal to use in breads. Other uses of the plant throughout history include as a fish intoxicant, in the preparation of gunpowder, as an ornamental tree, and in manufacturing furniture. It has also been used traditionally for treating congestion, backache, neuralgia, hemorrhoids, arthritis, strains, sports injuries, tendonitis, and rheumatism (McKenna et al., 2002).

In Europe, the extract form of horse chestnut is popular not only for the phytotherapy of chronic venous insufficiency but also for its topical use in cosmetics, lotions, and hand creams. A number of experimental models (preclinical) have supported its therapeutic benefits, such as antiedematous, anti-inflammatory, and venotonic properties (Sirtori, 2001).

COMMENTS

Horse chestnut has yet to gain popularity in the United States, but it has well-substantiated efficacy for treating chronic venous insufficiency (CVI), a condition for which few satisfactory treatment options exist.

SCIENTIFIC SUPPORT

Venous Insufficiency

In a review of the clinical studies on the efficacy of horse chestnut for chronic venous insufficiency, studies involving the oral use of horse chestnut monotherapy compared with a placebo were chosen. The reviewers found that horse chestnut appeared to be an efficacious and safe treatment for the short-term treatment of CVI (Pittler and Ernst, 2004). In an earlier meta-analysis, Pittler and Ernst (2002) came to the same conclusion.

In an even earlier systematic review of the literature, Pittler and Ernst (1998) included double-blind, randomized, controlled studies. All placebo-controlled studies found horse chestnut extract to be more effective than a placebo, and five studies found horse chestnut to be as effective as oxerutins.

Siebert et al. (2002) performed another systematic review of the literature on horse chestnut that included both randomized controlled trials and large-scale observational studies and compared outcomes and adverse effects. Included in the review were 13 randomized clinical trials and three observational studies. The authors found that horse chestnut extract appeared to be a safe and effective treatment for CVI. They noted that longer-term studies were needed to evaluate the safety and effectiveness of horse chestnut extract.

In a randomized, partially blinded, placebo-controlled, parallel study, the efficacy of horse chestnut seed extract was compared to compression stockings (Class 2). Both compression stockings and horse chestnut seed extract resulted in significant reductions in edema, and both therapies were shown to be equivalent (Diehm et al., 1996).

Rehn et al. (1996) conducted a double-blind, randomized, placebo-controlled, clinical study to compare oxerutins and horse chestnut extract for the treatment of CVI. The patients were treated with either 1,000 mg/day of oxerutins, 600 mg/day of horse chestnut, or 1,000 mg/day of oxerutins for 4 weeks, followed by 500 mg/day of oxerutins for 12 weeks. Horse chestnut was found to be equivalent or better than the oxerutins.

Hemorrhoids

In a placebo-controlled trial, patients with acute hemorrhoids were administered a saponin made from the seed of the horse chestnut, called escin (40 mg 2 times daily) or a placebo for 2 months. Improvements were reported after 6 days of treatment, and about 82% of patients receiving the escin treatment improved compared to 32% on the placebo (Pirard et al., 1976).

SAFETY/DOSAGE

The usual recommended dosage of escin from clinical studies is 50 mg 2–3 times daily. Therefore, in normal commercial extracts standardized to 16% triterpene glycosides, calculated as escin, the corresponding dosage is 300–900 mg/day (McKenna et al., 2002).

Because horse chestnut is considered toxic in its raw form, it is important to use only standardized extracts. Dosages equivalent to 100 mg of escin (250–313 mg of standardized extract) in a delayed-release form have been associated with few side effects. Side effects may include nausea, stomach discomfort, and itching (McKenna et al., 2002).

REFERENCES

Diehm C, Trampisch HJ, Lange S, Schmidt C. Comparison of leg compression stocking and oral horse-chestnut seed extract therapy in patients with chronic venous insufficiency. Lancet 1996;347(8997):292–294.

McKenna D, Jones K, Hughes K, eds. Botanical Medicines: The Desk Reference for Major Herbal Supplements. 2nd Ed. Binghamton, NY: Haworth Press, 2002.

Pirard J, Gillet P, Guffens JM, Defrance P. Double blind study of Reparil in proctology. Rev Med Liege 1976;31(10):343–345.

Pittler MH, Ernst E. Horse chestnut seed extract for chronic venous insufficiency. Cochrane Database Syst Rev 2002;(1):CD003230.

Pittler MH, Ernst E. Horse chestnut seed extract for chronic venous insufficiency. Cochrane Database Syst Rev 2004;(2):CD003230.

Pittler MH, Ernst E. Horse-chestnut seed extract for chronic venous insufficiency. A criteria-based systematic review. Arch Dermatol 1998;134(11):1356–1360.

Rehn D, Unkauf M, Klein P, Jost V, Lucker PW. Comparative clinical efficacy and tolerability of oxerutins and horse chestnut extract in patients with chronic venous insufficiency. Arzneimittelforschung 1996;46(5):483–487.

Siebert U, Brach M, Sroczynski G, Berla K. Efficacy, routine effectiveness, and safety of horse chestnut seed extract in the treatment of chronic venous insufficiency. A meta-analysis of randomized controlled trials and large observational studies. Int Angiol 2002;21(4):305–315.

Sirtori CR. Aescin: pharmacology, pharmacokinetics and therapeutic profile. Pharmacol Res 2001;44(3):183–193.

RED CLOVER (*TRIFOLIUM PRATENSE*)

Overall Rank

★★★★ for balancing hormones
★★★★ for reducing menopausal symptoms (hot flashes, loss of libido)
★★★ for balancing mood swings (associated with hormone imbalance)
★★★ for supporting cardiovascular health
★★★ for maintaining bone mass
★★ for treating and preventing prostate cancer

OVERVIEW

As a leguminous plant high in the plant phytoestrogens known as the isoflavones, red clover has gained popularity as a treatment for menopausal symptoms. The isoflavones are popular for balancing female hormones, especially during menopause, because they are thought to act like very weak estrogens. The isoflavones are able to interact with the estrogen receptors on cell surfaces, and in doing so are thought to very weakly mimic the effect of estrogen and, maybe more importantly, to compete with the more dangerous forms of estrogen in the body (higher levels of which cause the adverse effects of estrogen).

The difference between the soy isoflavones and those from red clover is that soy contains only two types of isoflavones, genistein and daidzein, whereas red clover contains four types, genistein, daidzein, biochanin, and formononetin. Studies on the soy isoflavones are more plentiful than those on the red clover isoflavones, but an increasing number of studies show that red clover may deliver the same if not better benefits.

COMMENTS

Red clover seems like another good source of isoflavones that is just starting to get clinical results. However, because half of its isoflavones are the same as those of soy, the benefits red clover should be similar to those of soy.

SCIENTIFIC SUPPORT

Menopausal Symptoms

Tice et al. (2003) conducted a randomized, double-blind, placebo-controlled study of the effect of two red clover products on menopausal women. The 252 participants were given either Promensil (82 mg/day of total isoflavones), Rimostil (57 mg/day of total isoflavones), or a matched placebo for 12 weeks. The primary outcome measure was the number of hot flashes, and the secondary outcome measure was adverse events and changes in quality of life. There were no significant differences found among the groups for any of the parameters measured. There was evidence, however, that Promensil reduced the frequency of hot flash faster than did either Rimostil or a placebo.

Red clover extract was clinically tested for its effect on hot-flash frequency in postmenopausal women in a randomized, double-blind, placebo-controlled study. The 30 participants were divided into two groups and given either 80 mg of isoflavones from red clover (Pomensil) or a placebo daily for 12 weeks. The treatment group resulted in a significant reduction (44%) in hot flashes at the end of the 12 weeks of Promensil treatment (van de Weijer and Barentsen, 2002).

Cholesterol and Insulin Resistance

To determine if isoflavones (from red clover) had an effect on cholesterol homeostasis or insulin resistance in premenopausal women, Blakesmith et al. (2003) conducted a randomized, double-blind, placebo-controlled, parallel, clinical study. The 25 participants were divided into two groups and given either (1) a placebo during one menstrual cycle and then red clover isoflavone supplement (86 mg/day of isoflavones) during three consecutive menstrual cycles or (2) a placebo during four consecutive menstrual cycles. Treatment 1 showed no significant effects on cholesterol homeostasis or insulin resistance.

Howes et al. (2000) studied the effect of a red clover isoflavone extract in 66 postmenopausal women with plasma cholesterol levels between 5.0 and 9.0 mmol/L in a placebo-controlled, randomized, double-blind, ascending-dose study. The isoflavone extract contained approximately 26 mg of biochanin, 16 mg of formononetin, 0.5 mg of daidzein, and 1 mg of genistein. The treatment period lasted 4 weeks. No significant difference in plasma lipids was found between treatment with isoflavones and a placebo for women with moderately high cholesterol levels.

Nestel et al. (1999) studied whether isoflavone intake could reduce the elevated risk of cardiovascular disease associated with menopause in a double-blind, placebo-controlled study. Two 5-week periods of active treatment consisted of the administration of 40 mg and then 80 mg of isoflavones derived from red clover. The effect on cardiovascular risk was determined by measuring arterial compliance (the elasticity of the large arteries). Treatment with isoflavones from red clover was found to significantly improve the arterial compliance and thus potentially reduce the risk of cardiovascular disease after menopause.

Isoflavone Absorption

In a clinical evaluation of the absorption of isoflavones from red clover versus those from soy, 14 subjects were studied in a single-blind, randomized, placebo-controlled, crossover, clinical trial. The soybean isoflavones and the red clover isoflavones were included in a breakfast cereal and administered as a meal for 2 weeks each. No significant difference was found between the two types of isoflavone sources in urinary excretion, signifying no difference in absorption (Tsunoda et al., 2002).

Prostate Cancer

Jarred et al. (2002) conducted a nonrandomized, nonblind study to assess if isoflavone consumption could be linked to prostate cancer incidence. Before surgery, 38 men who had been diagnosed with prostate cancer were given 160 mg/day of red clover–derived isoflavones. The tissue on radical prostatectomy was compared with historical specimens as a control. No differences were found for serum prostate-specific antigen, Gleason score, serum testosterone, and biochemical factors. There was, however, a significant increase in apoptosis in prostate tumor cells of treated patients, especially in regions of low- to moderate-grade cancer. The authors concluded that isoflavones may halt the progression of prostate cancer in low- to moderate-grade tumors, and that this may be a contributing factor in the lower incidence of prostate cancer in Asian men.

SAFETY/DOSAGE

The typical recommended dosage of isoflavones from red clover is 40–80 mg/day. No serious side effects are associated with red clover extract.

REFERENCES

Blakesmith SJ, Lyons-Wall PM, George C, Joannou GE, Petocz P, Samman S. Effects of supplementation with purified red clover (Trifolium pratense) isoflavones on plasma lipids and insulin resistance in healthy premenopausal women. Br J Nutr 2003;89(4):467–474.

Howes JB, Sullivan D, Lai N, Nestel P, Pomeroy S, West L, Eden JA, Howes LG. The effects of dietary supplementation with isoflavones from red clover on the lipoprotein profiles of post menopausal women with mild to moderate hypercholesterolaemia. Atherosclerosis 2000;152(1):143–147.

Jarred RA, Keikha M, Dowling C, McPherson SJ, Clare AM, Husband AJ, Pedersen JS, Frydenberg M, Risbridger GP. Induction of apoptosis in low to moderate-grade human prostate carcinoma by red clover-derived dietary isoflavones. Cancer Epidemiol Biomarkers Prev 2002;11(12):1689–1696.

Nestel PJ, Pomeroy S, Kay S, Komesaroff P, Behrsing J, Cameron JD, West L. Isoflavones from red clover improve systemic arterial compliance but not plasma lipids in menopausal women. J Clin Endocrinol Metab 1999;84(3):895–898.

Tice JA, Ettinger B, Ensrud K, Wallace R, Blackwell T, Cummings SR. Phytoestrogen supplements for the treatment of hot flashes: the Isoflavone Clover Extract (ICE) Study: a randomized controlled trial. JAMA 2003;290(2):207–214.

Tsunoda N, Pomeroy S, Nestel P. Absorption in humans of isoflavones from soy and red clover is similar. J Nutr 2002;132(8):2199–2201.

van de Weijer PH, Barentsen R. Isoflavones from red clover (Promensil) significantly reduce menopausal hot flush symptoms compared with placebo. Maturitas 2002;42(3):187–193.

Uva Ursi or Bearberry
(ARCTOSTAPHYLOS UVA-URSI)

Overall Rank

★★★ for urinary complaints and inflammation of the urinary tract
★ for treating and preventing kidney stone formation

OVERVIEW

Uva ursi is a small shrub found in North America, Canada, Europe and northern Asia. Long known as an astringent and diuretic, uva ursi has been used traditionally by Native Americans and other cultures to treat bladder and kidney diseases. Preparations of the leaves are also known to have antiseptic qualities. Many Native American tribes used uva ursi for treating inflammation of the genitourinary tract and for treating venereal disease; the plant was also used to control weight and treat stomach ailments, rheumatic conditions, and sprains. Today, uva ursi is most widely used for inflammatory conditions of the urinary tract, including urethritis, chronic cystitis, nephritis, and kidney stones (McKenna et al., 2002).

Uva ursi is known to contain several compounds thought to contribute to its therapeutic activity, including hydroquinone derivatives, often calculated as arbutin, and flavonoids, such as ursolic acid and quercetin. For treating urinary tract infections, the leaves are mostly used in extracts, normally in the form of an infusion, tea, or tincture (McKenna et al., 2002). Pharmacologically, uva ursi has been found to inhibit melanin synthesis and to have antiallergic, antiedemic, and anti-inflammatory activities. Additionally, it has been indicated to inhibit adjuvant-induced arthritis and immunoinflammation (Matsuda et al., 1990, 1991, 1992a, 1992b; Kubo et al., 1990).

COMMENTS

Uva ursi is used for various therapeutic complaints, but clinical validation exists only for urinary complaints, especially cystitis, although there is much more support needed to validate this use. Other purported uses for this herbal medicine include treating prostate problems, bronchitis, dysentery, dysmenorrhea, dysuria, hepatitis, hemorrhoids, rheumatism, ulcers, diabetes, dysentery, fever, and gonorrhea (McKenna et al., 2002).

SCIENTIFIC SUPPORT

Larsson et al. (1993) performed a randomized, double-blind, placebo-controlled, clinical study on the prophylactic effect of an uva ursi extract

(UVA-E, manufactured by Medic Herb AB in Sweden) on recurrent cystitis. For one month, the 57 women enrolled in the study were administered UVA-E (three tablets 2 times daily) or a placebo. Routine gynecological and bacteriological examinations were performed at 6 and 12 months. The study found that 23% of the women who were given the placebo had recurrences versus none in the UVA-E group; this was statistically significant. No side effects were noted in either group, and voiding patterns remained similar between groups.

SAFETY/DOSAGE

Uva ursi is normally recommended in the approximate dosage of 10 g of the cut or powdered herb, corresponding to 400–700 mg of arbutin in 150 mL (0.75 cup) water consumed as a tea or cold maceration. In Europe, uva ursi is used in the forms of infusions, cold macerates, or solid formulations. Assuming the extract of the herb is standardized to at least 6% hydroquinone derivatives, the usual recommendation is 1 g 3–6 times daily. The efficacy of uva ursi is said to depend on having alkaline urine, without which the uva ursi is not bioavailable (McKenna et al., 2002).

In the normal recommended dosages, uva ursi has shown no adverse effects. Excessive use of extracts may cause vomiting and diarrhea owing to the tannin content and can cause the urine to turn green, but that is harmless. One case of bull's eye maculopathy has been reported in women with long-term ingestion of uva ursi. As uva ursi is a known inhibitor of melanin synthesis, it may be capable of producing ocular damage (Wang and Del Priore, 2004).

REFERENCES

Kubo M, Ito M, Nakata H, Matsuda H. Pharmacological studies on leaf of Arctostaphylos uva-ursi (L.) Spreng. I. Combined effect of 50% methanolic extract from Arctostaphylos uva-ursi (L.) Spreng. (bearberry leaf) and prednisolone on immuno-inflammation. Yakugaku Zasshi 1990;110(1):59–67.

Larsson B, Jonasson A, Fianu S. Prophylactic effect of uva-e in women with recurrent cystitis: A preliminary report. Curr Ther Res 1993;53:441–443.

McKenna D, Jones K, Hughes K, eds. Botanical Medicines: The Desk Reference for Major Herbal Supplements. 2nd Ed. Binghamton, NY: Haworth Press, 2002.

Matsuda H, Nakamura S, Shiomoto H, Tanaka T, Kubo M. Pharmacological studies on leaf of Arctostaphylos uva-ursi (L.) Spreng. IV. Effect of 50% methanolic extract from Arctostaphylos uva-ursi (L.) Spreng. (bearberry leaf) on melanin synthesis. Yakugaku Zasshi 1992a;112(4):276–282.

Matsuda H, Nakamura S, Tanaka T, Kubo M. Pharmacological studies on leaf of Arctostaphylos uva-ursi (L.) Spreng, part V: effect of water extract from Arctostaphylos uva-ursi (L.) Spreng. (bearberry leaf) on the antiallergic and antiinflammatory activities of dexamethasone ointment. Yakugaku Zasshi 1992b;112(9):673–677.

Matsuda H, Nakata H, Tanaka T, Kubo M. Pharmacological study on Arctostaphylos uva-ursi (L.) Spreng, part II: combined effects of arbutin and prednisolone or dexamethazone on immuno-inflammation. Yakugaku Zasshi 1990;110(1):68–76.

Matsuda H, Tanaka T, Kubo M. Pharmacological studies on leaf of Arctostaphylos uva-ursi (L.) Spreng, part III: combined effect of arbutin and indomethacin on immuno-inflammation. Yakugaku Zasshi 1991;111(4–5):253–258.

Wang L, Del Priore LV. Bull's-eye maculopathy secondary to herbal toxicity from uva ursi. Am J Ophthalmol 2004;137(6):1135–1137.

VITEX OR CHASTEBERRY (*VITEX AGNUS-CASTUS* L.)

Overall Rank

★★★★★ for reducing and preventing PMS
★★★★★ for treating and preventing premenstrual tension syndrome (PMTS)
★★★★ for reducing and preventing breast pain
★★★★ for balancing hormones
★★★ for treating and preventing acne
★★ for menopausal complaints

OVERVIEW

Vitex or chasteberry is primarily used to treat PMS. However, some clinical evidence shows the efficacy of the herbal medicine for a list of conditions that includes hyperprolactinemia, corpus luteum insufficiency and associated infertility, mastodynia, PMTS, perimenopausal symptoms, uterine myomas, endometriosis (adjunctive therapy), Parkinson disease, lack of milk production, overproduction of milk in lactation, and acne (McKenna et al., 2001).

The chemistry of vitex (*Vitex agnus-castus*) is not yet fully understood, nor is the relationship of its chemical constituents to therapeutic use. Standardized extracts of vitex have had extensive clinical investigation. Standardization is normally to 0.5% agnusides of a 20:1 fruit extract. The fruit, leaves, and seeds of the vitex plant have had documented use in traditional medicine, but modern extracts focus only on the fruits. Known chemical compounds in the fruits are essential oils and flavonoids. The essential oils (0.15–1.0%) are made up of 73 identified compounds, including 4-terpinol, α pinene, β phellandrene, sabinene, β caryophyllene, E-β farnesene, caryophyllene oxide, alloaromadenedrene, and spathulenol. The flavonoids are orientin, iso-orientin, xyloside, vitexin, and isovitexin (McKenna et al., 2001).

Vitex exhibits a dopaminergic activity that inhibits prolactin activity. This is the activity to which its therapeutic applications are mostly attributed (McKenna et al., 2001). A few of the most notable preclinical studies are summarized here:

• Estrogenic activity has been reported by the equivalent of one-third the human dose administered to ovariectomized female rats (Eagon et al., 1997).

- Various parts of the vitex plant (mostly the leaves and fruits) have exhibited antimicrobial or growth-inhibitory activity against *Pseudomonas aeruginosa, Escherichia coli, Bacillus subtilis, Staphylococcus aureus, Aspergillus parasiticus, Candida krusei, C. albicans, Penicillium veredictum, Streptococcus faecalis, Trichophyton mentagrophytes, Microsporium gypseum, M. canis, Shigella sonnei,* and *Epidermophyton floccosum;* and common insect pests (Krustrak et al., 1992; Pepeljnjak et al., 1996; Snow, 1996).
- Vitex exhibits a dopamine-agonist action that causes an antiprolactin effect at the hypothalamus-pituitary axis. However, investigations have found that vitex does not increase the actual secretion of dopamine (McKenna et al., 2001; Wuttke et al., 1995).
- A concentration-dependent lowering of prolactin secretion in isolated rat pituitary cells in vitro was found using Agnolyt (Wuttke, 1992).

COMMENTS

Vitex is second in popularity only to black cohosh for women's health. Although vitex is generally thought of as a key phytotherapeutic for PMS, it also has good clinical support for menopausal symptoms, among other female complaints.

SCIENTIFIC SUPPORT

Clinical investigation of vitex has been ongoing since the 1930s. The early work, done by Madaus on their product Agnolyt , focused on the reputation of vitex as a galactogogue (McKenna et al., 2001).

Hormonal Balancing
Corpus luteum insufficiency is a condition in which serum progesterone levels are low 3 weeks after the onset of menstruation (less than 10–12 ng/mL). Symptoms can be long menstrual periods, anovulatory periods (with resultant infertility), PMS, and mastopathy. The underlying cause is thought to be hyperprolactinemia (McKenna et al., 2001). Clinical work has been performed with vitex on various menstrual symptoms, including PMS, PMTS, and corpus luteum insufficiency. Owing to the similarity between syndromes and symptoms, the participant groups may represent a mixture of those diagnoses.

The tolerance to and effect of high doses of vitex extract were studied in 20 healthy male subjects aged 20–32. Men were selected for this study, even though their prolactin levels are lower, because they have less hormonal variation than women. The extracts were described as mostly water- and alcohol-free "thick" extracts prepared from the ripe, dried fruits of *V. agnus-castus* (special extract BP1095E1). Analysis of the results found the lowest dose to decrease the 24-hour serum prolactin level by more than 15% and by 21% in the middle- and highest-dose extracts. Both dopamine antagonistic and agonistic actions were suspected, with the antagonistic actions taking place with the lower dosage of vitex. The extract was judged to be well tolerated because no significant effects were noted, and only temporary or idiosyncratic effects were found (Merz et al., 1996).

A study of 52 women with latent hyperprolactinemia found that therapy with vitex (20 mg/day) produced lower prolactin levels as well as a normalization of other hormone levels associated with the menstrual cycle. Vitex was also found to significantly reduce PMS symptoms in women who had presented with them in the beginning of the study. No side effects were found in the study, and 2 of the 17 women in the vitex group became pregnant (Milewicz et al., 1993).

In another study involving 13 women with hyperprolactinemia and cyclic disorders, a vitex product called Mastodynon was tested. At the end of the 3-month study, prolactin levels were measured and found to be reduced; some were within normal prolactin ranges. The menstrual cycles of the women on vitex therapy were also found to be normalized (Roeder, 1994).

The use of vitex (Agnolyt, 40 drops/day for 3 months) was tested in an open, noncontrolled study of 20 infertile women with no prolactin imbalance. Prolactin, thyroid and androgen hormones were within normal ranges in the women chosen for this study, but all had low levels of progesterone on day 20 of the menstrual cycle. At the end of the study, progesterone levels rose to normal ranges in seven of the women, and progesterone levels rose above normal in four women. In addition, basal body temperatures rose, and the women were found to have a longer, more normal hyperthermic phase in their cycles. Two of the women became pregnant, and no side effects were noted (Propping and Katzorke, 1987).

In one double-blind, placebo-controlled study of 52 women with corpus luteum insufficiency and abnormal menstrual cycles, vitex extract was administered over three cycles (Strotan, 20 mg/day). In the treatment group, the luteal phase changed from an average of 5.5 to 10.5 days, and the follicle phase was reduced from 23.8 to 18.5 days. In addition, prolactin levels were normalized (previously high), and there were significant increases in both progesterone and estrogen levels compared with the placebo. An added benefit from the study was that three women who previously could not conceive became pregnant (Bubenzer, 1983).

Several large drug-monitoring studies reported the use of vitex (in the form of Agnolyt drops; McKenna et al., 2001):

- The results of a questionnaire were reported on the use of vitex (various preparations) by 153 members of the National Institute of Medical Herbalists from England and Ireland. Treatments were reported for PMS (94.1%), perimenopausal complaints (86.3%), female infertility (89.5%), female acne (79.7%), and male acne (10.5%). Nearly all respondents (98.6%) believed vitex to be "very effective" or "effective" for hormonal imbalance syndromes. Mean length of treatment was 4.8 months for PMS and 7.1 months for menopausal complaints. The most common preparation used was tinctures (86.4%), followed by fluid extracts (28.1%) and powdered herb preparations (9.2%). Very few practitioners used standardized powdered extracts (Christie and Walker, 1997–1998).

- A multicenter study recorded the use of Agnolyt in 1,592 cases for menstrual disorders and PMS (usually with corpus luteum insufficiency). Mean treatment was 43 drops/day for 5 months. A good or satisfactory response was reported in 90% of cases. Of the 145 patients who had stated they wanted to become pregnant, 56 did. Side effects were reported in 2.4% of cases (Propping et al., 1991).

- In two drug-monitoring studies using Agnolyt drops, a total of 3,162 women, most with menstrual problems, were followed. Diagnoses included PMS (1,016 women), corpus luteum insufficiency (734 women), uterine myomas (320 women), and menopausal symptoms (167 women). Mean treatment was 153 days using 42 drops/ day of Agnolyt. The effectiveness of treatment was judged to be 90%, with 1% experiencing side effects (Loch et al., 1991).

- The use of Agnolyt was recorded in 1,571 women for menstrual problems associated with corpus luteum insufficiency or ovarian dysfunction. Average treatment was 40 drops/day, on an empty stomach, for 135 days. A response rate of almost 90% was recorded with adverse effects seen in only 1.9% of women (Feldmann et al., 1990).

- Attelman et al. (1972) wrote a drug-monitoring report on the use of vitex (Agnolyt) in the authors' general and consulting practices in Germany. In more than 2,000 cases, the authors used vitex for PMS, polymenorrhea, hypermenorrhea (due to uterine fibroids), headaches (from birth control pill use), mastopathia, amenorrhea (primary and secondary), uterine bleeding (juvenile), menopausal bleeding, and sterility. Most treatments for menopause used 40 drops/day, after meals. Side effects were reported as rare.

Premenstrual Syndrome

An extract of vitex (Ze 440; one dose daily of a 20-mg native extract over eight menstrual cycles) was administered to 50 patients with PMS in a prospective multicenter study. Results of the treatment were monitored using the validated Moos Menstrual Distress Questionnaire (MMDQ), a visual analogue scale (self-assessment), and a global impression scale. Lessening of PMS symptoms by treatment were indicated by a significant score reduction (42.5%) on the MMDQ. The global efficacy results were moderate to excellent (in 38 patients), and the number of days of the PMS symptoms was reduced slightly from 7.5 to 6.0. The results for patients on oral contraceptives were no different than those for the other patients, and no significant side effects were found (Berger et al., 2000).

A large multicenter study tested a new solid extract preparation of vitex over three menstrual cycles in women. The 1,634 patients were administered a questionnaire to follow common PMS symptoms, and 93% reported a decrease or cessation of PMS symptoms. Among the physicians, 85% reported the treatment efficacy as good or very good, while 81% of patients assessed treatment as very much or much better. No serious side effects were reported (Loch et al., 2000).

A double-blind, placebo-controlled, randomized trial of vitex included 600 women with PMS. Participants were judged using the MMDQ. Compared with the placebo group, women in the vitex group reported a significant improvement in the "feel jittery or restless" symptom; however, the authors concluded that otherwise the efficacy of vitex is no better than placebo (soy based). The authors also admitted that the design of the study could have unfairly biased the outcome of differences between the treatment and control groups (Turner and Mills, 1993).

A study comparing vitex with pyridoxine for treatment of PMTS was conducted in a multicenter, randomized, double-center manner involving 105 women. Efficacy was rated at 77.1% for vitex and 60.6% for pyridoxine (by the Clinical Global Impression Scale). Although the results were not statistically valid, the authors supported the overall beneficial results of Agnolyt (Lauritzen et al., 1997).

Another study examined the efficacy of Agnolyt capsules (a new preparation at the time) in PMTS. The study was randomized and double blind, using 175 mg/day of vitex or 200 mg/day of pyridoxine (vitamin B_6) in 175 women. Treatment lasted for three menstrual cycles and was ranked using the PMTS scale. In the treatment group, the PMTS rating fell from 15.2 to 5.1 points after treatment, and from 11.9 to 5.1 points in the pyridoxine group (reflecting a significant improvement in symptoms). Patient evaluations were 36.1% for vitex versus 21.3% for the pyridoxine; 24% of physicians rated vitex as excellent versus 12.1% for the pyridoxine (Reuter et al., 1995).

In a drug-monitoring study involving 1,542 women, vitex was used to treat various disorders, including PMS, corpus luteum insufficiency, uterine fibroids, and menopausal symptoms. Treatment consisted of 20–120 drops/day of Agnolyt (for an average of 42 drops/day) over a period of 7 days to 16 years. Symptom improvement began after an approximate mean of 25 days, and the dissatisfaction rate was only about 4.5% for both assessors and patients (Dittmar et al., 1992).

Acne

In the package insert for Agnolyt (1994), one of the most popular vitex preparations in Europe, the manufacturer (Madaus GmbH) describes several clinical studies. One use for Agnolyt recorded by the clinical studies was the treatment of acne. In one clinical study, Agnolyt was used to treat 118 patients for 12–24 months. The treatment group was compared with a group of 43 patients who received "conventional" treatment. At the end of the study, the vitex group was found to have healed more quickly and to have fewer recurrences than the conventional-therapy group. Men and women are both described as candidates for acne treatment by vitex in the package insert (McKenna et al., 2001).

Lactation

Vitex has historically been used for bringing on lactation in women who are having trouble producing milk. The exact mechanisms of the hormones involved in lactation are complex and not fully understood; similarly, the use of vitex for lactation has been controversial because the actions of the herbal medicine are not fully understood. Breastfeeding women with high prolactin levels and suppressed ovulatory function often show symptoms associated with disordered follicular development and corpus luteum insufficiency. More than half of all women with menstrual problems (62%) also have abnormally high levels of prolactin. The opposite is also true: women who are hyperprolactinemic almost always have menstrual disorders (Böhnert, 1997).

Breast Pain

Halaska et al. (1998) administered vitex extract to patients with mastodynia in a double-blind, placebo-controlled study. Two parallel groups of 50 patients were treated over three menstrual cycles (60 drops daily of vitex extract or placebo). The intensity of breast pain was found to diminish faster in the vitex treatment groups versus the placebo group, and the tolerability of treatment was found to be satisfactory.

In a randomized, double-blind, placebo-controlled, multicenter study, the use of vitex (Mastodynon N) was tested in women with cyclical mastalgia. The study included 120 women (ages 23–40) who had presented with breast pain for three or more menstrual cycles (for 3 or more days of the cycle). A parallel group design and double-dummy technique was used in the study, administering tablet and liquid extract forms of vitex and corresponding placebos. Prolactin levels were measured during the study, and the participants were scored using a linear analogue scale (VAS). Both the tablet form (3.7 ng/mL, $p = 0.015$) and the liquid form (4.35 ng/mL, $p = 0.039$) of vitex produced significant decreases in prolactin levels in subjects. The liquid vitex preparation was found to produce changes more quickly than the tablet, and neither preparation produced changes in FSH, LH, or progesterone. Symptoms of headache, abdominal pains, psychological symptoms, and a tendency to edemas were decreased in the treatment groups compared with the placebo group, and the number of pain-free days increased by 15% in the treatment groups compared with 8% in the placebo group. Estradiol levels were found to increase in the treatment groups (25.7 pg/mL for the tablet and 28.5 pg/mL for the liquid) compared with the placebo group (10.8 ng/mL). In addition to this study, small studies have reported good results for the use of vitex in mastalgia treatment (Kubista et al., 1983; Wuttke et al., 1997).

SAFETY/DOSAGE

Most studies of vitex have used brand names such as Agnolyt (liquids or capsules), Strotan, or Mastodyne. Dosage recommendations for the various preparations are as follows (McKenna et al., 2001):

- Agnolyt liquid (58% alcohol, 100 g of solution containing 9 g of 1:5 berry tincture): 40 drops/day after meals for several months.
- Agnolyt capsule (175 mg of dried berries, 1:5 alcoholic extract): one capsule daily with liquid for several months.
- Standardized powdered extract (175 mg of a 20:1 fruit extract, standardized to 0.5% agnusides): one capsule daily. This is a common preparation in the United States and is similar to the Agnolyt capsule formulation.
- Strotan capsule (20 mg of alcoholic extract containing 50–70% alcohol per volume): one capsule daily.
- Mastodyne (ethanol-water extract containing 55.4% ethanol by volume): 60 drops/day.

Serious side effects have not been cited for vitex, but skin rashes and itching have been reported. Although no contraindications are noted in the German Commission E monographs (Blumenthal et al., 1998), others have stated concern with using vitex along with oral contraceptives. Due to the discovery of vitex's dopamine agonist activityx, concern may be justified for those taking vitex who are also on dopamine antagonists (McKenna et al., 2001).

A review of the literature cites various opinions on the use of vitex with pregnancy (especially in the initial phase), but overall it is usually contraindicated. Possible reports of negative reactions to vitex in women undergoing in vitro fertilization have been cited. Vitex used during lactation has likewise been controversial (McKenna et al., 2001).

REFERENCES

Agnolyt. The Natural Way for Hormone Imbalance [Package insert and research summary]. Cologne, Germany: Madaus GmbH, 1994.

Attelman H, Bends K, Hellenkemper H, et al. Agnolyt® in the treatment of gynecological complaints. Zeitschrift für Praklinishche Geriatrie 1972;2:239.

Berger D, Schaffner W, Schrader E, Meier B, Brattstrom A. Efficacy of Vitex agnus castus L. extract Ze 440 in patients with pre-menstrual syndrome (PMS). Arch Gynecol Obstet 2000;264(3):150–153.

Blumenthal M, Busse WR, Goldberg A, Gruenwald J, Hall T, Riggins CW, Rister RS, eds. The Complete German Commission E Monographs. Austin, TX: American Botanical Council, 1998.

Böhnert KJ. Clinical study on chaste tree for menstrual disorders. Quart Rev Nat Med 1997;19–21.

Bubenzer RH. Therapy with Agnus Castus extract (strotan). Therapiewake 1993;43:32–33, 1705–1706.

Christie S, Walker, AF. Vitex agnus-castus L.: (1) a review of its traditional and modern therapeutic use; (2) current use from a survey of practitioners. Eur J Herb Med 1997–1998;3:29–45.

Dittmar FW, Bohnert KJ, Peeters M, et al. Premenstrual syndrome treatment with a phytopharmaceutical. Therapiewoche Gynäkologie 1992;5:60–68.

Eagon CL, Elm MS, Teepe AG, Eagon PK. Medicinal botanicals: estrogenicity in rat uterus and liver. Proceedings of the American Association for Cancer Research 1997;38:293.

Feldman HU, Albrechet M, Lamertz M, et al. The treatment of corpus luteum insufficiency and premenstrual syndrome. Experience in a multicenter study under clinical practice conditions. Gyne 1990;12:422–425.

Halaska M, Raus K, Beles P, Martan A, Paithner KG. Treatment of cyclical mastodynia using an extract of Vitex agnus castus: results of a double-blind comparison with a placebo. Ceska Gynekol 1998;63(5):388–392.

Krustrak D, Kuftinec J, Blazevic D. The composition of the essential oil of Vitex agnus-castus. Planta Medica 1992;58(suppl. 1):A681.

Kubista E, Muller G, Spona J. Conservative therapy of mastopathy. Zentralbl Gynakol 1983;105(18):1153–1162.

Lauritzen CH, Reuter HD, Repges R, Bohnert KJ, Schmidt U. Treatment of premenstrual tension syndrome with Vitex agnus-castus. Controlled, double-blind study versus pyridoxine. Phytomedicine 1997; 4: 183–189.

Loch EG, Bohnert KJ, Peeters M, et al. The treatment of menstrual disorders with Vitex agnus-castus tincture. Der Fraunarzt 1991; 32:867–870.

Loch EG, Selle H, Boblitz N. Treatment of premenstrual syndrome with a phytopharmaceutical formulation containing Vitex agnus castus. J Womens Health Gend Based Med 2000;9(3):315–320.

McKenna D, Jones K, Hughes K, eds. Botanical Medicines: The Desk Reference for Major Herbal Supplements. New York: Haworth Press, 2001.

Merz PG, Gorkow C, Schrodter A, Rietbrock S, Sieder C, Loew D, Dericks-Tan JS, Taubert HD. The effects of a special Agnus castus extract (BP1095E1) on prolactin secretion in healthy male subjects. Exp Clin Endocrinol Diabetes 1996;104(6):447–453.

Milewicz A, Gejdel E, Sworen H, Sienkiewicz K, Jedrzejak J, Teucher T, Schmitz H. Vitex agnus castus extract in the treatment of luteal phase defects due to latent hyperprolactinemia. Results of a randomized placebo-controlled double-blind study. Arzneimittelforschung 1993;43(7):752–756.

Pepeljnjak S, Antolic A. Kustrak D. Antibacterial and antifungal activities of the Vitex agnus-castus L. extracts. Acta Pharmaceutica (Zagreb) 1996;46:201–206.

Propping D, Bohnert KJ, Peeters M, et al. Vitex agnus-castus treatment of gynecological syndromes. Therapeutikon 1991;5:581–585.

Propping D, Katzorke T. Treatment of corpus luteum insufficiency. Zeitschrift für Allgemeinmedizin 1987;63:932–933.

Reuter HD, Bohnert KJ, Schmidt U. The therapy of the premenstrual syndrome with Vitex agnus castus: controlled double-blind study with pyridoxine [Abstract]. Zeitschrift für Phytotherapie 1995;7:7.

Roeder DA. Therapy of cyclic disorders with Vitex agnus-castus. Zeitschrift für Phytotherapie 1994;15:155–159.

Snow JM. Vitex agnus-castus L. (Verbenaceae). Protocol Journal of Botanical Medicine 1996;20–23.

Turner S, Mills S. A double-blind clinical trial on a herbal remedy for premenstrual syndrome: a case study. Complementary Therapies in Medicine 1993;1:73–77.

Wuttke, W. Zellbiologische untersuchungen mimt Agnolyt® –praparationen (NH 246, NH 247). Personlich Keit Mittleilung 1992;8.7.

Wuttke W, Gorkow C, Jarry H. Dopaminergic compounds in Vitex agnus-castus. In: Loew D, Rietbrock N, eds. Phytopharmaka un Forschung und Klinischer Anwendung Darmstatd, Germany: Steinkopff Verlag, 1995:81–91.

Wuttke W, Splitt G, Gorkow C, et al. Treatment of cyclical mastalgia with Agnus castus: results of a randomized, placebo-controlled, double-blind study. Geburtshilfe und Frauenheilkunde 1997;57:569–574.

12

Supplements for Diabetes and Blood Sugar Control

α-Lipoic Acid
Banaba (*Lagerstroemia speciosa*)
Chromium

Fenugreek (*Trigonella foenum-graecum*)
Gymnema (*Gymnema sylvestre*)
Vanadium

α-LIPOIC ACID

Overall Rank

★★★★ as an antioxidant
★★★★ for blood sugar control
★★ for antiaging benefits

OVERVIEW

α-Lipoic acid is a sulfur-containing fatty acid compound found in the mitochondria—the energy-producing structures found in our cells. As a dietary supplement, α-lipoic acid (also known as lipoic acid and thioctic acid) may act as a powerful antioxidant, possibly working in synergy with other nutritional antioxidants like vitamins C and E to help prevent cellular damage from free radicals. α-Lipoic acid has also been shown to help control blood sugar levels in patients with diabetes.

Although α-lipoic acid is involved in cellular energy production, its chief role as a dietary supplement may be as a powerful antioxidant. The body appears to be able to manufacture enough α-lipoic acid for its metabolic functions (as a cofactor for a number of enzymes involved in converting fat and sugar to energy), but the excess levels provided by supplements allow α-lipoic acid to circulate in a "free" state (outside the cells in which it is usually found). In this state, α-lipoic acid functions as a water- and fat-soluble antioxidant. The ability of α-lipoic acid to be active in both the water compartments and the lipid compartments of the body is important because most antioxidants, such as vitamins C and E, are effective in only one area. For instance, vitamin C is usually restricted to the interior compartment of cells and the aqueous (watery) portion of blood, while vitamin E embeds itself in the lipid (fatty) portion of cell membranes. Adding to the potential importance of α-lipoic acid is its role in the production of glutathione, one of the chief cellular antioxidants produced directly by the body.

COMMENTS

If α-lipoic acid were just another antioxidant, its value would be far less. After all, dozens of ingredients on the market have powerful antioxidant functions. The unique qualities of α-lipoic acid, functioning as both a water- and fat-soluble antioxidant as well as helping to increase the overall function of other dietary antioxidants, make it an intriguing supplement worthy of serious consideration. It may be especially useful for people with diabetes because of its potential benefits in preventing some forms of diabetic peripheral and autonomic neuropathy.

SCIENTIFIC SUPPORT

In animal studies and human trials, α-lipoic acid supplementation has been shown to improve several indices of metabolic activity and lower the degree of oxidative stress (Androne et al., 2000; Arivazhagan and Panneerselvam, 2000). α-Lipoic acid supplementation may also help to reverse the decline in mitochondrial energy production that is commonly observed during the "normal" aging process (Ames, 2003). Physical activity levels in animals can be increased by approximately threefold when supplemented with α-lipoic acid (Hagen et al., 1999), suggesting a beneficial effect on energy metabolism (Khanna et al., 1998). Levels of other antioxidants, such as glutathione and ascorbic acid, were also elevated in animals consuming α-lipoic acid, suggesting that the supplement may help protect and/or recycle these antioxidants and contribute to the overall capacity of the body to neutralize free-radical damage (Packer et al., 1995, 1997).

In conjunction with other antioxidants, such as vitamin E, α-lipoic acid may be particularly helpful in patients with diabetes. By promoting the production of energy from fat and sugar in the mitochondria, α-lipoic acid may enhance glucose removal from the bloodstream and improve insulin function. Indeed, α-lipoic acid has been shown to decrease insulin resistance and is prescribed frequently in Europe as a treatment for peripheral neuropathy (nerve damage) associated with diabetes. In the United States, the American Diabetes Association has suggested that α-lipoic acid plus vitamin E may be helpful in combating some of the health complications associated with diabetes, including heart disease, vision problems, nerve damage, and kidney disease. α-Lipoic acid has also been implicated in helping to protect the brain from damage following a stroke.

A consistent body of evidence shows that intravenous infusions of α-lipoic acid are associated with a reduction in sensory symptoms of diabetic neuropathy (Ametov et al., 2003; Ziegler et al., 2004) and that patients receiving α-lipoic acid supplements experience benefits within 8–14 days of treatment on measures of pain, burning, and numbness. In human feeding studies (as opposed to studies of intravenous infusions of α-lipoic acid, in which most of the positive results are for diabetic neuropathy), a handful of studies demonstrate that dietary supplementation with α-lipoic acid is able to help prevent hyperglycemia (Konrad et al., 1999) and improve energetic substrates in muscle cells (Burke et al., 2003).

SAFETY/DOSAGE

Despite relatively few feeding studies conducted with α-lipoic acid in humans, it appears to be safe as a dietary supplement. Intakes of as much as 600 mg/day have been used for treatment of diabetic neuropathy, with no serious side effects. For general antioxidant benefits, typical recommendations are for 50–100 mg/day, with higher levels of 300–600 mg/day for preventing and treating complications of diabetes.

REFERENCES

Ames BN. The metabolic tune-up: metabolic harmony and disease prevention. J Nutr 2003;133(5 suppl 1):1544S–1548S.

Ametov AS, Barinov A, Dyck PJ, Hermann R, Kozlova N, Litchy WJ, Low PA, Nehrdich D, Novosadova M, O'Brien PC, Reljanovic M, Samigullin R, Schuette K, Strokov I, Tritschler HJ, Wessel K, Yakhno N, Ziegler D; SYDNEY Trial Study Group. The sensory symptoms of diabetic polyneuropathy are improved with alpha-lipoic acid: the SYDNEY trial. Diabetes Care 2003;26(3):770–776.

Androne L, Gavan NA, Veresiu IA, Orasan R. In vivo effect of lipoic acid on lipid peroxidation in patients with diabetic neuropathy. In Vivo 2000;14(2):327–330.

Arivazhagan P, Panneerselvam C. Effect of DL - alpha -lipoic acid on neural antioxidants in aged rats. Pharmacol Res 2000;42(3):219–222.

Burke DG, Chilibeck PD, Parise G, Tarnopolsky MA, Candow DG. Effect of alpha-lipoic acid combined with creatine monohydrate on human skeletal muscle creatine and phosphagen concentration. Int J Sport Nutr Exerc Metab 2003;13(3):294–302.

Hagen TM, Ingersoll RT, Lykkesfeldt J, Liu J, Wehr CM, Vinarsky V, Bartholomew JC, Ames AB. (R)-alpha-lipoic acid-supplemented old rats have improved mitochondrial function, decreased oxidative damage, and increased metabolic rate. FASEB J 1999;13(2):411–418.

Khanna S, Atalay M, Lodge JK, Laaksonen DE, Roy S, Hanninen O, Packer L, Sen CK. Skeletal muscle and liver lipoyllysine content in response to exercise, training and dietary alpha-lipoic acid supplementation. Biochem Mol Biol Int 1998;46(2):297–306.

Konrad T, Vicini P, Kusterer K, Hoflich A, Assadkhani A, Bohles HJ, Sewell A, Tritschler HJ, Cobelli C, Usadel KH. alpha-Lipoic acid treatment decreases serum lactate and pyruvate concentrations and improves glucose effectiveness in lean and obese patients with type 2 diabetes. Diabetes Care 1999;22(2):280–287.

Packer L, Tritschler HJ, Wessel K. Neuroprotection by the metabolic antioxidant alpha-lipoic acid. Free Radic Biol Med 1997;22(1–2):359–378.

Packer L, Witt EH, Tritschler HJ. alpha-Lipoic acid as a biological antioxidant. Free Radic Biol Med 1995;19(2):227–250.

Ziegler D, Nowak H, Kempler P, Vargha P, Low PA. Treatment of symptomatic diabetic polyneuropathy with the antioxidant alpha-lipoic acid: a meta-analysis. Diabet Med 2004;21(2):114–121.

ADDITIONAL RESOURCES

Gualandri W, Gualandri L, Demartini G, Esposti R, Marthyn P, Volonte S, Stangoni L, Borgonovo M, Fraschini F. Redox balance in patients with Down's syndrome before and after dietary supplementation with alpha-lipoic acid and L-cysteine. Int J Clin Pharmacol Res 2003;23(1):23–30.

Haak E, Usadel KH, Kusterer K, Amini P, Frommeyer R, Tritschler HJ, Haak T. Effects of alpha-lipoic acid on microcirculation in patients with peripheral diabetic neuropathy. Exp Clin Endocrinol Diabetes 2000;108(3):168–174.

Jacob S, Ruus P, Hermann R, Tritschler HJ, Maerker E, Renn W, Augustin HJ, Dietze GJ, Rett K. Oral administration of RAC-alpha-lipoic acid modulates insulin sensitivity in patients with type-2 diabetes mellitus: a placebo-controlled pilot trial. Free Radic Biol Med 1999;27(3–4):309–314.

Marriage B, Clandinin MT, Glerum DM. Nutritional cofactor treatment in mitochondrial disorders. J Am Diet Assoc 2003;103(8):1029–1038.

Miquel J. Can antioxidant diet supplementation protect against age-related mitochondrial damage? Ann N Y Acad Sci 2002;959:508–516.

Morcos M, Borcea V, Isermann B, Gehrke S, Ehret T, Henkels M, Schiekofer S, Hofmann M, Amiral J, Tritschler H, Ziegler R, Wahl P, Nawroth PP. Effect of alpha-lipoic acid on the progression of endothelial cell damage and albuminuria in patients with diabetes mellitus: an exploratory study. Diabetes Res Clin Pract 2001;52(3):175–183.

Nickander KK, McPhee BR, Low PA, Tritschler H. Alpha-lipoic acid: antioxidant potency against lipid peroxidation of neural tissues in vitro and implications for diabetic neuropathy. Free Radic Biol Med 1996;21(5):631–639.

Podda M, Tritschler HJ, Ulrich H, Packer L. Alpha-lipoic acid supplementation prevents symptoms of vitamin E deficiency. Biochem Biophys Res Commun 1994;204(1):98–104.

Roy S, Sen CK, Tritschler HJ, Packer L. Modulation of cellular reducing equivalent homeostasis by alpha-lipoic acid. Mechanisms and implications for diabetes and ischemic injury. Biochem Pharmacol 1997;53(3):393–399.

Ruhe RC, McDonald RB. Use of antioxidant nutrients in the prevention and treatment of type 2 diabetes. J Am Coll Nutr 2001;20(5 suppl):363S–369S.

Ziegler D, Gries FA. Alpha-lipoic acid in the treatment of diabetic peripheral and cardiac autonomic neuropathy. Diabetes 1997;46(suppl 2):S62–S66.

Ziegler D, Hanefeld M, Ruhnau KJ, Hasche H, Lobisch M, Schutte K, Kerum G, Malessa R. Treatment of symptomatic diabetic polyneuropathy with the antioxidant alpha-lipoic acid: a 7-month multicenter randomized controlled trial (ALADIN III Study). ALADIN III Study Group. Alpha-Lipoic Acid in Diabetic Neuropathy. Diabetes Care 1999;22(8):1296–1301.

Ziegler D, Hanefeld M, Ruhnau KJ, Meissner HP, Lobisch M, Schutte K, Gries FA. Treatment of symptomatic diabetic peripheral neuropathy with the anti-oxidant alpha-lipoic acid. A 3-week multicentre randomized controlled trial (ALADIN Study). Diabetologia 1995;38(12):1425–1433.

Ziegler D, Reljanovic M, Mehnert H, Gries FA. Alpha-lipoic acid in the treatment of diabetic polyneuropathy in Germany: current evidence from clinical trials. Exp Clin Endocrinol Diabetes 1999;107(7):421–430.

BANABA (*LAGERSTROEMIA SPECIOSA*)

Overall Rank

★★★ for lowering blood sugar and controlling diabetes
★★ for controlling cravings for foods (especially carbohydrates)

OVERVIEW

As a traditional medicine from India, Southeast Asia, and the Philippines, banaba (*Lagerstroemia speciosa*) has been used for lowering blood sugar and controlling diabetes. The main active component in banaba has been thought to be corosolic acid, and typical formulations on the market are standardized to 1% corosolic acid. Some research has found another compound called lagerstroemin, an ellagitannin, which can cause insulin-like activity (Hattori et al., 2003; Hayashi et al., 2002). In animal studies and unpublished studies in humans, banaba has been found not only to regulate blood sugar but also to have the "side effect" of weight loss without dietary alterations (Suzuki et al., 1999). One hypothesis for moderate weight loss is lower fluctuations in blood sugar and thus fewer food cravings (for carbohydrates).

COMMENTS

Although published clinical studies are still lacking for banaba, the animal studies have shown good promise for using this herbal medicine to lower blood sugar levels in hyperglycemic states and diabetes (Kakuda et al., 1996; Liu et al., 2001; Murakami et al., 1993).

SCIENTIFIC SUPPORT

Banaba was studied in a randomized clinical trial for its effect on blood glucose levels in patients with type 2 diabetes. A standardized extract of banaba (Glucosol; *Lagerstroemia speciosa* standardized to 1% corosolic acid) was administered for 2 weeks in two different preparations: a softgel and a dry-powder hard gelatin capsule. Significant reductions in blood glucose levels were found at daily dosages of 32 mg and 48 mg from banaba administration, and the softgel preparation showed a larger (30% versus 20%) decrease in blood glucose, indicating a higher bioavailability in the softgel preparation (Judy et al., 2003).

SAFETY/DOSAGE

At the recommended dosages of 8–48 mg/day, no side effects have been found for banaba. At higher dosages, however, symptoms associated with low blood sugar (headache, dizziness, fatigue) may be expected.

REFERENCES

Hattori K, Sukenobu N, Sasaki T, Takasuga S, Hayashi T, Kasai R, Yamasaki K, Hazeki O. Activation of insulin receptors by lagerstroemin. J Pharmacol Sci 2003;93(1):69–73.

Hayashi T, Maruyama H, Kasai R, Hattori K, Takasuga S, Hazeki O, Yamasaki K, Tanaka T. Ellagitannins from Lagerstroemia speciosa as activators of glucose transport in fat cells. Planta Med 2002;68(2):173–175.

Judy WV, Hari SP, Stogsdill WW, Judy JS, Naguib YM, Passwater R. Antidiabetic activity of a standardized extract (Glucosol) from Lagerstroemia speciosa leaves in Type II diabetics. A dose-dependence study. J Ethnopharmacol 2003;87(1):115–117.

Kakuda T, Sakane I, Takihara T, Ozaki Y, Takeuchi H, Kuroyanagi M. Hypoglycemic effect of extracts from Lagerstroemia speciosa leaves in genetically diabetic KK-AY mice. Biosci Biotechnol Biochem 1996;60(2):204–208.

Liu F, Kim J, Li Y, Liu X, Li J, Chen X. An extract of Lagerstroemia speciosa L. has insulin-like glucose uptake-stimulatory and adipocyte differentiation-inhibitory activities in 3T3-L1 cells. J Nutr 2001;131(9):2242–2247.

Murakami C, Myoga K, Kasai R, Ohtani K, Kurokawa T, Ishibashi S, Dayrit F, Padolina WG, Yamasaki K. Screening of plant constituents for effect on glucose transport activity in Ehrlich ascites tumour cells. Chem Pharm Bull (Tokyo) 1993;41(12):2129–2131.

Suzuki Y, Unno T, Ushitani M, Hayashi K, Kakuda T. Antiobesity activity of extracts from Lagerstroemia speciosa L. leaves on female KK-Ay mice. J Nutr Sci Vitaminol (Tokyo) 1999;45(6):791–795.

CHROMIUM

Overall Rank

★★★★★   for correcting chromium deficiency
★★★★   for reducing blood sugar, improving activity of insulin
★★★   for reducing body fat and increasing lean muscle mass
★★   as an appetite suppressant
★★   for lowering cholesterol
★★   for enhancing exercise performance

OVERVIEW

Ninety percent of American diets are estimated to be deficient in chromium, and the general population is thought to show signs of marginal deficiencies, such as impaired glucose tolerance. Food sources of chromium include brewer's yeast, whole-grain cereals, broccoli, prunes, mushrooms, and beer. The typical American diet, however, is thought to exacerbate the problem of deficiency by the large-scale consumption of simple sugars in processed foods that may block chromium absorption. As part of a bioactive complex called glucose tolerance factor (GTF), brewer's yeast, also called nutritional yeast, is thought to be the most bioavailable form of chromium (Sterns et al., 1995).

Chromium is one of the essential trace minerals and is important for carbohydrate metabolism and the potentiation of insulin. Because the body absorbs only about 3% of the chromium consumed, supplementation is a viable option. Although many types of chromium supplements are on the market, concerns have arisen over the potential toxicity of chromium picolinate, one of the most studied supplemental forms of chromium. These concerns have not been validated. Chromium chloride, as well as some other forms of chromium (III) supplements, does not prompt this concern (Vincent, 2000, 2003).

COMMENTS

The evidence is still mounting for the use of chromium to normalize blood sugar and meet marginal deficiencies. Chromium's potential as a supplement seems great, however, because the American population is sorely in need of nutritional answers to its overweight and diabetic populations.

SCIENTIFIC SUPPORT

Athletic Performance
Chromium's clinical results so far for enhancing exercise performance have been limited. In a double-blind clinical study on the effects of chromium picolinate supplementation on football players, 200 µg/day was administered. The outcome measurements were urinary excretion, girth and skinfold measures, percentage of body fat, lean body mass, and isometric and dynamic strength. No changes in any of the parameters were found, except for an increase in urinary chromium output (Clancy et al., 1994).

In two earlier studies, 200 µg/day of chromium supplementation failed to show results. One study involved college students during weight training; the only group that showed a significant difference was the one composed of females, who had a significant increase in body weight (Hasten et al., 1992). In another double-blind, placebo-controlled study, no enhancement of athletic performance was found (Walker et al., 1998).

Weight Loss
Mixed results have been found clinically for chromium picolinate in weight loss. Pittler et al. (2003) performed a meta-analysis of chromium as it had been administered in randomized, double-blind, placebo controlled studies that reported on chromium picolinate's use in weight loss. Ten studies matched the criteria of the meta-analysis, and the

authors found a small benefit for the use of chromium picolinate in weight loss.

Volpe et al. (2001) tested the effects of chromium picolinate supplementation on body composition, resting metabolic rate, and zinc status in moderately obese women who underwent a prescribed exercise program. No changes in any of the measured outcomes were found except for a reduction in serum total cholesterol levels and total iron-building capacity in both groups resulting from the increase in exercise.

In a clinical study on the effects of chromium picolinate supplementation on the risk factors for coronary artery disease and type 2 diabetes in obese women, 400 µg/day was administered. In the groups that underwent exercise, chromium supplementation resulted in significant weight loss, whereas the groups that did not undergo exercise but used chromium had significant weight gain. The authors recommended chromium supplementation only for obese women who exercise regularly (Grant et al., 1997).

In an earlier double-blind, placebo-controlled study, chromium picolinate (400 µg/day) supplementation was administered and investigated for its effect on body composition in obese people undergoing an exercise program. The results of this study showed no difference between the placebo and chromium groups (Trent and Thieding-Cancel, 1995).

Blood Sugar Control and Controlling Diabetes

Ryan et al. (2003) performed a review of chromium supplements for diabetes type 2 and hyperlipidemia. It was found that chromium reduced blood glucose in hyperglycemia but not in people with normal blood glucose levels. Chromium was found to have variable effects on lipid levels. In another study, Keszthelyi et al. (2003) found that chromium supplementation used in diabetics for 6 months resulted in significant reductions in cholesterin levels, as well as a slight reduction in the HbA1c level.

Anderson et al. (2001) studied the effect of combined and individual zinc and chromium supplementation on oxidative stress and glucose homeostasis in people with type 2 diabetes. Diabetic subjects were supplemented with either 30 mg/day of zinc (as zinc gluconate), 400 µg/day of chromium (as chromium picolinate), a combination, or a placebo. The authors concluded that taking either the individual or combined supplementation of zinc or chromium led to potential beneficial antioxidant effects for patients with type 2 diabetes.

Bahijri (2000) found an improved lipid profile and glycemic control in a study on healthy adults given chromium tetrachloride daily. In this double-blind study, 200 µg or a placebo was given daily for 8 weeks. In a general study of urine and serum concentrations in diabetic and normal subjects, Ding et al. (1998) found that chromium loss is associated with aging and diabetes occurrence. Chromium supplementation on diabetic patients (with type 1 and type 2 diabetes) was investigated. Chromium supplementation (200 µg/day) produced beneficial results in reducing insulin sulfonylurea or metformin requirements. Greater results were found for type 2 diabetics, but type 1 diabetics also showed good results with supplementation (Ravina and Slezack, 1993).

SAFETY/DOSAGE

The recommended daily intake for chromium is 120 µg. Although numerous concerns have been raised about the toxicity of chromium picolinate, several recent studies have confirmed its safety (Campbell et al., 2004; Rhodes et al., 2005).

REFERENCES

Anderson RA, Roussel AM, Zouari N, Mahjoub S, Matheau JM, Kerkeni A. Potential antioxidant effects of zinc and chromium supplementation in people with type 2 diabetes mellitus. J Am Coll Nutr 2001;20(3):212–218.

Bahijri SM. Effect of chromium supplementation on glucose tolerance and lipid profile. Saudi Med J 2000;21(1):45–50.

Campbell WW, Joseph LJ, Ostlund RE Jr, Anderson RA, Farrell PA, Evans WJ. Resistive training and chromium picolinate: effects on inositols and liver and kidney functions in older adults. Int J Sport Nutr Exerc Metab 2004;14(4):430–442.

Clancy SP, Clarkson PM, DeCheke ME, Nosaka K, Freedson PS, Cunningham JJ, Valentine B. Effects of chromium picolinate supplementation on body composition, strength, and urinary chromium loss in football players. Int J Sport Nutr 1994;4(2):142–153.

Ding W, Chai Z, Duan P, Feng W, Qian Q. Serum and urine chromium concentrations in elderly diabetics. Biol Trace Elem Res 1998;63(3):231–237.

Grant KE, Chandler RM, Castle AL, Ivy JL. Chromium and exercise training: effect on obese women. Med Sci Sports Exerc 1997;29(8):992–998.

Hasten DL, Rome EP, Franks BD, Hegsted M. Effects of chromium picolinate on beginning weight training students. Int J Sport Nutr 1992;2(4):343–350.

Keszthelyi Z, Past T, Koltai K, Szabo L, Mozsik G. Chromium (III)-ion enhances the utilization of glucose in type-2 diabetes mellitus. Orv Hetil 2003;144(42):2073–2076.

Pittler MH, Stevinson C, Ernst E. Chromium picolinate for reducing body weight: meta-analysis of randomized trials. Int J Obes Relat Metab Disord 2003;27(4):522–529.

Ravina A, Slezack L. Chromium in the treatment of clinical diabetes mellitus. Harefuah 1993;125(5–6):142–145, 191.

Rhodes MC, Hebert CD, Herbert RA, Morinello EJ, Roycroft JH, Travlos GS, Abdo KM. Absence of toxic effects in F344/N rats and B6C3F1 mice following subchronic administration of chromium picolinate monohydrate. Food Chem Toxicol 2005;43(1):21–29.

Ryan GJ, Wanko NS, Redman AR, Cook CB. Chromium as adjunctive treatment for type 2 diabetes. Ann Pharmacother 2003;37(6):876–885.

Stearns DM, Belbruno JJ, Wetterhahn KE. A prediction of chromium(III) accumulation in humans from chromium dietary supplements. FASEB J 1995;9(15):1650–1657.

Trent LK, Thieding-Cancel D. Effects of chromium picolinate on body composition. J Sports Med Phys Fitness 1995;35(4):273–280.

Vincent JB. The potential value and toxicity of chromium picolinate as a nutritional supplement, weight loss agent and muscle development agent. Sports Med 2003;33(3):213–230.

Vincent JB. The biochemistry of chromium. J Nutr 2000;130(4):715-8.

Volpe SL, Huang HW, Larpadisorn K, Lesser II. Effect of chromium supplementation and exercise on body composition, resting metabolic rate and selected biochemical parameters in moderately obese women following an exercise program. J Am Coll Nutr 2001;20(4):293–306.

Walker LS, Bemben MG, Bemben DA, Knehans AW. Chromium picolinate effects on body composition and muscular performance in wrestlers. Med Sci Sports Exerc 1998;30(12):1730–1737.

FENUGREEK (*TRIGONELLA FOENUM-GRAECUM*)

Overall Rank

★★★★ for controlling blood sugar
★★★   for supporting cardiovascular health
★★   for suppressing appetite and promoting weight loss
★★   for inducing lactation

OVERVIEW

Fenugreek is a popular spice in Indian cuisine and has long been used in both ayurvedic and Chinese traditional medicine to induce labor and lactation, to aid in digestion, and as a general health and wellness tonic (Basch et al., 2003; Gabay, 2002). Both animal and human clinical studies are finding that fenugreek shows promising therapeutic activity as a hypoglycemic and hypocholesterolemic agent. Fenugreek's unique dietary fibers, high saponin content, and the possible presence of an amino acid (4-hydroxy-isoleucine) are thought to be responsible for its activities (Madar and Stark, 2002; Sauvaire et al., 1998).

COMMENTS

A study by Vajifdar et al. (2000) included fenugreek fiber in a dietary fiber mixture that had favorable results in lowering low-density lipoprotein (LDL) cholesterol, apolipoprotein A-1, body mass index, and waist circumference. As the mechanisms of action of dietary fiber are assumed to be similar, this study shows promise for the use of fenugreek fiber in treating ischemic heart disease. Likewise, another clinical study found fenugreek beneficial in the diabetic diet when combined with millet, legumes, and other herbs in (Bhardwaj et al., 1994; Pathak et al., 2000).

SCIENTIFIC SUPPORT

Type 1 and Type 2 Diabetes

Madar et al. (1988) tested the dietary effect of fenugreek in patients with type 2 diabetes (noninsulin dependent) following the meal tolerance test (MTT). Powdered fenugreek (15 g) was added to patients' diets and found to significantly reduce the postprandial glucose levels and to insignificantly lower the plasma insulin levels. There was no effect on the blood lipid levels 3 hours after the MTT.

Gupta et al. (2001) performed a double-blind, randomized, placebo-controlled study to determine the effect of fenugreek on glycemic control and insulin resistance in patients with type 2 diabetes. The participants were given either fenugreek extract (hydroalcoholic, 1 g/day) or a placebo for 2 months. The treatment group showed reduced serum triglycerides, greater insulin control, and a decrease in insulin resistance.

Sharma et al. (1990) tested the effect of fenugreek seeds on the blood glucose levels and serum lipid profiles of patients with type 1 diabetes in a placebo-controlled clinical study. Fenugreek seed was administered in the treatment group diet (100 g/day), and isocaloric diets without fenugreek served as the control; both diets were followed for 10 days. A 54% reduction in 24-hour urinary glucose excretion, along with significantly reduced serum total cholesterol, LDL and very low density lipoprotein (VLDL) cholesterol, and triglycerides were found in the treatment group. The high-density lipoprotein (HDL) levels remained unchanged in both groups. The authors concluded that fenugreek appears useful in the diets of diabetics.

Hypocholesterolemic Effect

Sowmya and Rajyalakshmi (1999) tested the effect of dietary germinated fenugreek seed powder on blood lipid levels in hypocholesterolemic adults. Twenty participants were divided into two groups and asked to add the fenugreek powder to their meals for one month, the groups differed in the amount of fenugreek in the packet: either 12.5 g or 18 g daily. Both treatment levels resulted in a hypocholesterolemic effect, but the 18 g dosage resulted in significant reductions in total and LDL cholesterol levels. There were no changes found between the groups in HDL, VLDL and triglyceride levels. The authors claimed that the germination of the seeds was able to increase the solubility of the fiber content of fenugreek.

SAFETY/DOSAGE

Fenugreek seed powder has been found to be beneficial in the typical dosages of 15–20 g/day or more for reducing serum cholesterol levels and improving blood sugar control in diabetics. Fenugreek is considered quite safe, even at the higher doses needed for therapeutic use (Muralidhara et al., 1999). As is the case with other botanicals with high coumarin contents, a potential adverse reaction is increased bleeding, and interaction with other blood-thinning drugs is also a concern (Abebe, 2002).

REFERENCES

Abebe W. Herbal medication: potential for adverse interactions with analgesic drugs. J Clin Pharm Ther 2002;27(6):391–401.

Basch E, Ulbricht C, Kuo G, Szapary P, Smith M. Therapeutic applications of fenugreek. Altern Med Rev 2003;8(1):20–27.

Bhardwaj PK, Dasgupta DJ, Prashar BS, Kaushal SS. Control of hyperglycaemia and hyperlipidaemia by plant product. J Assoc Physicians India 1994;42(1):33–35.

Gabay MP. Galactogogues: medications that induce lactation. J Hum Lact 2002;18(3):274–279.

Gupta A, Gupta R, Lal B. Effect of Trigonella foenum-graecum (fenugreek) seeds on glycaemic control and insulin resistance in type 2 diabetes mellitus: a double blind placebo controlled study. J Assoc Physicians India 2001;49:1057–1061.

Madar Z, Abel R, Samish S, Arad J. Glucose-lowering effect of fenugreek in non-insulin dependent diabetics. Eur J Clin Nutr 1988;42(1):51–54.

Madar Z, Stark AH. New legume sources as therapeutic agents. Br J Nutr 2002;88(suppl 3):S287–S292.

Muralidhara, Narasimhamurthy K, Viswanatha S, Ramesh BS. Acute and subchronic toxicity assessment of debitterized fenugreek powder in the mouse and rat. Food Chem Toxicol 1999;37(8):831–838.

Pathak P, Srivastava S, Grover S. Development of food products based on millets, legumes and fenugreek seeds and their suitability in the diabetic diet. Int J Food Sci Nutr 2000;51(5):409–414.

Sauvaire Y, Petit P, Broca C, Manteghetti M, Baissac Y, Fernandez-Alvarez J, Gross R, Roye M, Leconte A, Gomis R, Ribes G. 4-Hydroxyisoleucine: a novel amino acid potentiator of insulin secretion. Diabetes 1998;47(2):206–210.

Sharma RD, Raghuram TC, Rao NS. Effect of fenugreek seeds on blood glucose and serum lipids in type I diabetes. Eur J Clin Nutr 1990;44(4):301–306.

Sowmya P, Rajyalakshmi P. Hypocholesterolemic effect of germinated fenugreek seeds in human subjects. Plant Foods Hum Nutr 1999;53(4):359–365.

Vajifdar BU, Goyal VS, Lokhandwala YY, Mhamunkar SR, Mahadik SP, Gawad AK, Halankar SA, Kulkarni HL. Is dietary fiber beneficial in chronic ischemic heart disease? J Assoc Physicians India 2000;48(9):871–876.

ADDITIONAL RESOURCES

Hibasami H, Moteki H, Ishikawa K, Katsuzaki H, Imai K, Yoshioka K, Ishii Y, Komiya T. Protodioscin isolated from fenugreek (Trigonella foenumgraecum L.) induces cell death and morphological change indicative of apoptosis in leukemic cell line H-60, but not in gastric cancer cell line KATO III. Int J Mol Med 2003;11(1):23–26.

GYMNEMA (*GYMNEMA SYLVESTRE*)

Overall Rank

★★★★ for blood sugar control
★★ for appetite control and weight loss

OVERVIEW

Gymnema sylvestre is a plant used medicinally in India and Southeast Asia for treatment of "sweet urine," which in the West is referred to as diabetes or hyperglycemia. In ancient Indian texts on ayurvedic medicine, gymnema is referred to as gurmar, which means "sugar destroyer" in Sanskrit. Gymnema leaves, whether extracted or infused into a tea, suppress glucose absorption and reduce the sensation of sweetness in foods—effects that may deliver important health benefits for individuals who want to reduce blood sugar levels or body weight. Modern dietary supplements containing gymnema are typically intended for control of blood sugar and insulin levels, reduction of sugar cravings, and weight loss, particularly in patients with diabetes.

COMMENTS

As a dietary supplement to enhance control of blood glucose and insulin, *Gymnema sylvestre* appears to be effective, particularly for patients with diabetes or hyperglycemia (elevated blood sugar). As an agent to promote weight loss, gymnema may help control appetite and carbohydrate cravings.

SCIENTIFIC SUPPORT

Gymnema sylvestre leaves contain gymnemic acids, which are known to suppress transport of glucose from the intestine into the blood stream, and the small protein called gurmar, which interacts with receptors on the tongue to decrease the sensation of sweetness of many foods (Miyasaka and Imoto, 1995). This dual action has been shown to reduce blood sugar and cholesterol levels in diabetic animals and humans and may provide some benefits in terms of regulating appetite control and food cravings (Suttisri et al., 1995).

The hypoglycemic effect of gymnema has been known for centuries. Modern scientific methods have isolated at least nine different fractions of gymnemic acids that possess hypoglycemic activity (Chattopadhyay, 1998; Fushiki et al., 1992). The effect of gymnema extract on lowering blood levels of glucose, cholesterol, and triglycerides is fairly gradual, typically taking a few days to several weeks. Very high doses of the dried gymnema leaves may even help to repair the cellular damage that causes diabetes by helping to regenerate the insulin-producing β cells in the pancreas (Shanmugasundaram et al., 1990).

Several human studies conducted on gymnema for treatment of diabetes have shown significant reduction in blood glucose, glycosylated hemoglobin (an index of blood sugar control) and insulin requirements (Baskaran et al., 1990; Khare et al., 1983). Gymnema appears to increase the effectiveness of insulin rather than causing the body to produce more (Shanmugasundaram et al., 1981), although the precise mechanism by which this occurs remains unknown. As with other natural ingredients for control of blood sugar and insulin levels, such as banaba leaf, a common "side effect" is weight loss (Khare et al., 1983), probably owing to a combination of appetite suppression and control of food cravings (especially for carbohydrates and sweets).

SAFETY/DOSAGE

At typical recommended doses (see next paragraph), dietary supplements containing gymnema are not associated with significant adverse side effects. Mild gastrointestinal upset may occur if gymnema is taken on an empty stomach, so consumption with meals is recommended. Caution is urged, however, because of the potential to induce hypoglycemia in susceptible people. Patients with active diabetes should consult their personal physicians before and while using gymnema because alterations to dosages of insulin or other antidiabetic medications may be warranted. Certain medications, including antidepressants (St. John's wort) and salicylates (white willow and aspirin) can enhance the blood sugar-lowering effects of gymnema, whereas certain stimulants such as ephedra (ma huang) may reduce its effectiveness.

Most human studies have been conducted in diabetic patients and have used 400–600 mg/day of gymnema extract in conjunction with conventional oral antidiabetic medications to lower blood glucose and reduce insulin requirements. In patients who do not have diabetes, smaller doses may be effective in helping to control blood sugar and insulin fluctuations—and the associated swings in appetite and food cravings. Because it acts gradually, gymnema extract should be consumed regularly with meals for several days or weeks.

REFERENCES

Baskaran K, Kizar Ahamath B, Radha Shanmugasundaram K, Shanmugasundaram ER. Antidiabetic effect of a leaf extract from Gymnema sylvestre in non-insulin-dependent diabetes mellitus patients. J Ethnopharmacol 1990;30(3):295–300.

Chattopadhyay RR. Possible mechanism of antihyperglycemic effect of Gymnema sylvestre leaf extract. Gen Pharmacol 1998;31(3):495–496.

Fushiki T, Kojima A, Imoto T, Inoue K, Sugimoto E. An extract of Gymnema sylvestre leaves and purified gymnemic acid inhibits glucose-stimulated gastric inhibitory peptide secretion in rats. J Nutr 1992;122(12):2367–2373.

Khare AK, Tondon RN, Tewari JP. Hypoglycaemic activity of an indigenous drug (Gymnema sylvestre, 'gurmar') in normal and diabetic persons. Indian J Physiol Pharmacol 1983;27(3):257–258.

Miyasaka A, Imoto T. Electrophysiological characterization of the inhibitory effect of a novel peptide gurmarin on the sweet taste response in rats. Brain Res 1995;676(1):63–68.

Shanmugasundaram ER, Gopinath KL, Radha Shanmugasundaram K, Rajendran VM. Possible regeneration of the islets of Langerhans in streptozotocin-diabetic rats given Gymnema sylvestre leaf extracts. J Ethnopharmacol 1990;30(3):265–279.

Shanmugasundaram KR, Panneerselvam C, Samudram P, Shanmugasundaram ER. The insulinotropic activity of Gymnema sylvestre, R. Br. An Indian medical herb used in controlling diabetes mellitus. Pharmacol Res Commun 1981;13(5):475–486.

Suttisri R, Lee IS, Kinghorn AD. Plant-derived triterpenoid sweetness inhibitors. J Ethnopharmacol 1995;47(1):9–26.

ADDITIONAL RESOURCES

Murakami N, Murakami T, Kadoya M, Matsuda H, Yamahara J, Yoshikawa M. New hypoglycemic constituents in "gymnemic acid" from Gymnema sylvestre. Chem Pharm Bull (Tokyo) 1996;44(2):469–471.

Ota M, Shimizu Y, Tonosaki K, Ariyoshi Y. Role of hydrophobic amino acids in gurmarin, a sweetness-suppressing polypeptide. Biopolymers 1998;45(3):231–238.

Shanmugasundaram ER, Rajeswari G, Baskaran K, Rajesh Kumar BR, Radha Shanmugasundaram K, Kizar Ahmath B. Use of Gymnema sylvestre leaf extract in the control of blood glucose in insulin-dependent diabetes mellitus. J Ethnopharmacol 1990;30(3):281–294.

Shimizu K, Abe T, Nakajyo S, Urakawa N, Atsuchi M, Yamashita C. Inhibitory effects of glucose utilization by gymnema acids in the guinea-pig ileal longitudinal muscle. J Smooth Muscle Res 1996;32(5):219–228.

Shimizu K, Iino A, Nakajima J, Tanaka K, Nakajyo S, Urakawa N, Atsuchi M, Wada T, Yamashita C. Suppression of glucose absorption by some fractions extracted from Gymnema sylvestre leaves. J Vet Med Sci 1997;59(4):245–251.

Shimizu K, Ozeki M, Tanaka K, Itoh K, Nakajyo S, Urakawa N, Atsuchi M. Suppression of glucose absorption by extracts from the leaves of Gymnema inodorum. J Vet Med Sci 1997;59(9):753–757.

VANADIUM

Overall Rank

★★★ for controlling blood sugar
★ for reducing body fat and increasing lean muscle mass

OVERVIEW

Vanadium is an essential trace mineral that has only recently been identified as being truly essential in humans. A normal diet typically provides about 10–30 μg/ day of vanadium. This amount appears to be adequate for most healthy adults, although no recommended daily allowance has been established for vanadium. An upper-limit dosage of 1.8 mg/day has been established by the Food and Nutrition Board of the National Academy of Sciences.

Vanadium is thought to play a role in metabolism of carbohydrates and may have functions in cholesterol and blood lipid metabolism. Food sources of vanadium include seafood, mushrooms, some cereals, and soybeans. For people with diabetes, vanadium supplements may have a positive effect in regulating blood glucose levels. Supplements are usually in vanadyl or vanadate forms and are generally marketed with claims to mimic insulin action, reduce blood sugar levels, improve glycogen synthesis, and increase muscle size and vascularity.

COMMENTS

Vanadium is an essential trace mineral that is not contained in many multivitamin/mineral supplements. Although the average diet is thought to provide an adequate amount of vanadium, for people concerned with maintaining blood glucose levels—such as diabetics or people with hypoglycemia—a vanadium supplement may be beneficial. Some bodybuilding and diabetic dietary supplements contain vanadium at milligram levels, although dietary needs are likely to be only in microgram amounts (1,000 times lower). Prolonged consumption of high-dose vanadium supplements is not recommended and may cause serious kidney and liver toxicity.

SCIENTIFIC SUPPORT

Vanadium or its most common supplemental form, vanadyl sulfate, is thought to mimic the physiological effects of insulin by a mechanism that remains unclear (Cam et al., 2000). Through this insulin-like effect, vanadium is thought to promote glycogen synthesis, maintain blood glucose levels, and stimulate protein synthesis for muscle growth (Goldfine et al., 2000).

Vanadyl sulfate supplements have been shown to normalize blood glucose levels and reduce glycosylated hemoglobin levels (Boden et al., 1996) in patients with noninsulin-dependent diabetes mellitus (NIDDM). Also in NIDDM patients, vanadium sulfate (100 mg/day—a huge dose that is not suggested for long-term use) can reduce fasting glucose levels by about 20% and decrease hepatic insulin resistance (Cohen et al., 1995; Cusi et al., 2001). Nondiabetic subjects typically do not exhibit significant changes in glucose uptake or lipolysis, but vanadyl sulfate may acutely stimulate amino acid transport into skeletal muscle (Jandhyala and Hom, 1983). Studies of vanadyl sulfate for weight loss and exercise performance have been variable, with most showing only modest (if any) effects on body composition (Badmaev et al., 1999). Although vanadium has become a popular dietary supplement among bodybuilders, only limited data support claims of increased muscle mass and strength.

SAFETY/DOSAGE

Little information is available about vanadium toxicity. Traditionally, vanadium is considered quite safe in humans (because of its poor absorption), and an upper-limit dosage of 1.8 mg/day has been established by the Food and Nutrition Board of the National Academy of Sciences. In one safety study, 100 mg of vanadyl sulfate (close to 10,000 times higher than dietary needs) was given to NIDDM subjects for 4 weeks (50 mg twice daily). Gastrointestinal side effects were experienced by 75% of the subjects during the first week, but the supplements were well tolerated after that. The authors of the study concluded that vanadyl sulfate resulted in modest reductions of fasting plasma glucose, but they cautioned that the safety of large doses of vanadium supplements for long periods remained uncertain. It is thought that prolonged exposure to excessive vanadium could cause muscle cramps, emotional depression, and damage to the nervous system and other organs. Some animal studies have suggested the possibility of hematological and biochemical changes, reproductive and developmental toxicity, and pro-oxidative effects on glutathione, ascorbic acid, and lipids following prolonged vanadium use. Vanadium is now considered to be an essential trace mineral, and 10 µg/day is thought to satisfy the body's basic needs (our diets probably contain about 10–30 µg/day of vanadium).

REFERENCES

Badmaev V, Prakash S, Majeed M. Vanadium: a review of its potential role in the fight against diabetes. J Altern Complement Med 1999;5(3):273–291.

Boden G, Chen X, Ruiz J, van Rossum GD, Turco S. Effects of vanadyl sulfate on carbohydrate and lipid metabolism in patients with non-insulin-dependent diabetes mellitus. Metabolism 1996;45(9):1130–1135.

Cam MC, Brownsey RW, McNeill JH. Mechanisms of vanadium action: insulin-mimetic or insulin-enhancing agent? Can J Physiol Pharmacol 2000;78(10):829–847.

Cohen N, Halberstam M, Shlimovich P, Chang CJ, Shamoon H, Rossetti L. Oral vanadyl sulfate improves hepatic and peripheral insulin sensitivity in patients with non-insulin-dependent diabetes mellitus. J Clin Invest 1995;95(6):2501–2509.

Cusi K, Cukier S, DeFronzo RA, Torres M, Puchulu FM, Redondo JC. Vanadyl sulfate improves hepatic and muscle insulin sensitivity in type 2 diabetes. J Clin Endocrinol Metab 2001;86(3):1410–1417.

Goldfine AB, Patti ME, Zuberi L, Goldstein BJ, LeBlanc R, Landaker EJ, Jiang ZY, Willsky GR, Kahn CR. Metabolic effects of vanadyl sulfate in humans with non-insulin-dependent diabetes mellitus: in vivo and in vitro studies. Metabolism 2000;49(3):400–410.

Jandhyala BS, Hom GJ. Minireview: physiological and pharmacological properties of vanadium. Life Sci 1983;33(14):1325–1340.

ADDITIONAL RESOURCES

Aharon Y, Mevorach M, Shamoon H. Vanadyl sulfate does not enhance insulin action in patients with type 1 diabetes. Diabetes Care 1998;21(12):2194–2195.

Balasubramanyam M, Mohan V. Orally active insulin mimics: where do we stand now? J Biosci 2001;26(3):383–390.

Brichard SM, Henquin JC. The role of vanadium in the management of diabetes. Trends Pharmacol Sci 1995;16(8):265–270.

Cunningham JJ. Micronutrients as nutriceutical interventions in diabetes mellitus. J Am Coll Nutr 1998;17(1):7–10.

Goldwaser I, Gefel D, Gershonov E, Fridkin M, Shechter Y. Insulin-like effects of vanadium: basic and clinical implications. J Inorg Biochem 2000;80(1–2):21–25.

Halberstam M, Cohen N, Shlimovich P, Rossetti L, Shamoon H. Oral vanadyl sulfate improves insulin sensitivity in NIDDM but not in obese nondiabetic subjects. Diabetes 1996;45(5):659–666.

Poucheret P, Verma S, Grynpas MD, McNeill JH. Vanadium and diabetes. Mol Cell Biochem 1998;188(1–2):73–80.

Sakurai H, Yasui H, Adachi Y. The therapeutic potential of insulin-mimetic vanadium complexes. Expert Opin Investig Drugs 2003;12(7):1189–1203.

Sakurai H. A new concept: the use of vanadium complexes in the treatment of diabetes mellitus. Chem Rec 2002;2(4):237–248.

Srivastava AK. Anti-diabetic and toxic effects of vanadium compounds. Mol Cell Biochem 2000;206(1–2):177–182.

Supplements and Their Star Rankings

STAR RANKING SCALE

★★★★★ = Significant scientific agreement
★★★★ = Support, but not conclusive
★★★ = Some support, but limited and not conclusive
★★ = Very limited, preliminary support
★ = Theoretical basis, but scientific support nonexistent
ZERO = No scientific of theoretical support

SUPPLEMENT	STAR RANKING	
5-HTP (5-Hydroxy-Tryptophan)	★★★★	for alleviating depression
	★★★	for weight loss
	★★★	for treating fibromyalgia
	★★	for treating insomnia and sleep disorders
	★★	for preventing diabetes
	★★	for alleviating chronic headache
α-Lipoic Acid	★★★★	as an antioxidant
	★★★★	for blood sugar control
	★★	for antiaging benefits
Alfalfa (*Medicago sativa*)	★★★	for cholesterol reduction
	★★	for increasing energy levels
	★★	for liver health and detoxification
	★	for reducing the pain of arthritis
	★	for reducing hot flashes associated with menopause
Aloe (Aloe Vera)	★★★★	for healing wounds, burns, and minor skin irritations (topically)
	★★★	as a laxative
	★★	for blood sugar reduction
	★★	for immune system support
	★	for blood lipid reduction

SUPPLEMENT	STAR RANKING	
Amino Acids and Protein Supplements	★★★★★	for soy protein and heart health
	★★★★	for whey protein, muscle synthesis, and exercise recovery
	★★★★	for soy protein and menopausal benefits
	★★★★	for branched-chain amino acids (BCAAs) and endurance
	★★★	for colostrum and exercise recovery
	★★★	for hydrolyzed collagen protein (HCP) and joint health
	★★★	for glutamine and immune support
	★★★	for arginine and blood flow
Androstenedione **!** **WARNING:** *Banned for sale as a dietary supplement in the United States.*	★	for promoting muscle growth and accelerating fat loss
Antioxidants	★★★★★	for cellular protection
	★★★★	for antiaging benefits
Arginine	★★★★	for cardiovascular disease
	★★★	for sexual dysfunction
	★★★	for immune function
	★★	for high cholesterol
	★★	for high blood pressure
Astragalus	★★★	for stimulating the immune system
	★★★	for promoting resistance to stress (adaptogenic effect)
	★★	for cancer protection
β Carotene	★★★★★	for correcting vitamin A deficiency
	★★★★	for cellular protection (antioxidant effect)
	★★★	for anticancer effects
Banaba (*Lagerstroemia speciosa*)	★★★	for lowering blood sugar and controlling diabetes
	★★	for controlling cravings for foods (especially carbohydrates)
B-Complex Vitamins (B$_6$, B$_{12}$, Folic Acid, Niacin)	★★★★★	for folate to prevent neural tube defects during pregnancy
	★★★★★	for B$_6$, B$_{12}$, and folate to control homocysteine levels for heart health
	★★★★	for niacin to control cholesterol

SUPPLEMENT	STAR RANKING

Bee Products (Bee Pollen, Propolis, Royal Jelly)

★★★ for stimulating the immune system
★★★ for reducing cholesterol
★★★ as an overall tonic
★★ as an antibiotic
★★ for treating and preventing herpes
★★ for treating and preventing premenstrual syndrome (PMS)
★ for boosting energy levels

Bilberry (*Vaccinium myrtillus* L.)

★★★★ as an antioxidant
★★★★ for peripheral vascular disorders
★★★★ for eye health
★★★ for diabetic retinopathy
★★ for diarrhea

Black Cohosh (*Actaea racemosa* L., *Cimicifuga racemosa* [L.] Nutt)

★★★★★ for relief of menopausal symptoms
★★★★ for hormone balancing
★★★ for premenstrual syndrome (PMS)

Bladderwrack (*Fucus vesiculosis*)

★★★ as a dietary source of iodine
★ for weight loss and "fat burning"
★ for enhancing thyroid function

Blue Cohosh (*Caulophyllum thalictroides*)

★★ for inducing labor
★ for menstrual pain

> **WARNING:** Blue cohosh may be dangerous if used by the general public. Only qualified herbalists or midwives with the appropriate traditional training should administer blue cohosh, because no clinical evidence warrants or guides its use.

Boron

★★★★★ for correcting nutrient deficiency
★★★ for promoting bone and joint health
★★ for maintaining testosterone levels (in postmenopausal women)

Boswellia (*Boswellia serrata*)

★★★ for inflammatory diseases
★★ for joint pain and sports recovery

Branched-Chain Amino Acids (BCAAs)

★★★★ for enhancing endurance exercise performance
★★★★ for enhancing postexercise recovery

Brewer's Yeast (*Saccharomyces cerevisiae*)

★★★★ as a source of B vitamins
★★★★ as a source of "biologically active" chromium
★★★★ for reducing blood sugar
★★ for reducing cholesterol
★★ for preventing acne
★ for increasing energy
★ for enhancing exercise performance
★ for cardiovascular health

SUPPLEMENT	STAR RANKING
Calcium	★★★★★ for bone health ★★★ for blood pressure control ★★★ for maintaining metabolic rate ★★★ for alleviating symptoms of premenstrual syndrome (PMS) ★★ for reducing the risk of colon cancer
Carnitine	★★★ for enhancing general heart function (in congestive heart failure and post–myocardial infarction when combined with coenzyme Q_{10}) ★★ for weight loss and "fat burning" ★★ for endurance
Carnosine	★★ as a broad-spectrum antioxidant ★ for enhancing exercise performance
Cat's Claw (*Uncaria tomentosa*)	★★★★ for immune modulation ★★★ as an anti-inflammatory ★★★ for treating infections ★★★ for osteoarthritis ★★ as an antioxidant ★★ for cancer treatment
Cayenne or Chili (*Capsicum annuum, C. frutescens*)	★★★ for digestive health ★★★ for pain (internally and topically) ★★ for headache ★★ for skin health (topically) ★★ for incontinence
Cetyl Myristoleate	★★★ for joint pain
Chitosan	★★ for fat absorption ★★ for cholesterol reduction ★ for weight loss
Choline	★★★★ for general nutritional support ★★★ for memory support ★ as a fat burner
Chondroitin Sulfate	★★★★ for joint health
Chromium	★★★★★ for correcting chromium deficiency ★★★★ for reducing blood sugar, improving activity of insulin ★★★ for reducing body fat and increasing lean muscle mass ★★ as an appetite suppressant ★★ for lowering cholesterol ★★ for enhancing exercise performance
***Citrus aurantium* (Synephrine)**	★★★ for weight loss ★★ for thermogenesis ★ for athletic performance

SUPPLEMENT	STAR RANKING	
Coenzyme Q$_{10}$ (CoQ$_{10}$)	★★★★	for heart patients, especially in conjunction with statins
	★★★★	as an antioxidant
	★★	for endurance performance
	★★	for energy and chronic fatigue
Colostrum	★★★★	for boosting gastrointestinal immunity
	★★★	for boosting systemic immune function
Conjugated Linoleic Acid (CLA)	★★★★	for fat loss in moderately overweight adults
	★	for control of blood lipids
	ZERO	for fat loss in trained athletes
	ZERO	for anticancer effects in humans
Cordyceps Mushroom (*Cordyceps sinensis*)	★★★★	for enhancing endurance and exercise performance
	★★★★	for enhancing overall lung function (measured by maximal oxygen consumption)
	★★★	for direct energy-promoting and antifatigue benefits
Cranberry (*Vaccinium macrocarpon*)	★★★★★	for urinary tract infections (UTIs)
	★★★★	for antioxidant activity
	★★★★	as an antibacterial
Creatine	★★★★★	for enhancing muscle building and improving muscular power
	★★	for enhancing endurance exercise performance (by enhancing glycogen storage)
Damiana (*Turnera diffusa*)	★★	for enhancing sexual performance and desire
	★★	for inducing relaxation and decreasing anxiety
	★	for alleviating depression
	★	for promoting blood sugar regulation and weight loss
Devil's Claw (*Harpagophytum procumbens*)	★★★★	for joint, low back, and arthritis pain
DHEA (Dehydroepiandrosterone)	★★★★	for restoring DHEA and DHEA-S levels in elderly men and women and in overtrained athletes
	★★	for building muscle and reducing fat in healthy young athletes
	★★	for boosting testosterone levels and enhancing sexual function
Dong Quai (*Angelica sinensis*)	★★★	for hormonal balance and easing symptoms of menopause and PMS
	★	for increasing libido

SUPPLEMENT	STAR RANKING

Echinacea (*Echinacea angustifolia, E. pallida, E. purpurea*)

★★★★★ for prophylaxis and treatment of cold and flu symptoms

★★★★★ to increase resistance to colds, influenza, and other infections (oral formulations)

★★★ for wounds and inflammatory skin conditions (topical formulations)

★★★ for vaginal candidiasis

★★ for urinary tract infections

★★ for genital herpes (herpes simplex virus types 1 and 2)

★★ as an antimicrobial

Essential Fatty Acids (ω-3, ω-6, Fish Oil, Evening Primrose Oil, Borage Seed Oil, Flaxseed Oil)

★★★★★ for correcting essential fatty acid deficiency

★★★★★ for general heart health

★★★★ for controlling inflammation

Evening Primrose Oil

★★★★ for alleviating symptoms of PMS

Fenugreek (*Trigonella foenum-graecum*)

★★★★ for controlling blood sugar

★★★ for supporting cardiovascular health

★★ for suppressing appetite and promoting weight loss

★★ for inducing lactation

Feverfew

★★★★ for migraine prevention

Fiber

★★★★★ for gut health

★★★★★ for cholesterol control

★★★★ for gut regularity and constipation

Flaxseed Oil and Linseed Oil

★★★★ for treating inflammatory conditions

★★★★ for promoting heart health

Garlic

★★★★ for blood pressure control

★★★ for cholesterol control

Ginger (*Zingiber officinale*)

★★★★ for nausea prevention

★★★★ for control of inflammation

★★★ for pain relief

as an antioxidant

Ginkgo biloba

★★★★★ for improving cognitive function (senile dementia)

★★★★ for improving systemic blood flow

★★★★ for intermittent claudication

★★ for asthma

SUPPLEMENT	STAR RANKING

Ginseng

★★★★ for increasing energy levels
★★★★ for relieving stress (adaptogenic effect)
★★★★ for enhancing athletic performance
★★★ for controlling blood sugar
★★★ for improving mental function
★★★ for promoting general well-being (tonic effect)
★★ for enhancing sexual performance
★★ for enhancing immune system function

Glucosamine

★★★★★ for joint health

Glutamine

★★★★ to promote tissue repair
★★★★ to reduce muscle catabolism
★★★★ to prevent infections and boost immune system function

Glycerol

★★★ for enhancing hydration status
★★★ for improving endurance performance in hot environments

Goldenseal (*Hydrastis canadensis*)

★★★ for diarrhea (as a source of berberine)
★★★ for immune system support (as a source of berberine)
★★★ as an antimicrobial (as a source of berberine)

Gotu Kola

★★★ for enhancing wound healing
★★★ for treating and preventing varicose veins and hemorrhoids
★★ for antianxiety effects
★★ for enhancing memory and cognitive function

Grape Seed (*Vitis vinifera*)

★★★★ as an antioxidant
★★★★ for cardioprotective and circulatory benefits (capillary reinforcement, collagen protection, vasorelaxation)
★★★★ for treating and preventing varicose veins

Green Tea (*Camellia sinensis*)

★★★★★ as an antioxidant
★★★★ for anticancer effects
★★★★ for thermogenic benefits (weight loss)
★★★ for energy (as a source of caffeine)

Green-Lipped Mussel (*Perna canaliculus*)

★★★ arthritis, joint pain and stiffness
★★ inflammatory conditions
★★ promoting postexercise recovery

Guarana (*Paullinia cupana*)

★★★ for energy
★★ for athletic and mental performance
★★ for weight loss
★ for aphrodisiac properties

SUPPLEMENT

STAR RANKING

Gymnema (*Gymnema sylvestre*)

★★★★ for blood sugar control
★★ for appetite control and weight loss

Hawthorn (*Crataegus oxyacantha* L.)

★★★★ for cardiovascular health
★★★★ as an antioxidant
★★★ for high blood pressure
★★★ for arteriosclerosis

HMB (ß-Hydroxy-ß-Methylbutyrate)

★★★★ for reducing muscle catabolism during intense exercise training
★★★★ for slowing muscle loss from wasting associated with cancer or AIDS

Horse Chestnut (*Aesculus hippocastanum* L.)

★★★★★ for vein health (venotonic)
★★★ for treating and preventing hemorrhoids
★★ for treating and preventing inflammatory conditions
★★ for reducing and preventing postoperative edema

Hydrolyzed Collagen Protein (HCP, Gelatin)

★★★ for joint health
★★★ for wound healing

Hydroxycitric Acid (HCA, *Garcinia cambogia*)

★★★ for appetite suppression
★★ for weight loss and "fat burning"

Inosine

★★ for improving energy metabolism and endurance performance

Kava Kava (*Piper methysticum*)

WARNING: *Some contaminated kava supplements have been implicated in isolated cases of hepatotoxicity. Readers are referred to the "Safety/Dosage" subsection of this section for a discussion.*

★★★★ for anxiety and stress
★★★ for insomnia
★★★ for reducing musculoskeletal pain
★★ for reducing menstrual discomfort and anxiety
★★ for benzodiazepine withdrawal
★★ for attention-deficit/hyperactivity disorder (ADHD)
★★ for headaches and migraines
★ as an aphrodisiac
★ as an analgesic
ZERO for treating or preventing upper respiratory infection (URI)
ZERO for treating or preventing urinary tract infections (UTI)

Lutein and Zeaxanthin

★★★★ for general eye health
★★★★ for prevention of age-related macular degeneration (ARMD)

Lycopene

★★★★★ as an antioxidant
★★★★ for reducing the risk of prostate and cervical cancers
★★ for skin health

SUPPLEMENT	STAR RANKING	
Ma Huang (*Ephedra sinensis*, Ephedrine)	★★★★	for weight loss
	★★★	for thermogenesis
	★★	for athletic performance
! **WARNING:** Banned for sale as a dietary supplement in the United States.		
Maca (*Lepidium meyenii*)	★★	for sexual performance and libido
	★★	for increasing energy and endurance
	★★	for increasing memory and mood
Magnesium	★★★★★	for bone health
	★★★	for blood pressure control
	★★★	for alleviating PMS
	★★★	for alleviating anxiety
Mastic (from *Pistacia lentiscus*)	★★	for treating and preventing ulcers
	★★	for alleviating gastrointestinal discomfort (heartburn)
	★★	for treating and preventing bad breath
Medium-Chain Triglycerides (MCTs)	★★★	for modestly increasing metabolic rate compared with long-chain triglycerides
	★★	for promoting weight loss
	★	for enhancing endurance exercise performance
Melatonin	★★★★	as a sleep aid
	★★★★	for alleviating jet lag
	★★★	as an antioxidant
	★	for antiaging effects
	★	for depression
Milk Thistle (*Silybum marianum*)	★★★★★	for detoxification and liver health
	★★★★★	for liver protection (against toxins)
	★★★★	as a restorative from liver disorders
MSM (Methylsulfonylmethane)	★★★★	as a sulfur supplement
	★★	for treating athletic injuries
	★★	for treating or preventing arthritis and joint pain
	★★	for treating or preventing seasonal allergic rhinitis
	★	for preventing cancer
	★	for treating bladder disorders
N-Acetylcysteine (NAC)	★★★★	for antioxidant benefits (glutathione related)
	★★★	for general immune support
NADH (Nicotinamide Adenine Dinucleotide)	★★★	for jet lag
	★★	for chronic fatigue syndrome (CFS)
	★	for increased energy levels

SUPPLEMENT	STAR RANKING
Perilla Seed Oil (*Perilla frutescens*)	★★★ for asthma and allergy ★★★ for inflammatory conditions ★★★ for cardiovascular health ★★ for immune function
Phosphatidylserine	★★★★ for cognitive function ★★★ for anti-stress effects
Pine Bark (*Pinus* spp.)	★★★★ as an antioxidant ★★★★ for cardiovascular health ★★★★ for venous health (venous insufficiency and capillary health) ★★★ for complications of diabetes (diabetic retinopathy) ★★ for asthma ★★ for skin health ★★ for improving cognitive function
Prebiotics or Fructo-Oligosaccharides (FOS)	★★★ for gut health ★★ for immune system support
Probiotics (Acidophilus, Bifidus)	★★★★ for gut health ★★★★ for gut immunity ★★★ for systemic immunity ★★★ for reducing the risk of colon cancer
Protein (Casein, Whey, Soy, Collagen, Colostrum)	*See "Amino Acids and Protein Supplements."*
Proteolytic Enzymes	★★★★ for reducing inflammation and pain associated with tissue trauma and injury ★★★★ for enhancing postexercise recovery
Pygeum	★★★★ for alleviating symptoms of benign prostatic hyperplasia (BPH)
Pyruvate	★★★ for weight loss ★★ for athletic performance
Quercetin	★★★★ as an antioxidant ★★★★ for cardiovascular disease ★★★★ for venous and capillary health ★★ to support eye health (antioxidant) ★ to enhance thermogenesis
Red Clover (*Trifolium pratense*)	★★★★ for balancing hormones ★★★★ for reducing menopausal symptoms (hot flashes, loss of libido) ★★★ for balancing mood swings (associated with hormone imbalance) ★★★ for supporting cardiovascular health ★★★ for maintaining bone mass ★★ for treating and preventing prostate cancer

SUPPLEMENT	STAR RANKING

Red Yeast Rice

★★★★★ for cholesterol control

 WARNING: *Banned for sale as a dietary supplement in the United States.*

Rhodiola

★★★ for stress control (adaptogenic effects)
★★★ for endurance performance
★★★ as a physical and mental tonic (adaptogenic effects)

Ribose

★★★★ for prevention of exercise-induced ischemia in cardiac disease
★★★ for enhancement of endurance exercise performance
★★ for improvement of muscle strength and power

SAMe (S-Adenosyl-L-Methionine)

★★★★ for depression
★★★★ for liver disease
★★★ for osteoarthritis
★ for fibromyalgia

Saw Palmetto

★★★★★ for alleviating symptoms of BPH
★★ for treating male-pattern baldness
★★ for enhancing sexual performance

Schisandra (*Schisandra chinensis*)

★★★★ as an antioxidant
★★★ for cardiovascular disease
★★★ as an adaptogen
★★★ for liver support
★★ for central nervous system (CNS) dysfunctions related to old age
★★ for treating and preventing diabetes
★★ for treating and preventing cancer

Sea Buckthorn (*Hippophae rhamnoides*)

★★★ as an antioxidant
★★★ for cardiovascular health
★★★ for wound healing and dermatitis
★ as an energizer

Sea Cucumber (*Stichopus japonicus*, Other Genera Depending on Location)

★ for joint pain
★ for fibromyalgia

Selenium

★★★★★ for correcting selenium deficiency
★★★★ as an antioxidant
★★★★ for anticancer effects

Shark Cartilage and Bovine Cartilage (Tracheal)

★ for anticancer effects (antiangiogenesis)

SUPPLEMENT	STAR RANKING
Slippery Elm (*Ulmus rubra, U. fulva*)	★★★ for soothing effect on mucous membranes (sore throat) ★★ for digestive health ★ for dry coughs ★ as a skin moisturizer in minor skin irritations
Soy	★★★★★ for cardiovascular disease ★★★★ for menopausal symptoms ★★★ for osteoporosis ★★★ for cancer prevention
Spirulina (*Spirulina maxima, S. platensis*)	★★★ as an antioxidant ★★★ to stimulate the immune system ★★ as a "holistic" vitamin or nutritional supplement ★★ for heart disease prevention (cholesterol lowering) ★ for promoting healthy energy levels and mood ★ for promoting weight loss
St. John's Wort	★★★★★ for mild-to-moderate depression or anxiety
Tribulus (*Tribulus terrestris*)	★★★ for sexual performance ★★ for athletic performance
Uva Ursi or Bearberry (*Arctostaphylos uva-ursi*)	★★★ for urinary complaints and inflammation of the urinary tract ★ for treating and preventing kidney stone formation
Valerian	★★★★★ as a sleep aid ★★★★ for anxiety
Vanadium	★★★ for controlling blood sugar ★ for reducing body fat and increasing lean muscle mass
Vinpocetine (from *Vinca minor*)	★★★★ for cerebrovascular disease ★★ as a memory enhancer ★★ for dementia
Vitamin A	★★★★★ for correcting vitamin A deficiency ★★★ for supporting immune function ★★★ for eye health
Vitamin B$_1$ (Thiamin)	★★★★★ for correcting nutrient deficiency ★★★ during stress ★★ for an energy boost

SUPPLEMENT	STAR RANKING	
Vitamin B₂ (Riboflavin)	★★★★★	for correcting nutrient deficiency
	★★★	during stress
	★★	for an energy boost
Vitamin C	★★★★★	for correcting vitamin C deficiency
	★★★★	for preventing and treating colds and flu
	★★★★	for antioxidant support
Vitamin D (Calciferol, Cholecalciferol)	★★★★★	for correcting nutrient deficiency
	★★★★★	for bone health
	★★	for anticancer effects
Vitamin E	★★★★★	for correcting vitamin E deficiency
	★★★★	for heart health
	★★★★	for antioxidant support
Vitamin K (Phylloquinone, Menaquinone)	★★★★★	for correcting nutrient deficiency
	★★★★	for bone health
Vitex or Chasteberry (*Vitex agnus-castus* L.)	★★★★★	for reducing and preventing PMS
	★★★★★	for treating and preventing premenstrual tension syndrome (PMTS)
	★★★★	for reducing and preventing breast pain
	★★★★	for balancing hormones
	★★★	for treating and preventing acne
	★★	for menopausal complaints
White Willow Bark (*Salix alba*)	★	for weight loss (when combined with ephedrine and caffeine as the *A* in ECA stacks)
	★	for pain control
	ZERO	for weight loss (as a stand-alone supplement)
Yellow Dock (*Rumex crispus*)	★★	as a laxative
	★	for digestive health
	★	for liver support (to stimulate bile flow)
	★	for skin conditions
Yohimbine from Yohimbe and Quebracho (*Pausinystalia yohimbe, Aspidosperma quebracho-blanco*)	★★★★	for enhancing sexual performance
	★★★★	for improving erectile dysfunction (ED)
	★★★	as a stimulant
	★★	as an aphrodisiac
	★★	for increasing muscle mass (by increasing testosterone)
	★★	for promoting weight loss
	★	for alleviating depression
Zinc	★★★★★	for correcting zinc deficiency
	★★★★	for support of immune function
	★★★★	for treating colds (lozenge form)
	★★★★	as a general antioxidant
	★★★	for enhancing testosterone and sexual performance

Index

Note: Page numbers followed by "t" denote tables.